Atlas of
HEART DISEASES

VALVULAR HEART DISEASE

Volume XI

Atlas of HEART DISEASES

VALVULAR HEART DISEASE

Volume XI

VOLUME EDITOR

Shahbudin H. Rahimtoola, MB, FRCP, MACP

Distinguished Professor
George C. Griffith Professor of Cardiology
Chairman, Griffith Center
Professor of Medicine
University of Southern California
Los Angeles, California

SERIES EDITOR

Eugene Braunwald, MD, MD (Hon), ScD (Hon)

Hersey Professor of the Theory and Practice of Medicine
Harvard Medical School
Chairman, Department of Medicine
Brigham and Women's Hospital
Boston, Massachusetts

Mosby

St. Louis Baltimore Boston Carlsbad Chicago Naples New York Philadelphia Portland
London Madrid Mexico City Singapore Sydney Tokyo Toronto Wiesbaden

Developed by Current Medicine Inc., Philadelphia

CURRENT MEDICINE

400 MARKET STREET, SUITE 700 • PHILADELPHIA, PA 19106

Development Editor .... *Marian Bellus*

Editorial Assistant .... *Charlene French*

Design .... *Lisa Caro*

Layout .... *Jerilyn Bockorick, Lisa Weischedel*

Illustrators .... *Marie Dean, Sue Ann Fung-Ho, Wendy Jackelow, Lisa Antonucci Messina*

Managing Editor .... *Lori Bainbridge*

Art Director .... *Paul Fennessy*

Illustration Director .... *Ann Saydlowski*

Production .... *David Myers, Lori Holland*

Indexing .... *Alexandra Nickerson*

Distribution rights for North America
and territories not listed below:
MOSBY-YEAR BOOK, INC.
11830 Westline Industrial Drive
St. Louis, MO 63146

In Canada: TIMES MIRROR
PROFESSIONAL PUBLISHING LTD.
130 Flaska Drive • Markham, Ontario
Canada L6G 1B8

Distribution rights for Central and
South America: NUEVA EDITORIAL
INTERAMERICANA, SA DE CV.

Distribution rights for Japan:
NANKODO CO LTD.

Distribution rights for Indian Subcontinent
and South East Asia (except Japan):
TIMES MIRROR INTERNATIONAL
PUBLISHERS, LTD.

Library of Congress Cataloging-in-Publication Data
Valvular heart disease /
volume editor, Shahbudin H. Rahimtoola.
p. cm.—(Atlas of heart diseases; v. 11)
Includes bibliographical references and index.
ISBN 1-878132-30-X (hard cover :alk. paper)
1. Heart valves—Diseases—Atlases. 2. Endocarditis—Atlases.
I. Rahimtoola, Shahbudin H. II. Series.
[DNLM: 1. Heart Valve Diseases—atlases. 2. Endocarditis—atlases.
WG 17 A8816 1997 v.11]
RC682.A818 1997 vol. 11
[RC685.V2]
616.1′25—dc20
DNLM/DLC 95-42589
for Library of Congress CIP

Library of Congress Cataloging-in-Publication Data
ISBN 1-878132-30-X

Printed in Singapore by Imago Productions (FE) Ltd.

10 9 8 7 6 5 4 3 2 1

SERIES PREFACE

Disorders of the cardiovascular system are the most common causes of death and serious morbidity in the industrialized world. In 1991, more than 40% of all deaths in the United States were attributed to cardiac and vascular diseases. These conditions accounted for almost 5 million years of potential life lost.

Despite these sobering statistics, progress in cardiovascular medicine has been immense, and is, in fact, accelerating. Our understanding of the pathobiology of most forms of heart disease has advanced steadily and there have been enormous advances in the diagnosis, treatment, and prevention of cardiovascular disorders. For example, during just one decade, from 1981 to 1991, the overall death rates from cardiovascular disease declined by 26% and death rates from acute myocardial infarction and stroke declined by 32%. Similar progress has been made in other major cardiovascular disorders, including hypertension, valvular and congenital heart disease, congestive heart failure, and the arrhythmias.

The physician responsible for the care of patients with cardiovascular disease now has a number of vehicles available for obtaining up-to-date information, including excellent journals and textbooks of every conceivable size, scope, and depth. In developing new strategies for transmitting information about these conditions, it is important to consider that cardiovascular medicine is the most "visual" of medical specialties. Cardiovascular diagnosis is based on the recognition and understanding of a variety of graphic waveforms, images, decision trees, and microscopic sections. Treatment increasingly involves the intelligent use of algorithms, which are most effectively portrayed visually. Likewise, mechanical correction of cardiovascular disorders, whether catheter-based or surgical, can best be described pictorially. This *Atlas of Heart Diseases* has been designed to provide a detailed and comprehensive visual exposition of all aspects of cardiovascular medicine. Several thousand images, accompanied by detailed captions, have been carefully selected by expert authors and reviewed by the distinguished Volume Editors. These images are now available separately in print and slide form and also have been formatted for CD-ROM use.

Many people deserve credit for the successful completion of this ambitious effort. The expertise and hard work of the authors and the devoted efforts of the volume editors naturally form the foundation of the *Atlas of Heart Diseases*. Great credit is also due to Abe Krieger, President of Current Medicine, who conceived the *Atlas* series; to Maureen McNally, the extremely effective Developmental Editor, and to Kathryn Saxon, who coordinated the efforts in my office.

All of us who have been engaged in this project hope that each individual volume, and the entire *Atlas*, will be useful to physicians of all specialties who are responsible for the care of patients with cardiovascular disorders, to investigators and teachers of cardiovascular medicine, and ultimately to the millions of patients worldwide with disorders of the heart and circulation.

Eugene Braunwald, MD

PREFACE

With the decline of rheumatic fever and rheumatic heart disease in the United States and other developed and affluent countries, the incidence of rheumatic valvular heart disease has declined significantly. However, it is still very common in the less well developed and less affluent parts of the world. In the United States, valvular heart disease due to other etiologies such as "degenerative," myxomatous involvement of valves and coronary artery disease has increased significantly. As a result, valvular heart disease is still common and is the second most frequent form of heart disease for use of interventional diagnostic studies and interventional therapies.

The clinical examination (history, physical examination, electrocardiogram, and chest roentgenogram) is the initial and most important tool in diagnosing and assessing the severity of valve disease. Cardiac catheterization/angiography, including coronary arteriography, is an extremely important test in the assessment of valvular heart disease and is still needed in most patients being considered for interventional therapy. Echocardiography/Doppler ultrasound studies, both transthoracic and transesophageal, are extremely useful in providing knowledge about the anatomy and function of valves, in diagnosing and assessing the severity of valve disease, and in determining cardiac chamber sizes and left ventricular function.

Other tests are performed as needed. Vasodilator therapy has proven to be useful in certain subgroups of patients with severe valve regurgitation. Prophylactic antibiotic therapy in appropriate patients has stood the test of time.

Valve surgery is the single most important therapeutic modality available for patients with severe valve disease. Mitral valve commissurotomy has stood the test of time. Valve replacement is needed in most patients with severe disease, and has been performed using mechanical, xenograft, autograft, and homograft valves. However, with valve replacement the patient all too commonly exchanges one disease for another; therefore, there is an increased tendency to perform valve repair whenever it is feasible to do so. More recently, catheter interventional therapy for stenotic valves has been shown to be useful, particularly in those with noncalcified, mobile valves.

This volume of the *Atlas of Heart Diseases* covers all aspects relevant to an understanding of valve disease, its pathogenesis, pathology, pathophysiology, diagnosis, and management. It will be useful to clinicians, teachers, investigators, and "students" at all levels of experience.

Shahbudin H. Rahimtoola, MB, FRCP, MACP

CONTRIBUTORS

MANUEL J. ANTUNES, MD, PhD, DSc
Professor
Cardiothoracic Surgery
University of Coimbra
Professor and Head
University Hospital
Coimbra, Portugal

GERALD G. BLACKWELL, MD
Cardiovascular Associates, PC
Kingsport, Tennessee

ALLEN P. BURKE, MD
Adjunct Professor
Department of Pathology
Georgetown University
Staff Pathologist
Armed Forces Institute of Pathology
Washington, District of Columbia

BLASE A. CARABELLO, MD
Charles Ezra Daniel Professor of Cardiology
Department of Medicine
Gazes Cardiac Research Institute
Medical University of South Carolina
Ralph H. Johnson Department of Veterans Affairs Medical Center
Charleston, South Carolina

JOHN D. CARROLL, MD
Associate Professor
Department of Medicine
Pritzker School of Medicine
University of Chicago
Director, Hans Hecht Cardiac Catheterization Laboratory
University of Chicago Hospitals
Chicago, Illinois

MELVIN D. CHEITLIN, MD
Professor of Medicine
Department of Medicine
University of California, San Francisco
Chief, Cardiology Division
San Francisco General Hospital
San Francisco, California

ADNAN S. DAJANI, MD
Professor of Pediatrics
Department of Pediatrics
Wayne State University
Chief, Infectious Diseases
Children's Hospital of Michigan
Detroit, Michigan

ANDREW FARB, MD
Clinical Assistant Professor
Department of Medicine
Georgetown University
Staff Cardiologist
Armed Forces Institute of Pathology
Washington, District of Columbia

GARY L. GRUNKEMEIER, PhD
Director, Medical Data Research Center
Providence Health System
Portland, Oregon

DAVID T. KAWANISHI, MD
Associate Professor
Department of Internal Medicine/Cardiology
University of Southern California
Director, Cardiac Catheterization Laboratory
Los Angeles California & University of Southern California Medical Center
University of Southern California University Hospital
Los Angeles, California

MORTON J. KERN, MD
Professor of Medicine
Department of Internal Medicine
St. Louis University
Director, JG Mudd Cardiac Catheterization Laboratory
St. Louis University Medical Center
St. Louis, Missouri

CONTRIBUTORS

JOHN S. MacGREGOR, PhD, MD
Assistant Clinical Professor of Medicine
Department of Medicine
University of California, San Francisco
Director, Cardiac Catheterization Laboratory
San Francisco General Hospital
San Francisco, California

PETER C. NISHAN, MD, FACC
LeBauer Research Institute
Cone Memorial Hospital
Greensboro, North Carolina

RICK A. NISHIMURA, MD, FACC
Professor of Medicine
Consultant
Division of Cardiovascular Diseases and Internal Medicine
Mayo Clinic
Rochester, Minnesota

ROBERT A. O'ROURKE, MD
Charles Conrad Brown Distinguished Professor in Cardiovascular Disease
Department of Medicine
Division of Cardiology
University of Texas Health Science Center
Staff Attending Physician
University Hospital and South Texas Veterans Health Care System
San Antonio, Texas

GERALD M. POHOST, MD
Professor of Medicine
Professor of Radiology
Department of Medicine
Division of Cardiovascular Disease
University of Alabama, Birmingham, School of Medicine
Director, Division of Cardiovascular Disease
University Hospital
Birmingham, Alabama

SUMANTH D. PRABHU, MD
Assistant Professor
Department of Medicine
Division of Cardiology
University of Texas Health Science Center at San Antonio
Staff Physician
University Hospital and South Texas Veterans Health Care System
San Antonio, Texas

SHAHBUDIN H. RAHIMTOOLA, MB FRCP, MACP
Distinguished Professor
George C. Griffith Professor of Cardiology
Chairman, Griffith Center
Professor of Medicine
University of Southern California
Los Angeles, California

ALBERT STARR, MD
Professor of Surgery
Oregon Health Sciences University
Director of the Heart Institute
Providence Health System
Portland, Oregon

KATHRYN A. TAUBERT, PhD
Adjunct Associate Professor
Department of Physiology
University of Texas Southwestern Medical School
Senior Science Consultant
American Heart Association
Dallas, Texas

RENU VIRMANI, MD
Adjunct Research Professor
Department of Pathology
Vanderbilt University
Nashville, Tennessee
Chairperson
Department of Cardiovascular Pathology
Armed Forces Institute of Pathology
Washington, District of Columbia

CONTENTS

CHAPTER 1

Pathology of Valvular Heart Disease

Renu Virmani, Allen P. Burke, and Andrew Farb

CHAPTER 2

Effects of Pressure and Volume Overload on Left and Right Ventricles

John D. Carroll

CHAPTER 3

Role of Two-Dimensional Echocardiography and Doppler Ultrasound

Peter C. Nishan and Rick A. Nishimura

CONTENTS

CONTENTS

CONTENTS

CHAPTER 12

Repair for Acquired Valvular Heart Disease

Manuel J. Antunes

CHAPTER 13

Prosthetic Heart Valves

Gary L. Grunkemeier, Shahbudin H. Rahimtoola, and Albert Starr

CHAPTER 14

Antibiotic Prophylaxis for Rheumatic Fever and Endocarditis

Kathryn A. Taubert, Adnan S. Dajani, and Shahbudin H. Rahimtoola

PATHOLOGY OF VALVULAR HEART DISEASE

1

CHAPTER

Renu Virmani,
Allen P. Burke,
and Andrew Farb

In the Western world, the incidence of the various forms of cardiac valve disease has changed markedly in the latter half of this century. Until 1960, virtually all acquired valve disease was considered rheumatic in origin [1]. However, it is now well appreciated that isolated aortic valve (AV) disease is usually nonrheumatic [2,3]. Mitral valve prolapse (MVP) is currently the most common cause of mitral regurgitation (MR). Ischemic papillary muscle dysfunction has only recently been recognized as a surgically correctable cause of MR. Finally, in the last four decades there has been an explosion of surgical treatments for valve disease, including the introduction of prosthetic heart valves, which themselves undergo unique pathologic changes.

In patients younger than 15 years, most AV disease results in stenosis. The most frequent causes of aortic stenosis (AS) are dysplastic unicuspid or bicuspid valves, subvalvular stenosis, and supravalvular stenosis. In patients aged 15 to 70 years, the common etiologies of AS are calcification of nondysplastic congenital bicuspid AV and chronic rheumatic disease. The most important cause of AS in patients 70 years or older is degenerative AS. Mediastinal irradiation may result in AS that requires valve replacement [4]. Pure aortic regurgitation (AR) is most frequently due to aortic root dilatation, followed by congenitally bicuspid valve, chronic rheumatic valvulitis, and regurgitation resulting from valvuloplasty. Combined AS and insufficiency is infrequent and results from degenerative AV disease, bicuspid AV, chronic rheumatic valvulitis, and posttherapeutic disease.

Current trends indicate that the age of patients undergoing AV replacement is increasing [3]. This has led to a proportional increase in surgical cases of AV disease secondary to degenerative calcification and aortic root dilatation.

Since 1965, the frequency of pure MR has increased [5–7], mirroring an increase in the frequency of MVP. In contrast, the relative frequency of mitral stenosis (MS) has decreased to less than 50% of excised valves in 1990, reflecting a continuing decline in the relative frequency of chronic rheumatic mitral valve disease.

The etiology of 99% of pure MS remains chronic rheumatic heart disease; congenital MS is rare [8]. Two thirds of mitral valve excisions for MR are currently performed for MVP. Another reason for the reduction in mitral valve excision is the increased performance of mitral valve repair. MVP is congenital in origin but is most often recognized only in adult life [9,10]. The second most common cause of MR is papillary muscle dysfunction from coronary heart disease. Endocarditis is an infrequent cause of MR in the general population.

Tricuspid valve (TV) disease generally manifests as pure tricuspid regurgitation (TR) or TR with tricuspid stenosis (TS) [11,12]. A variety of congenital disorders may result in TR; the most common acquired causes are postrheumatic disease and pulmonary venous hypertension.

Isolated pulmonary stenosis is one of the most frequent congenital cardiac defects in which survival to adult age is expected [13]. Pulmonary outflow stenosis, which is often associated with tetralogy of Fallot, may be at the level of the valve, which is dysplastic, hypoplastic, or atretic. Alternatively, there may be subvalvular obstruction in the form of fibrous bands, short segments of muscular impingement on the lumen, or long narrowed segments of the infundibulum. Acquired lesions of the pulmonary valve (PV) include chronic rheumatic valvulitis and carcinoid syndrome. Cardiac tumors, most of which are metastatic to the heart, are a rare cause of obstruction of the outflow tract.

The pathologic processes that affect heart valve prostheses are best approached by type of valve (bioprosthetic versus mechanical). Bioprosthetic porcine valves, bovine pericardial bioprosthetic valves, and cadaver-derived homograft valves undergo gradual tissue degeneration but are relatively resistant to thrombosis. Mechanical valves have the advantage of greater durability than bioprosthetic valves, but they require continuous anticoagulation.

Mechanical and bioprosthetic valves may become infected, usually in the form of a ring abscess, although bioprosthetic valves may also become infected on the cusp surface.

Native Valves

AORTIC VALVE DISEASE

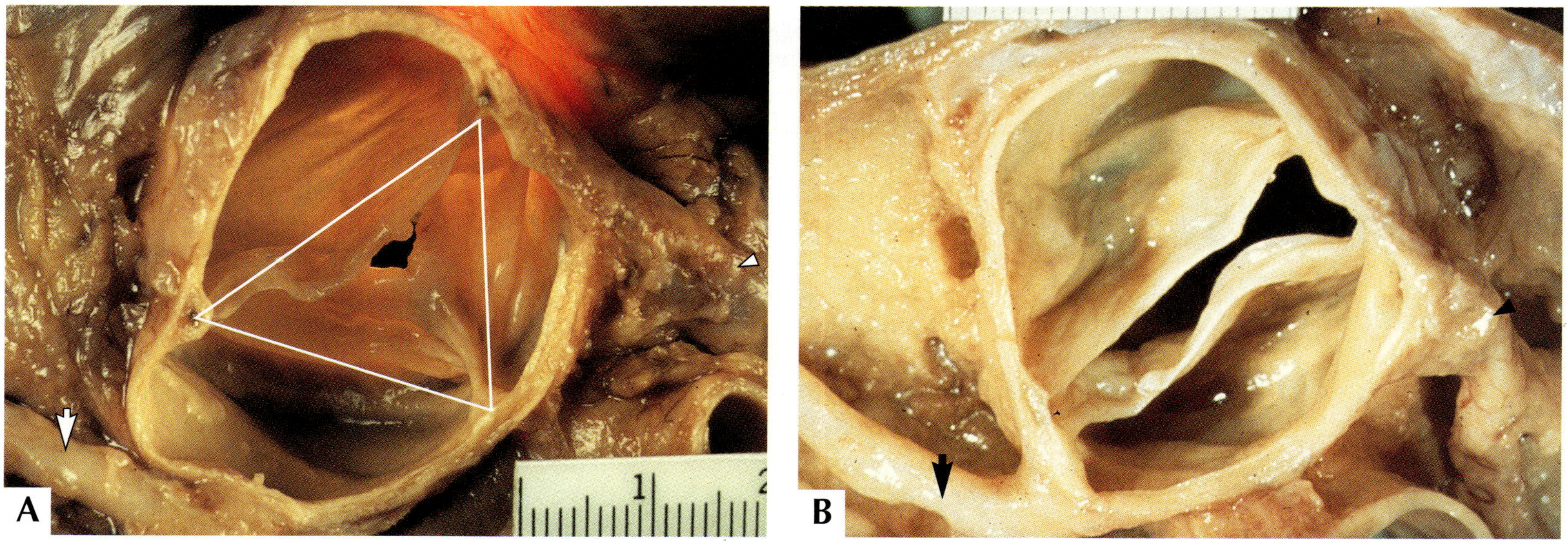

FIGURE 1-1. Congenital aortic valve (AV) disease. **A,** A normal aortic three-cuspid valve viewed from the superior aspect with the aorta cut transversely at the sinotubular junction. The three commissures are equidistant from one another (*sides of triangle*) and the three cusps are similar in size. The right coronary artery is denoted by an *arrow;* the left coronary artery is denoted by an *arrowhead*.

B, A normally functioning bicuspid AV with two commissures and the two leaflets, which are almost equal in size in a 58-year-old man who died of metastatic lung carcinoma. The commissures are located right and left and both coronary ostia arise from the anterior aortic sinus. Note the absence of raphe in either leaflet. The right coronary artery is denoted by an *arrow;* the left coronary artery is denoted by an *arrowhead*.

C, A mildly calcified congenitally bicuspid AV in a 69-year-old man. Note a nonstenotic functionally normal bicuspid valve with mild calcification (*arrows*) and a raphe (*arrowhead*) in the anterior leaflet. (*continued*)

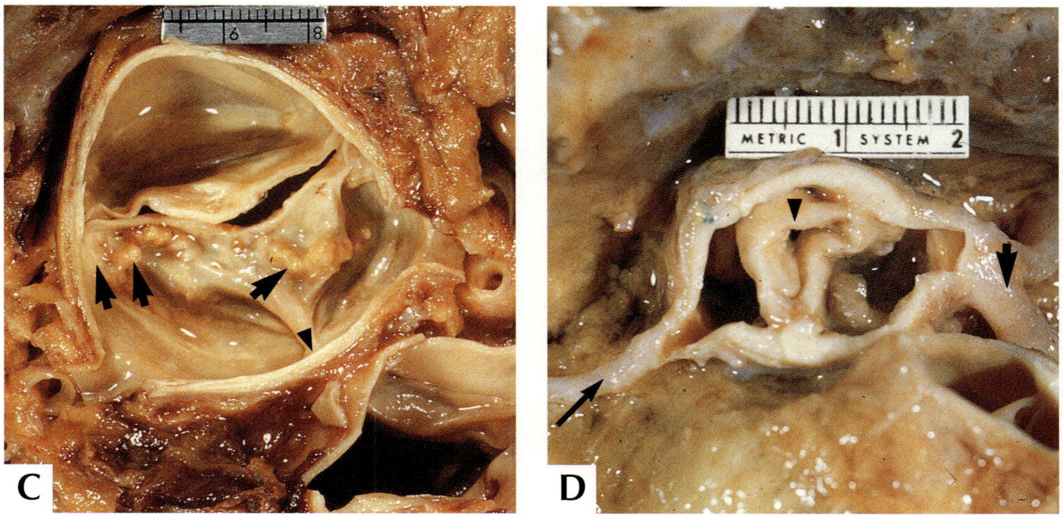

FIGURE 1-1. (*continued*) **D,** A bicuspid dysplastic and fibrotic AV (*arrowhead*) from a 24-year-old woman who had a commissurotomy 5 years before death. She was found dead in the hospital while awaiting repeat surgery. The commissures are located anterior and posterior and the leaflets are right and left with the right coronary artery (*long arrow*) and the left coronary artery (*short arrow*) arising from the right and left coronary sinuses. Patients with dysplastic bicuspid valves usually become symptomatic early in life, whereas those with calcified and fibrotic bicuspid valves usually present in the fifth to seventh decade.

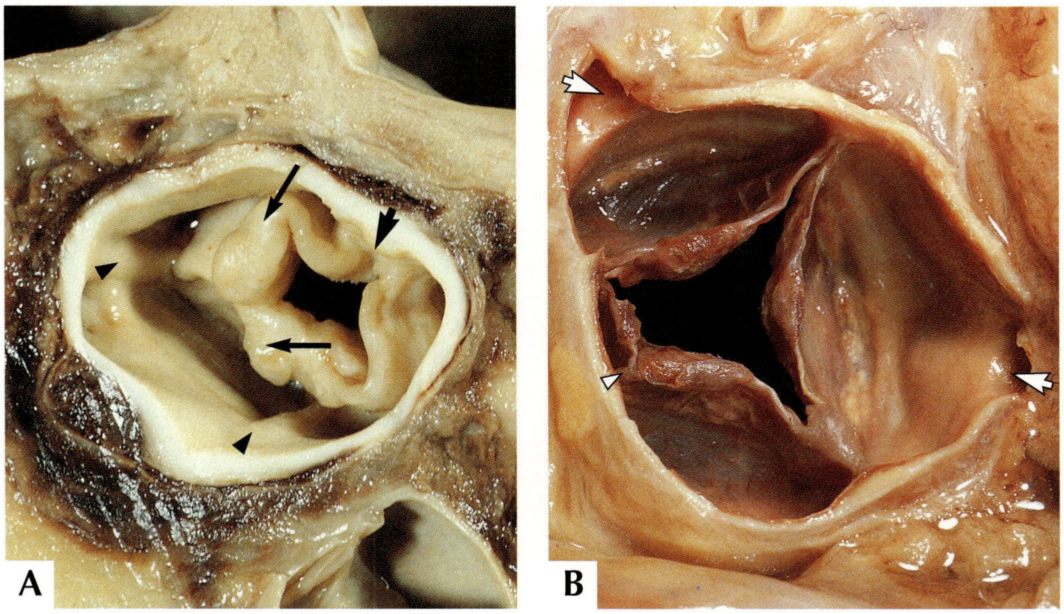

FIGURE 1-2. **A,** A unicuspid dysplastic AV (*long arrows*) in a 23-year-old woman who died suddenly while dancing. Note eccentric orifice of the dysplastic valve (*short arrow*) with two rudimentary raphes (*arrowheads*). The patient died from aortic dissection.

B, A quadricuspid AV from a 52-year-old woman on chronic hemodialysis. The four cusps are dissimilar in size. The right and left sinuses are normal, and the posterior sinus contains two cusps, with a smaller left posterior cusp. The incidence of quadricuspid valve is low in the general population (0.008% to 0.014%) and is more frequent in men [14]. Usually, there are no symptoms; occasionally, calcification or fibrosis of a quadricuspid AV results in aortic incompetence. *Top left arrow* shows right coronary ostium; *lower right arrow* shows left coronary ostium; *arrowhead* shows accessory commissure.

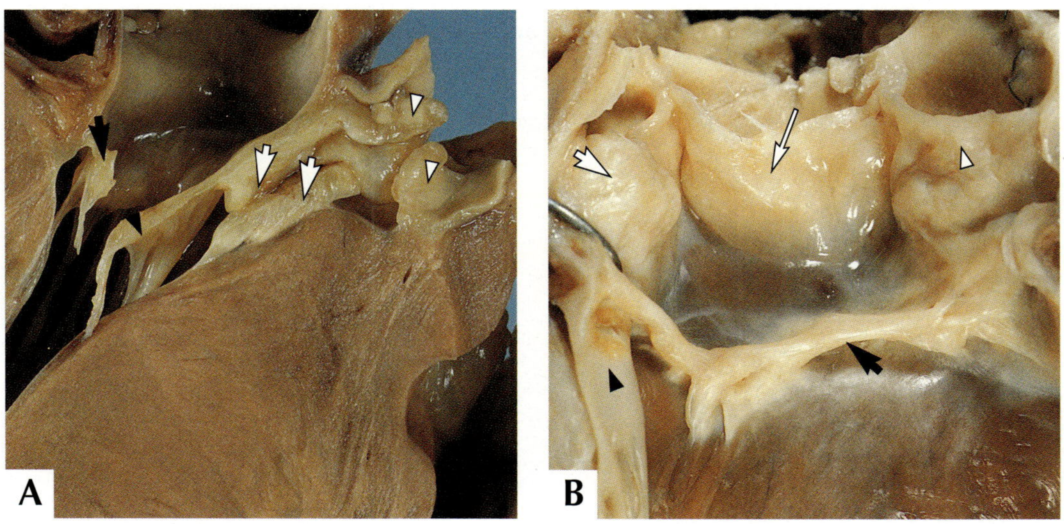

FIGURE 1-3. Subaortic stenosis, tunnel. Aortic stenosis (AS) is not limited to the valve but may involve the subvalvular outflow tract. Discrete subvalvular AS may be due to either a short localized fibrous ridge or, less commonly, a longer diffuse fibrous tunnel. A complete fibrous diaphragm may rarely be present. In tunneled subvalvular AS, fibrous thickening starts close to the AV and extends downward for 1 to 3 cm. The AV may be normal, tricuspid, dysplastic, or bicuspid, and most frequently the valve is only mildly incompetent. **A,** The heart of a 12-year-old girl who had a commissurotomy for AS 2 years before death. One week before death, a ventricular aortic conduit was placed. The patient died postoperatively of sepsis.

The dysplastic AV (*white arrowheads*) and the fibrous subaortic tunnel (*white arrows*) can be seen. Operative repair requires generous myectomy to prevent recurrence, or atrioventriculoplasty with or without valve replacement (Konno and modified Konno operation). Eighty percent of patients live 15 years after surgery. Surgery is indicated between the ages of 3 and 6 years and is uncommon beyond 20 years of age [15]. *Black arrow,* posterior mitral leaflet; *black arrowhead,* anterior mitral leaflet.

B, Subaortic stenosis, fibrous ridge (*black arrow*). Note discrete band underlying the AV in a boy aged 15 years who died suddenly. The valve had three leaflets and was dysplastic. The patient underwent unsuccessful open valvuloplasty 10 years previously. Severe left ventricular hypertrophy was noted at autopsy. Currently, the preferred surgery is removal of the fibrous band with myectomy. *Short white arrow,* posterior coronary cusp; *long white arrow,* right coronary cusp; *white arrowhead,* left coronary cusp; *black arrowhead,* anterior mitral leaflet.

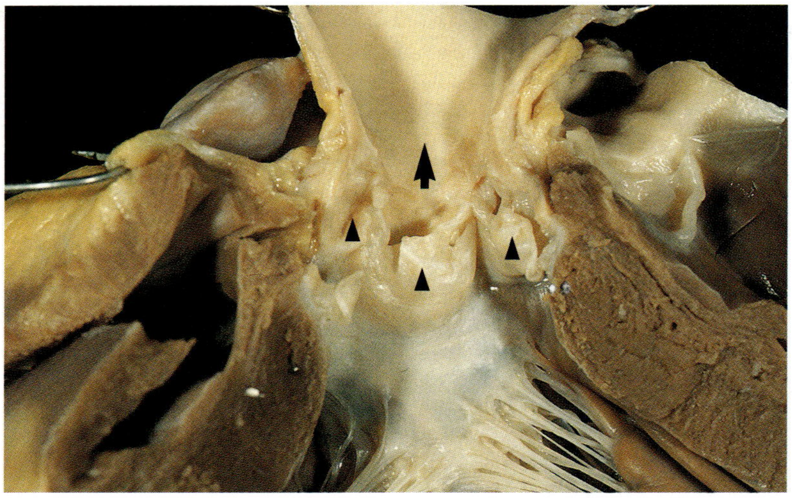

FIGURE 1-4. Supravalvular AS. Note irregular constricted area at the sinotubular junction distal to the valve (*arrow*), which is composed of three dysplastic leaflets (*arrowheads*). The patient was a 14-year-old boy with Williams syndrome who died suddenly. Associated cardiac defects in supravalvular AS include coronary artery dysplasia.

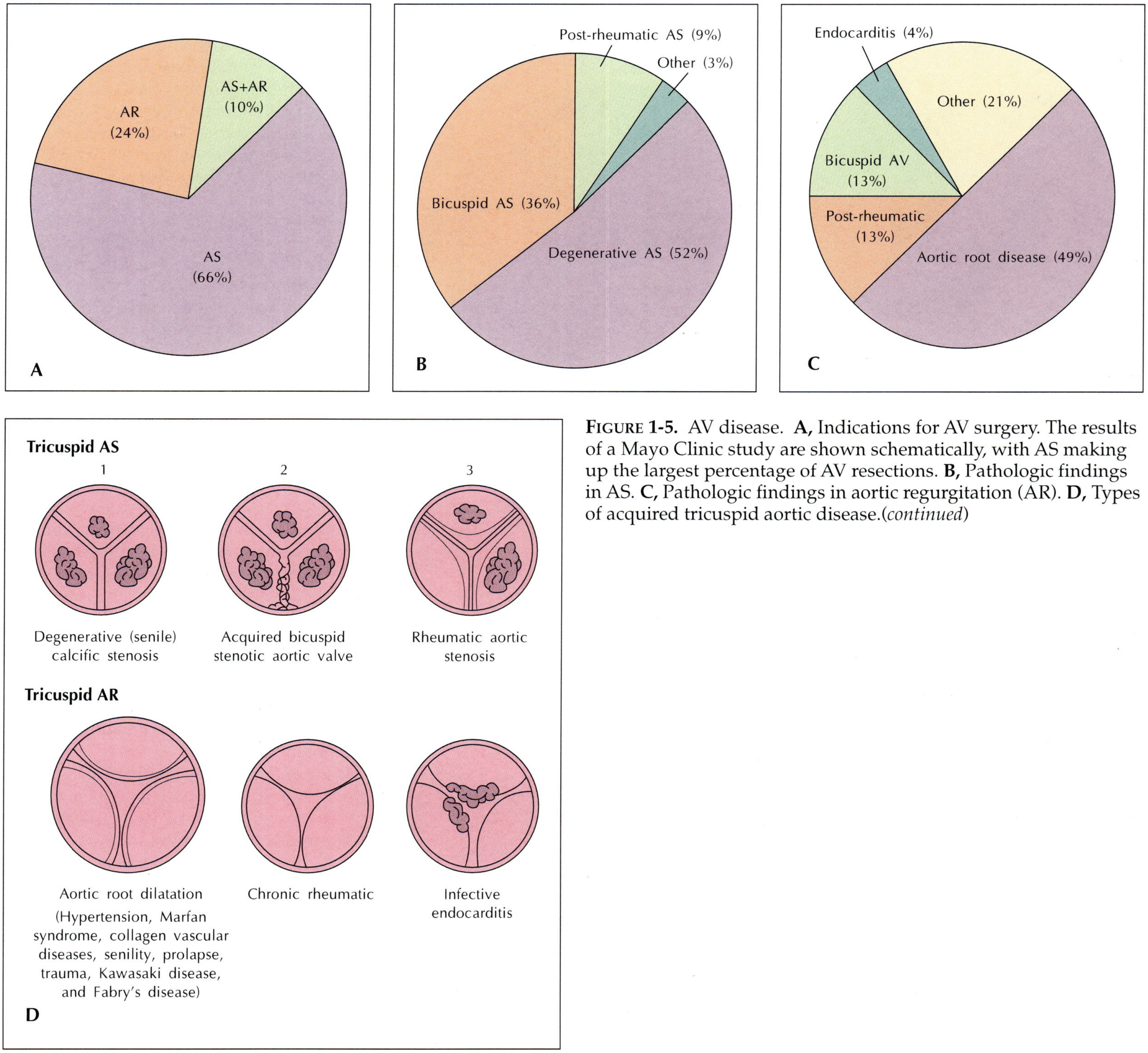

FIGURE 1-5. AV disease. **A,** Indications for AV surgery. The results of a Mayo Clinic study are shown schematically, with AS making up the largest percentage of AV resections. **B,** Pathologic findings in AS. **C,** Pathologic findings in aortic regurgitation (AR). **D,** Types of acquired tricuspid aortic disease.(*continued*)

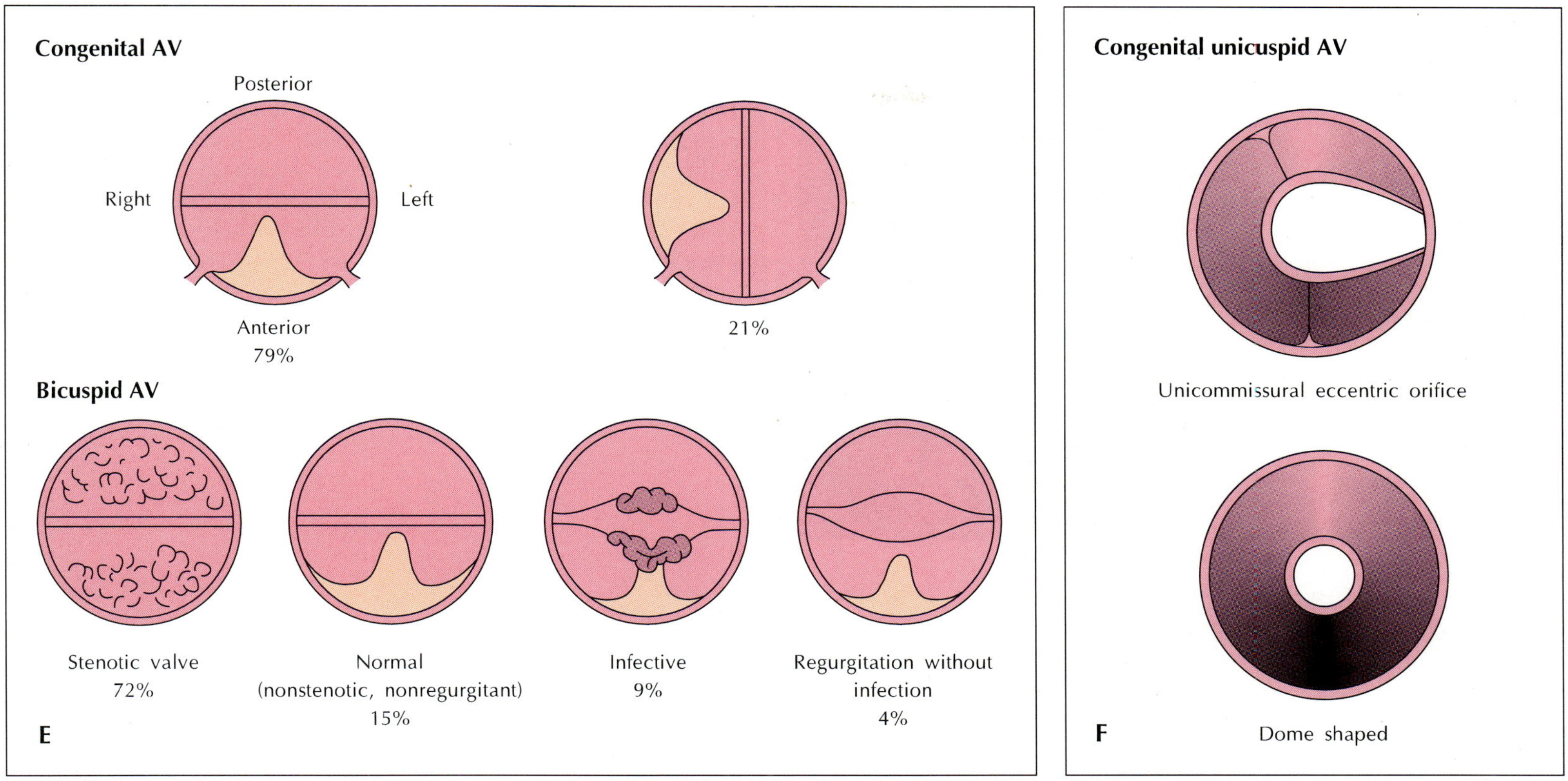

FIGURE 1-5. (*continued*) **E,** Congenital bicuspid (nondysplastic) AV. **F,** Unicuspid AV. (Parts A, B, and C *adapted from* Dare and coworkers [3].)

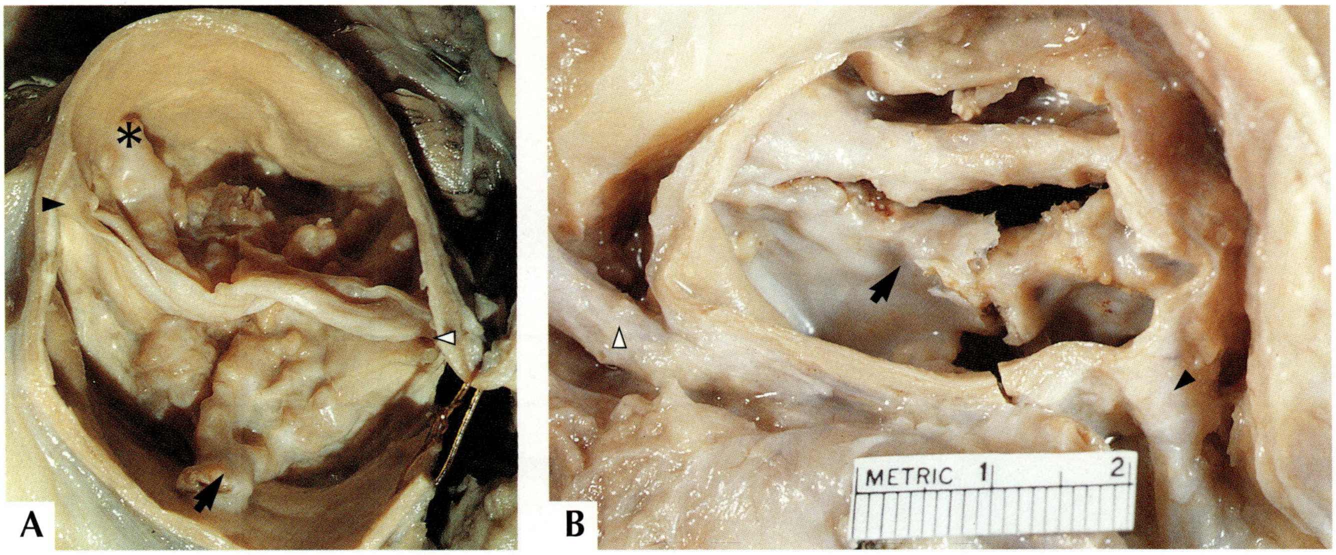

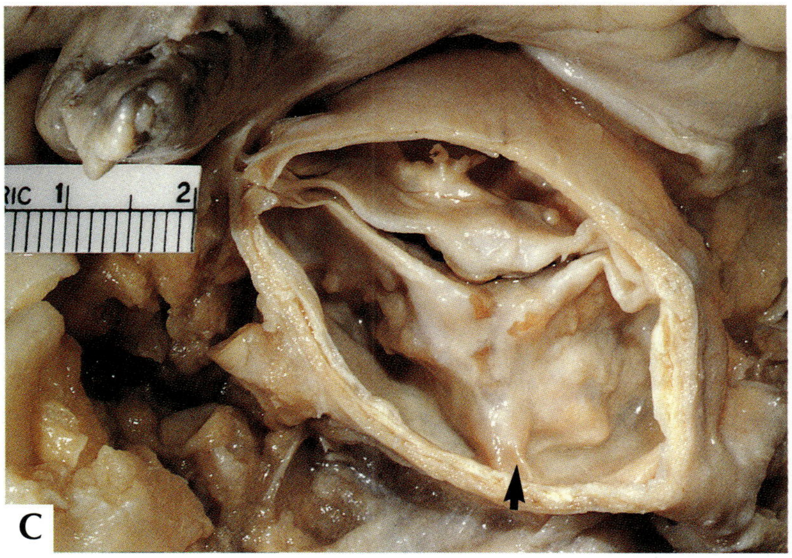

FIGURE 1-6. Bicuspid AV: congenital versus acquired. **A,** Congenital bicuspid stenotic AV with calcified and fibrotic raphe (*arrow*). The patient was in his fifth decade. Note that leaflets are anterior and posterior, and there is a rudimentary commissure in the anterior leaflet that does not reach the level of the true commissures. *Asterisk* shows calcified nodules; *black arrowhead* shows right commissure; *white arrowhead* shows left commissure.

B, Calcified fibrotic congenital bicuspid AS (*arrow*). No raphe is identified. Note the marked thickening of the valve leaflets, which are similar in size. The patient was a woman in her forties with symptomatic AS. *White arrowhead* shows right coronary artery; *black arrowhead* shows left coronary artery.

C, Acquired bicuspid stenotic AV. A 65-year-old man died suddenly while awaiting valve replacement surgery. Note the presence of three commissures that are equidistant. The anterior commissure is fused (*arrow*), and the commissure is at the same level as the other two nonfused commissures. (*continued*)

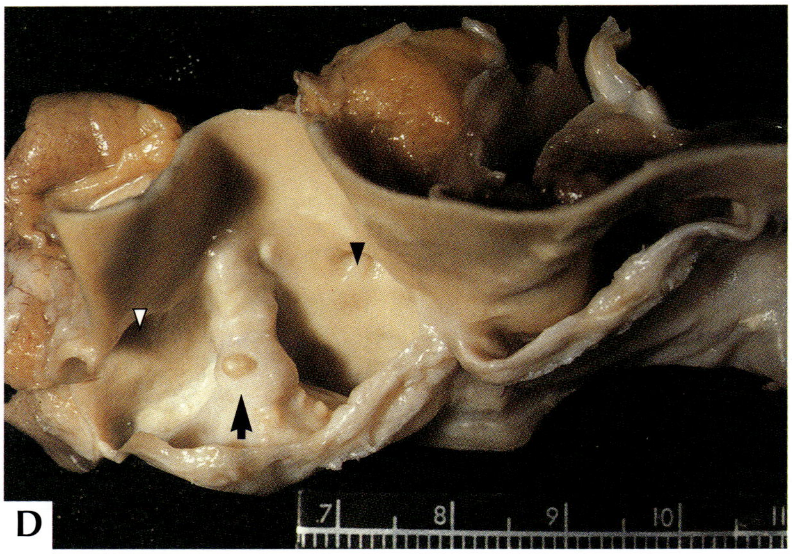

FIGURE 1-6. (*continued*) **D,** Congenital bicuspid AV. The AV is viewed from the superior aspect after opening the valve along the left ventricular outflow tract. There are two functional leaflets, with a raphe (*arrow*) situated between the left (*white arrowhead*) and right (*black arrowhead*) coronary ostia. The raphe is calcified, and the valve margin beyond the raphe is smooth.

The cause of acquired fusion of AV leaflets is often obscure but may be related to healed endocarditis or rheumatic valve disease limited to one commissure.

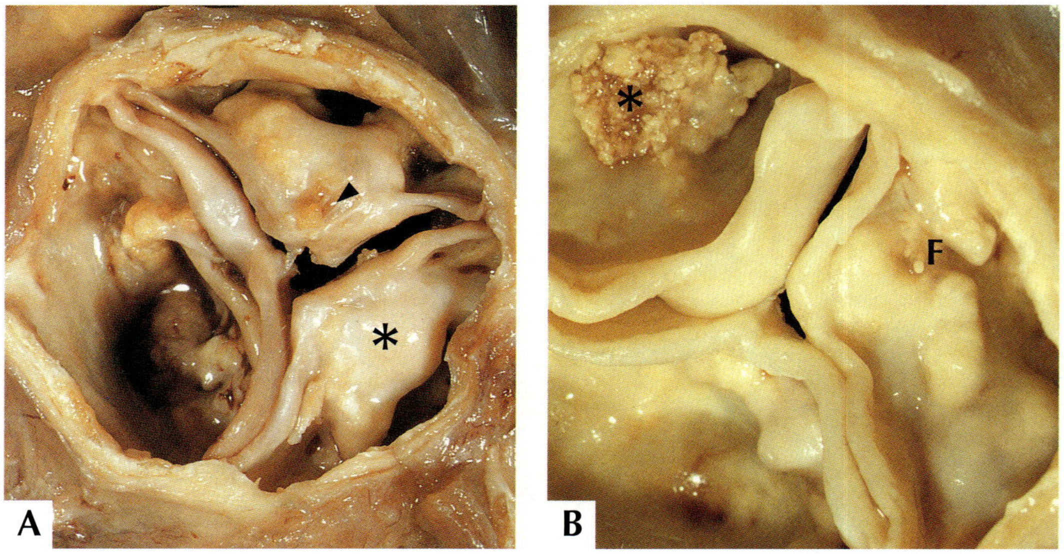

FIGURE 1-7. Degenerative AV disease. **A,** Tricuspid stenotic AV in an 81-year-old man who died suddenly. At autopsy the heart weighed 675 g, and there was severe stenosis of the AV with marked calcific deposits on the left (*asterisk*) and the posterior noncoronary (*arrowhead*) cusps without commissural fusion. **B,** A close view of the AV shows extruding calcific material in the posterior noncoronary cusp and a fracture (F) in the calcific nodule in the left coronary cusp secondary to the balloon valvuloplasty.

MITRAL VALVE DISEASE

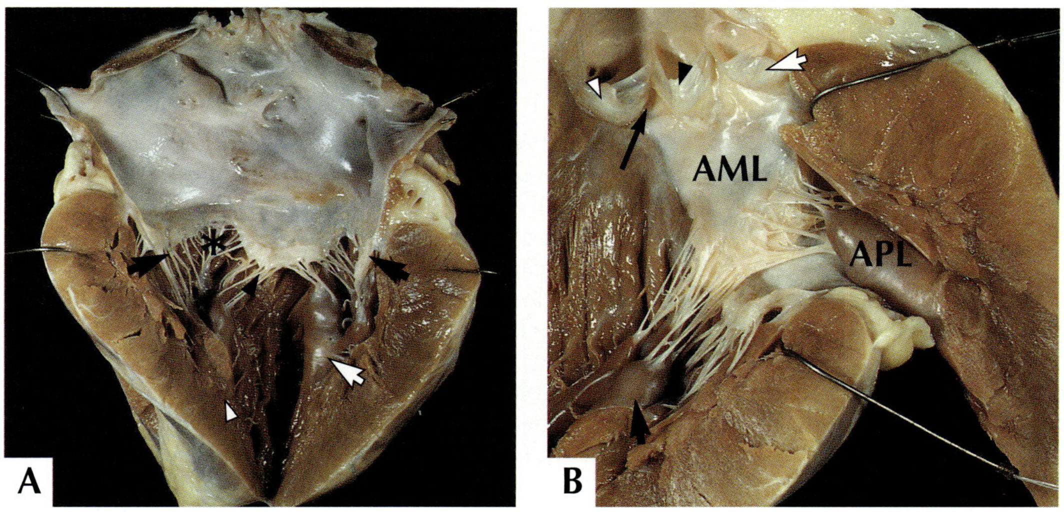

FIGURE 1-8. Normal mitral valve (MV). **A,** A normal heart after opening the left atrium (LA) and left ventricle along the left lateral border of the heart. The MV consists of an anterior mitral leaflet (AML) (*black arrowhead*) connected by the commissures to the posterior mitral leaflet (PML) (*black arrows*). The AML is longer than the PML and the chordae arise at 45° from the AML on the ventricular surface. The chordae insert into the anterolateral (*white arrow*) and the posteromedial (*white arrowhead*) papillary muscles. The commissural chordae (*asterisk*) fan out from the papillary muscle, whereas leaflet chordae are usually single and fan near the insertion site. **B,** The heart has been further opened by extending the left ventricular apex incision through the left ventricular outflow tract into the AV and aorta. Note the three AV leaflets, and the membranous septum (*long black arrow*) separating the posterior noncoronary cusp (*black arrowhead*) from the right coronary cusp (*white arrowhead*). The AML is in direct continuity with the posterior noncoronary cusp. *White arrow* signifies the left coronary cusp. *Short black arrow* shows the posteromedial papillary muscle. APL—anterolateral papillary muscle.

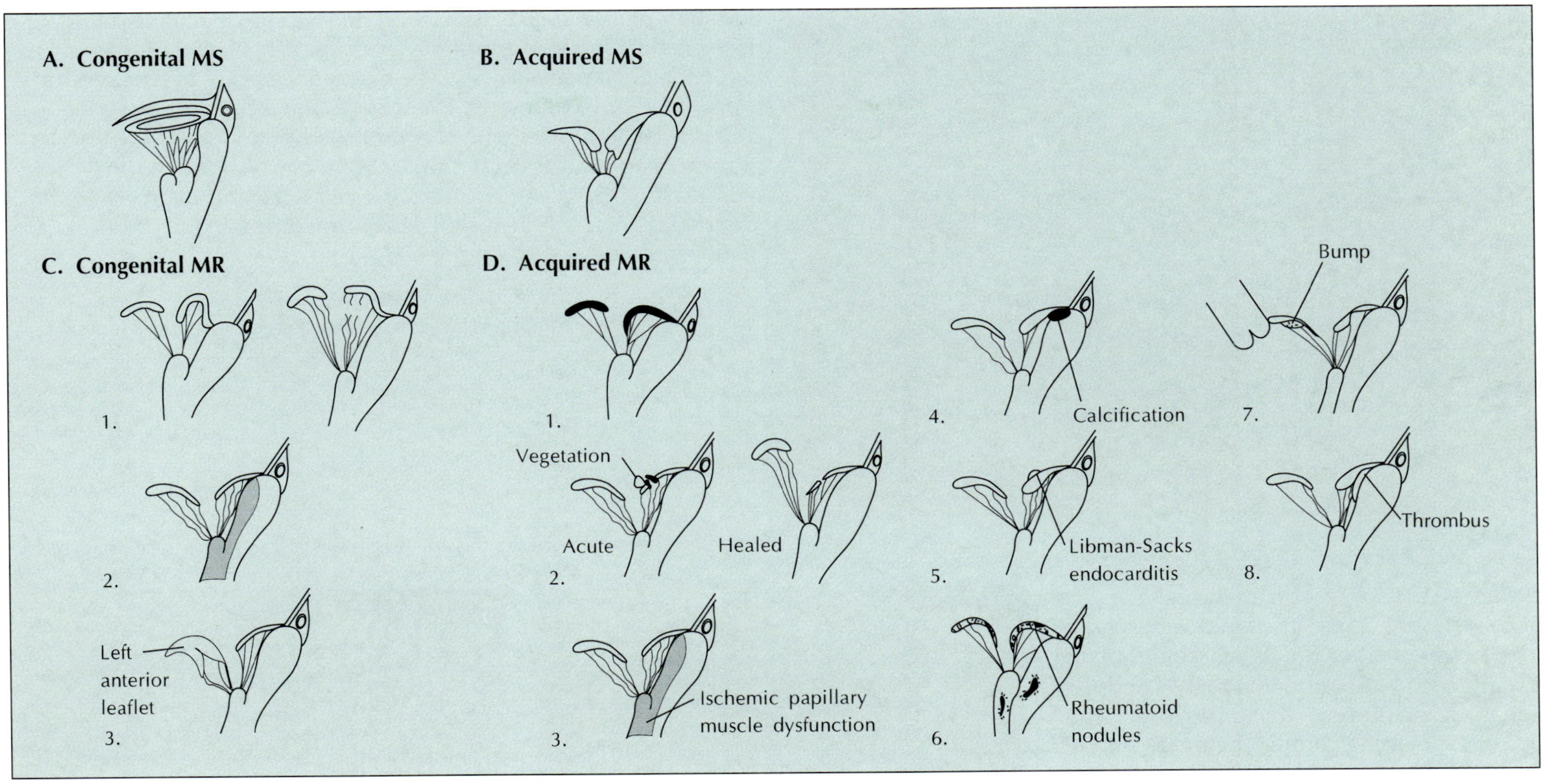

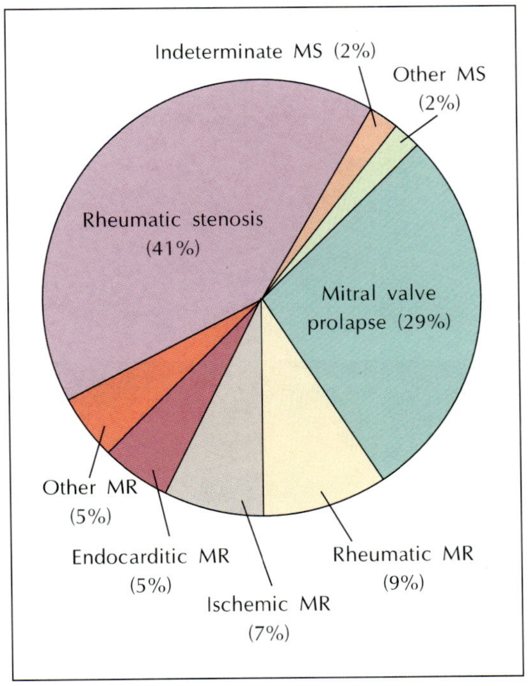

Figure 1-9. Causes of congenital and acquired MV disease. **A**, Congenital mitral stenosis (MS) (parachute MS). **B**, Acquired MS (chronic rheumatic valvulitis). **C,** Congenital mitral regurgitation [MR], resulting from a prolapsed MV (Marfan syndrome, Ehlers-Danlos syndrome, and pseudoxanthoma elasticum) (*1*), anomalous origin of the left coronary artery from the pulmonary trunk (*2*), and cleft MV (*3*). **D,** Acquired MR , resulting from chronic rheumatic valvulitis (*1*), infective endocarditis (*2*), ischemic heart disease with MR (*3*), degenerative annular calcification (*4*), systemic lupus erythematosus (*5*), rheumatoid arthritis (*6*), ankylosing spondylitis (*7*), and hypereosinophilic syndrome (*8*). **E**, Pathologic findings noted in MV excisions. (Part E *adapted from* Dare and coworkers [5].)

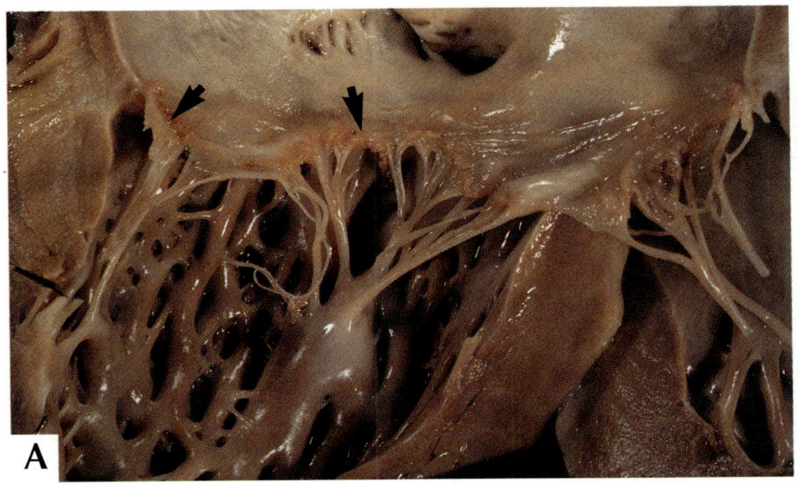

FIGURE 1-10. Acute rheumatic fever. This inflammatory disease affects principally children with recent group A streptococcal pharyngitis. It is characterized by fever, migratory polyarthritis of the large joints, carditis, subcutaneous nodules, and erythema marginatum of the skin and chorea. On gross inspection, the heart is slightly enlarged and flabby and fibrinous pericarditis is present. Verrucal lesions are most frequently seen on the MV and AV and rarely on the tricuspid and pulmonic valves.

A, MV shows small 1- to 2-mm friable vegetations (verrucae) along the lines of closure (*arrows*). The patient was an 18-year-old mentally retarded man with cardiac arrest and a recent history of fever and diarrhea of unknown duration. The underlying endocardium demonstrated mixed acute and chronic inflammatory infiltrates with occasional macrophages and even Aschoff bodies. (*continued*)

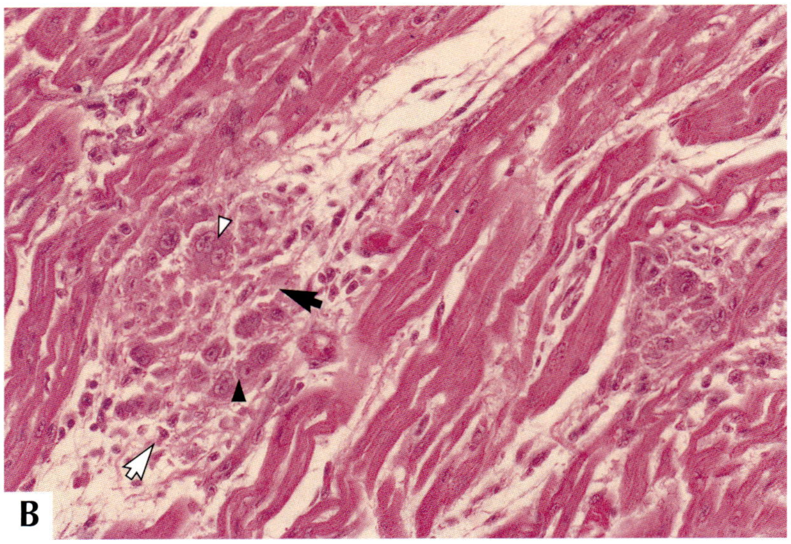

FIGURE 1-10. (*continued*) **B,** Aschoff nodules are foci of fibrinoid necrosis (*black arrow*), lymphocytes (*white arrow*), macrophages, and occasional plasma cells. The macrophages are of two specific types. The Anitschkow cell (*black arrowhead*, or Aschoff cell) has round to ovoid nuclei with chromatin condensation at the nuclear periphery and in the center; this feature has resulted in the designations "owl-eyed" and "caterpillar cell." Aschoff giant cells (*white arrowhead*) are multinucleated cells formed from Antischkow's histiocytes.

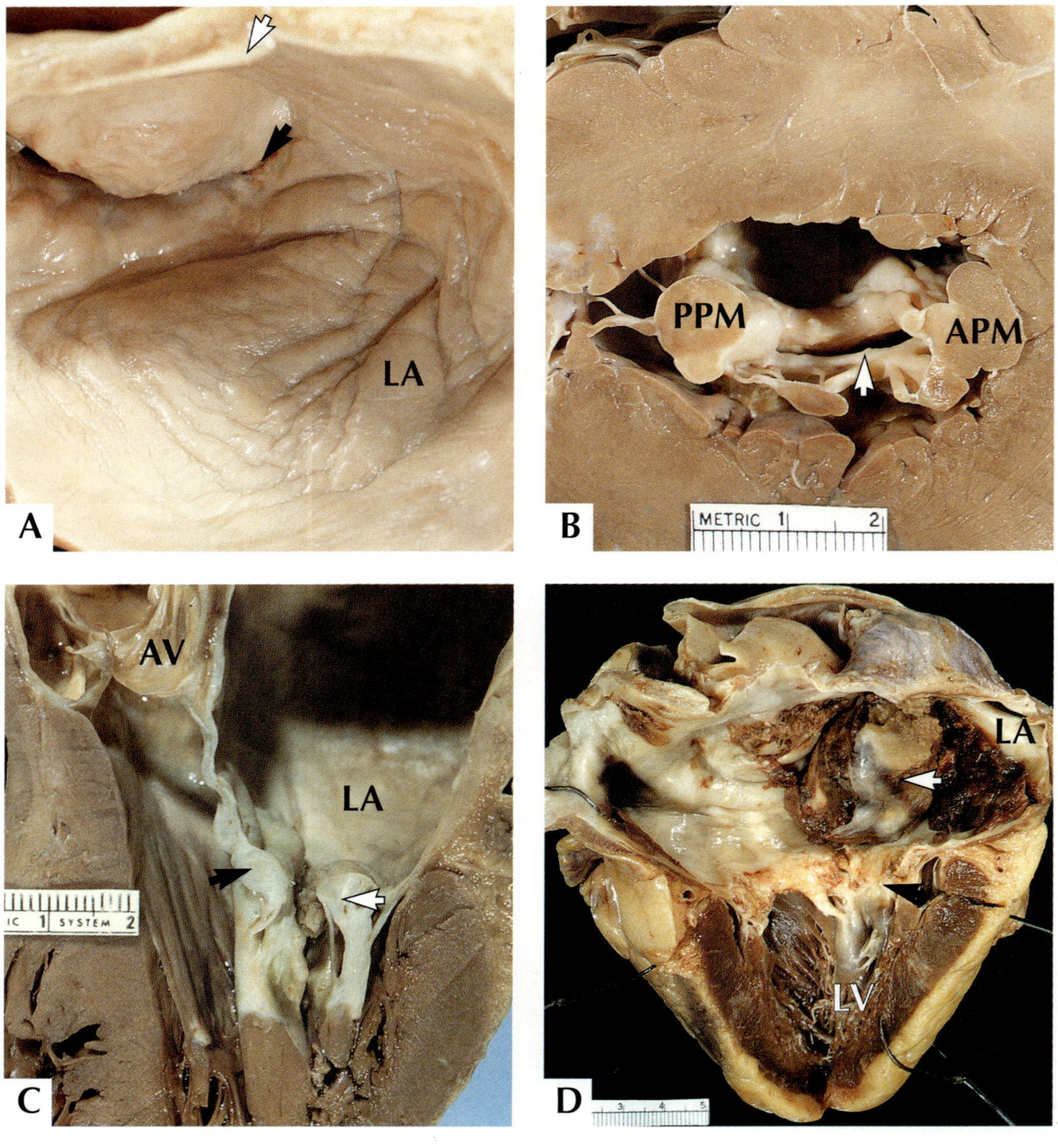

FIGURE 1-11. Chronic rheumatic valve disease (mitral, aortic, tricuspid valves). Chronic rheumatic valvulitis becomes manifest after a latent period that ranges in duration from 5 to 30 years (mean 19 years). The risk of developing chronic rheumatic valvulitis after an episode of acute rheumatic fever is 18% to 65% and is highest in patients with rheumatic carditis that results in congestive heart failure [16]. In the industrialized world, the incidence of rheumatic fever has declined dramatically, but in recent years, there has been a resurgence in military and civilian populations in the United States. A correlation has been found with the appearance of the virulent, encapsulated, M protein–rich strain, which is referred to as "rheumatogenic" group A *Streptococcus* [17]. Chronic rheumatic disease affects only the MV in two thirds of the patients, and both the MV and AV in one third; tricuspid and pulmonary valve involvement is rare.

A, A 68-year-old white man, with history of acute rheumatic fever at age 14 and a long-standing heart murmur, had remained asymptomatic from age 14 to 61 years when he developed dyspnea on exertion and paroxysmal nocturnal dyspnea. Significant MS was documented with an MV area of 0.67 cm^2, a mitral gradient of 14 mm Hg, and mild MR. Note a markedly dilated left atrium (LA) and MS (*black arrow*). *White arrow* indicates the intra-atrial septum.

B, The ventricular surface of the MV shows a markedly stenotic MV orifice ("fish-mouth") (*arrow*) with chordal fusion and thickening of the valve leaflets. There is fibrosis and thickening with retraction of leaflets. The commisures are fused and the chordae tendineae are thickened, fibrotic, matted, and shortened.

C, Long-axis view of left ventricular (LV) outflow tract from a 64-year-old woman with isolated severe MS and a peak transmitral gradient of 18 mm Hg. The patient had a closed mitral commissurotomy 3 years before death from progressive congestive heart failure. Note dilated LA and markedly fibrotic MV leaflets, with mild calcification, and severe chordal thickening with total chordal fusion into pillars of fibrous tissue (*white arrow*). The AV was unaffected. *Black arrow* denotes the anterior mitral leaflet.

D, MS. Another 64-year-old woman had severe isolated MS and congestive heart failure with marked deformity of the mitral valve, which was thickened, fibrotic, and fused (*black arrow*). Note LA dilatation and presence of a thrombus in the LA (*white arrow*). APM—anterolateral papillary muscle; PPM—posteromedial papillary muscle.(Part C *adapted from* Roberts [18]; with permission)

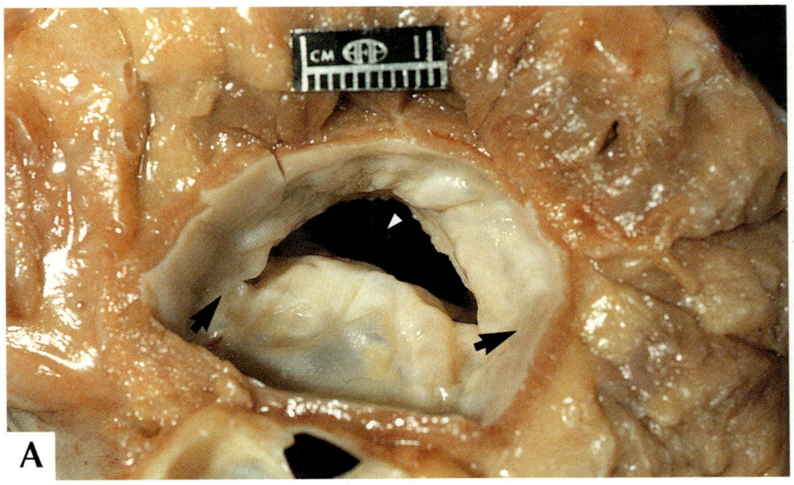

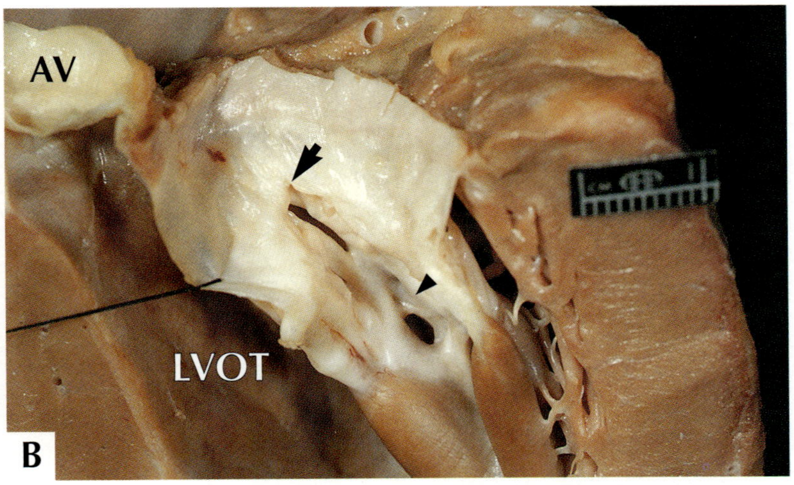

Figure 1-12. MR. **A,** A 66-year-old woman had a history of shortness of breath and MR. Note regurgitant, nonstenotic MV with fibrosis. Commissures are fused and fibrotic and valve leaflets are retracted (*arrows*). The MV orifice (*arrowhead*) remains open during systole, producing MR.

B, Long-axis view of the left ventricular outflow tract (LVOT) of the heart illustrated in *A* demonstrates commissural fusion (*arrow*) and chordal thickening with fusion (*arrowhead*).

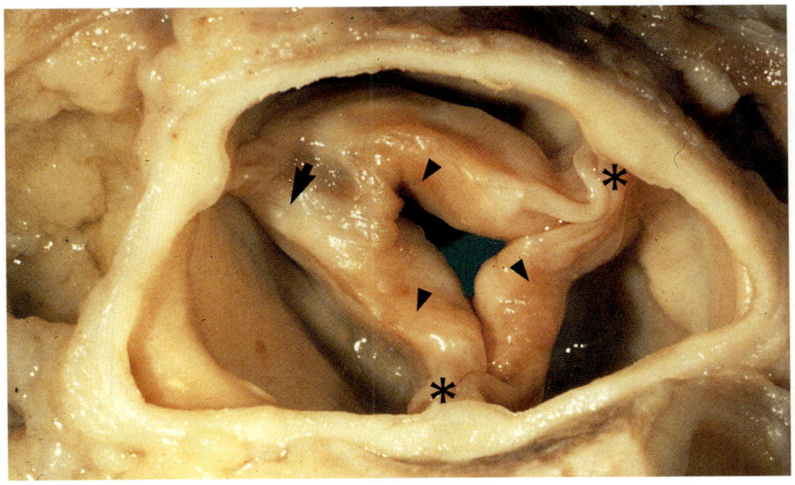

Figure 1-13. AS. This AV is from a 24-year-old woman who had undergone bioprosthetic MV replacement 5 years before death. One week before death she experienced progressive dyspnea. At autopsy, a large linear tear in one of the leaflets of the bioprosthetic valve was found. The AV is illustrated and shows fusion of the right posterior commissure (*arrow*) and marked AV leaflet thickening (*arrowheads*) consistent with mild to moderate AS. *Asterisks* denote nonfused commissures.

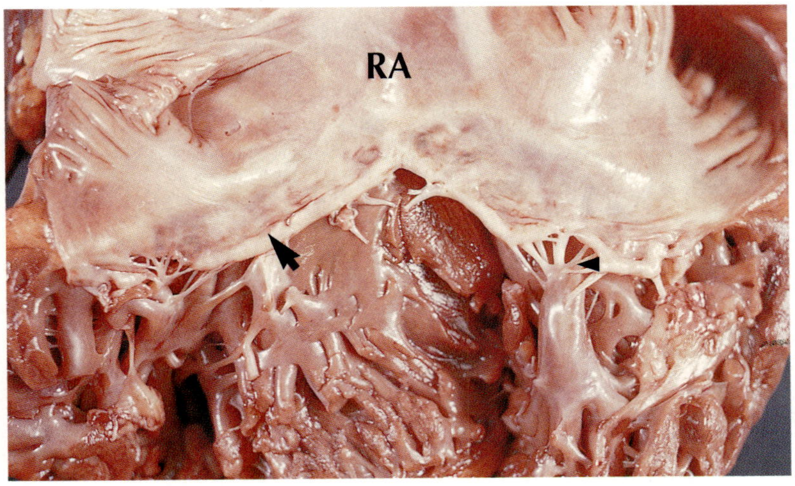

Figure 1-14. Tricuspid valve (TV). The patient had mitral, aortic, and tricuspid involvement with chronic rheumatic valvulitis. Note thickened and rolled free margins of the TV margins (*arrow*) along with thickened and retracted chordae tendineae (*arrowhead*). RA—right atrium.

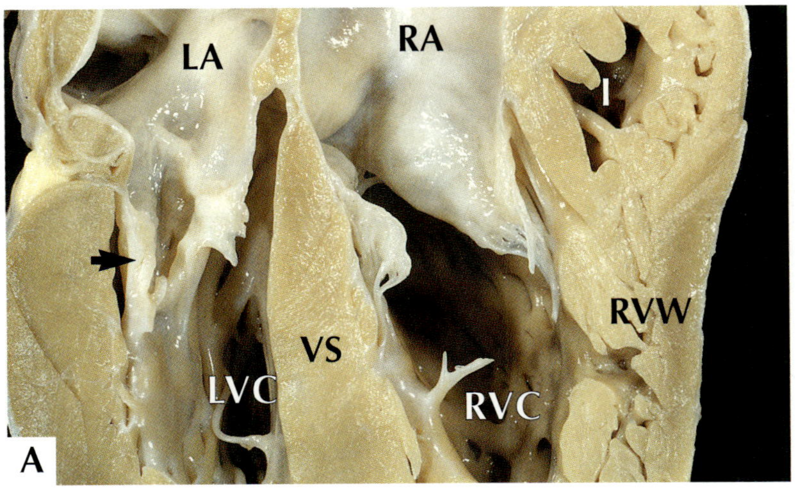

Figure 1-15. Congenital MV disease. **A,** Parachute MV is a rare congenital anomaly. There is close apposition or fusion of the papillary muscles into one structure. The MV leaflets either directly or via thickened chordae insert into a single papillary muscle (*arrow*), which results in a stenotic mitral orifice. Parachute MV is associated with the supravalvular mitral ring; the combination of parachute MV, supravalvular ring of left atrium (LA), subaortic stenosis, and coarctation of the aorta constitute the classic Shone's syndrome. Shone complex refers to coarctation of the aorta and multiple left-sided obstructive lesions. (*continued*)

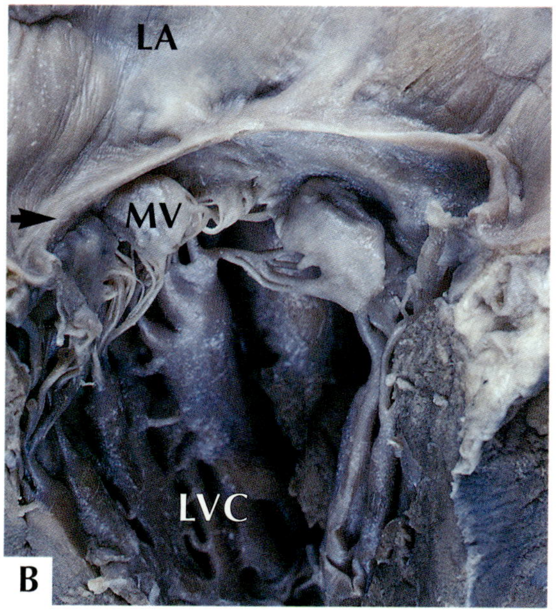

Figure 1-15. *(continued)* **B,** A supravalvular mitral ring (*arrow*) in a child with double inlet left ventricular and ventricular septal defect in the absence of parachute MV. I—infundibulum; LVC—left ventricular cavity; RA—right atrium; RVC—right ventricular cavity; RVW—right ventricular wall; VS–ventricular septum.

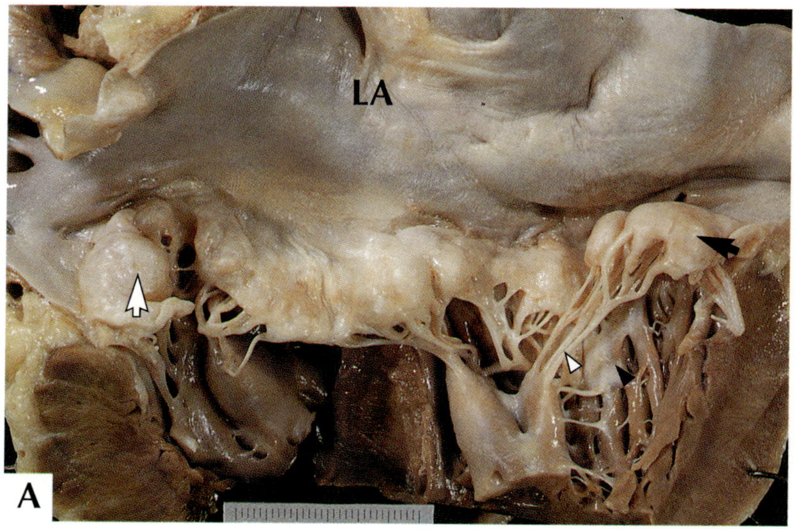

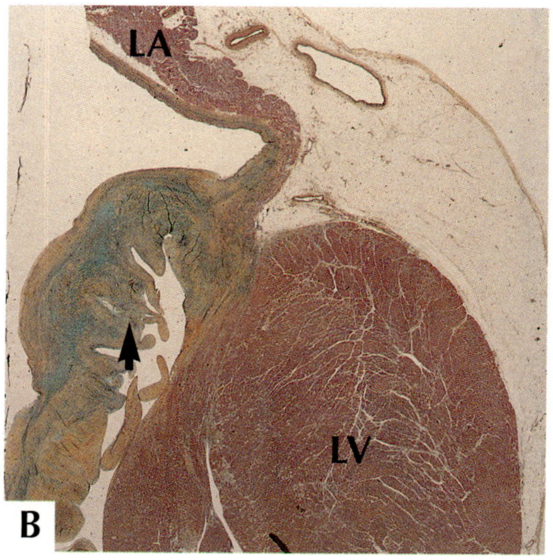

Figure 1-16. Mitral valve prolapse (MVP). The incidence of MVP in the general population is 3% to 5% and is higher in women. The majority of patients are asymptomatic. Symptomatic MR occurs in 10% to 15% of patients and is more common in men older than 50 years [19].

A, A 54-year old white man died suddenly without previous cardiac history. Note the enlarged and billowing intermediate (*black arrow*) and medial (*white arrow*) scallop of the posterior mitral valve leaflet. *White arrowhead* denotes elongated chordal tendinae and *black arrowhead* denotes endocardial plaque.

B, Histologic section of the MV shown in *panel A*. Note proteoglycan deposits (*green staining*) expanding the spongiosa and extending into the fibrosa. This Movat pentachrome stain demonstrates elastic tissue (*black*), fibrous tissue (*yellow*), and proteoglycans (*blue-green*). *Arrow* denotes fibrosa. (Part A *adapted from* Farb and coworkers [19]; with permission.)

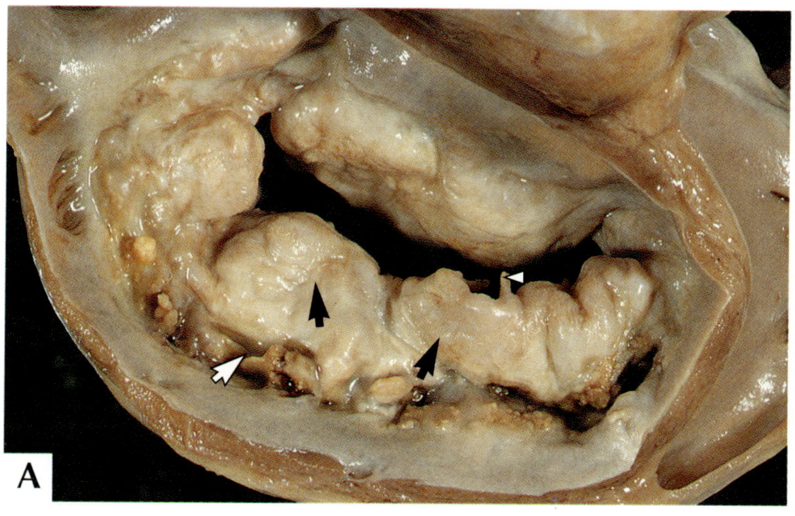

Figure 1-17. Severe MR. **A,** A 48-year-old white woman had severe MR and congestive heart failure secondary to mitral valve prolapse (MVP) with extensive calcification of the mitral annulus (*white arrow*). The patient died while awaiting surgery. The mitral valve is viewed from the left atrium. Note prolapsing posterior mitral leaflet (PML) with involvement of the intermediate and lateral scallops (*black arrows*). *Arrowhead* denotes ruptured chordae tendineae. (*continued*)

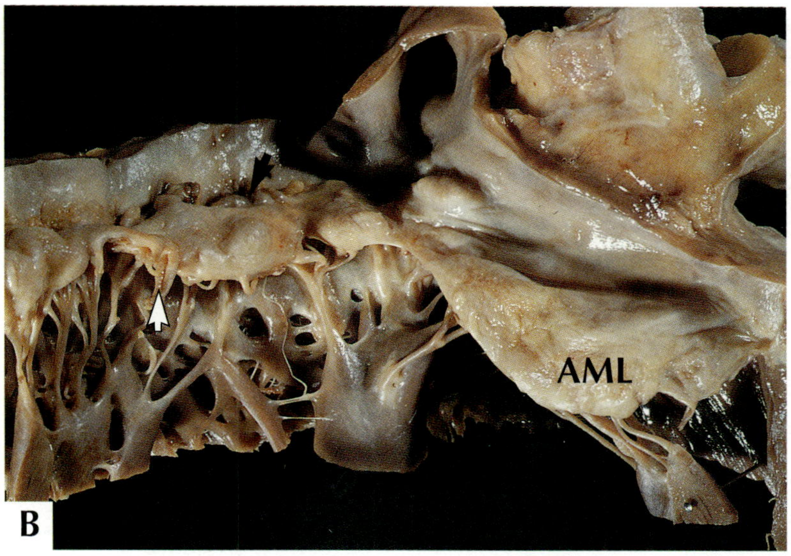

FIGURE 1-17. (*continued*) **B,** The MV is opened and the intermediate scallop of the PML is hooded and flail. Note ruptured chordae tendineae (*white arrow*). Mitral annular calcification (*black arrow*) is accelerated in patients with MVP.

C, Histologic section of PML shows increased proteoglycan deposition (*arrowhead*) and marked annular calcification (*arrow*). AML–anterior mitral leaflet.(Parts A and C *adapted from* Virmani and coworkers [10]; with permission.)

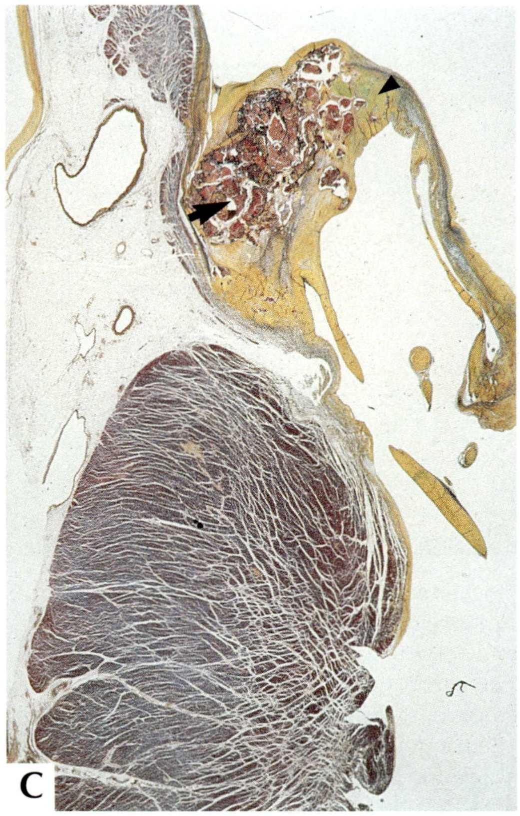

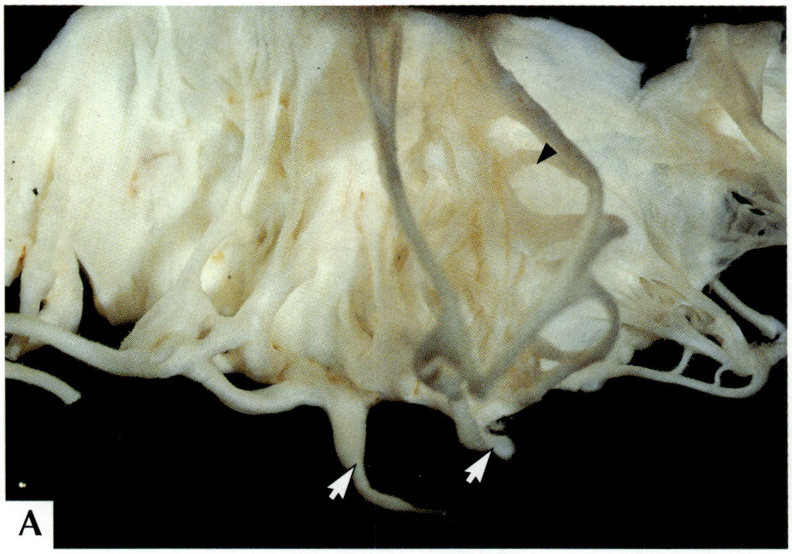

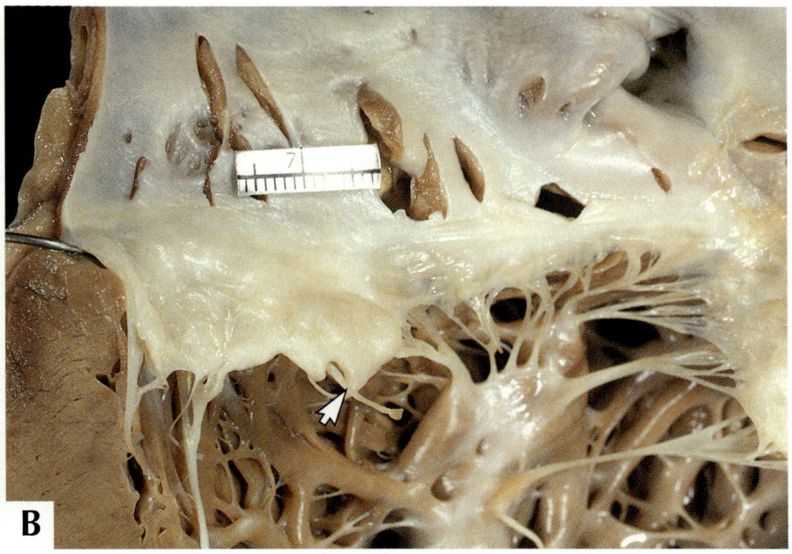

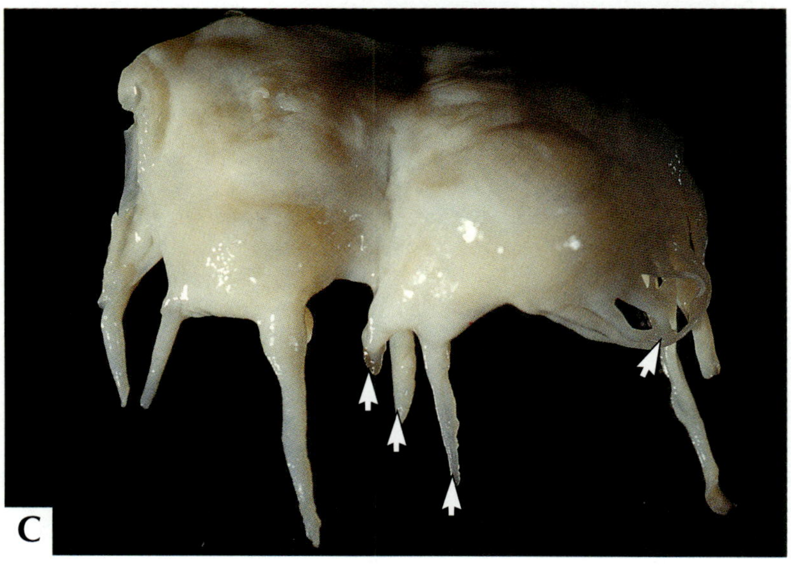

FIGURE 1-18. Severe MR. **A,** Surgically removed mitral valve from a patient with severe MR secondary to MVP. Note excessive chordal insertion and ruptured chordae (*arrows*). The gross appearance of surgically excised prolapsed mitral valve is typically glistening whitish blue. *Arrowhead* denotes excessive length and branching of the chordae tendineae.

B, A 30-year-old woman died suddenly. At autopsy, the only significant pathologic finding was prolapse of the posterior mitral valve leaflet and ruptured chordae tendineae (*arrow*). The risk of sudden death in patients with MVP is low, and the mechanism of ventricular arrhythmias is yet unexplained.

C, Atrial view of a portion of the posterior mitral leaflet removed at surgery from a patient who underwent mitral valve reconstructive surgery. Chordae tendineae are torn, and the free edges of the chordae are tapered (*arrows*).

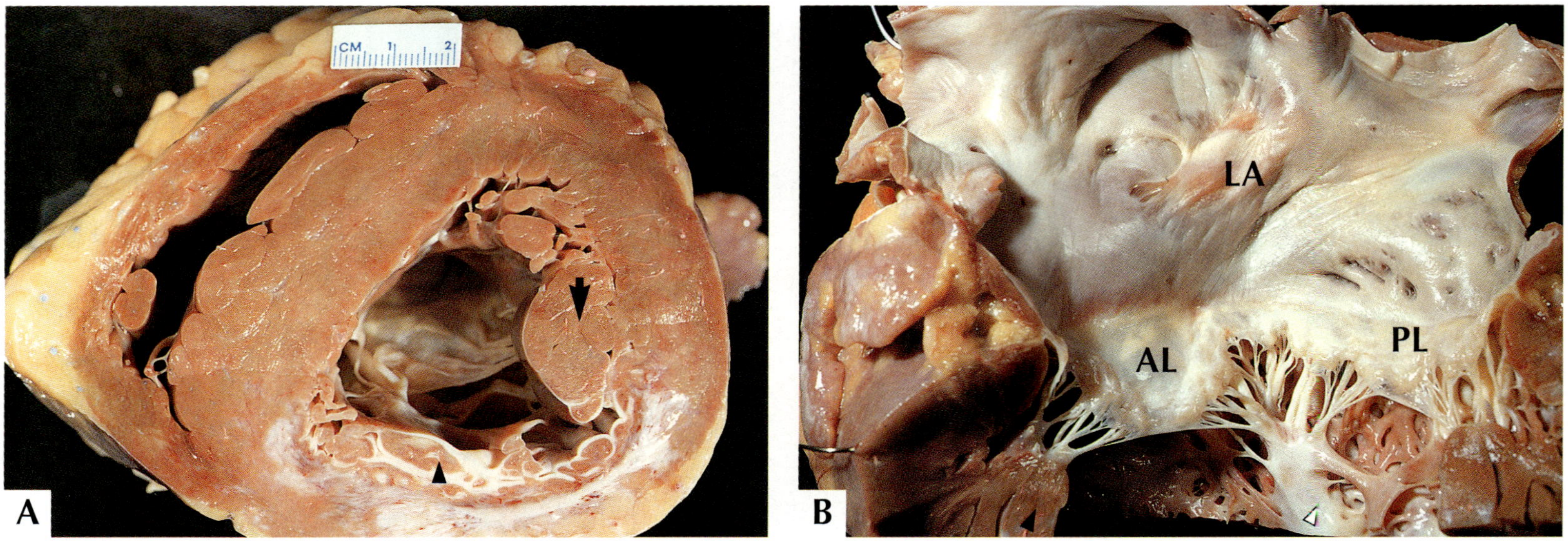

FIGURE 1-19. Ischemic MR. Papillary muscle dysfunction in the absence of papillary muscle rupture occurs frequently in patients with coronary artery disease (CAD) and results in MR. The papillary muscles are perfused by endarteries of the coronary vascular bed and are therefore most vulnerable to ischemic injury. In acute myocardial infarction (MI), the papillary muscles undergo necrosis with eventual healing and fibrosis. The posteromedial papillary muscle (PPM) is supplied by the posterior descending branch of the right coronary artery (RCA). It is more vulnerable to ischemic injury than the anterolateral papillary muscle (APM), which has a dual blood supply (left diagonal branches of the left anterior descending coronary artery and the left obtuse marginal branches of the left circumflex coronary artery. The increased relative susceptibility of the PPM to ischemic injury may also occur because the distance from the origin of the RCA to its distal branches is greater than the distance between the origin of the left coronary artery and the APM, resulting in a lower perfusion pressure.

A, PPM scarring (*arrowhead*) in a patient with severe (greater than 75% luminal narrowing) coronary atherosclerosis of the RCA and left circumflex coronary arteries. The APM (*arrow*) appears normal.

B, A 60-year-old man with congestive heart failure and MR secondary to CAD had a healed MI of the left ventricle at autopsy. Note scarred and thinned PPM (*white arrowhead*) whereas the APM is hypertrophied (*black arrowhead*). Note dilated left atrium (LA). AL—anterior leaflet; PL—posterior leaflet.

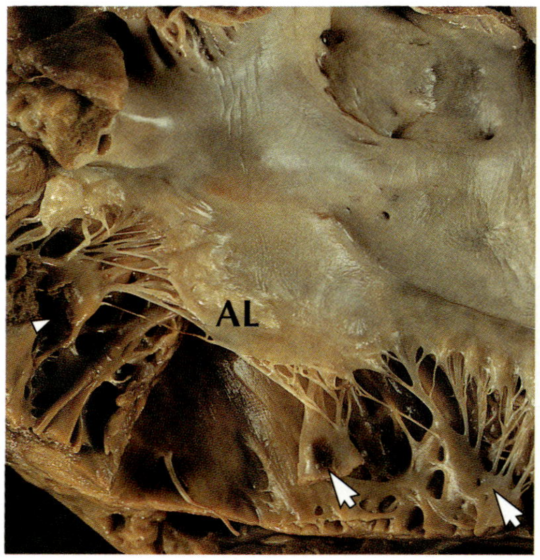

FIGURE 1-20. Papillary muscle rupture. A 58-year-old man admitted with chest pain had electrocardiographic evidence of subendocardial ischemia and died suddenly in the coronary care unit. Note rupture of one head of the anterolateral papillary muscle (*arrowhead*), which accompanied a subendocardial acute myocardial infarction. *Arrows* denote posteromedial papillary muscles. AL–anterior leaflet.

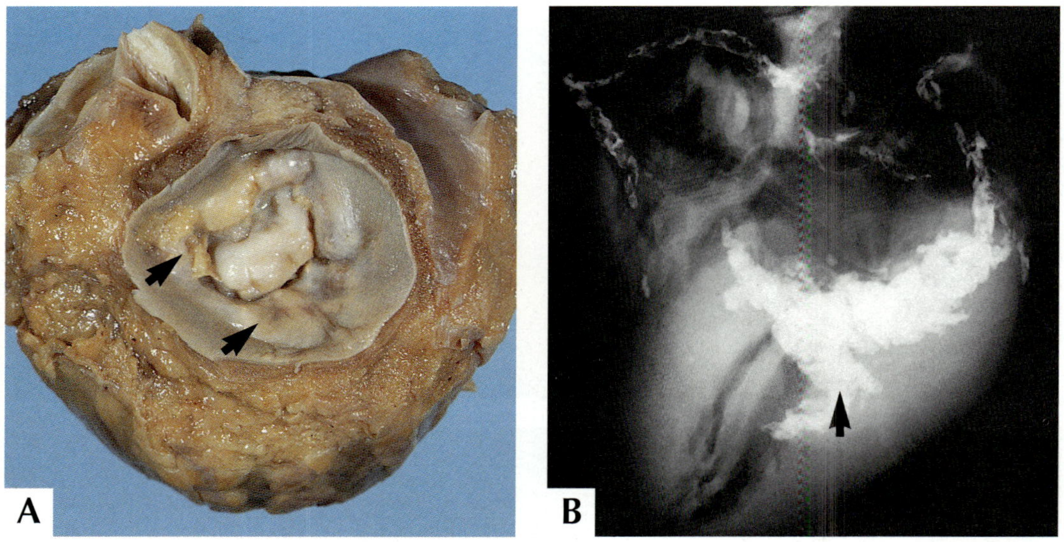

FIGURE 1-21. Mitral annular calcification (MAC). Seen primarily in patients older than 70 years and four times more common in women than men, MAC usually occurs at the angle between the base of the posterior MV where it meets the left ventricular endocardium. MAC may be only barely detectable grossly or may involve the entire posterior leaflet and extend onto the anterior leaflet forming a "D." The AV is also calcified in approximately 50% of cases [19]. Advanced degrees of MAC may result in MR.

A, An atrial view of the MV shows extensive calcification in the annular region with supravalvular extension (*arrows*) in a 72-year-old woman with mitral incompetence.

B, A postmortem radiograph shows extensive annular calcification that has extended into the left ventricular myocardium (*arrow*). Occasionally, mitral annular calcification can result in nodules that extend to the epicardial surface.

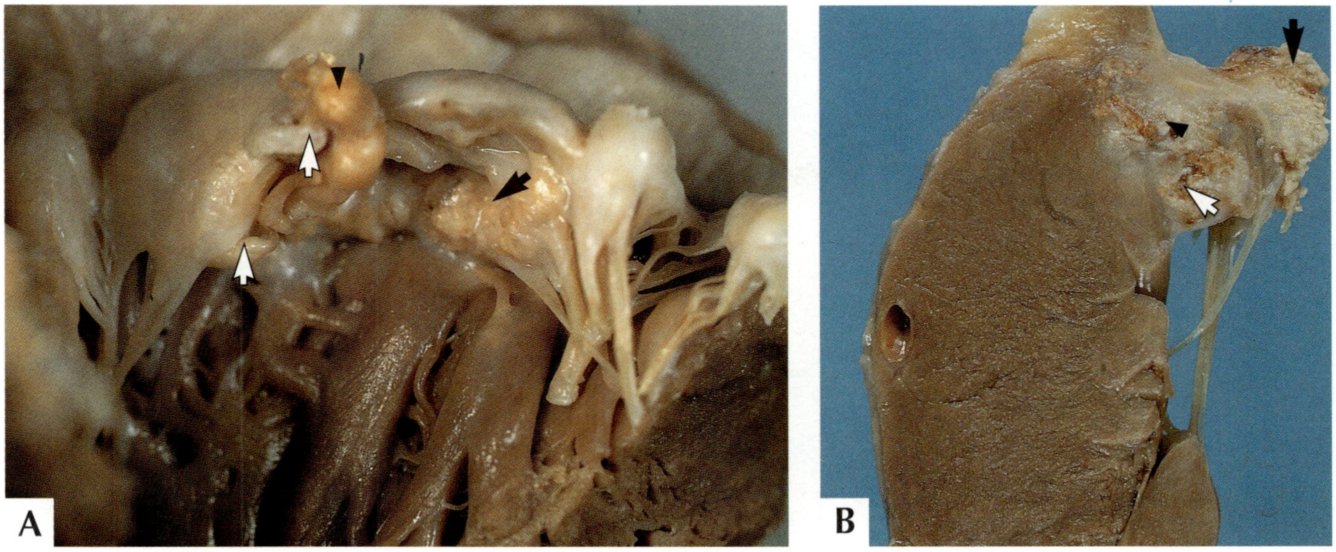

FIGURE 1-22 Mitral annular calcification. **A,** An elderly woman had a diagnosis of MR. At autopsy, there were calcific nodules in the annulus of the mitral valve. Annular calcification was located at the angle formed by the base of the mitral valve and the left ventricular endocardium (*black arrow*). A bar of calcium extended to the free margin of the MV (*arrowhead*), causing chordal rupture (*white arrows*).

B, A cut section of the left ventricular free wall shows the calcific nodule in the angle of the posterior leaflet and the left ventricular endocardium (*white arrow*). Center of the calcific nodule is yellow and pultaceous (*arrowhead*); this type of necrosis is seen in 10% of the cases. Histologically, at the periphery of the calcified area, there may be a giant cell reaction. The calcific nodules may also protrude onto the atrial surface, resulting in surface thrombosis and thromboembolism, including transient ischemic attacks. *Black arrow* demonstrates area of nonbacterial thrombotic endocarditis.

CONNECTIVE TISSUE DISEASE

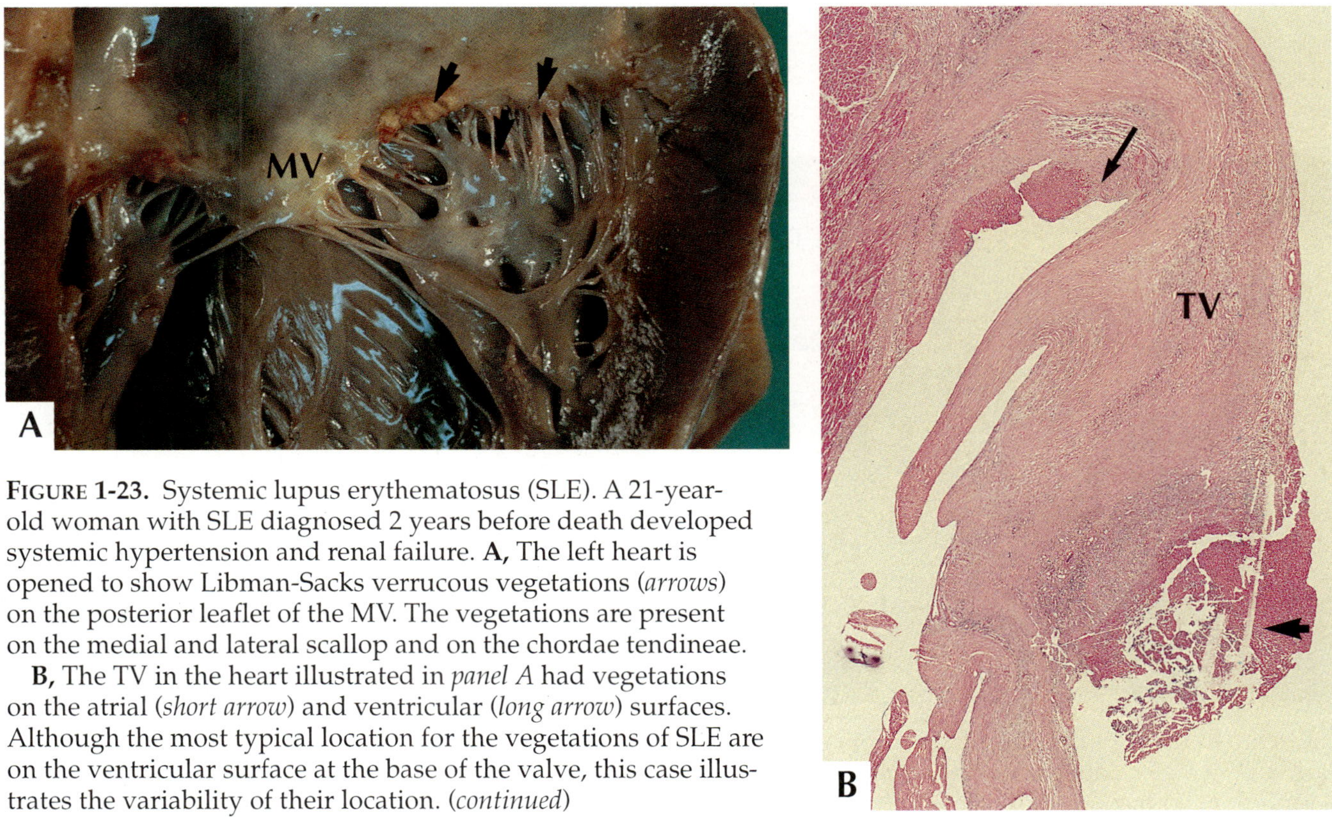

FIGURE 1-23. Systemic lupus erythematosus (SLE). A 21-year-old woman with SLE diagnosed 2 years before death developed systemic hypertension and renal failure. **A,** The left heart is opened to show Libman-Sacks verrucous vegetations (*arrows*) on the posterior leaflet of the MV. The vegetations are present on the medial and lateral scallop and on the chordae tendineae.

B, The TV in the heart illustrated in *panel A* had vegetations on the atrial (*short arrow*) and ventricular (*long arrow*) surfaces. Although the most typical location for the vegetations of SLE are on the ventricular surface at the base of the valve, this case illustrates the variability of their location. (*continued*)

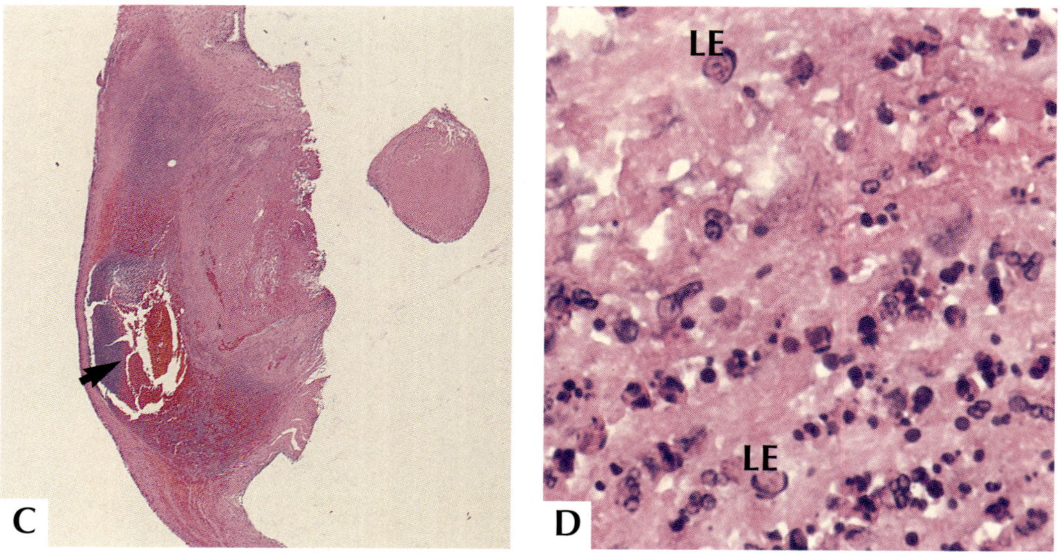

Figure 1-23. *(continued)* **C,** Low-power view of a histologic section of the MV shows central area of polymorphonuclear leukocyte infiltration and hemorrhage (*arrow*), which accounts for the vegetation seen grossly.

D, A high magnification of the histologic findings demonstrates lupus erythematosus (LE) cells in the acute inflammatory infiltrate.

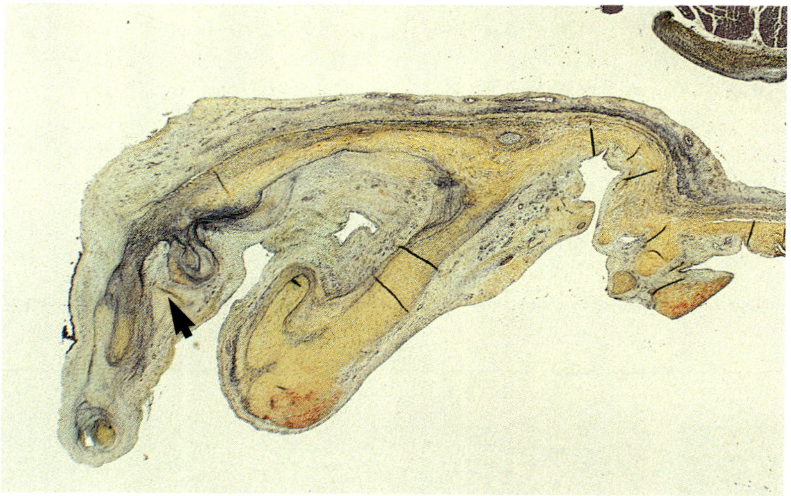

Figure 1-24. Systemic lupus erythematosus (SLE). Histologic section of the posterior mitral leaflet from a 42-year-old woman with a long history of SLE complicated by congestive heart failure. The patient was treated with glucorticosteroids and cyclophosphamide (Cytoxan). Note fibrosis of the atrial and ventricular surface of the mitral valve (*arrow*). Libman-Sacks vegetations are not seen.

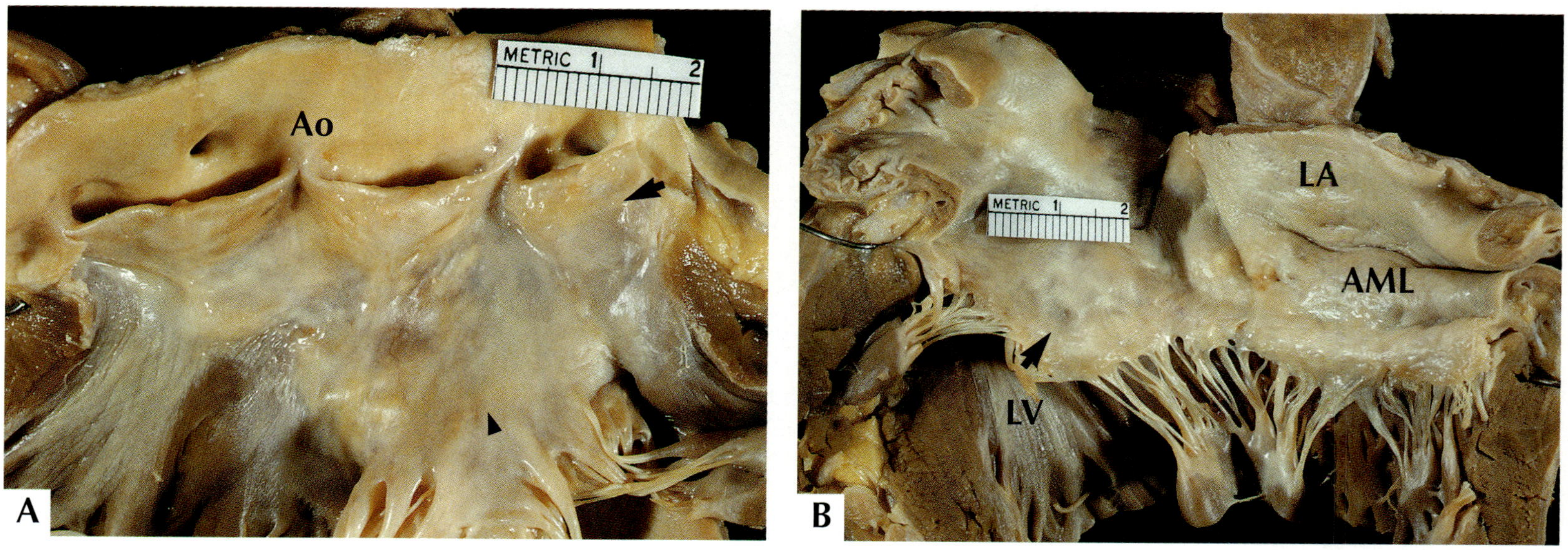

Figure 1-25. Rheumatoid valve disease. Rheumatoid cardiac involvement occurs in 5% of patients with rheumatoid arthritis. Rheumatoid granulomata may occur in the pericardium, myocardium, endocardium, and the valves. The extent of cardiac involvement is proportional to the severity of the disease. Most frequently the aortic and mitral valves are involved; valve dysfunction is extremely unusual, and if present, is usually regurgitant.

A, A 56-year-old white woman had a 10-year history of severe rheumatoid arthritis. At autopsy, rheumatoid nodes were present in the joints, lung, pericardium, myocardium, and AVs and MVs. AV and anterior mitral leaflets (AML) are shown. Note marked thickening of the AV leaflets (*arrow*) and scarring and thickening of the AMLs (*arrowhead*).

B, The MV from the same heart illustrated in *A*. Note thickened posterior leaflet (*arrow*) and left atrial (LA) endocardial thickening. *(continued)*

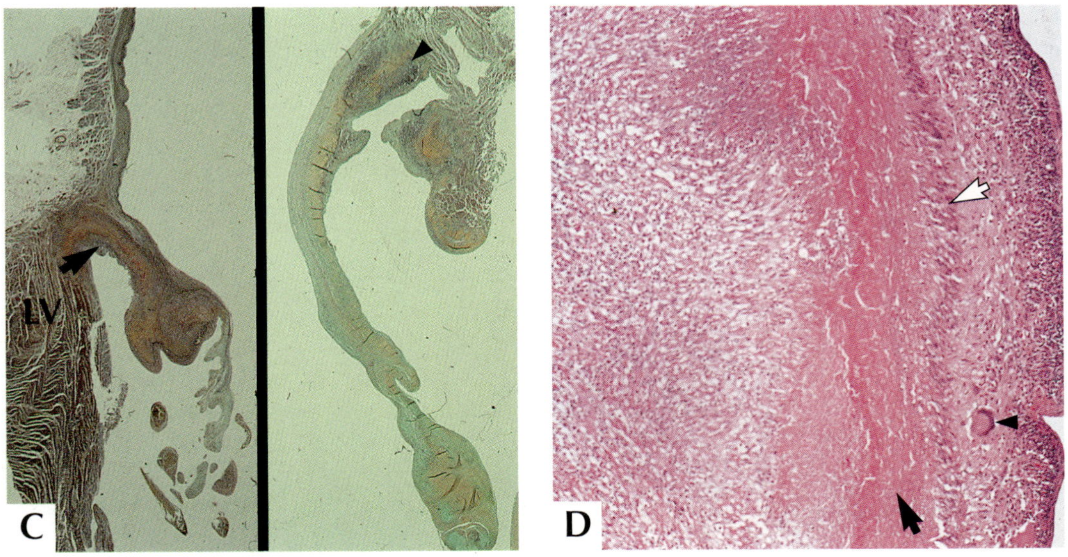

FIGURE 1-25. *(continued)* **C,** Histologic section of the MV (*left panel*) shows marked thickening and rheumatoid nodules in the valve leaflet and the left ventricular (LV) endocardium (*arrow*). The AML (*right panel*) contains a rheumatoid nodule at the basal attachment (*arrowhead*).

D, A histologic section of the endocardium near the valve insertion shows a rheumatoid nodule (*black arrow*) with central necrosis, surrounding palisading histiocytes (*white arrow*) and giant cells (*arrowhead*) and extensive chronic inflammation. Ao—aorta.

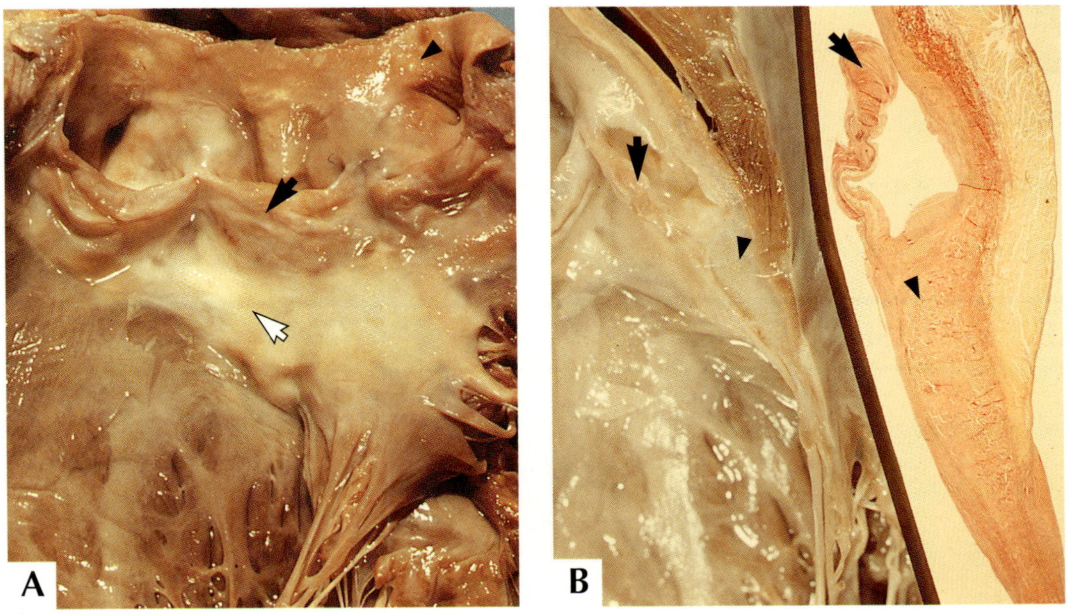

FIGURE 1-26. Ankylosing spondylitis. **A,** The incidence of cardiac involvement in ankylosing spondylitis is 3.5% to 10% (with duration of disease 10 to 30 years, respectively). Ankylosing spondylitis causes dilatation of the aortic annulus, fibrosis and inflammation of the aortic wall (*arrowhead*) and valve cusps, AR, and rarely mitral insufficiency. This gross photograph demonstrates thickening of the AV leaflets (*black arrow*) and a bump on the anterior leaflet of the MV (*white arrow*).

B, The inflammation and scarring extend below the AV to involve the anterior mitral leaflet resulting in a bump on the anterior leaflet (*arrowheads*) [20]. The gross heart (*left side of panel B*) shows cut section view of bump, with corresponding histologic section (*right side of panel B*). *Arrows* denote left aortic cusp. (Courtesy of Dr. William C. Roberts, Houston, Tx)

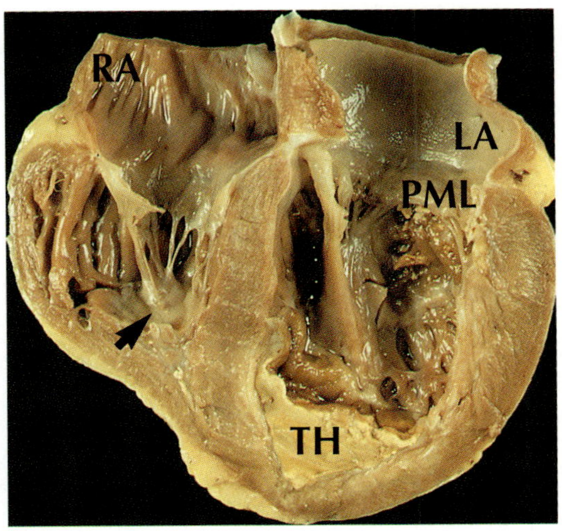

FIGURE 1-27. Hypereosinophilic syndrome. This syndrome is characterized by chronic eosinophilia of greater than 1500 eosinophils/mm^3, thromboembolic phenomena, and generalized arteritis. It typically occurs in middle-aged men. Cardiac dysfunction is responsible for a high morbidity and mortality. In the acute phase, the heart may be enlarged, and there are apical and inflow biventricular mural thrombi on the ventricular surfaces of the atrioventricular valves. Eosinophils are present within the thrombi, which may involve small intramural coronary arteries, and eosinophilic myocarditis may be present.

In this figure, the heart from a 9-year-old boy with eosinophilic leukemia of 9 months' duration shows biventricular dilatation and hypertrophy (four-chamber view). *Arrow* denotes apical endocardial fibrosis in the right ventricle. LA—left atrium; PML—posterior mitral leaflet; RA—right atrium; TH—thrombus.

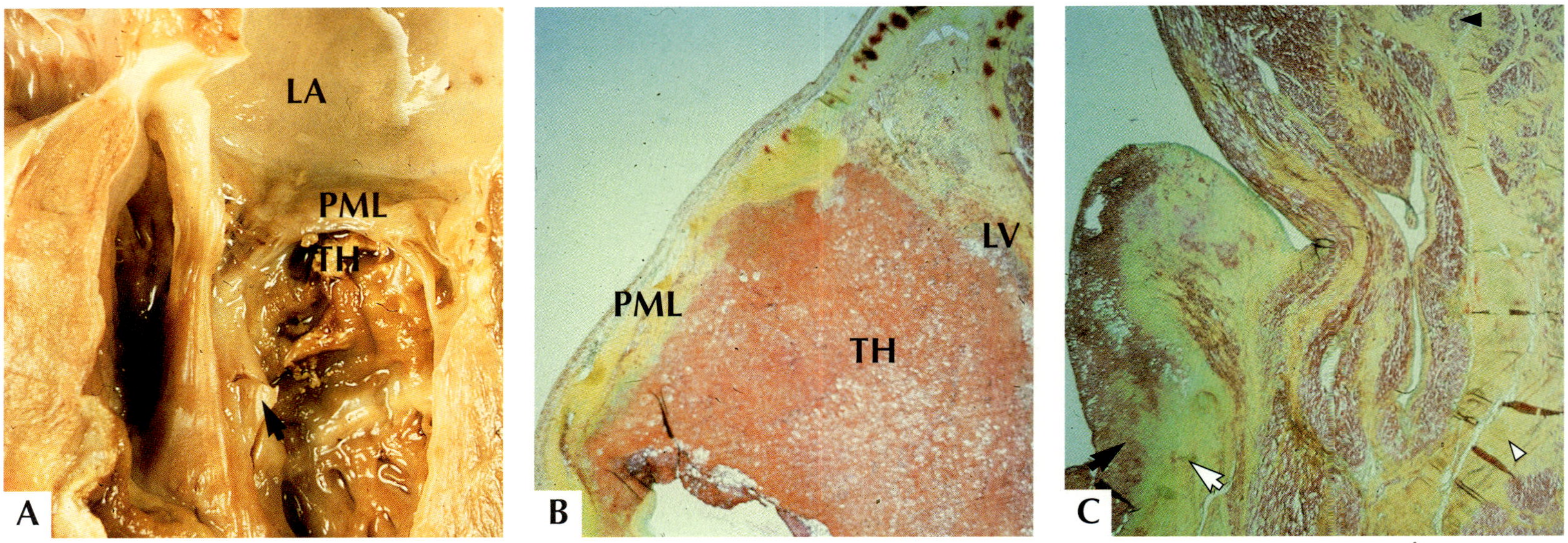

FIGURE 1-28. Hypereosinophilic syndrome. **A,** In the chronic phase, mural thrombi (TH) become organized resulting in endocardial thickening and restrictive cardiomyopathy [21]. Mural thrombi are present in the apex of the left ventricle (LV) and behind the posterior mitral leaflet (PML) causing adherence of the PML to the LV free wall. *Arrow* denotes endocardial fibrosis of the posteromedial papillary muscle.

B, Histologic section of the MV from the heart illustrated in *panel A* demonstrates organizing thrombus underneath the PML.

C, Microscopic examination of the LV from the heart illustrated in *panel A* reveals endocardial fibrosis (*white arrow*) with a superimposed organizing thrombus (*black arrow*). The myocardium shows that extensive subendocardial scarring and an organized thrombus (multiluminal channels) (*black arrowhead*) are present within intramural coronary arteries. Focal fibrosis is present within the myocardium (*white arrowhead*). LA—left atrium. (*Adapted from* Olson and coworkers [21]; with permission.)

TRICUSPID AND PULMONARY VALVE DISEASE

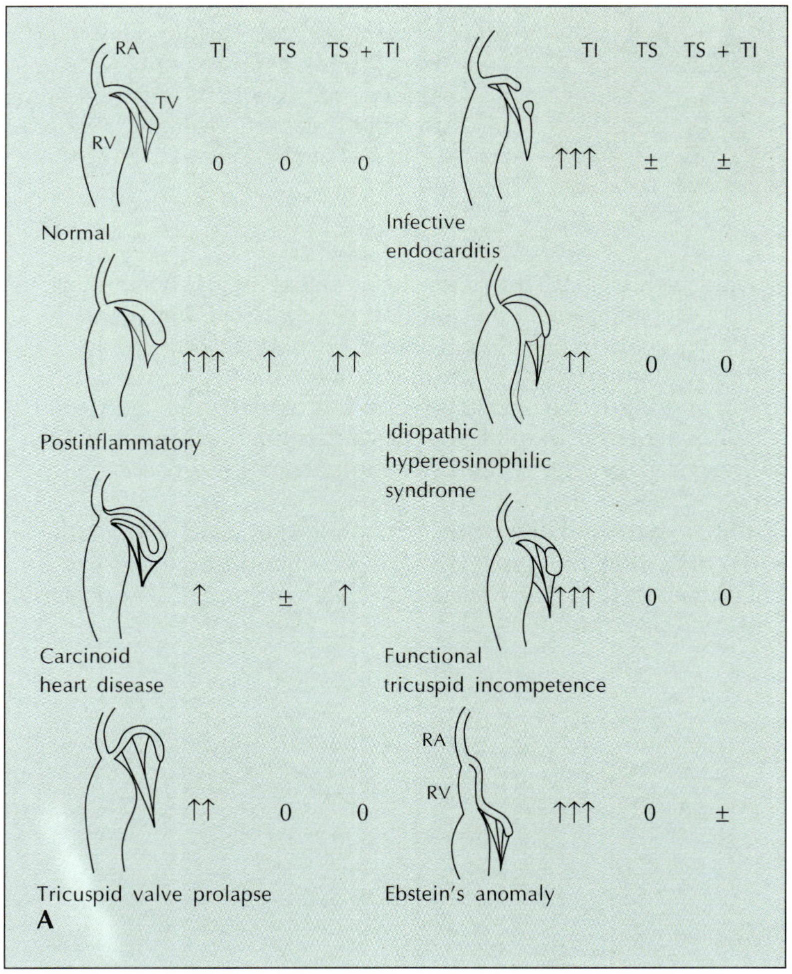

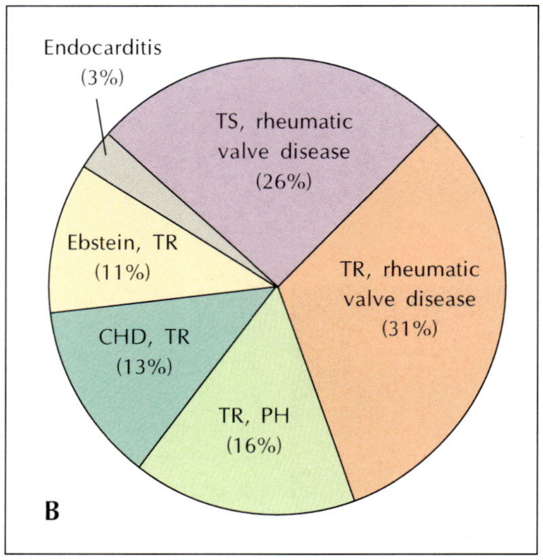

FIGURE 1-29. Tricuspid valve (TV) disease. **A,** Diagrammatic illustration of TV. **B,** Pathologic findings in TV. (*continued*)

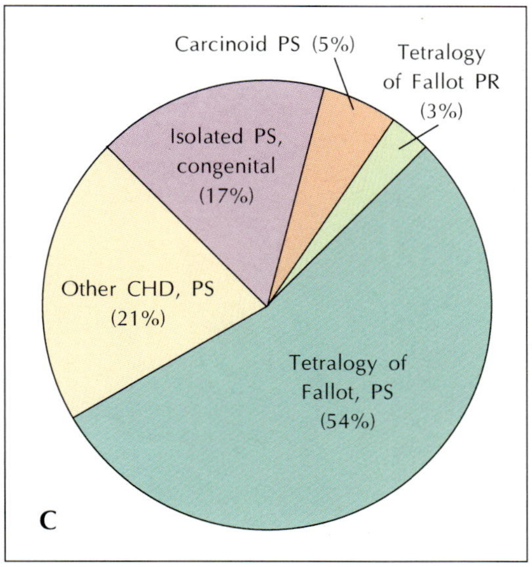

FIGURE 1-29. *(continued)* **C,** Pathologic findings in pulmonary valve (PV) replacement. CHD—congenital heart disease; PH—pulmonary hypertension; PR—pulmonary regurgitation; PS—pulmonary stenosis; TR—tricuspid regurgitation; TS—tricuspid stenosis (Part A *adapted from* Virmani [22]; part B *adapted from* Hauck and coworkers [11]; and part C *adapted from* Altrichter and coworkers [23].)

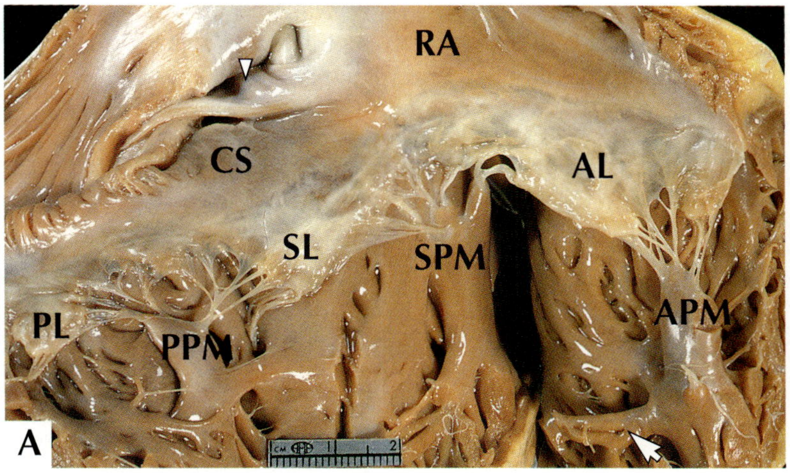

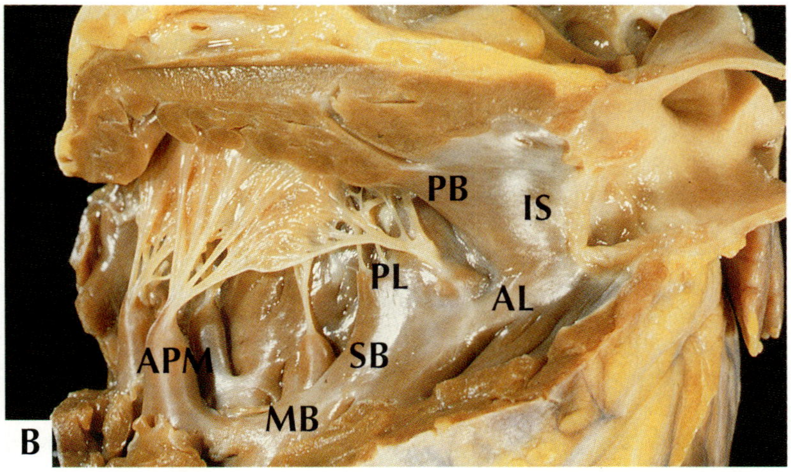

FIGURE 1-30. Normal TV. **A,** A right lateral incision exposes the right atrium (RA) and the coronary sinus (CS) situated just above the septal leaflet (SL) of the TV. The atrioventricular node is located on the right atrial wall within the triangle of Koch, defined by the coronary sinus posteriorly, the TV annulus inferiorly, and the tendon of Todaro superiorly. The tendon of Todaro is the continuation of the Eustachian valve of the inferior vena cava. The TV consists of the anterior (AL), posterior (PL), and septal leaflets, separated by commissures. Chordae tendineae from the AL and PL attach to a large single anterior papillary muscle (APM), which arises from the anterior free wall of the right ventricle (RV) and fuses with the moderator band (MB;*arrow*). Multiple small PPMs receive chordae from the posterior and septal leaflets and are attached to the free wall of the RV. The septal papillary muscle (SPM) may be rudimentary or absent, and chordae from the AL and SL insert directly into the ventricular septum. *Arrowhead* denotes the inferior vena cava orifice.

B, The RV is divided into the inflow region consisting of the TV, chordae tendineae, papillary muscle, and the heavily trabeculated myocardium; and a smooth myocardial outflow infundibulum. The inflow and outflow are separated by four muscular bands: the infundibular septum (IS), the parietal band (PB), the septal band (SB) (with its anterior [AL] and posterior limb [PL]), and the MB. The IS and the PB form the crista supraventricularis. The septal band extends apically to become continuous with the MB. The MB is an important anatomic landmark in echocardiography because it assists in the identification of the RV in cases of RV hypertrophy and dilatation.

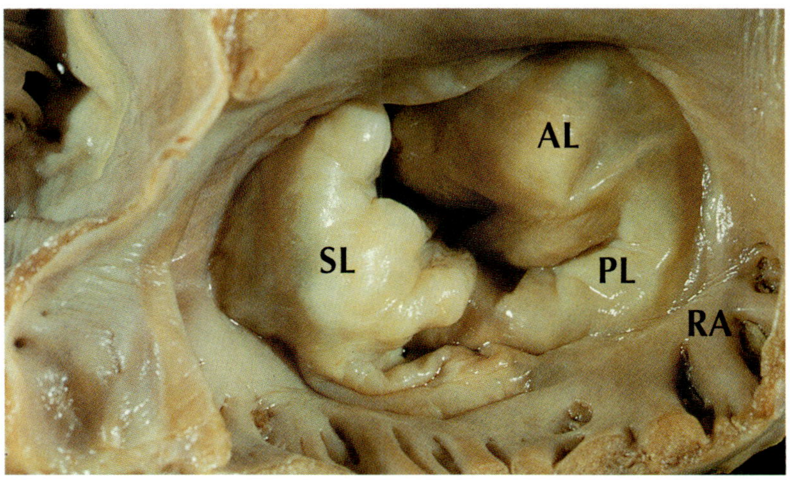

FIGURE 1-31. Tricuspid valve prolapse (TVP). TVP is present in 0.1% to 5.5% of the general population and in about 22% of patients with MVP. Tricuspid regurgitation (TR) is usually mild and does not correlate with the severity of the prolapse. TVP usually involves the septal leaflet (SL) alone or both the septal and the anterior leaflets (AL) [24]. Note redundancy of the AL and SL; the posterior leaflet (PL) is normal. RA—right atrium.

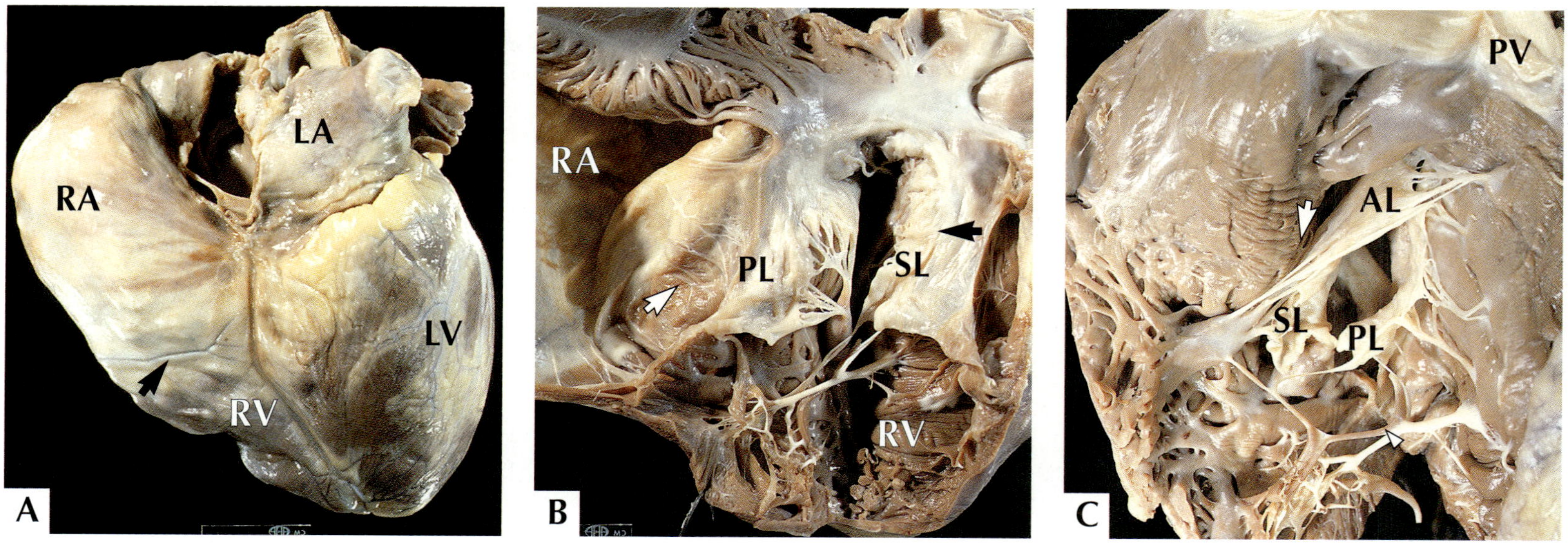

FIGURE 1-32. Ebstein's anomaly. **A,** Ebstein's anomaly is an uncommon congenital cause of TR and, rarely, TS. There is downward displacement of the functional valve annulus (*arrow*) of a portion of the septal leaflet (SL) or the posterior leaflet (PL) such that there is apposition of leaflet tissue against the right ventricle (RV). This area becomes markedly thinned and dilated, or "atrialized."

B, The anterior tricuspid leaflet is often large and "sail-like" with its annular attachment normally placed at the true atrioventricular junction. The anterior leaflet (AL) may contain abnormal fibrous strands and may be focally muscularized and fenestrated. Both the SL (*black arrow*) and the PL (*white arrow*) are displaced inferiorly toward the apex of the heart. These leaflets typically have abnormal chordal attachment and are tethered to the RV wall. The RV is anatomically divided into the atrialized proximal chamber and a distal "true" ventricular chamber.

C, At its free edge, the AL may attach directly into the RV wall or via abnormal papillary muscles; its attachment to the crista supraventricularis (*arrow*) is always directly chordal. The proximal chamber may be large or small depending on the extent of downward displacement of the TV. The endocardium of the atrialized RV is fibrotic with poorly developed trabeculae. The distal chamber is located behind the anterior tricuspid leaflet. *Arrowhead* denotes abnormal chordae. LA—left atrium; LV—left ventricle; PV—pulmonary valve. (Parts B and C *adapted from* Farb and coworkers [24]; with permission.)

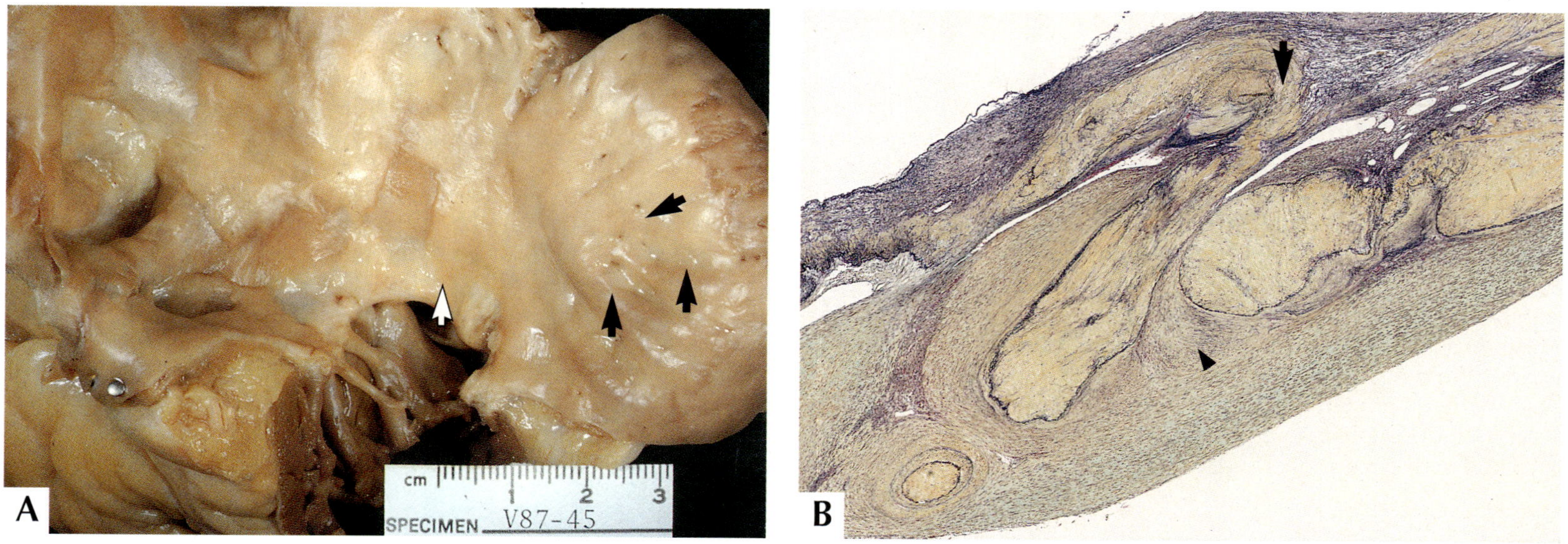

FIGURE 1-33. Carcinoid heart disease. **A,** The right atrium (RA) from a patient with carcinoid heart disease and combined TR and TS. Note raised white plaques (*black arrow*) on the endocardial surface of the dilated RA and TV (*white arrow*). Carcinoid heart disease occurs in 19% to 53% of patients with carcinoid syndrome and is an important cause of morbidity and mortality.

B, Section of a TV shows carcinoid plaque (*arrowhead*) composed of smooth muscle cells in a proteoglycan matrix overlying a normal TV (*arrow*). Carcinoid endocardial plaques superimposed on the normal RA, right ventricle, and right-sided valves. Carcinoid lesions rarely involve the MV or AV. (Part A courtesy of J.B. Atkinson, MD, PhD; part B *adapted from* Farb and coworkers [24]; with permission.)

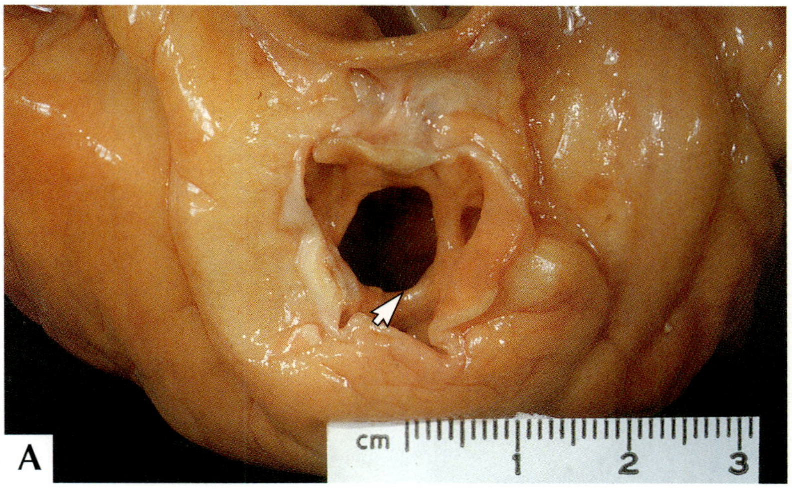

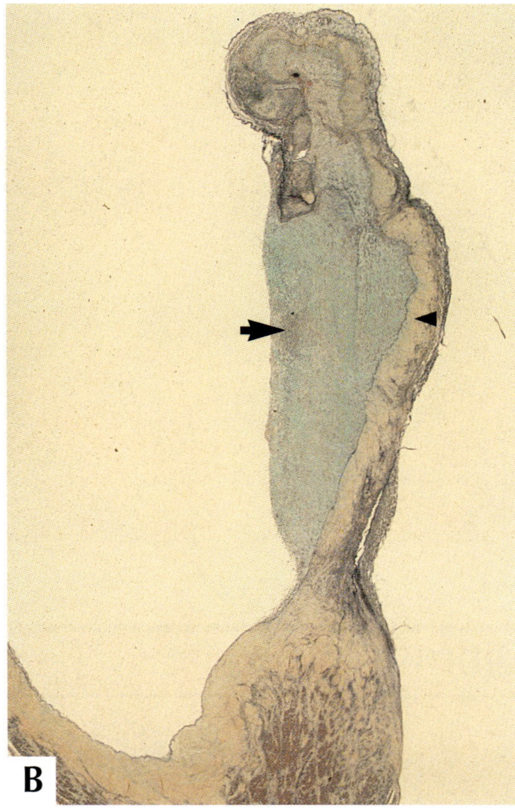

FIGURE 1-34. Carcinoid heart disease. **A,** PV leaflets are markedly thickened and fibrotic (*arrow*) from a patient with pulmonary regurgitation (PR) and pulmonary stenosis (PS). Carcinoid involvement of the TV usually causes insufficiency, while involvement of the PV typically causes PS [24].

B, Carcinoid plaque (*arrow*) on the arterial surface of a pulmonic valve cusp (*arrowhead*). Lesions reminiscent of carcinoid plaques have been described in patients on methylsergide and ergotamine treatment [25]. (Part A courtesy of J.B. Atkinson, MD, PhD; Part B *Adapted from* Farb and coworkers [24]; with permission.)

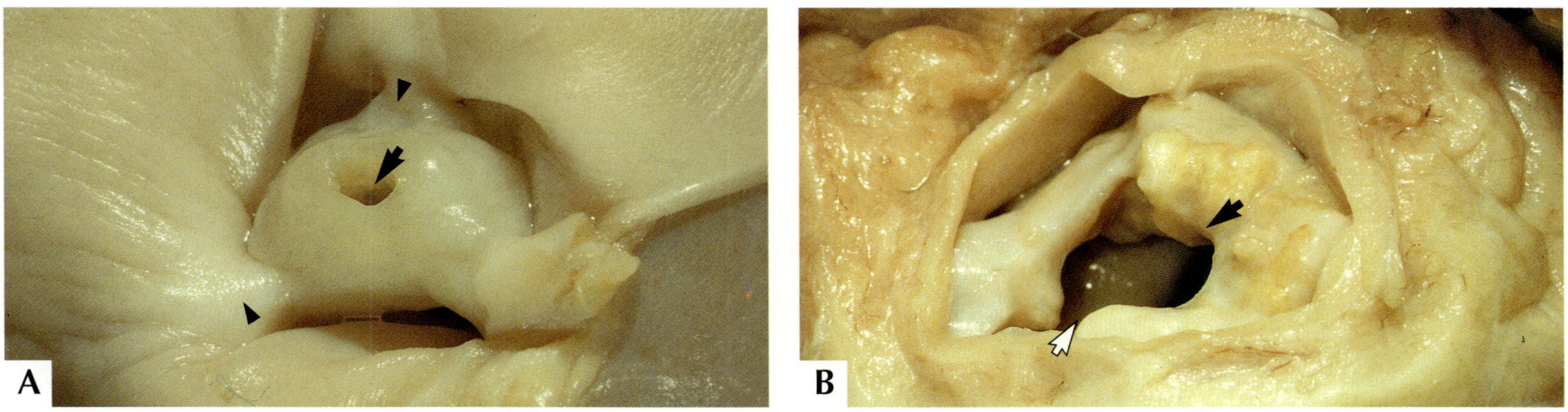

FIGURE 1-35. Pulmonary stenosis. (PS) **A,** PS occurs as an isolated congenital anomaly, and the stenosis is usually valvular or both valvular and infundibular. The PV shown is that of a neonate with a dome- or funnel-shaped myxomatous PV (*arrow*) with fibrosis and a small outlet at the apex of the cone with two ridges (*arrowheads*) on the pulmonary arterial side of the unicuspid valve. Excellent results have been reported with surgical correction (valvotomy with or without infundibular resection); balloon dilatation is now the procedure of choice.

B, PS in 58-year-old man with history of PS and open valvotomy. At autopsy, there was right ventricular hypertrophy and dilatation. PS is associated with right ventricular hypertrophy, which is dependent on the severity of the obstruction. The TV was normal, and the ventricular septum was intact. Note the PV is markedly thickened with fibrosis and calcification (*black arrow*) with an eccentric opening (*white arrow*).

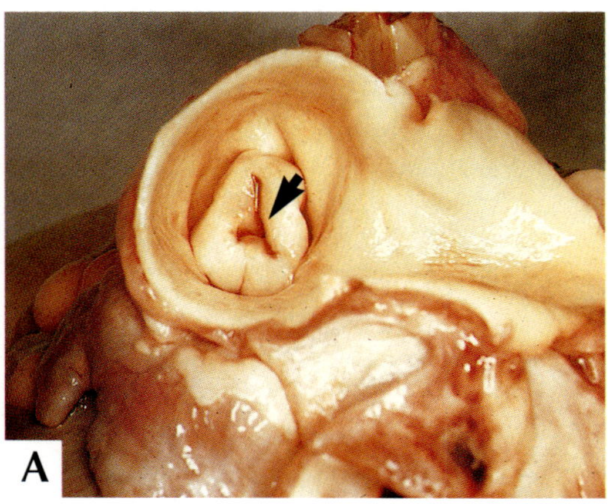

FIGURE 1-36. Pulmonary stenosis. (PS). **A,** PS secondary to mucopolysaccharidosis (Hurler syndrome). The valves are markedly thickened, and the valve thickening is most pronounced at the free margins (*arrow*); there is no fusion of the commissures. Usually there is involvement of the left-sided valves (especially mitral) and, infrequently, the right-sided valves (the PV is shown). (*continued*)

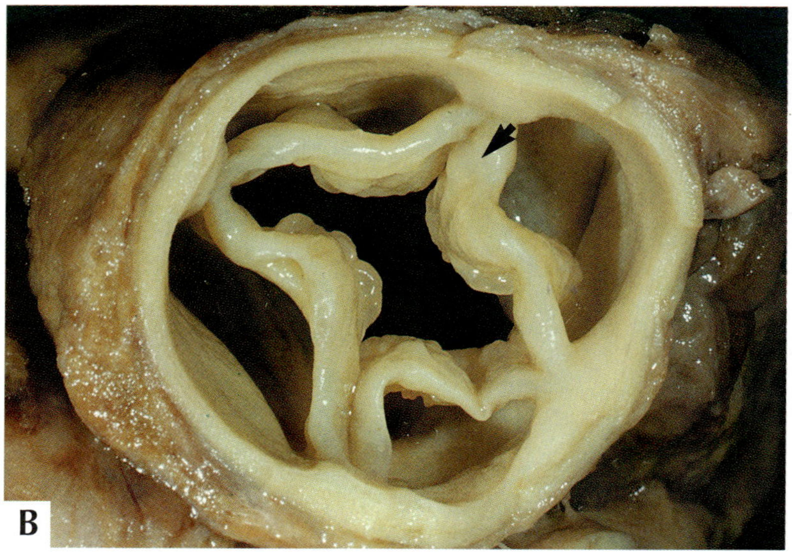

FIGURE 1-36. (*continued*) **B,** Quadricuspid PV with mild dysplasia. This patient was a 12-year-old girl with tunnel subaortic stenosis who at autopsy had a mildly dysplastic quadricuspid PV (*arrow*). Quadricuspid PV is more frequent than quadricuspid AV and is usually an incidental finding. (Part A *adapted from* Farb and coworkers [24]; with permission.)

ENDOCARDITIS

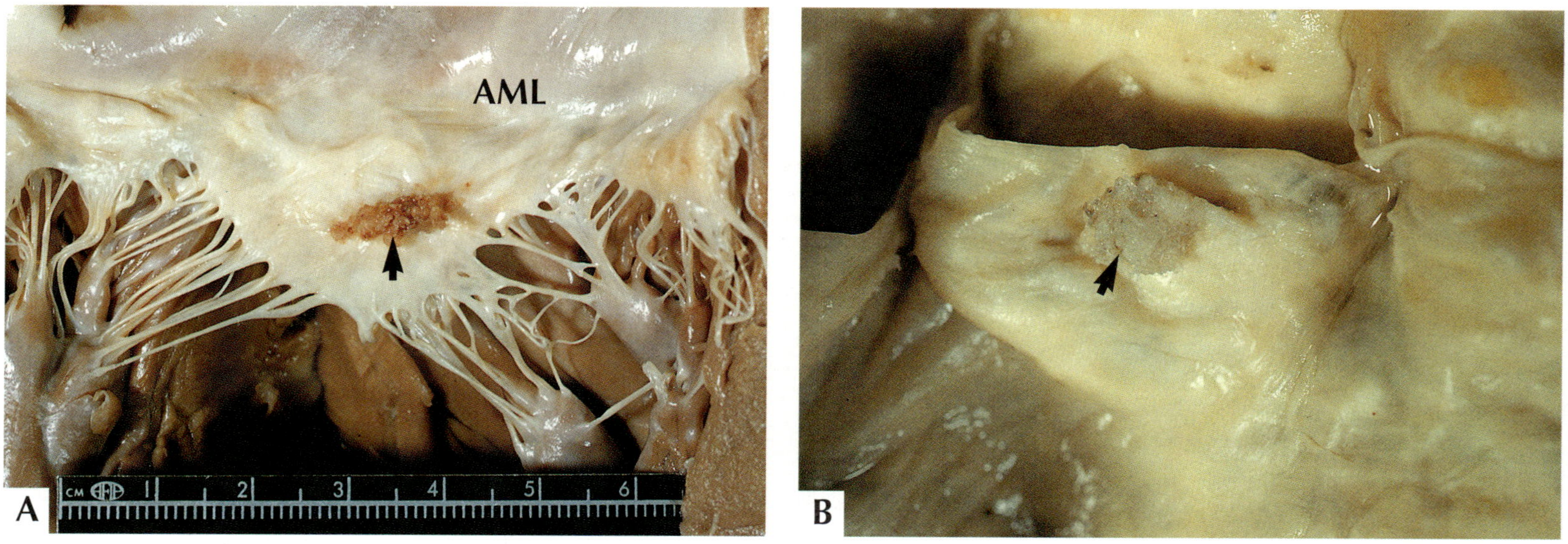

FIGURE 1-37. Endocarditis. **A,** Marantic endocarditis. Marantic endocarditis usually occurs in patients with an underlying chronic inflammatory condition or malignancy. This MV shows nonbacterial thrombotic endocarditis (*arrow*) on the anterior mitral leaflet (AML) in a patient who initially survived injuries incurred in a motor vehicle accident but died 7 days after injury.

B, AV shows a 0.5-cm papillary fibroelastoma (*arrow*) that echocardiographically can be mistaken for bacterial endocarditis.

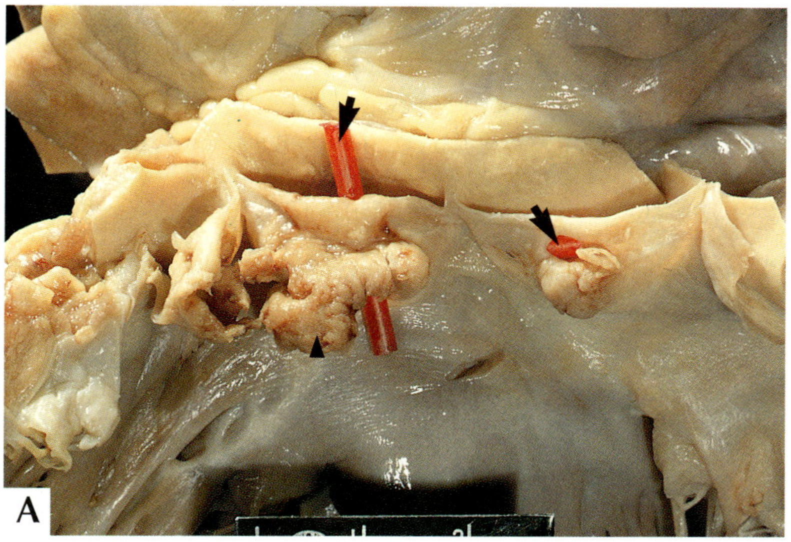

FIGURE 1-38. Infective endocarditis (IE). This infection usually occurs on congenitally malformed valves, on valves with acquired disease, or on normal valves in intravenous drug abusers or immunocompromised patients. However, the incidence of IE on anatomically normal heart valves is increasing. **A,** This AV shows large friable vegetations of IE (*arrowhead*) caused by *Staphylococcus aureus* in a 62-year-old man with a normal tricuspid AV. The *left arrow* denotes a probe through the perforation. The *right arrow* denotes another perforation. (*continued*)

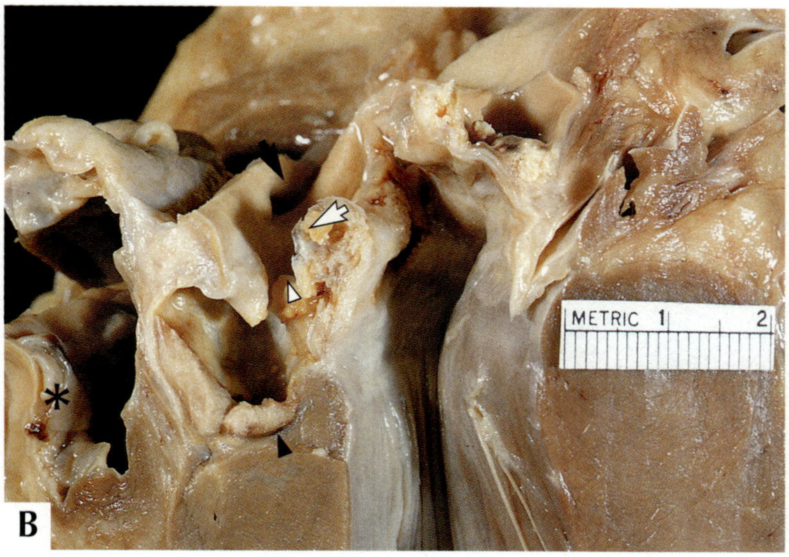

FIGURE 1-38. *(continued)* **B,** A bicuspid stenotic valve shows a ring abscess (*black arrowhead*) located in the sinus of Valsalva (*white arrowhead*) with extension into the myocardium in a 58-year-old man with recurrent fever. The organism was *Streptococcus bovis*. Thickened and calcified anterior and posterior AV leaflets are denoted by the *black* and *white arrows*, respectively. *Asterisk* denotes anterior MV. (Part B *adapted from* Atkinson and Virmani [26]; with permission.)

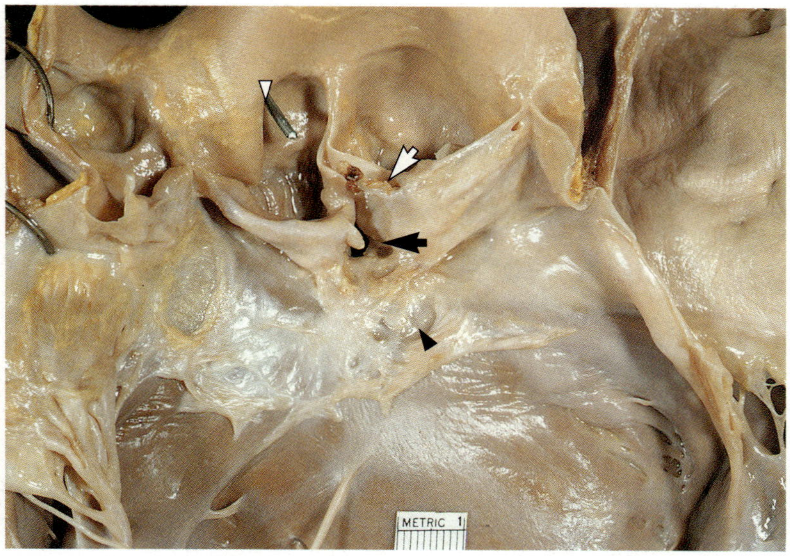

FIGURE 1-39. Endocarditis. A 42-year-old man known to have a murmur since childhood died suddenly. At autopsy a membranous ventricular septal defect (*black arrow*) with superimposed endocardial thickening and irregularities of the free margins of the AV from a healed endocarditis were present. The right coronary cusp is thickened and retracted, whereas the posterior noncoronary cusp shows superficial ulceration and thickening (*white arrow*). Note presence of endocardial plaque on the septal wall from AR (*black arrowhead*). The right coronary ostium is marked by the *white arrowhead*. (*Adapted from* Atkinson and Virmani [26]; with permission.)

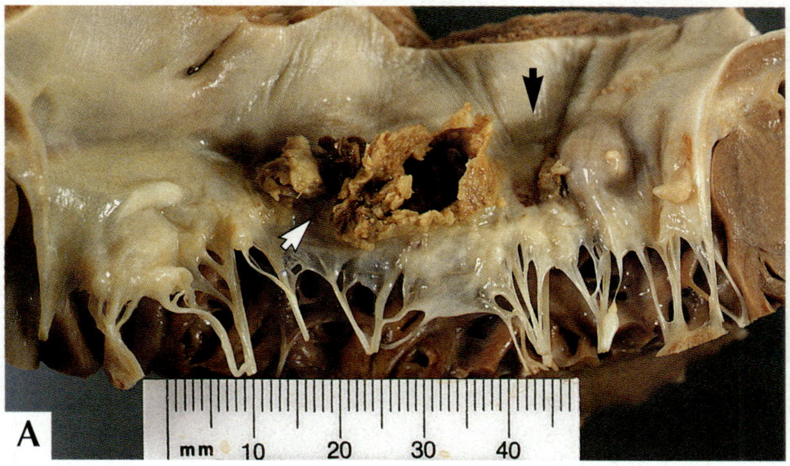

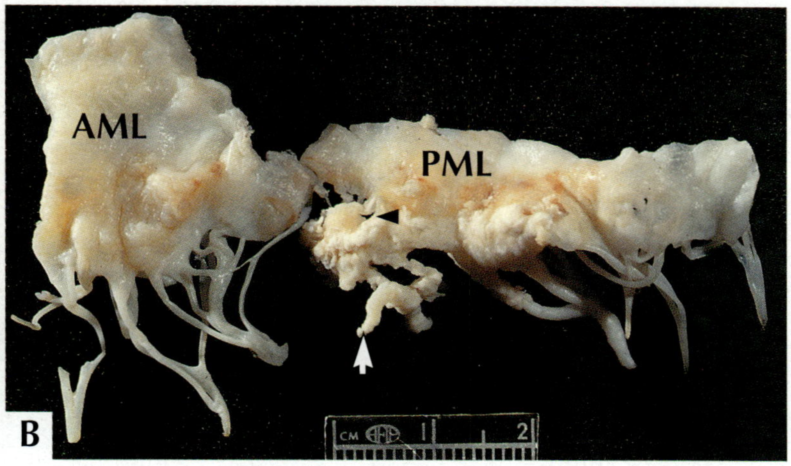

FIGURE 1-40. Mitral annular ring abscess. **A,** A 56-year-old man with chronic renal failure, pericardial friction rub, gallop rhythm, and systolic murmur died of septic shock. At autopsy, the heart was enlarged and the anterior mitral leaflet (AML) was perforated by a large vegetation (*white arrow*). A mitral annular ring abscess extended into but did not perforate the endocardium of the left atrium (*black arrow*). Microscopic sections showed gram-positive cocci.

B, Mitral valve prolapse (MVP) seen in a patient with superimposed bacterial endocarditis and worsening MR. Note vegetations (*arrowhead*) on the posterior mitral leaflet (PML), on an operatively excised MV, with rupture of chordae (*arrow*) of the PML. MVP is now the most common condition associated with infective endocarditis (IE) (up to 54% of cases). Degenerative aortic and mitral disease (degenerative AS, mitral annular calcification) are also conditions that predispose to IE, are increasing in prevalence, and account for an increase in the age of patients with IE.

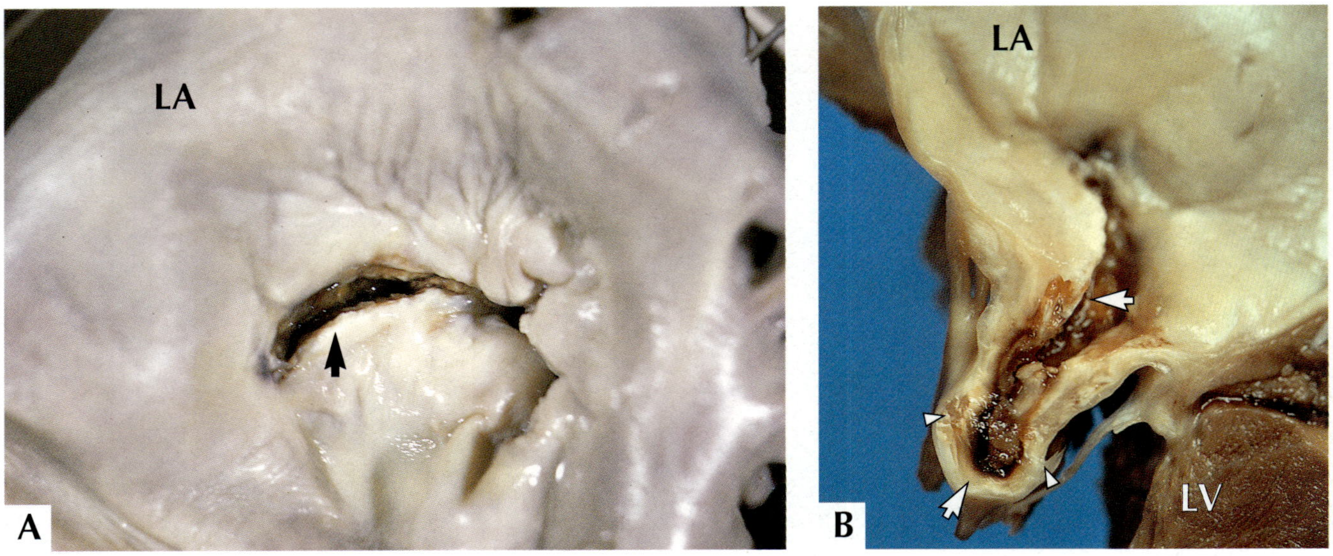

FIGURE 1-41. Infective endocarditis (IE). **A,** Atrial view of the MV in a 56-year-old woman with rheumatic MS who had sudden onset of transient ischemic attacks. Note the vegetation on the valve margins of a stenotic valve secondary to rheumatic heart disease (*arrow*).

B, Anterior (*white arrowhead*) and posterior (*black arrowhead*) cut surface of the valve illustrated in *panel A* shows vegetations (*black arrow*) in the fused fibrotic MV leaflet (*white arrow*). Rheumatic heart disease is a frequent condition predisposing to IE and accounts for about 30% of cases, down from between 37% to 76% in the past.

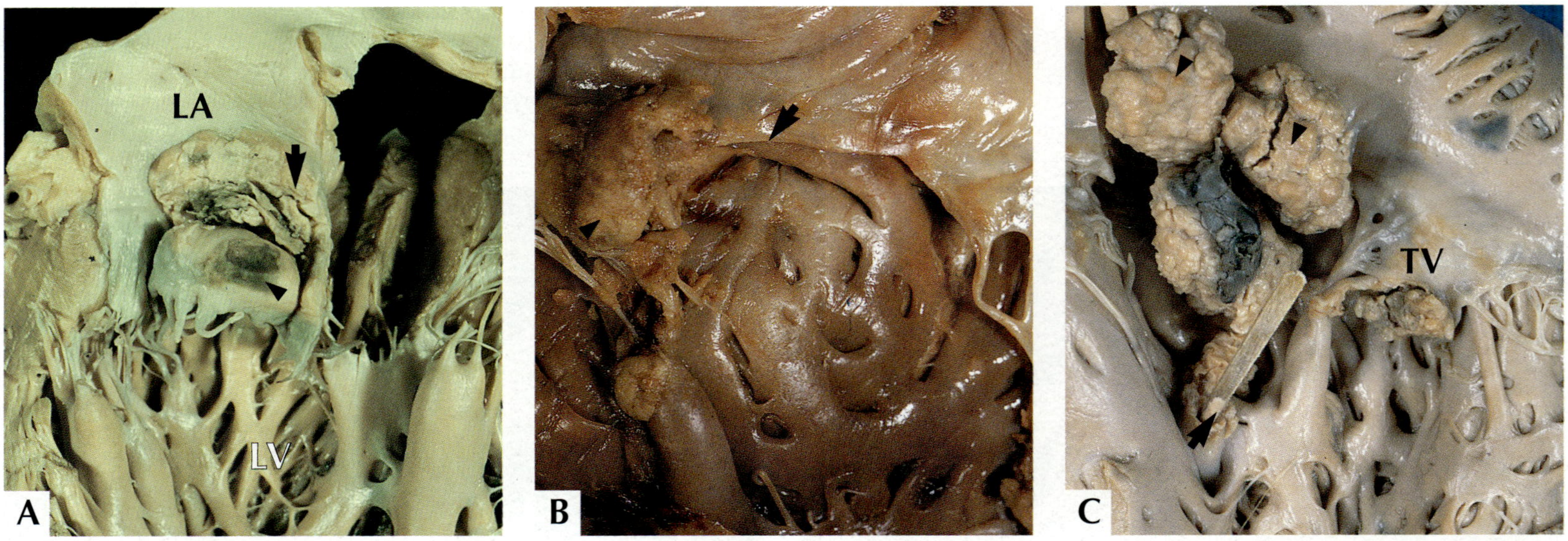

FIGURE 1-42. Infective endocarditis. **A,** A 53-year-old woman was admitted with acute myocardial infarction and died 3 days after admission. At autopsy, there was MVP (*arrowhead*) with superimposed friable infectious endocarditis (*arrow*) and embolic obstruction of the left anterior descending coronary artery.

B, A 28-year-old male intravenous drug abuser with a history of recurrent fever and multiple admissions for *Staphylococcus aureus* sepsis. The edge of the TV has been eroded (*arrow*) and a portion of the leaflet is absent. The adjacent TV shows bulky and friable bacterial vegetations (*arrowhead*).

C, Foreign body endocarditis. A 58-year-old woman had abdominal pain for 1 year and recurrent pulmonary infarcts beginning 6 months prior to death. At autopsy, a toothpick (*arrow*) protruded through the TV into the right ventricle, and the TV was surrounded by large polypoid vegetations (*arrowheads*). Microscopic examination showed the large vegetations were formed by budding yeast consistent with *Candida*. LA—left atrium; LV—left ventricle. (Part C *adapted from* Atkinson and Virmani [26]; with permission.)

Prosthetic Valves

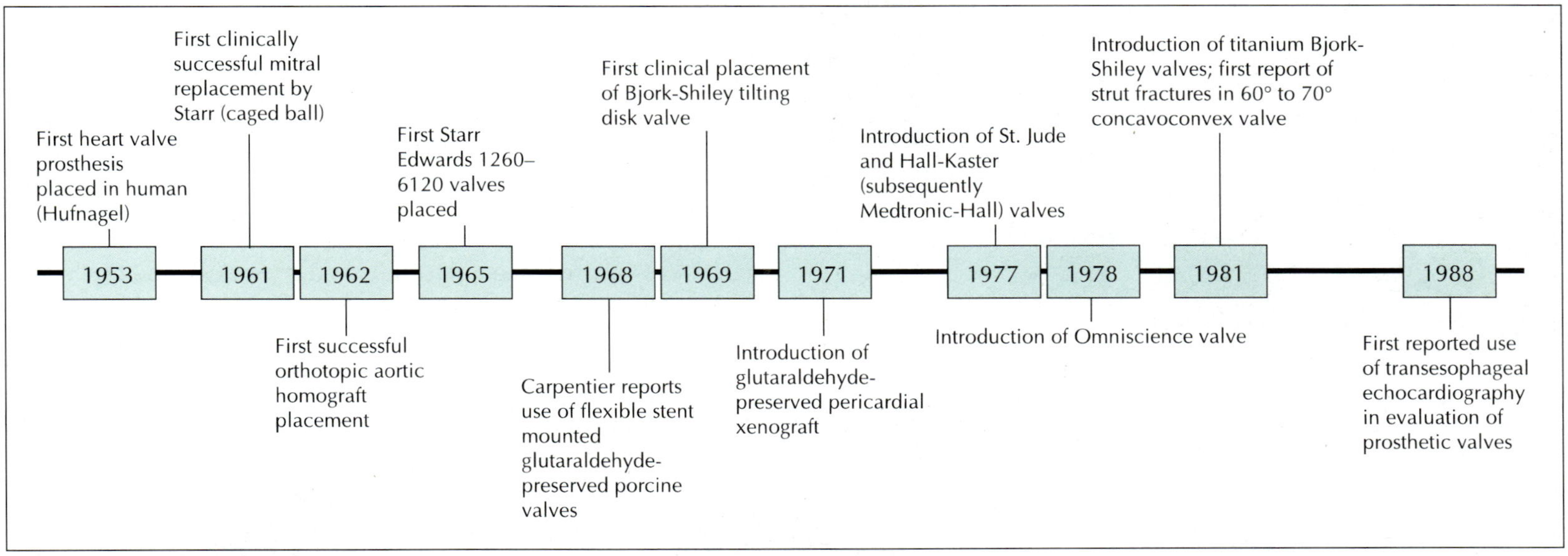

Figure 1-43. Major milestones in the development of prosthetic heart valves. Of the dozens of prosthetic valves that have been developed, four mechanical valves are approved for use in the United States [27]: Starr-Edwards caged-ball (Baxter Healthcare Corporation, Edwards Division, Irvine, CA), Medtronic-Hall and Omniscience tilting disk (Medtronic, Inc., Minneapolis, MN, and Medical Inc., Inver Grove Heights, Minneapolis, MN), and St. Jude bileaflet (St. Jude Medical, Inc., St. Paul, MN) valves. The Bjork-Shiley (Shiley, Inc., Irvine, CA) valves have been removed from the market. Two xenograft valves are also approved for routine clinical use. Although homografts were first used in the early 1960s, widespread use was not attained until more recently with the development of improved preservation.

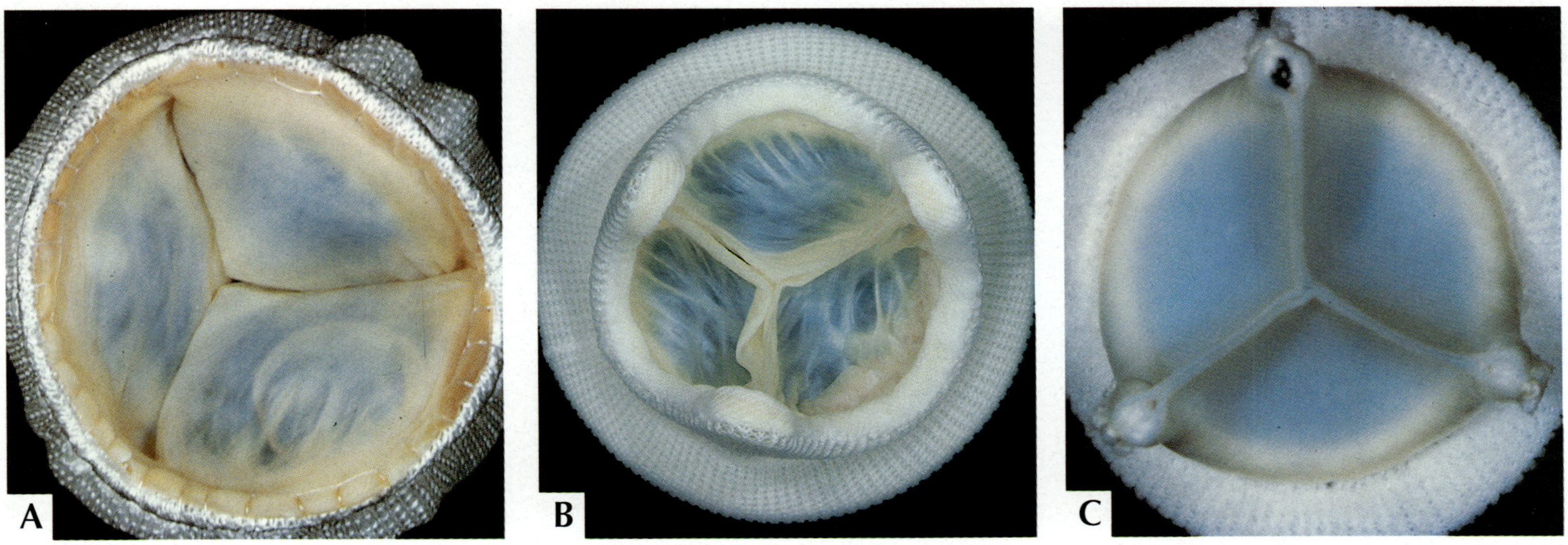

Figure 1-44. Bioprosthetic valves. **A,** Carpentier-Edwards porcine bioprosthesis (Baxter Healthcare Corporation, Irvine, CA), ventricular view. The stent is made of Elgiloy and is slightly noncircular to allow for the muscular shelf attached to the right coronary cusp in the native porcine AV. Glutaraldehyde (0.2% to 0.6%) is used for preservation.

B, Hancock porcine bioprosthesis (Medtronic, Inc, Minneapolis, MN), aortic view. The stents are circular and made of polypropylene. In general, bioprosthetic valves are indicated in patients over 65 years of age for AV replacement, in patients over 70 years of age for mitral valve replacement, in women of childbearing age, in patients in whom anticoagulation is contraindicated, and as replacements for thrombosed mechanical valves [27,28].

C, Bovine pericardial valve, Ionescu-Shiley. Introduced in the mid-1970s, these valves had a higher rate of tissue failure than porcine valves and are no longer approved for use in the United States. New generation bioprosthetic valves are not yet approved for general use and are undergoing clinical trials. These models have tissue preservation at low or zero pressure in the presence of calcium mitigative agents, may have altered stent profiles that are reduced or even absent, and, in the case of the Hancock II valve, a Delrin ring replacing polypropylene [27]. These investigational valves include the Hancock II porcine, Carpentier-Edwards Supra Annular porcine, St. Jude-BioImplant porcine, Medtronic Intact porcine, Mitroflow pericardial (Mitroflow, International, Inc., Richmond, BC, Canada), and Carpentier-Edwards stentless porcine. The Carpentier-Edwards pericardial valve is now approved by the FDA for clinical use.

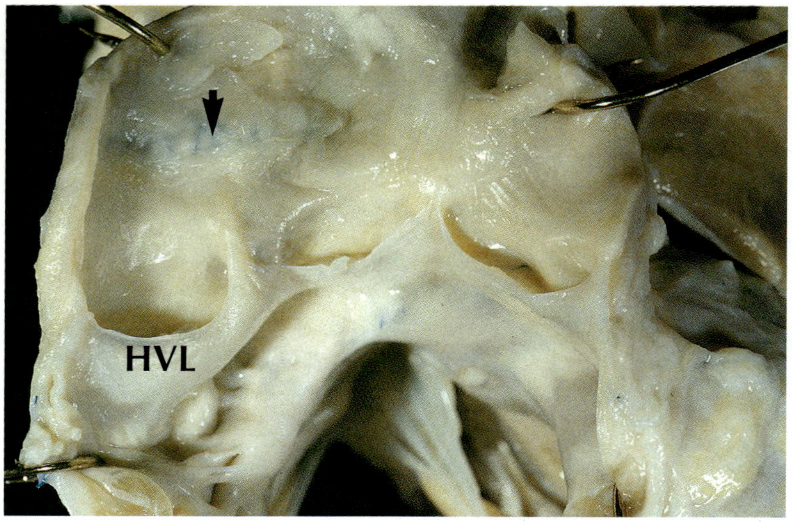

FIGURE 1-45. Aortic homografts. Cryopreserved valves have a long shelf-life and are preferentially harvested from donors with a warm ischemic time of less than 12 to 24 hours [29,30]. Fresh valves may be harvested from beating heart donors or transplant recipients, are usually stored in nutrient media with low concentrations of antibiotics, and must be used soon after harvesting.

The figure shows an aortic homograft, pulmonary position, from a patient with truncus arteriosus. Death was secondary to complications of obstruction at distal sewing ring. Use of these valves in the semilunar position is largely limited by supply [30,31]. They are indicated for use in children, in adults for reimplantation of an infected prosthetic AV, and as a possible alternative to mechanical valves in AV replacement in adults under 50 years of age. Irradiation and higher concentrations of antibiotics during preservation in the 1960s led to a high rate of valve degeneration. Improved cryopreservation techniques developed in the 1970s have led to a resurgence of their use. Distal anastomosis is shown by *arrow*. HVL–homograft value leaflets.

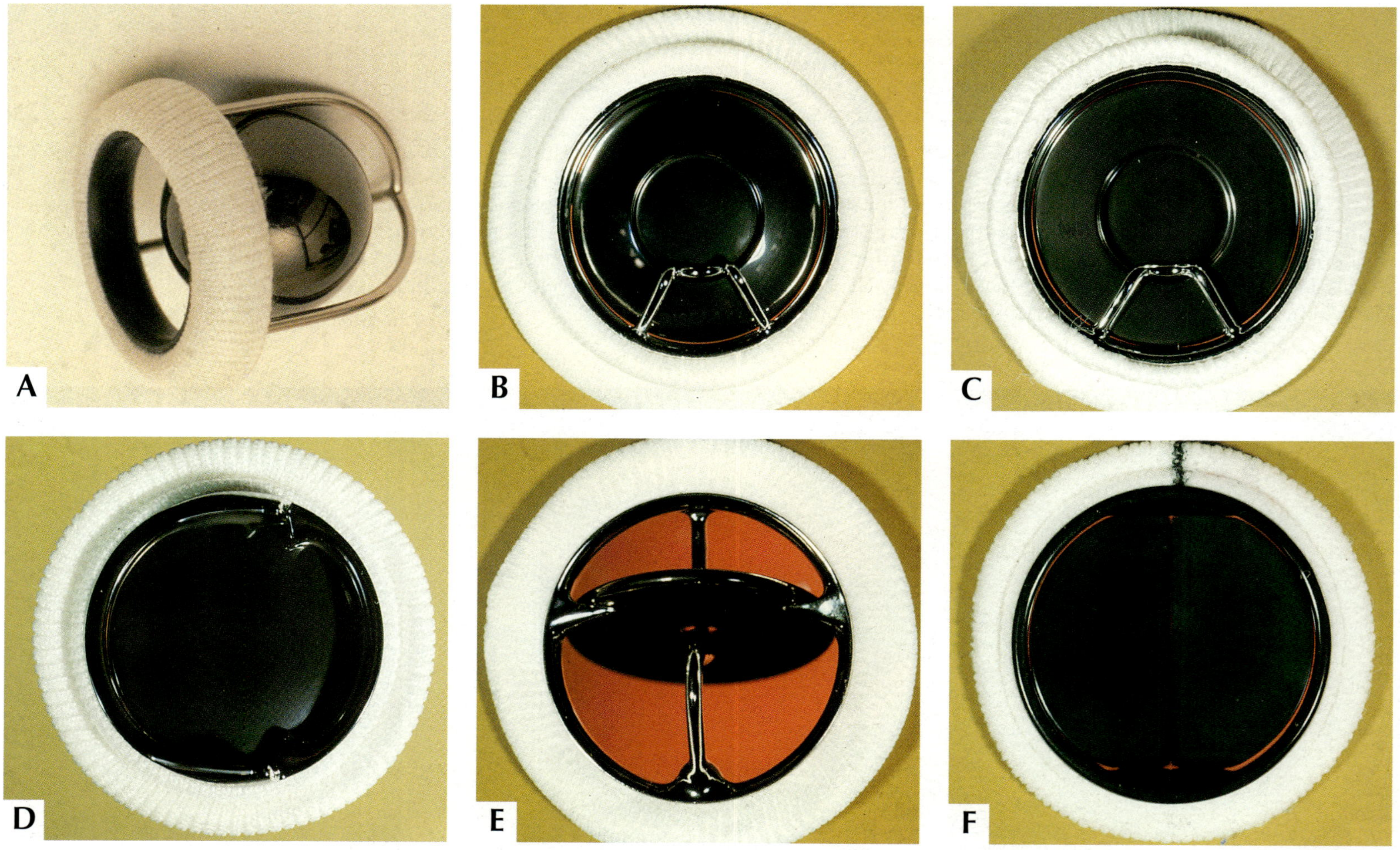

FIGURE 1-46. Mechanical valves. Of the dozens of mechanical valves that have been implanted in human hearts, six are chosen for illustration.

A, Starr-Edwards caged-ball valve. These valves have separate models for aortic and mitral positions and have been in longest continuous clinical use. They have a relatively high rate of thromboembolic complications and have high pressure gradients in small sizes.

B, Bjork-Shiley convexoconcave valve. These valves were extremely popular tilting disk valves but are no longer in use because of problems with strut fractures.

C, Bjork-Shiley spherical valve. In contrast to the convexoconcave valve, the spherical valve had a flat surface. The Bjork-Shiley Monostrut prosthesis (not shown) is in clinical trials.

D, Omniscience tilting disk valve is a monoleaflet prosthesis with a titanium orifice ring and a pyrolytic carbon disc controlled by short struts. The opening angle is 80°.

E, The Medtronic-Hall pyrolytic carbon disk opens to 70° (mitral) and 75° (aortic), and the ring and strut combination is machined from a single piece of titanium. The strut passes through a hole in the center of the disk. The valve is rotatable within the sewing ring.

F, St. Jude bileaflet valve is composed of pyrolytic carbon-coated graphite; the leaflets open to 85°. The St. Jude bileaflet valve is one of the most popular mechanical valves in use today. (Part A courtesy of Baxter Healthcare Corporation, Edwards Division, Irvine, CA; parts B and C courtesy of Shiley Inc., Irvine, CA; part D courtesy of Medical, Inc., Inver Grove Heights, Minneapolis, MN; part E courtesy of Medtronic, Inc., Minneapolis, MN; part F courtesy of St. Jude Medical, Inc., St. Paul, MN.)

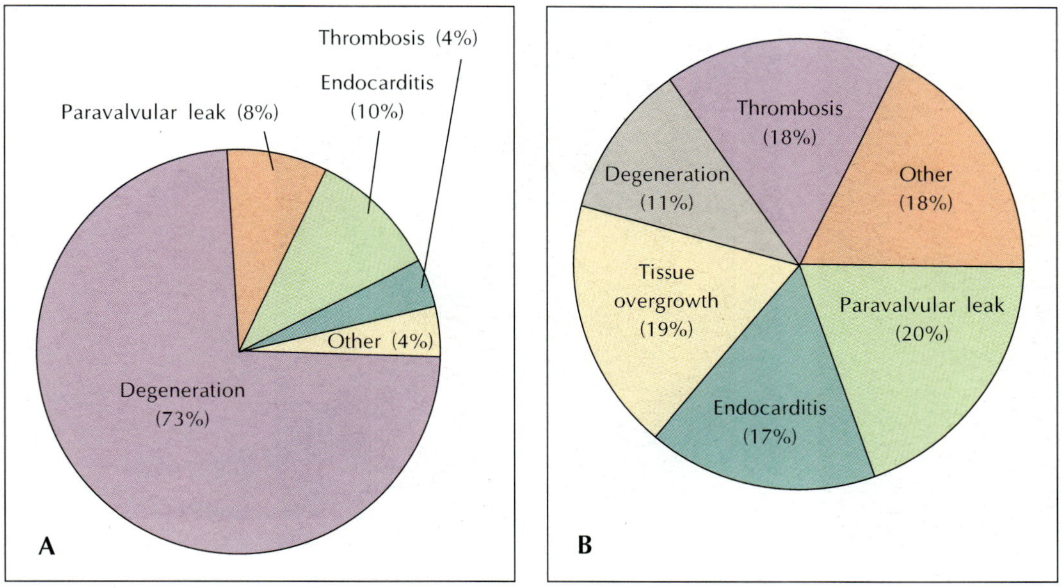

FIGURE 1-47. Causes of valve failure, bioprosthetic versus mechanical valves. **A,** Bioprosthetic valves are almost always removed because of tissue degeneration. **B,** Causes of failure of mechanical valves are more diverse. (*Adapted from* Schoen and coworkers [32].)

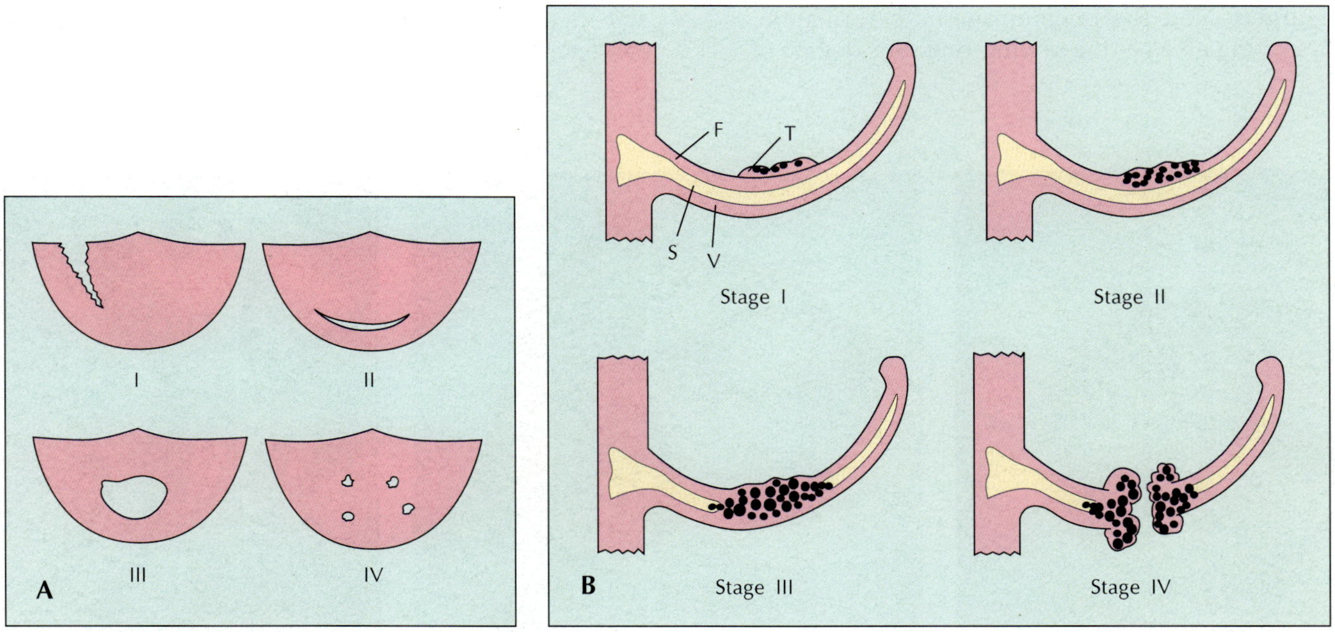

FIGURE 1-48. Schematic diagram of bioprosthetic degeneration and infection. **A,** Types of degeneration include cuspal tears (type I), crescentic tears at the bases of the sinus not involving the free margin (type II), irregular tears in the center of the valve cusp (type III), and multiple small perforations (type IV) [33]. Type III degeneration is often caused by infection. Bioprosthetic valves are prone to gradual tissue degeneration or primary tissue failure related to cuspal mineralization. This complication occurs at a rate of about 50% at 15 years in adults [34] and at a much faster rate in children.

B, Stages of infection of bioprosthetic valves. In contrast to mechanical valves, which become infected exclusively at the sewing ring, bioprosthetic valves may become infected either at the sewing ring or, as illustrated, on the cuspal surface. Later stages may result in perforation and type III tears. F—fibrosa; S—spongiosa; T—thrombus; V—ventricularis. (*Adapted from* Ishihara and coworkers [33].)

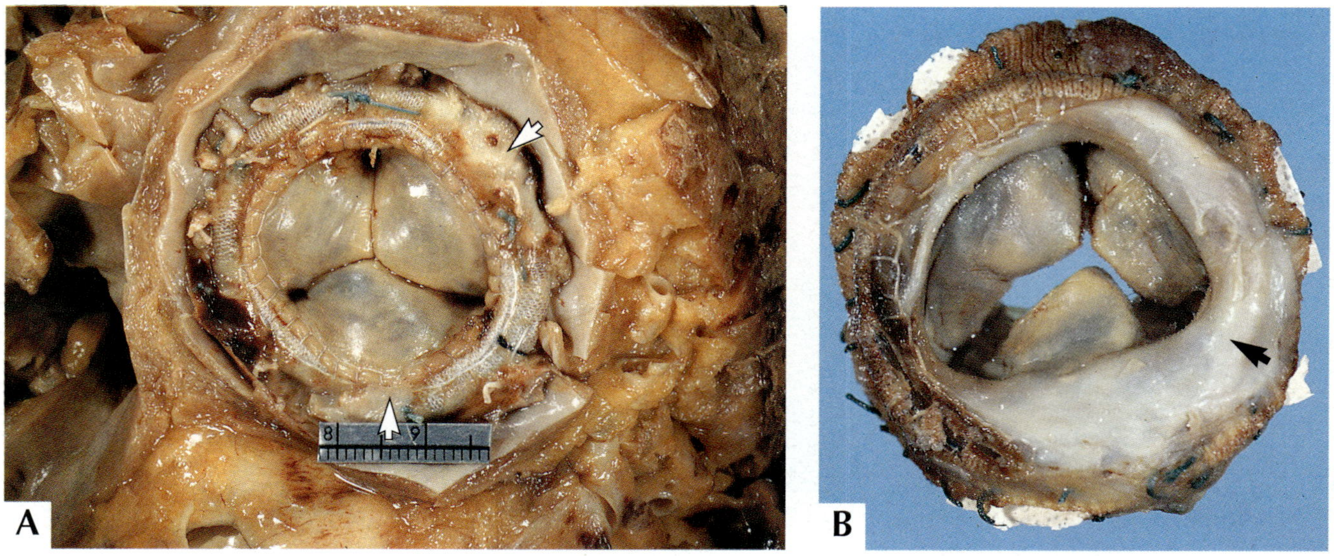

FIGURE 1-49. Bioprosthetic valves, pannus growth. **A,** Normal Carpentier-Edwards valve in situ, mitral position, viewed from the atrium. This patient died of nonvalvular complications 1 month after surgery. Note foci of pannus (*arrows*) formation (neointima) covering areas of the sewing ring; this degree of overgrowth is normal and does not interfere with valve function. **B,** Tissue overgrowth (arrow shows exaggerated neointima [pannus]) can result in increased pressure gradients and is moderatate in this example. There is also degenerative change as evidenced by thickening of valve leaflets

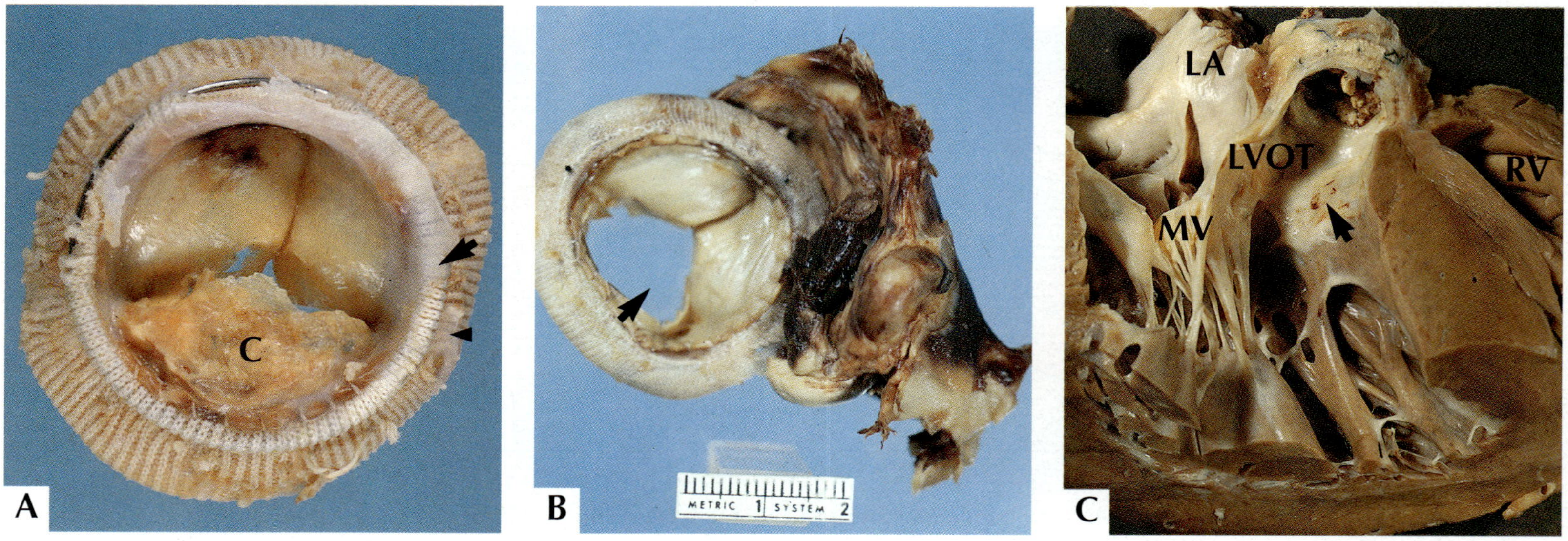

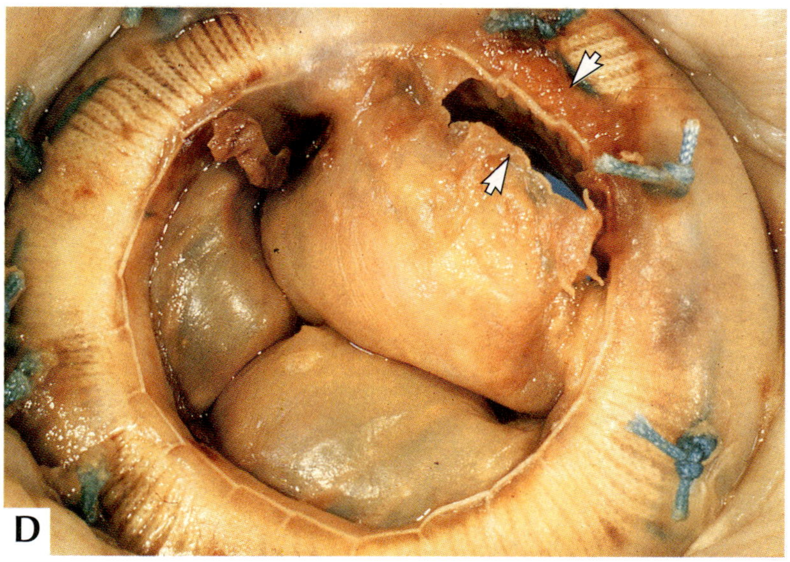

FIGURE 1-50. Bioprosthetic valves, degenerative changes. **A,** Mineralization occurs in virtually all bioprosthetic valves, especially in children and young adults. In this case calcification (C) was limited primarily to one cusp. The porcine AV is asymmetric, the right coronary cusp being larger, with a muscle shelf that results in less complete opening and accelerated calcification after xenotransplantation. The stent and sewing ring are denoted by the *arrow* and *arrowhead*, respectively.

B, A calcified porcine cusp can occasionally dislodge completely and embolize (*arrow*). Embolization, although a rare complication of bioprosthetic valves, may result in catastrophic complications, including stroke and sudden death.

C, A 42-year-old man had congenital AS treated with valvulotomy and valve replacement 11 years before death. Note left ventricular outflow tract (LVOT) regurgitant jet lesion. *Arrow* denotes endocardial fibrosis from aortic regurgitation.

D, Perforation, bioprosthetic valve. This Hancock valve had been in the mitral position for 5 years. The patient died soon after

(*continued*)

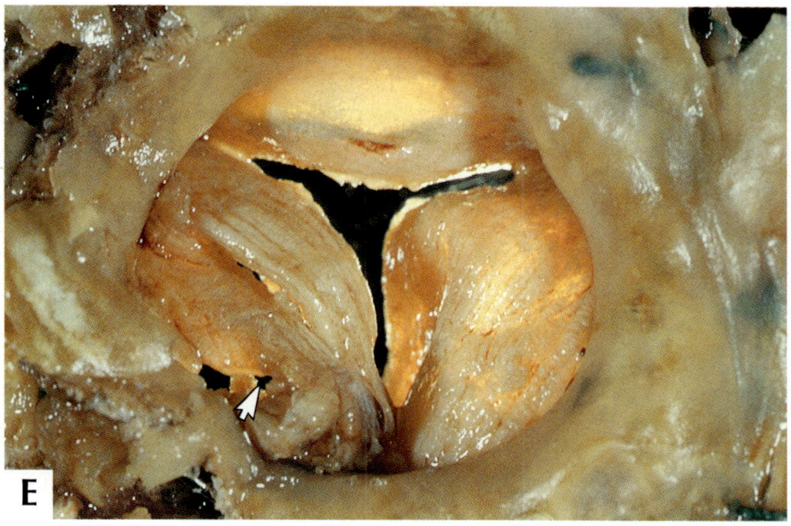

FIGURE 1-50. (*continued*) hospitalization for sudden-onset congestive heart failure. There is a linear type II perforation (*arrows*) at the base of the cusp that does not involve the free edge. **E,** Type II tear (*arrow*) in a fascia lata bioprosthetic valve. Valves constructed of autologous fascia lata mounted on a stent have been discontinued due to overgrowth of fibrous sheath and disintegration of cuspal connective tissue. LA—left atrium; MV—mitral valve; RV—right ventricle.

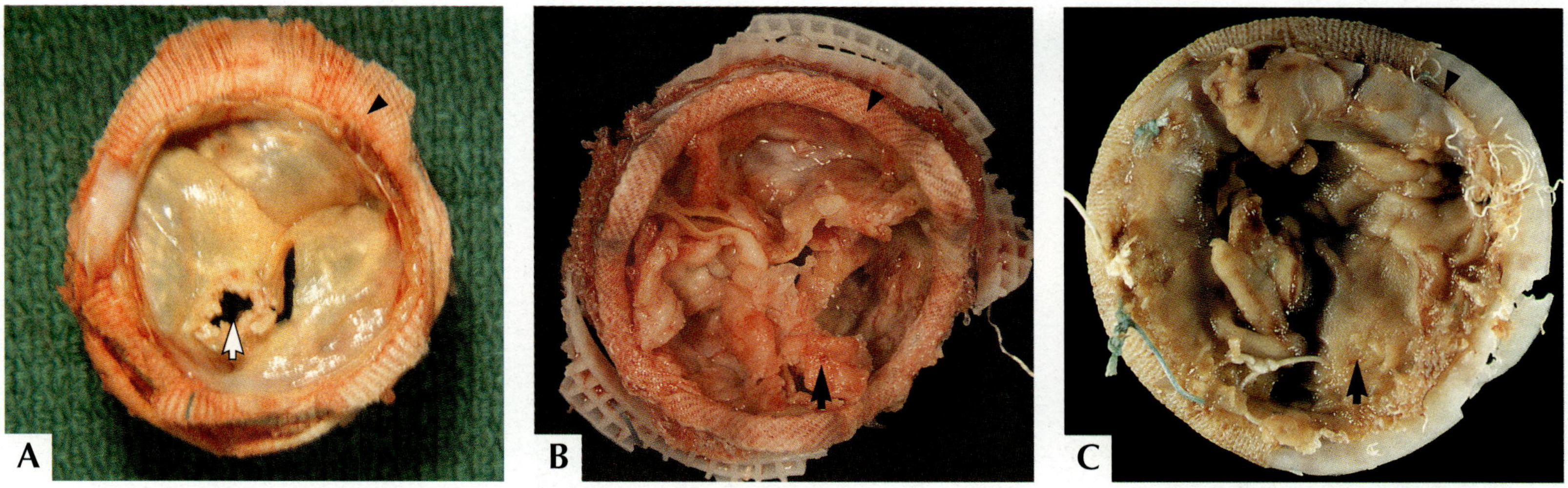

FIGURE 1-51. Bioprosthetic valve, endocarditis. **A,** Type III tear (*arrow*) in a Hancock valve with infective endocarditis. Endocarditis is a potentially disastrous complication of valve replacement. In bioprosthetic valves, it takes one of two forms: infection of valve leaflet and sewing ring abscess; in this example, the infection is localized to the leaflet. *Arrowhead* denotes stent.

B, Porcine valve viewed from aortic aspect. Note destruction of valve leaflets by infectious vegetation (*arrow*). The infectious agent was *Staphylococcus epidermidis*; the valve was moved 1 month after insertion. Endocarditis occurs at a rate of about 5% at 5 years, and up to five times this rate in patients originally operated for endocarditis. Early infections are usually secondary to perioperative contaminants, whereas infections after 60 days result from bacteremic seeding. *Arrowhead* denotes cloth-covered stent.

C, A 45-year-old woman had severe MVP treated with mitral valve replacement. Clinical symptoms of endocarditis and congestive failure occurred 2.5 years later. The photograph demonstrates a Carpentier-Edwards valve infected by *Staphylococcus aureus*, with cuspal tissue destroyed by vegetation (*arrow*). Staphylococci are extremely destructive to bioprosthetic tissues and are the most common cause of infections involving either mechanical or bioprosthetic valves. *Arrowhead* denotes stent.

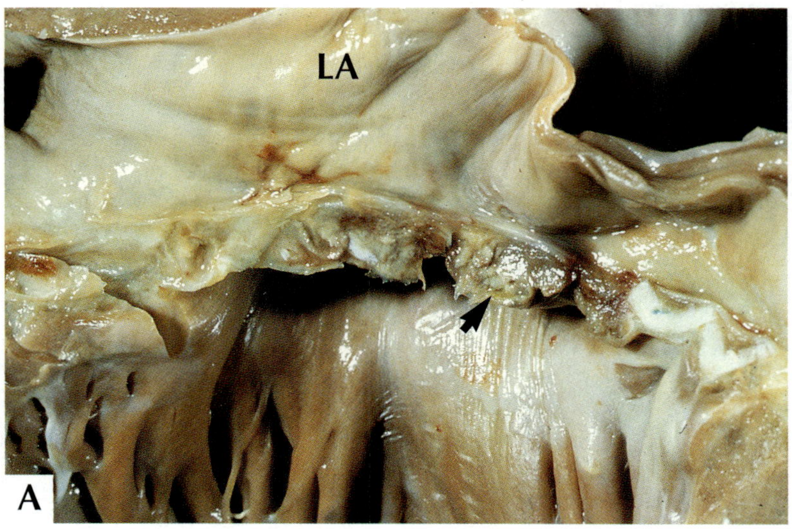

FIGURE 1-52. Carpentier-Edwards valve, mitral position. No abnormality was originally noted in this patient. Ring abscesses may be difficult to identify on cursory examination of the valve itself.

A, After postmortem removal of the valve, a ring abscess (*arrow*) is evident as friable excrescences along the mitral annulus. Histologic section (not shown) demonstrated *Aspergillus* species. (*continued*)

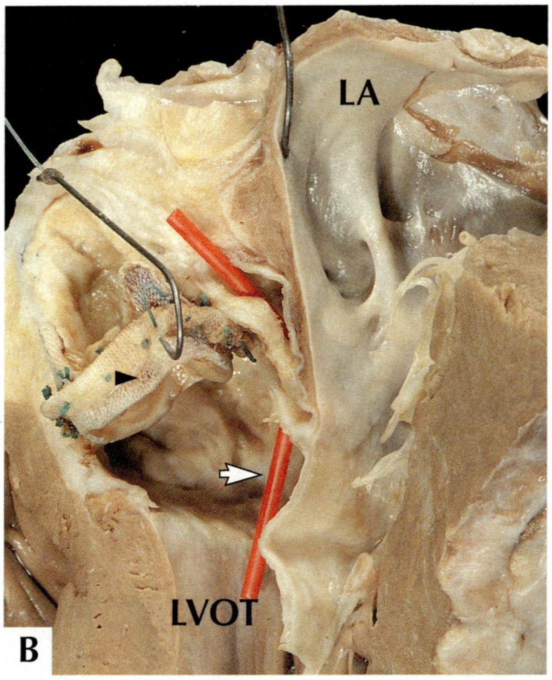

FIGURE 1-52. (*continued*) **B,** Healed endocarditis. A 34-year-old drug addict with recurrent bacterial endocarditis and AV replacement died of narcotic intoxication. A long-axis cut through the heart demonstrates the aortic outflow, porcine valve in aortic position.

A healed ring abscess (a colored probe [*arrow*]) is present, demonstrating the perivalvular leak. No active endocarditis was present on histologic examination. Perivalvular leaks can be a result in noninfectious tissue retraction, incomplete surgical seating, or endocarditis. *Arrowhead* denotes prosthetic valve. LA—left atrium, LVOT—left ventricular outflow tract.

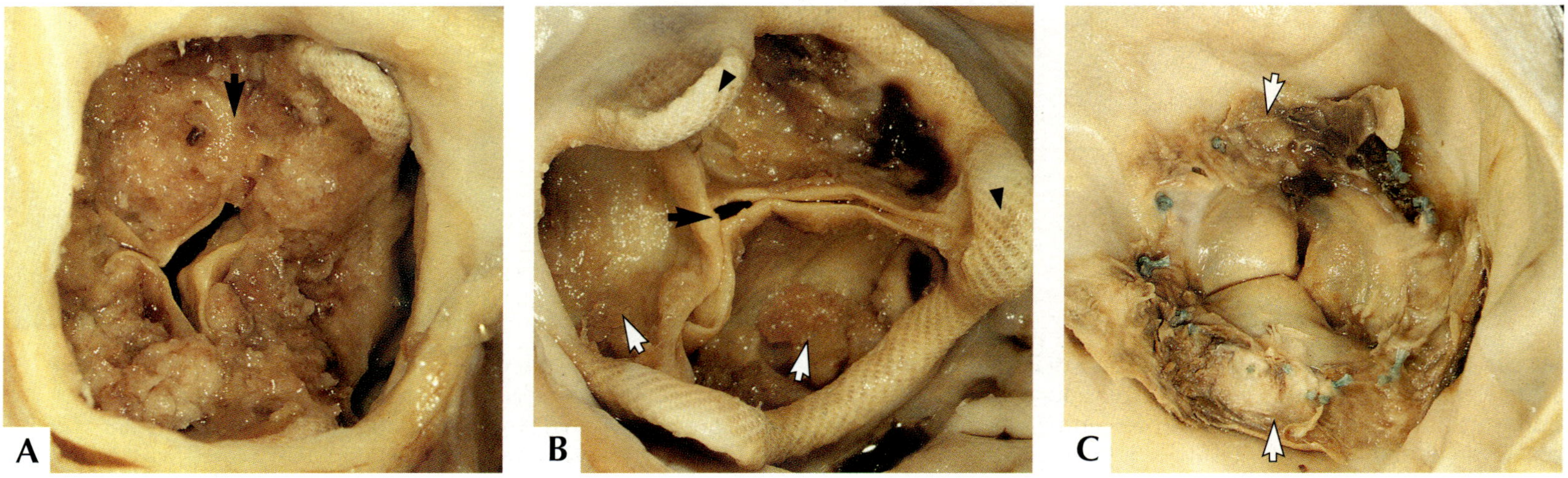

FIGURE 1-53. Bioprosthetic valves, thrombosis. Thrombosis on prosthetic valves results in thrombotic closure or thromboembolism. It is a major complication of prosthetic valves and occurs at a rate of 1% to 4% annually in the average patient and at a higher rate in patients with atrial fibrillation or heart block.

A, Thrombotic closure (*arrow*), porcine valve. The patient was a 66-year-old man with AV replacement 7 years prior to sudden death. Thrombotic closure is relatively uncommon in bioprosthetic valves compared with mechanical valves [36].

B, Thrombotic vegetations (*white arrows*), Carpentier-Edwards valve. The patient was a 55-year-old woman 2 years after placement of prosthetic valve in the mitral position. The free edges of the valve leaflet are shown by the *black arrow*. She died of complications of chronic cerebral thromboembolism. *Arrowheads* indicate the stent.

C, Organizing thrombi (*arrows*) were also attached to the sewing ring on the atrial surface of the valve. The valve illustrated is that shown in *panel B*.

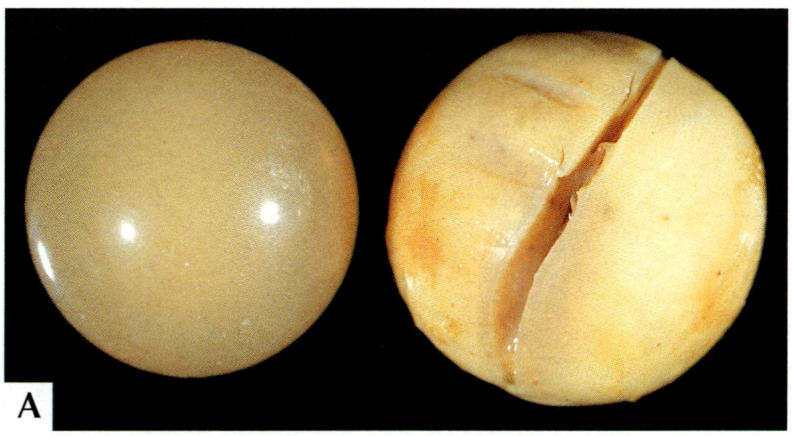

FIGURE 1-54. Degenerative changes, mechanical valves. **A,** Ball variance. A normal poppet from a Starr-Edwards adjacent to a swollen, cracked poppet from a Starr-Edwards valve removed for ball variance. With current generation Silastic poppets this complication is virtually no longer seen. Today, the occluders are made of pyrolytic carbon, which has high strength and is fatigue and wear resistant. (*continued*)

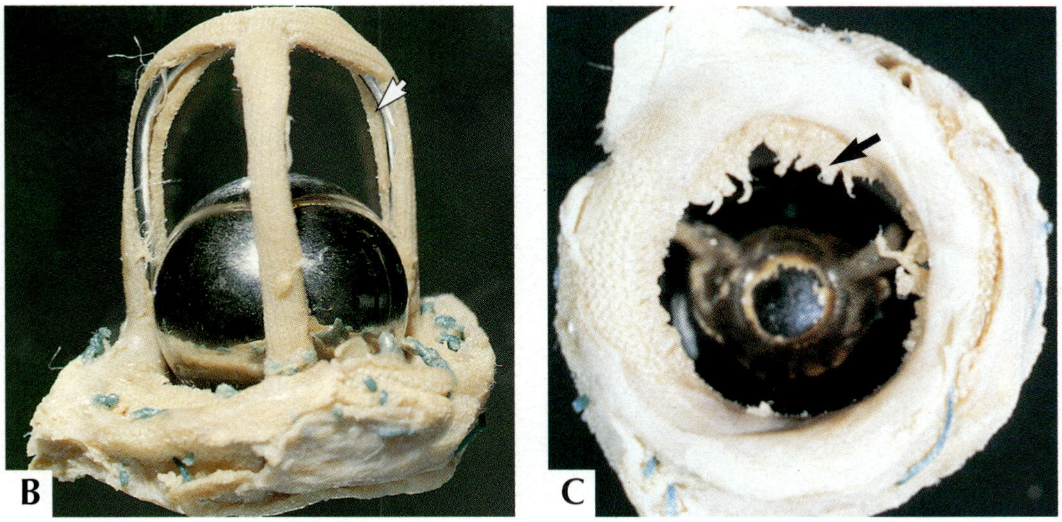

FIGURE 1-54. (*continued*) **B,** Cloth wear, mechanical valves. Starr-Edwards aortic prosthesis, model 2310, shows cloth wear with exposure of metal cage bars (*arrow*). Because of such complications and the introduction of newer materials, current valves have minimal cloth coverings over metal surfaces.

C, Cloth wear, mechanical valves. An undersurface view of the same valve shown in *panel B* demonstrates cloth wear with ragged edges (*arrow*).

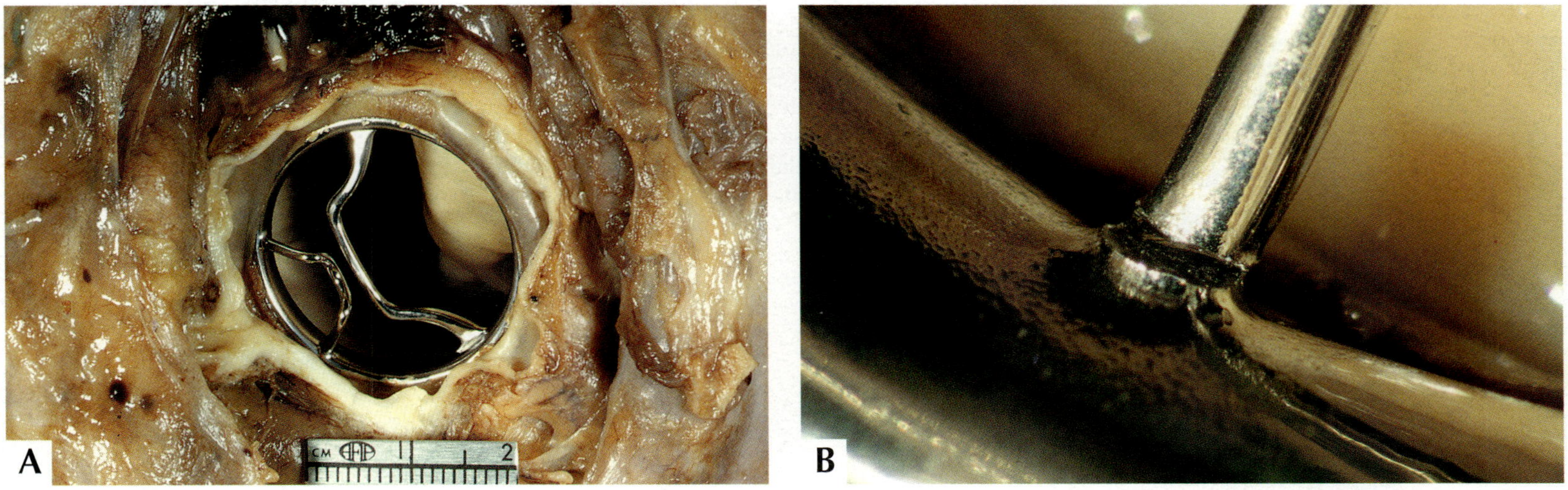

FIGURE 1-55. Strut fracture, Bjork-Shiley valve. Early versions of the 60° to 70° concavoconvex valves were prone to strut fracture (**A**) and disk embolization due to improper welds. A 34-year-old man died suddenly 1 year after AV replacement. The disk was found at the iliac bifurcation (not shown).

B, Strut fracture, Bjork-Shiley valve. A closer view of the valve shown in *panel A* demonstrates fracture of one weld of the minor strut. The identification of strut fractures is difficult *in vivo;* early fractures of postmortem specimens are best detected by special techniques such as scanning electron microscopy.

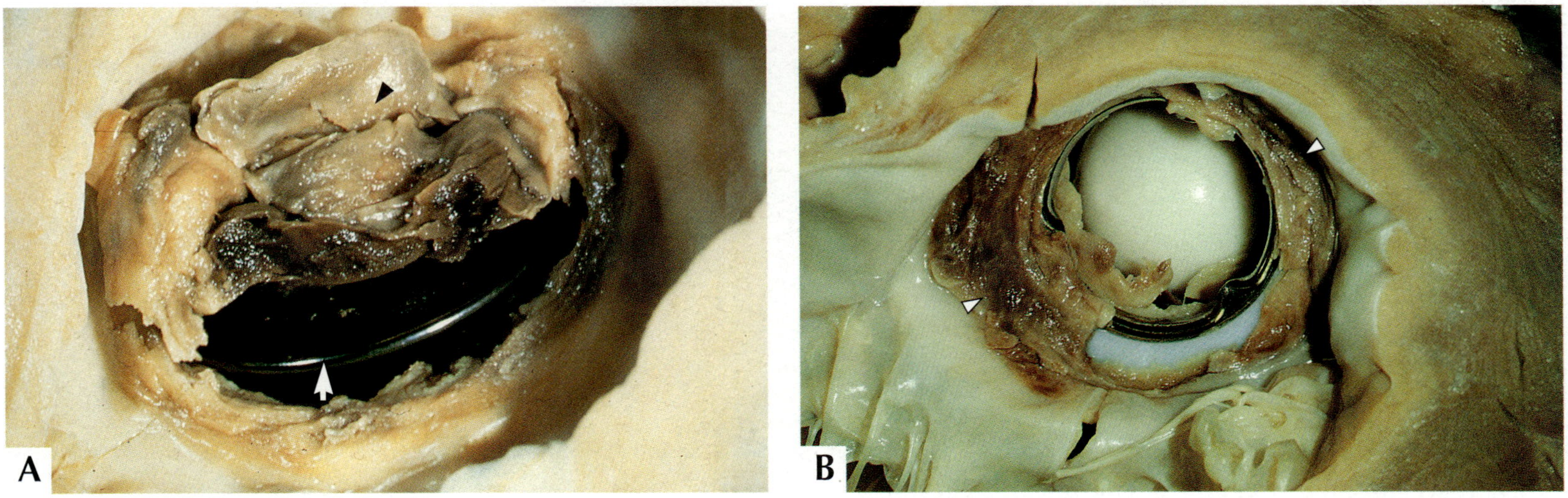

FIGURE 1-56. Thrombosis, mechanical valves. **A,** Obstructive thrombosis (*arrowhead*), Bjork-Shiley valve (*arrow*) in mitral position, resulted in sudden death. The patient was a middle-aged woman who was inadvertently given vitamin K in the emergency room to reverse anticoagulation.

B, Obstructive thrombosis, Starr-Edwards valve. Thrombus (*arrowheads*) has formed around the sewing ring of a Starr-Edwards valve impeding the full range of motion of the poppet, resulting in incompetence.

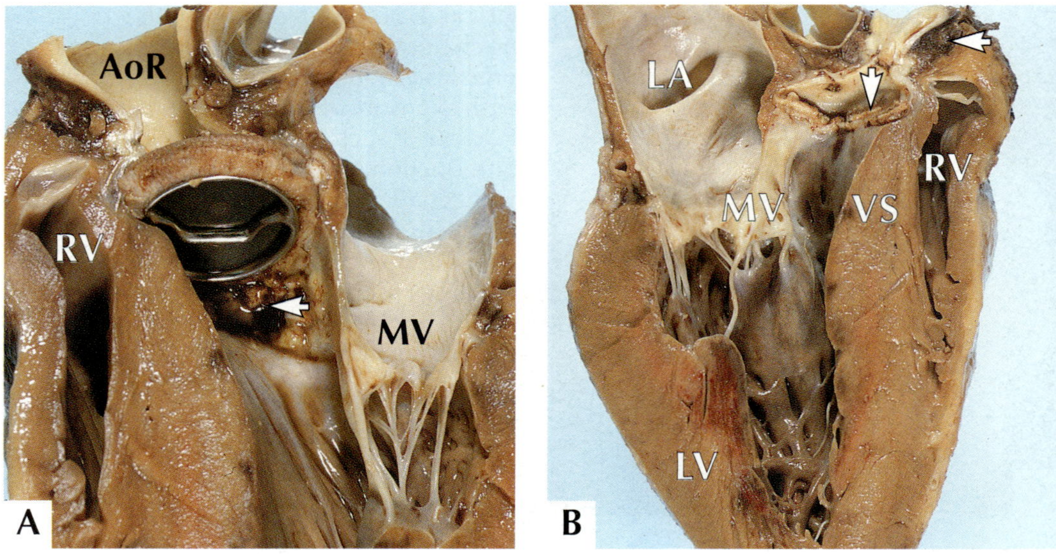

FIGURE 1-57. Infections, mechanical valves. **A,** Ring abscess (*arrow*) posterior to a Bjork-Shiley valve in the aortic position. Endocarditis of mechanical valves is generally limited to the sewing ring (ring abscess). **B,** Ring abscess, Bjork-Shiley valve. Same heart illustrated in *panel A* shows the opposite half of the heart. Ring of infected granulation tissue is evident (*arrows*). AoR—aortic root; LA—left atrium; LV—left ventricle; MV— mitral valve; RV—right ventricle; VS—ventricular septum.

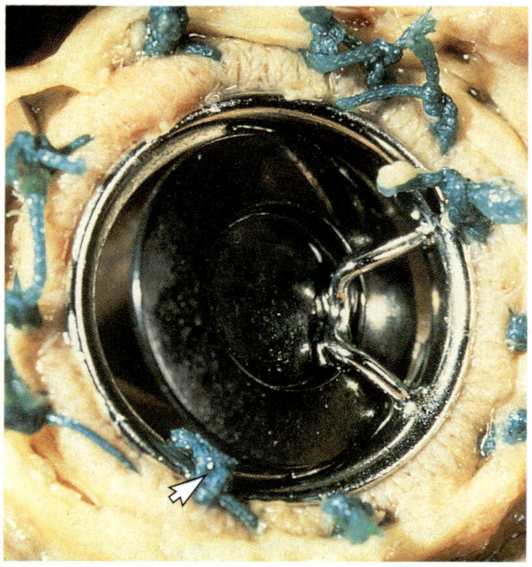

FIGURE 1-58. Miscellaneous cause of failure, mechanical valve. Surgical knot (*arrow*) overhanging sewing ring resulted in reduced excursion of the disk and valvular incompetence. The patient died suddenly 6 hours after replacement of the valve. Sudden cardiac death occurs as a late complication in 0.2% to 0.9% of patients with heart valve prostheses per year and is directly related to the valve in about 50% of cases [37]. Arrhythmias secondary to cardiomegaly or atherosclerotic disease cause the majority of the remaining deaths.

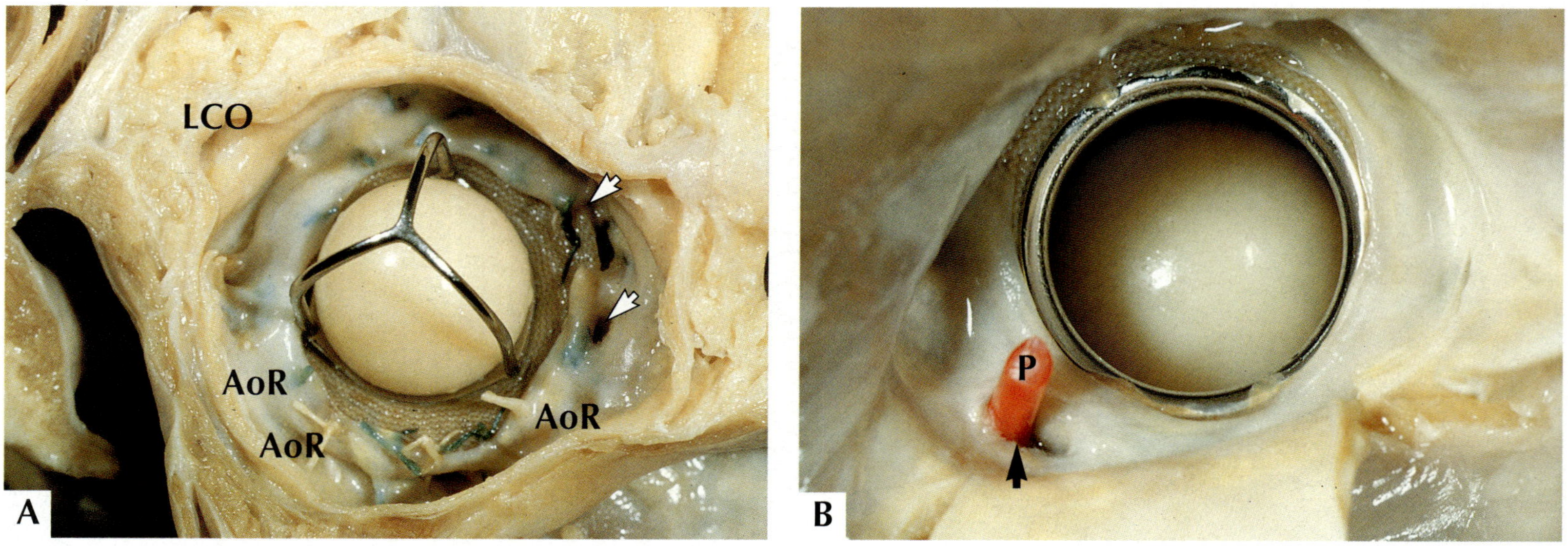

FIGURE 1-59. Perivalvular leak, Starr-Edwards valve in aortic position. Perivalvular leaks (*arrows* in **A**) may form from tissue retraction or a ring abscess and occur as a complication in fewer than 1% of replaced valves.

B, The same valve illustrated in *panel A*, from the ventricular aspect, with the probe (P) emanating through the perivalvular leak (*arrow*). Other complications of mechanical valves include some degree of hemolysis and renal hemosiderosis caused by the flow gradient across the prosthesis. (*continued*)

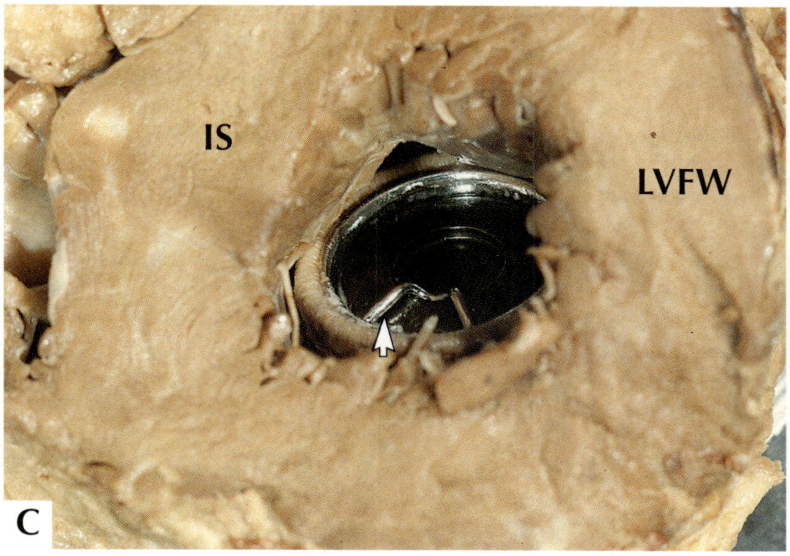

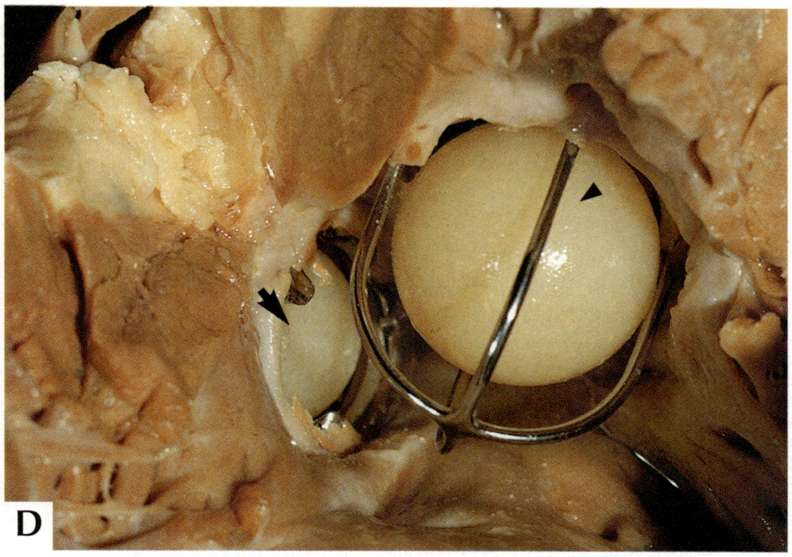

FIGURE 1-59. (*continued*) **C,** Size disproportion, Bjork-Shiley valve, mitral position. Size disproportion (valve prosthesis–patient mismatch [38]) is usually due to inappropriately large valves, especially in the mitral position with a small ventricular cavity (*eg*, MS). In this case there was a very small ventricular cavity with incomplete excursion of the disproportionately large disk. Valves that rotate within the sewing ring, such as Medtronic-Hall valves, are especially suited for small ventricular cavities with septal hypertrophy. *Arrow* denotes minor strut.

D, Size disproportion, Starr Edwards-valve, mitral (*arrowhead*) and aortic (*arrow*) positions. Valves with a high profile, such as Starr-Edwards valves, are currently not recommended for use in the mitral position with small ventricular cavity. Prosthetic disproportion by the placement of inappropriately large valves may result in septal irritation, interference to left ventricular emptying, and decreased occluder motion. AoR—cut surface of aortic root; IS—interventricular septum; LCO—left coronary ostium; LVFW—left ventricular free wall; RCO—right coronary ostium.

REFERENCES

1. Besterman E: The changing face of acute rheumatic fever. *Br Heart J* 1970, 32:579–582.
2. Peterson MD, Roach RM, Edwards JE: Types of aortic stenosis in surgically removed valves. *Arch Pathol Lab Med* 1985, 109:829–832.
3. Dare AJ, Veinot JP, Edwards WE, *et al.*: New observations on the etiology of aortic valve disease: a surgical pathology study of 236 cases from 1990. *Hum Pathol* 1993, 24:1330–1338.
4. Carlson RG, Mayfield WR, Normann S, Alexander JA: Radiation associated valvular disease. *Chest* 1991, 99:538–545.
5. Dare AJ, Harrity PJ, Tazelaar HD, *et al.*: Evaluation of surgically excised mitral valves: revised recommendations based on changing operative procedures in the 1990s. *Hum Pathol* 1993, 24:1286–1293.
6. Olson LT, Subramanian R, Ackerman DM, *et al.*: Surgical pathology of the mitral valve: a study of 712 cases spanning 21 years. *Mayo Clin Proc* 1987, 62:22–34.
7. Waller BF, Morrow AG, Maron BJ, *et al.*: Etiology of clinically isolated, severe, chronic pure mitral regurgitation: analysis of 97 patients over 30 years of age having mitral valve replacement. *Am Heart J* 1982, 104:276–288.
8. Moore P, Adatia I, Spevak PJ, *et al.*: Severe congenital mitral stenosis in infants. *Circulation* 1994, 89:2099–2106.
9. Virmani R, Atkinson JB, Forman MB, Robinowitz M: Mitral valve prolapse. *Hum Pathol* 1987, 18:596–602.
10. Virmani R, Atkinson JB, Forman MD: Mitral valve prolapse. *Herz* 1988, 13:215–226.
11. Hauck AJ, Freeman DP, Ackermann DM, *et al.*: Surgical pathology of the tricuspid valve: a study of 363 cases spanning 25 years. *Mayo Clin Proc* 1988, 63:851–863.
12. Waller BF, Block T, Eble JN, *et al.*: Etiology of tricuspid stenosis and pure tricuspid regurgitation. In *Pathology of the Heart and Great Vessels*. Edited by Waller BF. New York: Churchill Livingstone; 1988:149–189.
13. Waller BF, Howard J, Fess S: Pathology of pulmonic valve stenosis and pure regurgitation. *Clin Cardiol* 1995, 18:45–50.
14. Fischler D, Fitzmaurice M, Ratliff NB Jr: Quadricuspid aortic valve. *Am J Cardiovasc Pathol* 1990, 3:91–94.
15. Kirklin JW, Barratt-Boyes BG, eds.: *Cardiac Surgery*, New York: John Wiley & Sons; 1986:972–987.
16. Davies JW: *Pathology of Cardiac Valves*, London-Boston: Butterworths; 1980, 100–123.
17. Stollerman GH: Rheumatogenic group A streptococci and the return of rheumatic fever. *Adv Intern Med* 1990, 35:1–25.
18. Roberts WC: Morphologic features of the normal and abnormal mitral valve. *Am J Cardiol* 1983, 51:1005–1028.
19. Farb A, Tang AL, Atkinson JB, *et al.*: Comparison of cardiac findings in patients with mitral valve prolapse who die suddenly to those who have congestive heart failure from mitral regurgitation and to those with fatal noncardiac conditions. *Am J Cardiol* 1992, 70:234–239.
20. Roberts WC, Hollingsworth JF, Bulkley BH, *et al.*: Combined mitral and aortic regurgitation in ankylosing spondylitis. Angiographic and anatomic features. *Am J Med* 1974, 56:237–243.
21. Olson TA, Virmani R, Ansinelli RA, *et al.*: Cardiomyopathy in a child with hypereosinophilic syndrome. *Pediatr Cardiol* 1982, 3:161–169.
22. Virmani R: The tricuspid valve. *Mayo Clin Proc* 1989, 63:943–945.
23. Altrichter PM, Olson LJ, Edwards WD, *et al.*: Surgical pathology of the pulmonary valve; a study of 116 cases spanning 15 years. *Mayo Clin Proc* 1989, 64:1352–1360.
24. Farb A, Burke AP, Virmani R: Anatomy and pathology of the right ventricle (including acquired tricuspid and pulmonic valve disease). *Cardiol Clin North Am* 1992, 10:1–21.

25. Hauck AJ, Edwards WD, Danielson GK, *et al.*: Mitral and aortic valve disease associated with ergotamine therapy for migraine. Report of two cases and review of literature. *Arch Pathol Lab Med* 1990, 114:62–64.
26. Atkinson JB, Virmani R: Infective endocarditis: changing trends and general approach for examination. In *Cardiovascular Pathology. Major Problems in Pathology Series.* Edited by Virmani R, Atkinson JB, Fenoglio J. Philadelphia: WB Saunders; 1992:435–450.
27. Jamieson WR: Modern cardiac valve devices—bioprostheses and mechanical prostheses: state of the art. *J Card Surg* 1993, 8:89–98.
28. Turina J, Hess OM, Turina M, Krayenbuehl HP: Cardiac bioprostheses in the 1990s. *Circulation* 1993, 88:775–781.
29. Kirklin JK, Smith D, Novick W, *et al.*: Long-term function of cryopreserved aortic homografts. A ten-year study. *J Thorac Cardiovasc Surg* 1993, 106:154–165.
30. Crescenzo DG, Hilbert SL, Messier RH Jr, *et al*: Human cryopreserved homografts: electron microscopic analysis of cellular injury. *Ann Thorac Surg* 1993, 55:25–30.
31. Albertucci M, Wong K, Petrou M, *et al.*:The use of unstented homograft valves for aortic valve reoperations. Review of a twenty-three-year experience. *J Thorac Cardiovasc Surg* 1994, 107:152–161.
32. Schoen FJ, Titus JL, Lawrie GM: Autopsy-determined causes of death after cardiac valve replacement. *JAMA* 1983, 249:899–902.
33. Ishihara T, Ferrans VJ, Boyce SW, *et al.*: Structure and classification of cuspal tears and perforations in porcine bioprosthetic cardiac valves implanted in patients. *Am J Cardiol* 1981, 48:665–678.
34. Brudon RA, Miller DC, Oyer PE, *et al.*: Durability of porcine valves at fifteen years in a representative North American patient population. *J Thorac Cardiovasc Surg* 1992, 103:238–251.
35. Willerson JT: Marked thrombosis and calcification of procine heterograft valves. *Circulation* 1980, 62:862–869.
36. Grunkemeier GL, Rahimtoola SH: Artificial heart valves. *Annu Rev Med* 1990, 41:251–263.
37. Burke AP, Farb AF, Sessums L, Virmani R: Sudden cardiac death in patients with heart valve prostheses: an autopsy study. *J Heart Valve Dis* 1994, 3:10–16.
38. Rahmitoola SH: The problem of the valve prosthesis–patient mismatch. *Circulation* 1978, 58:20–24.

Effects of Pressure and Volume Overload on Left and Right Ventricles

2
CHAPTER

John D. Carroll

In this chapter the effects of pressure and volume overload on the ventricles are presented. The first series of figures deals with background issues such as the intellectual and clinical framework needed to understand how the heart adapts to these abnormal states. The nature of pressure and volume overload is illustrated, the stages of adaptation are outlined, and the pathophysiologic viewpoints of the engineer and the molecular biologist are given to broaden the reader's perspective.

The altered structure and function of the myocardium is critical to an understanding of adaptation to pressure and volume overload. Therefore a series of illustrations demonstrate what happens at the myocyte, the sarcomere, and the chamber level of myocardial organization. In brief, the hypertrophied muscle unit is much more than an enlarged version of the normal unit.

Between myocytes and encircling the vasculature is the cardiac interstitium. These illustrations explore the reconfiguration of the interstitium during pressure and volume overload. Extracellular material is altered, including the normal collagen matrix, as is the appearance of pathologic fibrosis. The biochemical and cellular elements are reviewed and related to the chamber properties that result from these hemodynamic overloads.

Next a series of figures demonstrates the important alterations in the coronary vasculature that occur in response to pressure-volume overload. Anatomic alterations are illustrated and important physiologic consequences that have an impact on ventricular function are discussed. Coronary pathophysiology in the severely hypertrophied heart is presented.

Altered myocardial oxygen demand and reduced supply from a compromised coronary vasculature lead to ischemia. It is now appreciated that the pressure-overloaded heart, in particular, exhibits ischemia even in the absence of atherosclerotic coronary artery abnormalities. This series of figures explores findings from experimental studies.

Altered cardiac function leads to activation of systemic and local neuroendocrine mechanisms. These mechanisms must be considered in pressure and overload lesions.

An understanding of myocardial hypertrophy, interstitial matrix reconfiguration, coronary vascular adaptation, and neurohumoral activation provides a framework for the next series of figures. Diastolic function is first explored with figures on the diastolic pressure-volume relationship emphasizing mechanisms and evolution with prototypical valve lesions. The important mechanisms of abnormal myocardial relaxation and diastolic suction are illustrated. Chamber and myocardial stiffness and chamber geometry are described in the different overloaded states. Filling dynamics are illustrated and discussed.

Systolic function in response to pressure and volume overload is also described in this chapter. The hyperdynamic left ventricle in compensated mitral regurgitation and in some cases of aortic stenosis is contrasted with the myopathic heart requiring transplantation and leading to cardiogenic shock.

Finally, all the detrimental consequences of ventricular adaptation to pressure and volume overload are reviewed. This summarizes important pathophysiologic features that are further discussed in subsequent chapters on specific valve lesions.

Clinical Framework

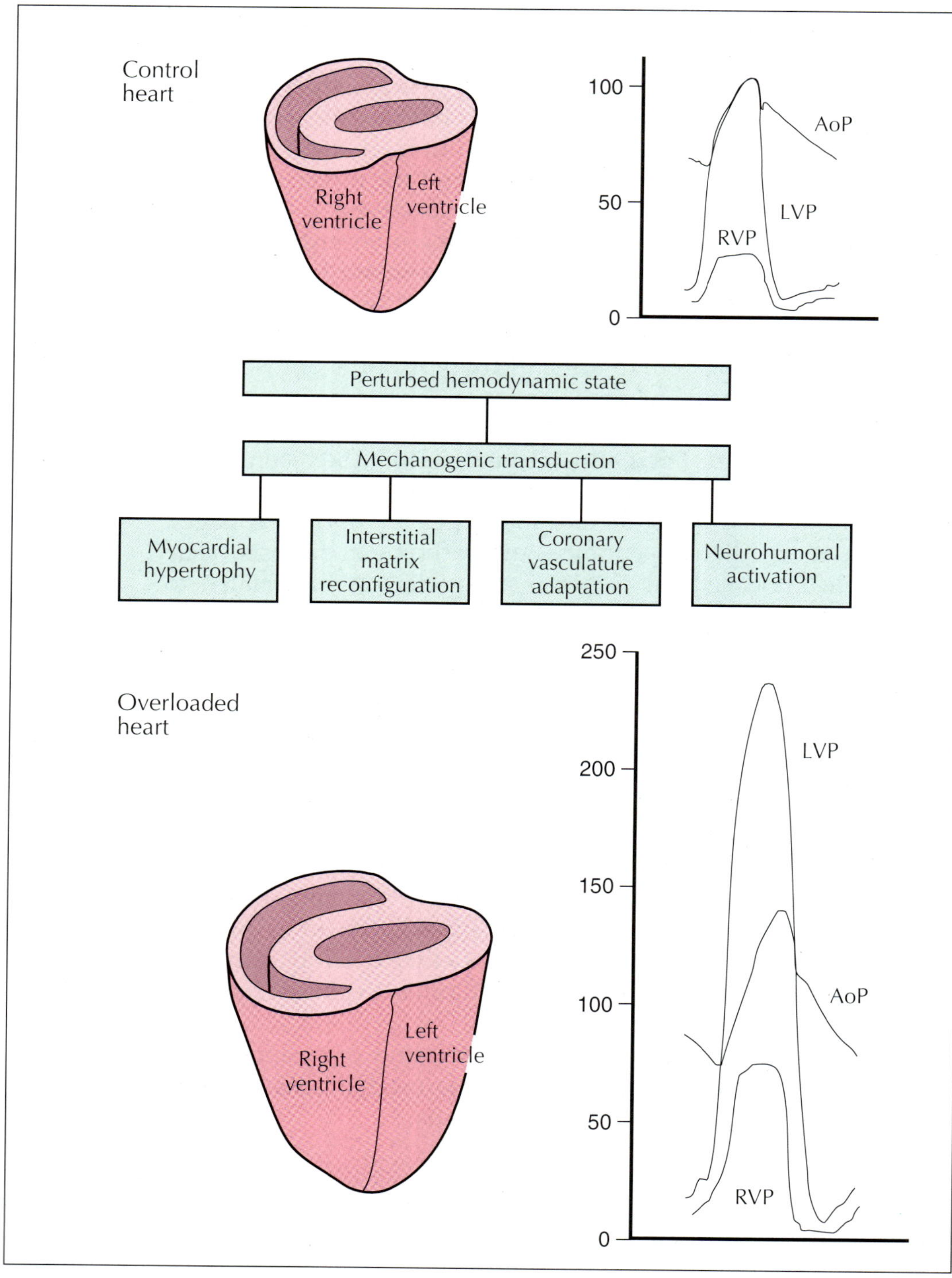

Figure 2-1. An overview of the pathophysiology of valvular heart disease. A transformation of the right and left ventricles unfolds after exposure to either an abnormal pressure or volume load, that is, a hemodynamic overload. Stenotic or incompetent cardiac valves are common etiologies. The characteristics of the hemodynamic load (*ie*, pressure versus volume) and the responses of the major subsystems of the cardiovascular system (*ie*, the myocardium, the interstitium, the vasculature, and the neuroendocrine axis) define the nature of this transformation in structure and function. The *left upper quadrant icon* represents right and left ventricular size and shape under baseline conditions. In the *right upper quadrant* the ventricular pressure waveforms depict normal ventricular function. The perturbed hemodynamic state must first be sensed and translated into a genetic/cellular activation—mechanogenic transduction. Four major processes—myocardial hypertrophy, interstitial matrix reconfiguration, coronary vascular adaptation, and neurohumoral activation—subsequently generate these transformations of structure and function. The transformations in right and left ventricular chamber properties induced by these abnormal hemodynamic conditions are symbolized in the *lower quadrants*. This chapter sequentially examines the characteristics of the hemodynamic load, the major processes unfolding in reaction to the load, and the resultant transformations in ventricular structure and function. AoP—aortic pressure; LVP—left ventricular pressure; RVP—right ventricular pressure.

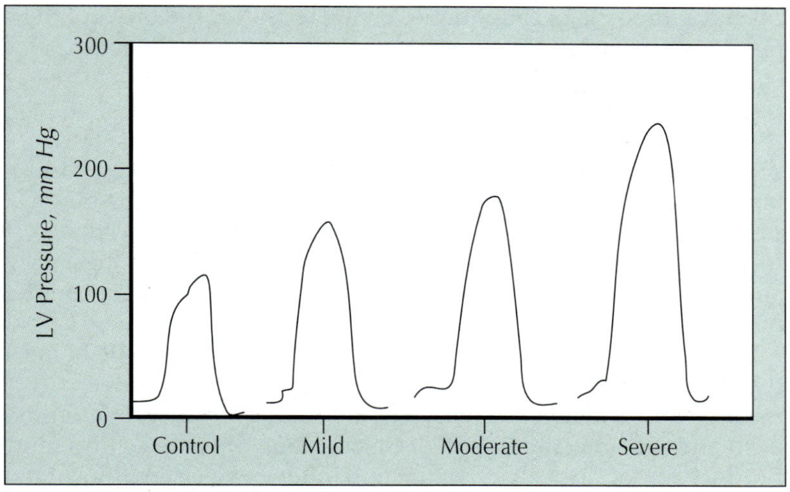

FIGURE 2-2. The prototypes of hemodynamic overloads produced by valvular heart disease: pressure overload. The nature, degree, and duration of the abnormal load determine in large part the clinical and hemodynamic presentation of valvular disease. The prototype of *pressure overload*, aortic stenosis, is displayed in this figure with left ventricular (LV) waveforms.

Four subjects had these high-fidelity pressure waveforms recorded at the time of cardiac catheterization. One subject had no cardiac abnormality and three patients had progressively more severe pressure overload due to narrowing of the aortic valve. Myocardial hypertrophy transforms the pressure-overloaded ventricle so it can produce an increased systolic pressure to surmount this hemodynamic load. Pressure overload of either ventricle is a chronic abnormality with a slow progression in the severity of the stenosis paralleled by increased myocardial mass. Often chamber size is normal and wall thickness increases, producing a concentric pattern of chamber hypertrophy. These pressure tracings come from patients with hypertrophied myocardium with normal contractile strength. Myocardial failure reduces the pressure generation ability of the ventricle. Thus, systolic pressure is not always an indicator of the severity of the hemodynamic load.

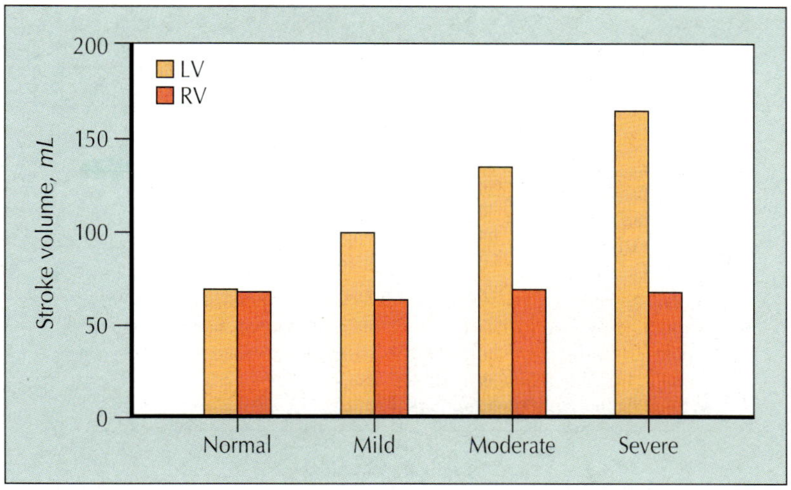

FIGURE 2-3. The prototypes of hemodynamic overloads produced by valvular heart disease: volume overload. A prototype of *volume overload* is aortic regurgitation. Right ventricular (RV) stroke volume is compared with left ventricular (LV) stroke volume in four groups of individuals [1]. The RV and LV stroke volumes are equal in normal subjects. Patients with three progressive degrees of aortic valve regurgitation display a greater and greater mismatch of RV and LV stroke volumes. The difference between RV and LV stroke volume represents the amount of regurgitation (regurgitant fraction = [LV - RV stroke volume]/RV stroke volume × 100). Cine magnetic resonance images were used in the calculation of stroke volume from measured ventricular volume at end-diastole and end-systole for each chamber.

Volume overload of the RV or LV is typically a chronic abnormality. The ventricle adapts by chamber dilatation and wall thickening, a so-called eccentric pattern of chamber hypertrophy. The compensated ventricle maintains a normal forward stroke volume, but at the expense of wasted work dealing with the regurgitant portion of the total stroke volume. With severe regurgitation it may be impossible for even the otherwise healthy myocardium to maintain a normal forward stroke volume. Both the forward stroke volume and the absolute regurgitant volume decline with myocardial failure.

Regurgitant lesions such as aortic regurtgitation are not pure volume overloads for the ventricle because higher systolic pressures are often produced. The hemodynamic load is more complex.

The categories of pressure and volume overloads are, therefore, simplifications. Also, myocardial failure reduces the pressure and flow-generating ability of the RV and LV used to quantify the severity of the lesion. Therefore, quantification of the load severity cannot be accomplished without commenting on ventricular function. (*Adapted from* Pflugfelder and coworkers [1].)

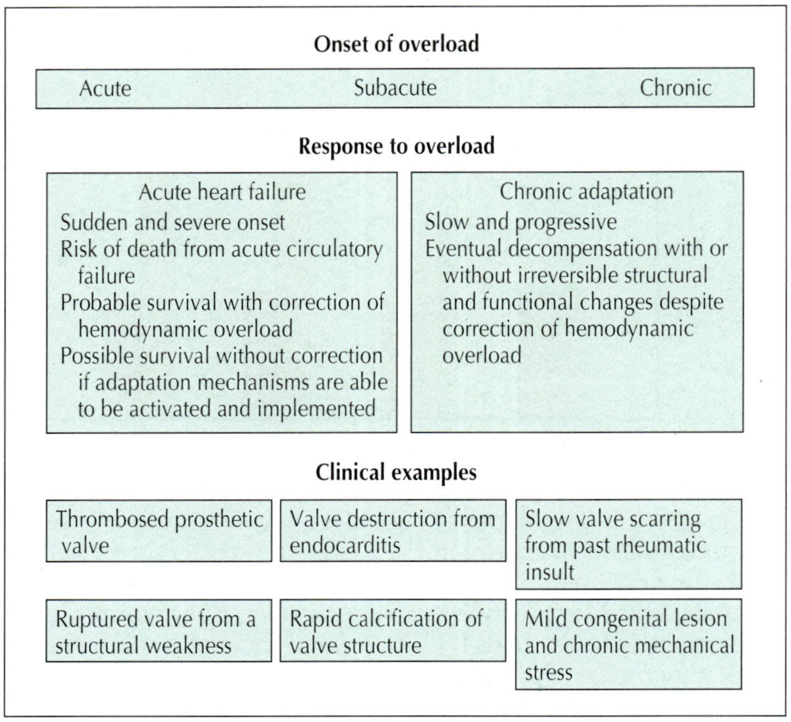

FIGURE 2-4. A clinical overview of pressure and volume overload. Broad and complex is the clinical context for right and left ventricular pressure and volume overload. The time bar at the top displays three major time frames characteristic of the onset of the overload. The middle shows the spectrum of the clinical and compensatory responses. Clinical examples in the bottom boxes portray these features.

A thrombosed prosthetic valve produces a sudden and severe pressure load to the upstream cardiac chamber. A ruptured papillary muscle during myocardial infarction results in acute volume overload with heart failure. These lesions rapidly lead to circulatory collapse and death without correction, stressing the measurable time necessary for the circulatory system to produce a condition of stable function.

Endocarditis destroys the integrity of cardiac valves. The hemodynamic severity of the hemodynamic lesion, usually valve incompetence, increases often over the course of weeks to months even after the infection is cured. Calcification of valve leaflets may produce important valve dysfunction, often stenosis, within a few years. These are clinical examples of the subacute onset of volume and pressure overload.

Rheumatically scarred valves and congenitally abnormal valves, such as a bicuspid aortic valve, often produce a gradually worsening hemodynamic overload. A testament to the plasticity of the cardiovascular system is the long period of a clinically and hemodynamically successful adaptation to a severe hemodynamic load. The right and left ventricular adaptation, though, has limits and irreversible structural and functional abnormalities eventually emerge. Clinical status deteriorates, although occasionally asymptomatic individuals harbor irreversible abnormalities.

STAGES OF ADAPTATION TO PRESSURE AND VOLUME OVERLOAD

STAGE	OSLER [4]	MEERSON [5]	KATZ [2]	ROSS [3]
1	Development	Transient breakdown	Developing hypertrophy	Early hypertrophy
2	Full compensation	Stable hyperfunction	Compensatory hypertrophy	Compensated hypertrophy
3	Broken compensation	Progressive cardiosclerosis	Heart failure	Impaired performance with load-mismatch
				Irreversible myocardial depression

FIGURE 2-5. Stages in the adaptation to pressure overload. The fundamental process of cardiovascular adaptation is a dynamic one. The stages or phases of adaptation have been outlined by clinical and basic science investigators [2–4].

All schemes include a compensatory period when the hemodynamic load is counterbalanced or neutralized by adaptive processes and a period when clinical symptoms emerge and mechanical adaptation fails. (*Adapted from* Katz [2].)

MECHANISTIC VIEWPOINTS ON CARDIAC ADAPTATION

MECHANICS VIEWPOINT

Hypertrophy may help to compensate for excessive afterload by increasing the myocardial mass in turn reducing the stress per unit area of muscle [6].

MOLECULAR VIEWPOINT

Hypertrophy is accompanied by a dissociated and complex modulation of a battery of genes responsible for contraction and relaxation [7].

FIGURE 2-6. Mechanistic viewpoints on cardiac adaptation. The adaptation of the right and left ventricles to the pressure and volume overloaded state is frequently studied and expressed as a mechanical problem with a mechanical solution [6]. More physical work must be done in a state of hemodynamic overload. More work-producing units (*ie*, sarcomeres) are developed to regain a balance. Clinical compensation is thus equated with the degree of hypertrophy returning elevated wall stresses to normal. Decompensation signals the inability of the hypertrophic process to match the increased load. Elevated systolic and diastolic wall stresses typically accompany the onset of heart failure.

Currently the molecular viewpoint is the perspective being used to focus investigation on the underlying biologic mechanisms. Molecular pathways are responsible for the translation of the sensed, abnormal hemodynamic load and for the initiation of cellular machinery to produce a remodeled organ [7]. The diverse battery of gene expression also emphasizes the complexities of the process. Our understanding must go beyond the simple concept of an increase in cardiac mass to balance the workload.

A synthesis of all viewpoints is needed to understand the adaptive and maladaptive processes [8] leading to a heart that is not simply an enlarged version of the normal heart [9]. Therefore, starting at the onset of the abnormal load, it is necessary to understand the sequence of events from the gene to the organ level.

ALTERED MYOCARDIAL STRUCTURE AND FUNCTION

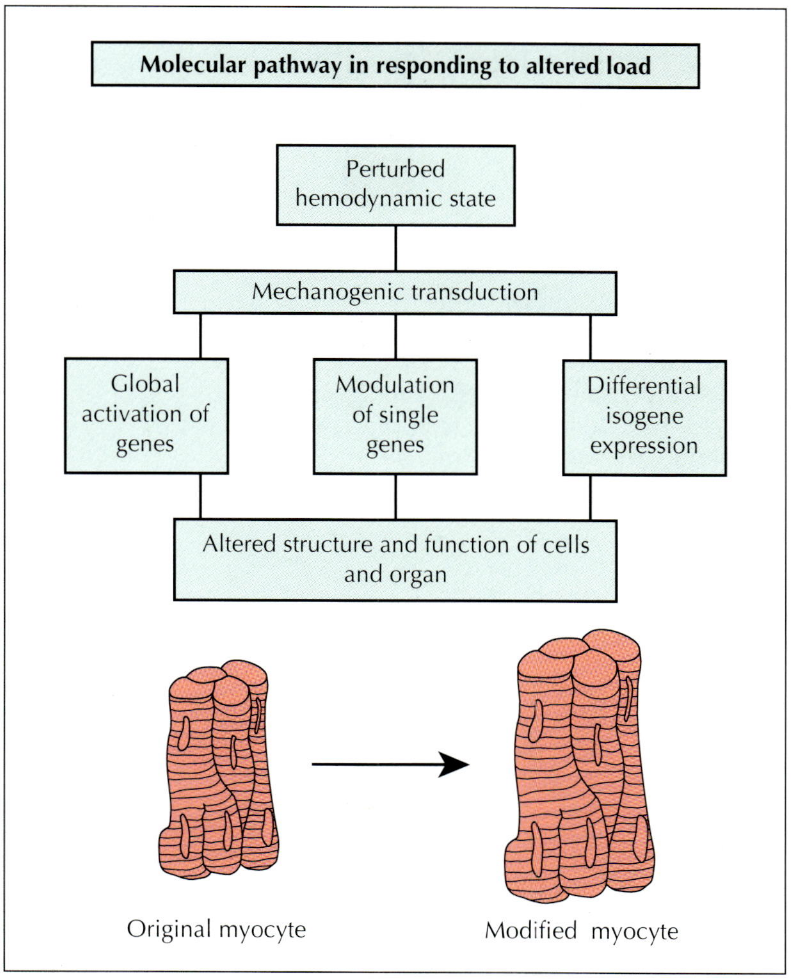

FIGURE 2-7. The molecular pathway in responding to altered load. The initial event in the adaptation to a valvular abnormality is the transduction of hemodynamic load to altered gene expression, mechanogenic transduction [9]. This key event remains poorly understood [10,11]. Subsequently the response of a variety of cell types in the heart may involve a variety of molecular strategies [7]. A global activation of genes results in hypertrophy. The modulation of a single gene results in, for example, increased production of atrial natriuretic factor. Finally, differential isogene expression occurs for proteins such as myosin, actin, and tropomyosin [7]. The end point of these molecular pathways is phenoconversion–the net alterations in cardiac structure and function [9]. The cell populations, which are exposed to the transduced hemodynamic signal, are diverse. The myocyte, the interstitial fibroblast, and the endothelial cell of the coronary vessel are some major cell types. The myocyte, though not the most numerous cell type, accounts for most of the mass of the heart and is discussed in detail next. (*Adapted from* Schwartz and coworkers [7].)

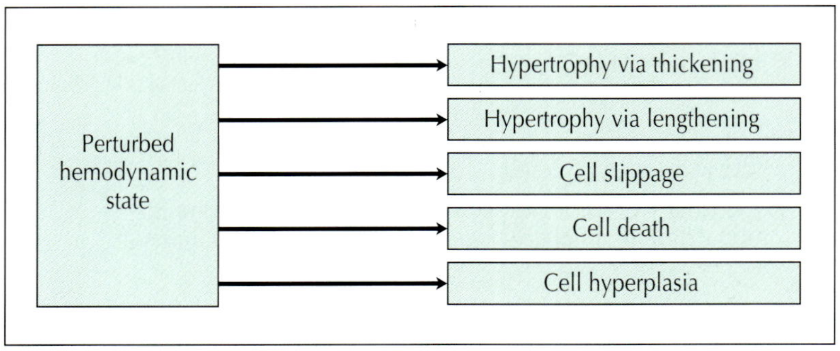

Figure 2-8. Myoctye alterations in hypertrophy. After the transduction of the hemodynamic load has caused gene expression and protein production, the myocyte emerges with a new cellular morphology. Five paradigms for myocyte transformation are listed and have a variable contribution in individual patients.

The cell growth from additional sarcomeres being added in series results in a longer myocyte. Cell growth from sarcomere addition in parallel with existing units results in a thicker myocyte. As a consequence, the wall thickness of the cardiac chamber increases. Animal models and human diseases of pressure and volume overload have consistently shown the increase in cell diameter, length being a more difficult parameter to measure [12,13]. In aortic stenosis and aortic insufficiency the average myocyte diameter increases from a normal value of 14±1 µm to 31±1 µm [14].

The increased chamber diameter and reduced number of cells across the wall observed in volume-overloaded hearts imply that the myocytes can slip in relation to each other. This side-to-side slippage is an important component of the architectural rearrangement of myocytes throughout the wall of the ventricles. Slippage allows chronic chamber enlargement to occur without overstretching of individual cells and sarcomeres [13].

Cell death is probably a common event in the decompensated late state of pressure and volume overload. Cell hyperplasia, that is, true division of the myocyte, is not thought to occur in the adult heart, although this dogma has been recently challenged [13].

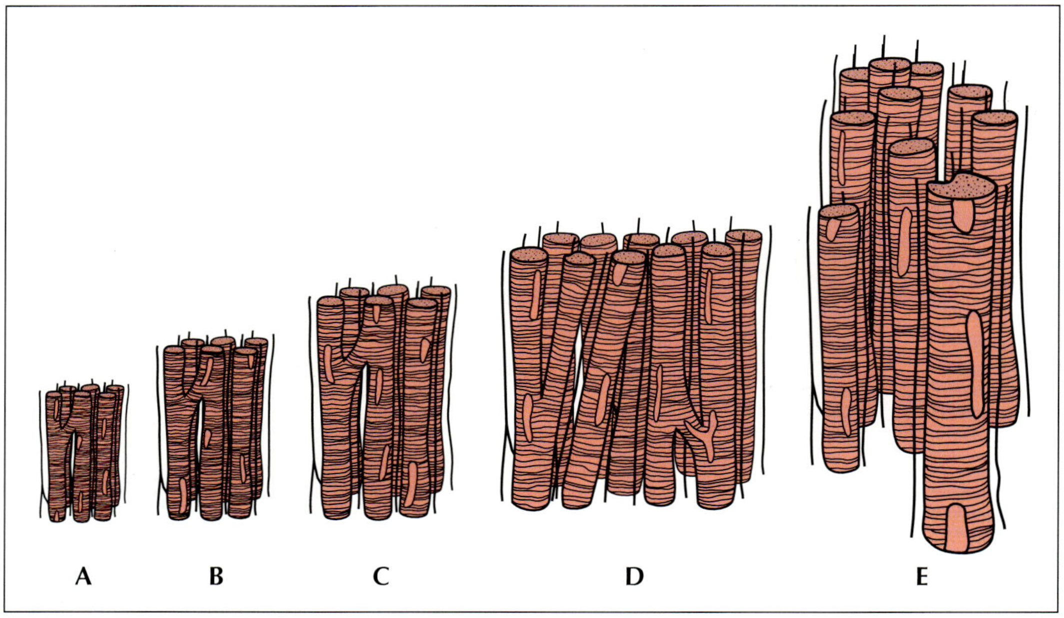

Figure 2-9. Examples of myocyte alterations in hypertrophy. Examples of the morphology produced by the five paradigms for myocyte transformations include an infant's heart (**A**), a 300-g normal adult heart (**B**), a 500-g athlete's heart (**C**), a 650-g pressure-overloaded heart (**D**), and a 900-g dilated decompensated heart (**E**) [15]. Other important modifiers of the cellular hypertrophic process need to be added to appreciate variability in the heart's response to pressure and volume overload. (*Adapted from* Linzbach [15].)

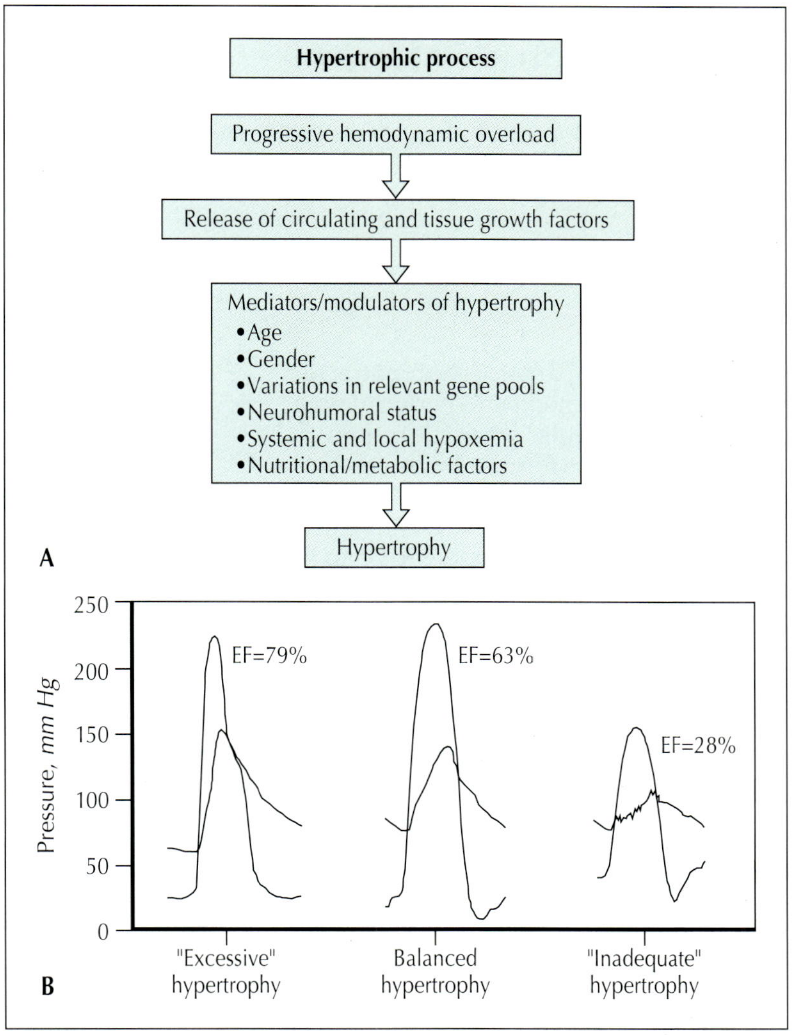

Figure 2-10. Mediators/modulators of hypertrophy. Why do cardiac structure, function, and clinical presentation differ so much in patients with the same valvular abnormality? Mediators/modulators of the hypertrophic process (**A**) are identified demographic, genetic, and biochemical factors that alter the transformation involved in response to a pressure or volume overload [16]. Following the transduction of the abnormal hemodynamic load, multiple growth factors propel a cascade of events leading to hypertrophy. But the qualitative characteristics of the hypertrophied myocyte and cardiac chamber are strongly influenced by these mediators/moderators.

For example, the progressive narrowing of the aortic valve produces a spectrum of chamber function, as represented by the three patterns illustrated in **B** [17]. Variations in left ventricular mass do not explain these different outcomes. Qualitative and not simply quantitative issues are important in hypertrophy. Chamber geometry plays an additional role. The hypertrophic process appears "excessive" in some patients with hyperdynamic chamber shortening, lower than normal wall stresses, and markedly abnormal myocardial relaxation and left ventricular pressure decay (*left side*). On a mechanical level the excessive hypertrophic response with supranormal systolic chamber performance does not mean the myocyte is stronger or that the adaptation is clinically successful. These patients often are very symptomatic [17]. On the other hand, the hypertrophic process may be inadequate to normalize wall stresses, ejection performance fails, and diastolic pressures and volumes increase (*right side*). EF—ejection fraction.

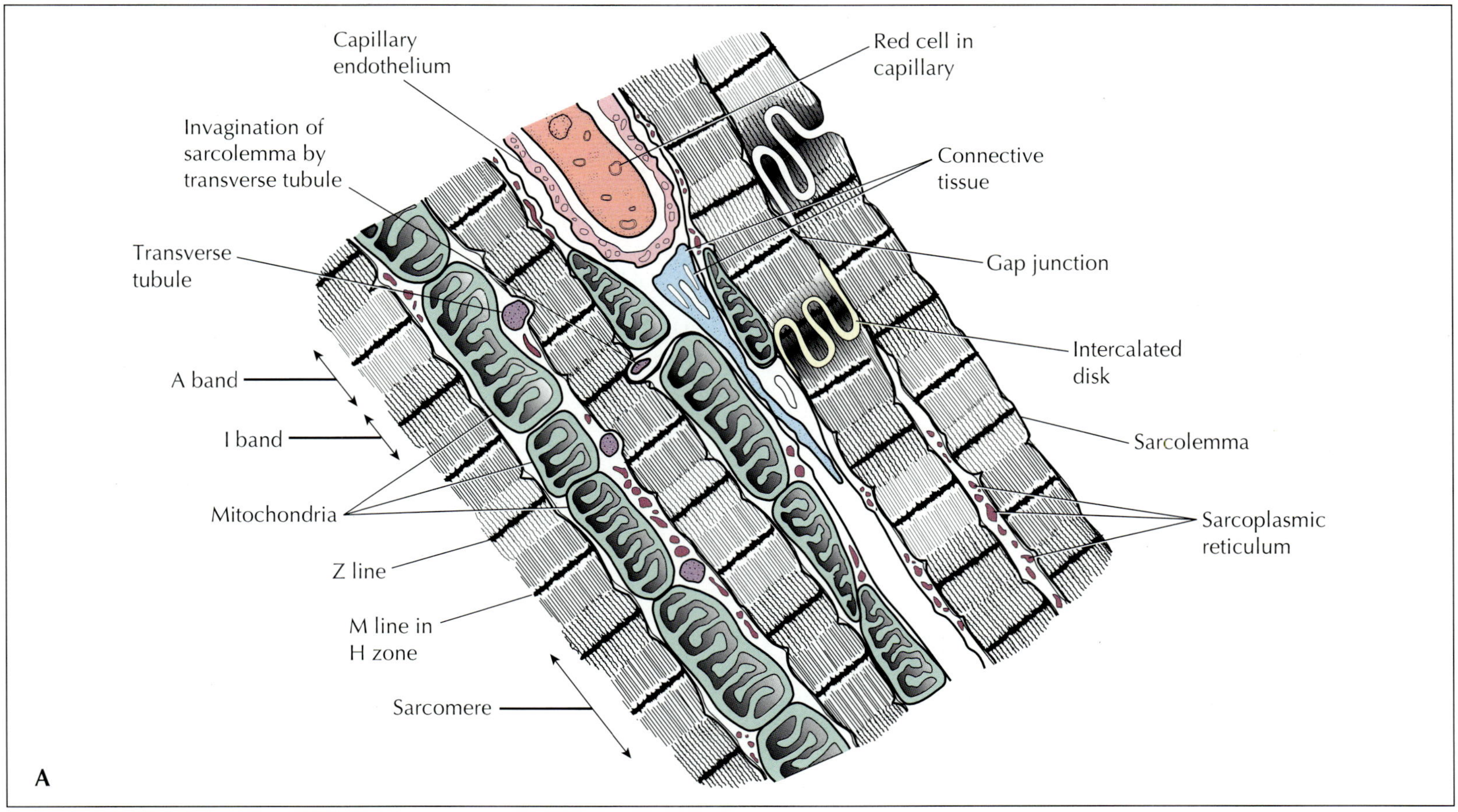

Figure 2-11. Change in cardiac myocyte composition with hypertrophy. The hypertrophied cardiac myocyte is not simply an enlarged version of the normal myocyte (**A**). The composition is altered by a relatively greater increase in the number of myofibrils than mitochondria and by a greater average distance from a capillary [11]. As the cell lengthens and becomes thicker, (*continued*)

B. CHANGES IN CARDIAC MYOCYTE COMPOSITION WITH HYPERTROPHY

STRUCTURE	CONTROL HEART	OVERLOADED HEART	PERCENT CHANGE
Mitochondria, μm^3	2620	3510	+34
Myofibrils, μm^3	3700	6290	+67
Intercapillary distance, μm	15.6	17.9	+15

FIGURE 2-11. (*continued*) an increased number of sarcomeres is apparent. These contractile units provide the individual cell and the whole organ with the potential to perform more work. Yet the relatively smaller increase in mitochondria, the cellular organelle responsible for energy production, and the greater distance to capillaries for nutrient exchange may become problematic as the process progresses [11]. Thus, the hypertrophied myocyte has quantitative differences in these and other important parameters determining function (**B**). Furthermore, changes in the protein building blocks of the sarcomere have an impact on function [18]. (Part A *adapted from* Berne and Levy [18]; part B *adapted from* Bugaisky and coworkers [11].)

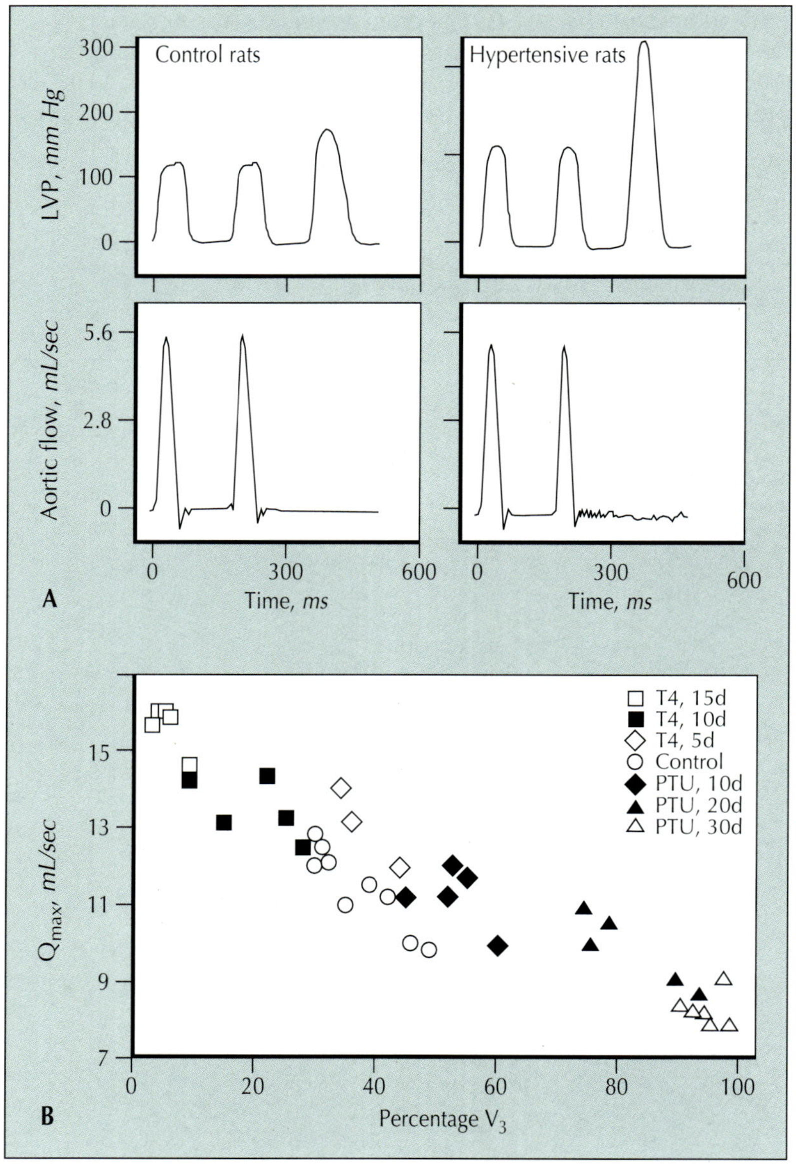

FIGURE 2-12. Structure and function alterations of the sarcomere in hypertrophy. Myocardial hypertrophy leads to more mass capable of performing more work to effectively deal with the increased hemodynamic load. The response of the myocyte also involves alterations in the dynamic properties of the contractile unit and alterations in biochemical processes (*ie*, availability of Ca^{++}) [11,19].

A, Experimental records from control rats and hypertensive rats with a chronically pressure overloaded ventricle [20]. The pressure and flow signals represent the two forms of work the ventricle performs. The third beat of each panel shows the response to sudden clamping of the aorta to prevent ejection. Analysis of these data revealed that the left ventricle (LV) of the hypertensive rats was a stronger pressure generator but weaker flow generator. Thus the effects on contractility are not unidimensional. Descriptors of the physiologic versus pathologic may be a gross oversimplification. The LV is neither stronger nor weaker; it has simply adapted in a unique fashion.

B, Q_{max} is an index inversely related to LV systolic resistance and percentage V_3 is the isomyosin composition that has been experimentally altered in groups of rats, each group noted by different symbols [21]. Note how the modification of one protein that is a building block of the sarcomere affects the mechanical performance of the entire unit.

Therefore, the myocyte's response to altered hemodynamic loads is modulated for the type of load and by changes in composition and function of the contractile unit, not just by the addition of more units. Alterations in other components of the contractile unit and related intracelluar biochemical processes have been shown to influence mechanical performance, perhaps even responsible for decompensation [22–26]. (Part A *adapted from* Shroff and Motz [20]; part B *adapted from* Shroff and coworkers [21].)

Cardiac Interstitium

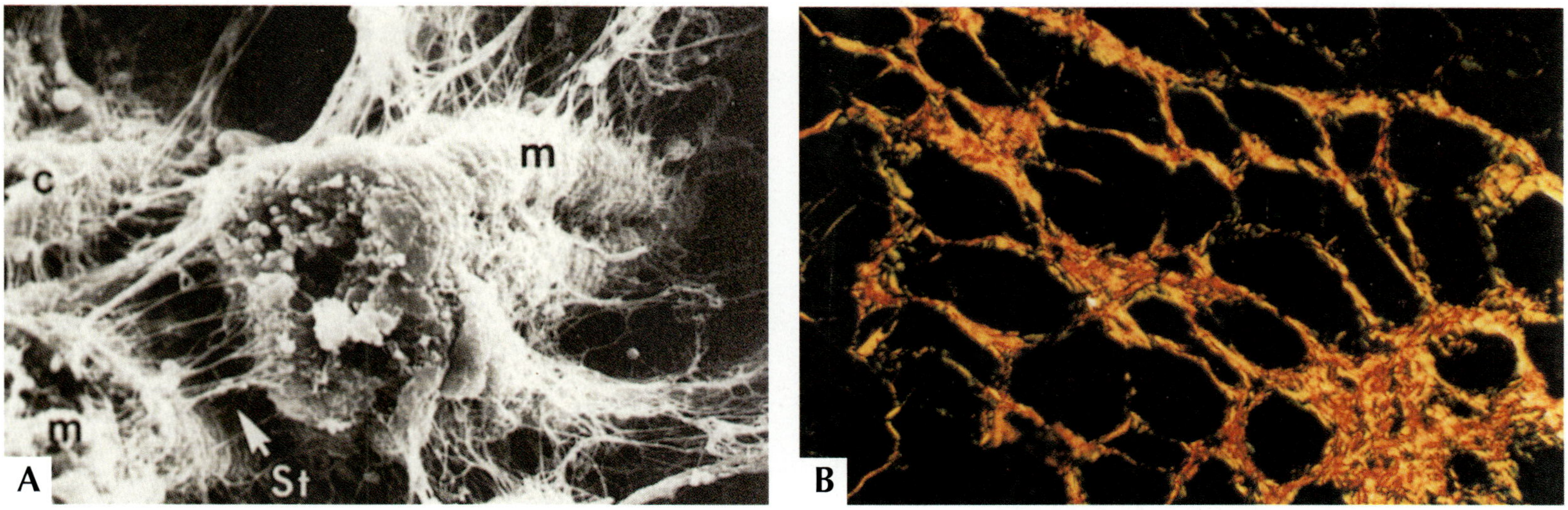

Figure 2-13. Interstitial matrix (m) reconfiguration versus pathologic fibrosis. Invisible to conventional histologic staining and microscopy, the normal interstitial matrix of the heart was studied in detail only recently [23,27]. The struts (*arrow* near St), weaves, and coils are composed of collagen types I and III. **A**, Scanning electron microscopy shows an intricate, highly organized matrix that surrounds individual cells (c), connects them to each other, and provides a framework for other interstitial occupants such as the coronary vasculature [28,29].

Dense, extensive interstitial fibrosis has always been recognized as pathologic. **B**, The fibrotic scarring seen by picrosirius red staining and polarization microscopy is a reaction to injury that is permanent and is proportional to the extent of injury. Reparative or replacement fibrosis represents a scar such as after myocyte loss in myocardial infarction [30]. Neurohumoral activation promotes a reactive fibrosis that may occur after inflammation from diverse etiologies [31]. (Part A *adapted from* Weber and coworkers [32]; part B *adapted from* Carroll and coworkers [30]; with permission.)

EFFECTS OF NORMAL AND ABNORMAL INTERSTITIAL MATRIX

EFFECTS OF NORMAL COLLAGEN MATRIX	DETRIMENTAL EFFECTS OF INTERSTITIAL FIBROSIS
Prevention of sarcomere overdistention	Impaired utilization of Starling mechanism
Storage of energy and release as elastic recoil	Reduction in elastic recoil
Structural intergrity without reduction in organ compliance	Diastolic dysfunction
Mediation of cell-to-cell slippage for chamber remodeling	Fixation of cell-to-cell relations
Scaffolding for coronary vasculature	Encroachment on vasculature and nutrient barrier
Enhancement of mechanical/electrical syncytium	Mechanical tethering and electrical inhomogeneity/instability

Figure 2-14. Function of the normal and abnormal cardiac interstitium. Mechanical effects are the major influences of the normal and abnormal interstitial matrix. In this table the mechanical effects are apparent on the cellular and organ level and influence the entire cardiac cycle including systole and diastole [27].

Collagen is the major protein composing the matrix and has the tensile strength of steel [30]. Yet the normal configuration of collagen in the interstitial matrix preserves the compliant nature of the cardiovascular system [27,28].

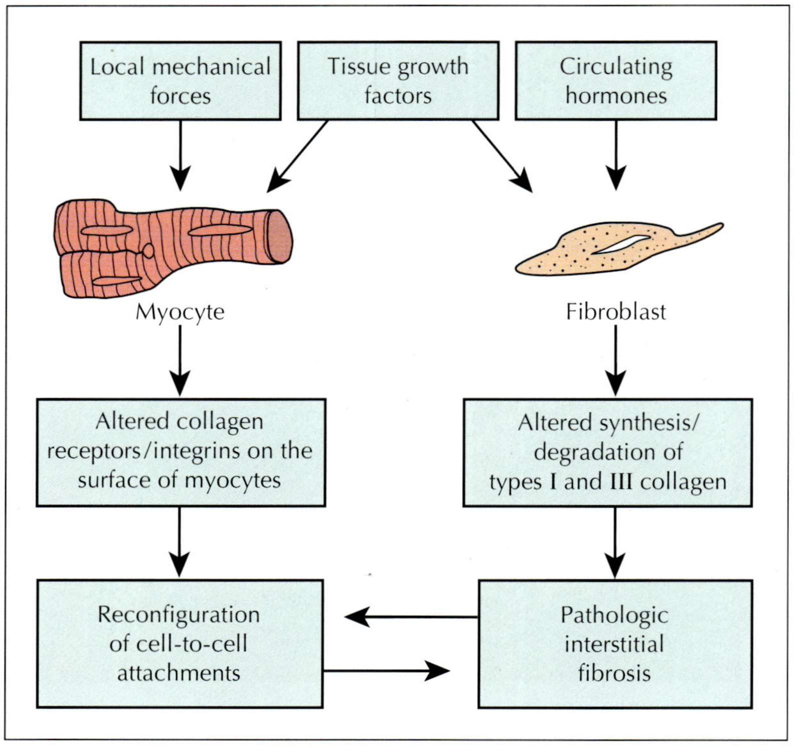

FIGURE 2-15. Modulation of the reconfiguration of the interstitial matrix. Pressure and volume overload of the ventricles sets off a cascade of events that not only produces myocardial hypertrophy but alters the interstitium. Cell-to-cell attachments are disconnected and reconnected allowing for cell slippage. New sets of cell membrane sites of collagen attachment are produced and are composed of integrins [33]. These are modified with the development of hypertrophy [33]. The interstitial matrix is reconfigured as the fibroblasts degrade and renew the intricate collagen network. In advanced hemodynamic overload the extracellular space expands with broad, less organized bands of collagen [28].

This flow sheet emphasizes that both the myocyte and fibroblast participate in this process. Local and circulating humoral factors and mechanical stresses appear to command these cellular elements [28,34,35].

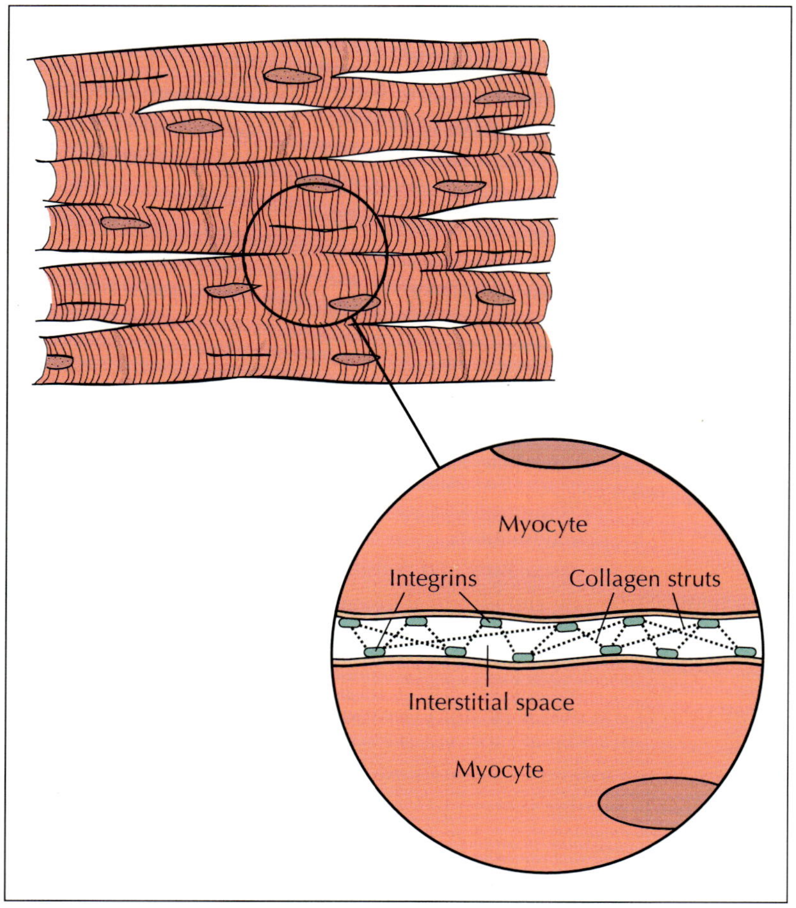

FIGURE 2-16. Cell-to-cell connections. The movement of myocytes relative to each other is fixed, as illustrated here by the collagen struts binding to cell surface receptors called integrins [27,33]. The response of the ventricle to volume overload involves considerable chamber dilatation without an increase in the number of myocytes from the endocardial to the epicardial layer [12]. Successful adaptation to volume overload must involve the release and attachment of these cell-to-cell connections (*inset*).

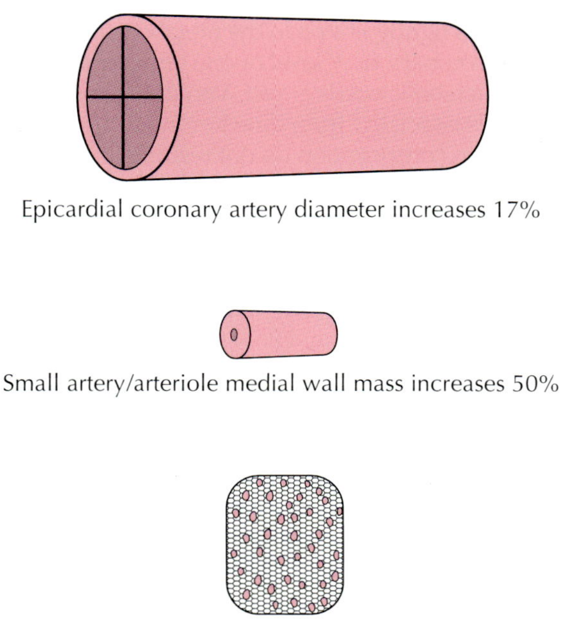

FIGURE 2-17. Anatomic alterations in the coronary circulation. Alterations in the coronary circulation also occur when the muscle hypertrophies and the interstitium is reconfigured. In this figure three sites of anatomic changes are described.

The epicardial coronary arteries are larger in diameter in the setting of hypertrophy of many causes [36–38]. This adaptation probably does not influence the mean coronary flow because these large vessels have more of a capacitance and distributive function than resistance effect.

Small artery and arteriolar medial wall areas are increased and may play an important role in modifying the maximum coronary flow [39–41]. Medial hypertrophy is especially marked when the coronary circulation is exposed to hypertension.

Finally, microcirculatory alteration, particularly an increased intercapillary distance, occurs in hypertrophy, including adult aortic stenosis [11,41]. The impact on the exchange processes between the vasculature and the myocardium may be sufficient to limit myocardial oxygen supply. Angiogenesis in infants and children appears to be adequate to prevent any mismatching of the size of the microcirculation when myocardial mass is increasing due to aortic stenosis [40, 42].

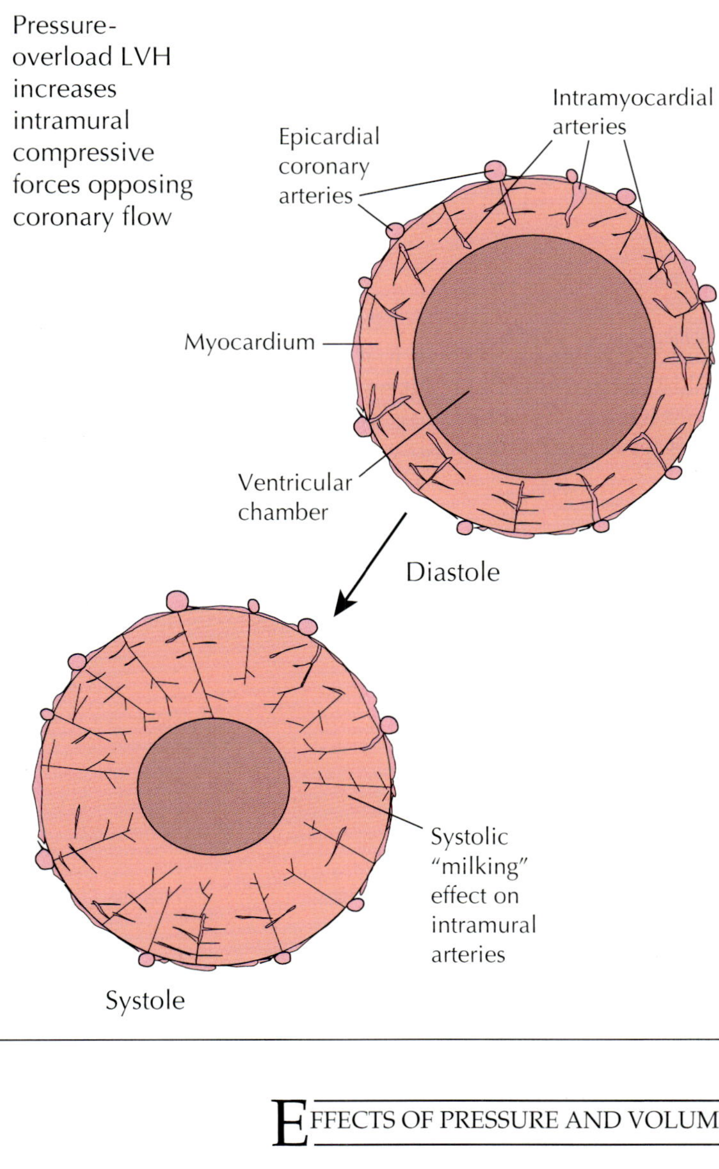

FIGURE 2-18. Intramyocardial forces modify coronary flow. The coronary circulation in the pressure- and volume-overloaded heart must not only supply a greater mass of myocardium but also must operate in an environment where compressive and other forces may modify coronary flow patterns. During systole a rising intramyocardial pressure and other torsional forces normally reduce and often stop antegrade flow in intramural coronary arteries [43]. This effect may be exaggerated when there is myocardial hypertrophy and when intramural pressures are elevated as in aortic stenosis. Often the septal perforating arteries in hypertrophic cardiomyopathy disappear during systole (*ie*, a milking effect).

Additionally, during diastole the elevated intracavitary pressure exerts a force that retards coronary flow particularly into the endocardial layer of the wall [43].

Phasic flow patterns in the large coronary arteries on the surface of the heart are also influenced by the direct effects of a valvular abnormality, as well as these intramyocardial forces. In aortic regurgitation the torrential flow of blood back into the ventricle through the incompetent valve may reduce forward flow in the coronary artery during diastole [44]. LVH—left ventricular hypertrophy.

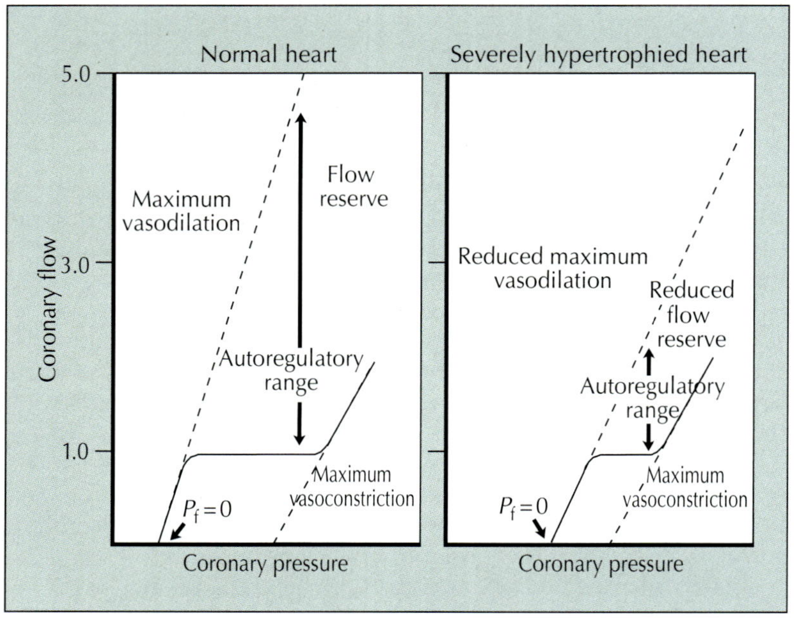

FIGURE 2-19. Coronary pressure-flow relationship in left ventricular hypertrophy (LVH). The coronary pressure-flow relationship is useful in understanding coronary physiology and the impact of modifications of anatomy that occur with hypertrophy [45].

The perfusion pressure at which coronary flow stops is denoted as $P_f = 0$. This pressure is normally greater than right atrial pressure and is increased in the severely hypertrophied heart.

Coronary flow is tightly linked to the metabolic needs of the myocardium. A coronary flow level of one represents the amount of flow to handle metabolic needs at rest. Variations in perfusion pressure that are totally disassociated from direct or indirect alterations in myocardial oxygen consumption do not result in altered coronary flow due to autoregulatory adjustments in coronary vascular resistance. The range of autoregulatory control is reduced in the severely hypertrophied heart, in part due to the reduced maximum vasodilation capacity [40].

There is a substantial increase in flow with increased physiologic needs or after pharmacologic induction of coronary vasodilation. A five-fold increase in flow is the normal flow reserve available to meet metabolic needs. Coronary flow reserve is markedly reduced in the severely hypertrophied heart [40]. (*Adapted from* Klocke [43].)

CORONARY CIRCULATION ADAPTATIONS TO PRESSURE AND VOLUME OVERLOADED STATES

ANATOMICAL	EARLY COMPENSATED	LATE DECOMPENSATED
Epicardial coronary artery cross-sectional area	Slightly increased	Moderately increased
Intramyocardial artery medial wall thickness mass	Slightly increased	Moderately increased
Perivascular collagen	Minimally increased	Markedly increased
Intercapillary distances	Minimally increased	Moderately increased
Myocardial cell size	Moderately increased	Markedly increased
PHYSIOLOGIC		
Resting coronary vascular resistance	Normal	Moderately increased
Minimum coronary vascular resistance	Normal	Increased
Coronary vasodilator reserve	Normal	Decreased
Myocardial-capillary diffusion capacity	Normal	Decreased

FIGURE 2-20. Summary of anatomic and physiologic alterations in the coronary circulation. This table summarizes the important modifications in coronary anatomy and physiology that occur in early compensated and late decompensated states of pressure and volume overload. The pressure overloads of aortic stenosis and systemic hypertension appear to exert the greatest effects on the coronary circulation [40,41]. Abnormalities of coronary function may not have an important role in the pathophysiology of the diseases associated with volume overload.

Myocardial Ischemia

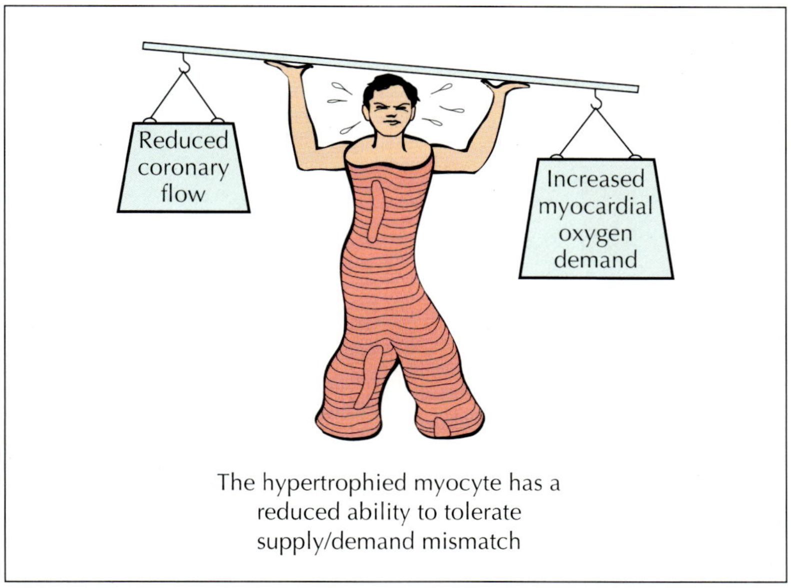

Figure 2-21. Ischemia in the setting of hypertrophy. Myocardial ischemia results when there is a mismatch between myocardial oxygen supply and demand. The manifestations of ischemia include mechanical dysfunction and electrical instability. The hypertrophied myocyte appears more susceptible to the metabolic stress of ischemia, showing more severe and prolonged manifestations. And, as previously discussed, the hypertrophied heart has important modifications in coronary flow that limit oxygen delivery. This susceptible myocardium also has greatly augmented metabolic needs due to its increased mass. Therefore, the important role of myocardial ischemia in these disorders of loading conditions and valve function needs to be further clarified.

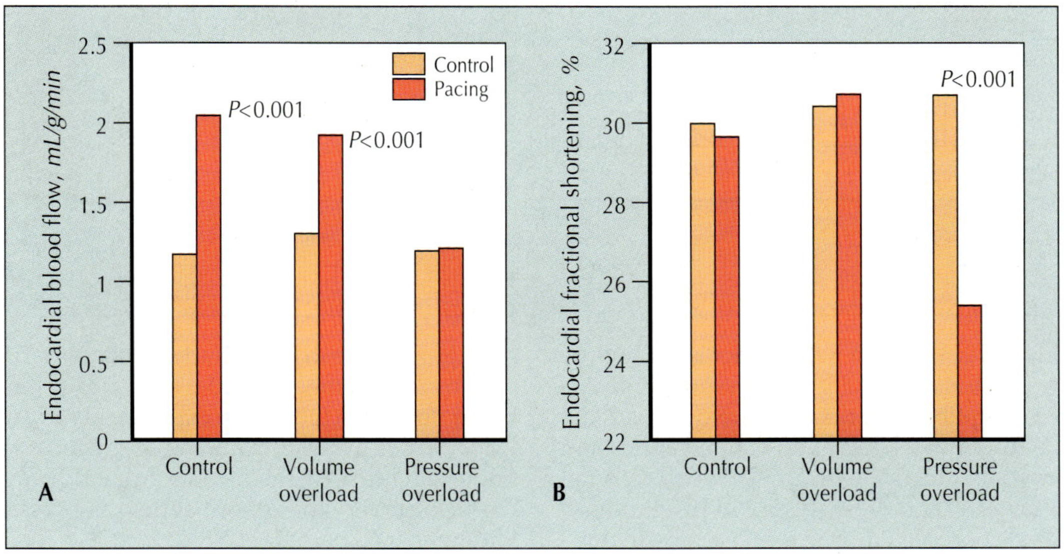

Figure 2-22. Pacing-induced coronary flow abnormalities. Atrial pacing is a useful means to test the ability of the overloaded heart to tolerate tachycardia. Pacing reduces the time in diastole for coronary flow and generally increases myocardial oxygen consumption. In this series of dog experiments control animals were compared to those with a pressure overload from aortic banding and volume overload from mitral regurgitation [46,47]. Pacing increased coronary endocardial blood flow above baseline values for the control and volume-overload animals but not the pressure-overload group (**A**). As a consequence endocardial shortening fraction fell (**B**). Therefore the modest stress of pacing produced systolic dysfunction due to the development of ischemia in animals with pressure but not volume overload. (*Adapted from* Nakano and coworkers [46] and Carabello and coworkers [47].)

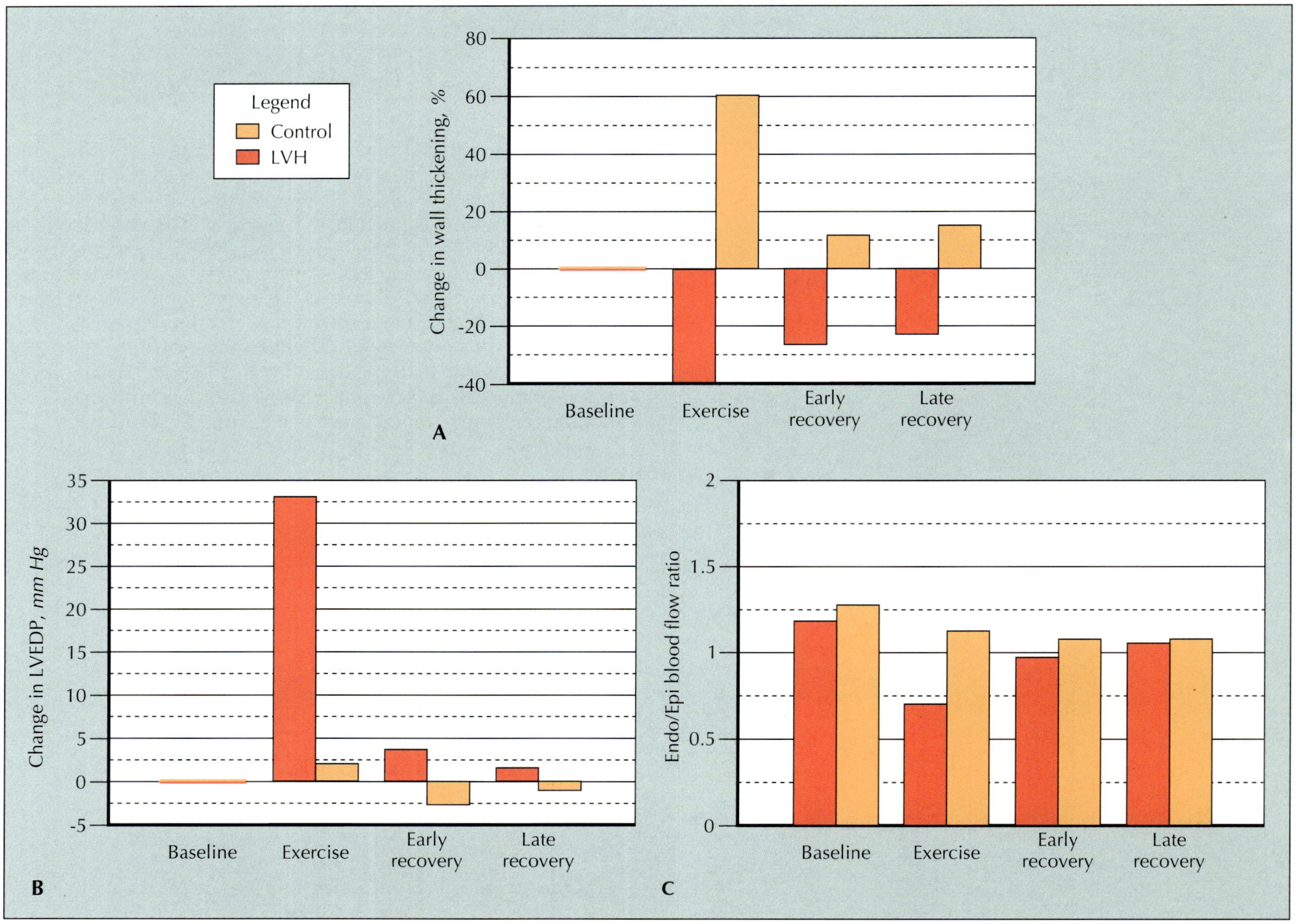

Figure 2-23. Exercise-induced ischemia in left ventricular hypertrophy (LVH). Dynamic exercise is a clinically *and* physiologically relevant means to test the susceptibility of the pressure-overloaded heart to ischemia. In these experiments dogs with banded aortas and resultant LVH were exercised and then allowed to recover [48]. A fall in endocardial wall thickening (**A**) and dramatic rise in LV end-diastolic pressure (LVEDP) (**B**) are observed during exercise only in the LVH group. The diastolic and systolic abnormalities were accompanied by a sustantial fall in the endocardial (endo) to epicardial (epi) blood flow ratio (**C**). These experiments reveal that the pressure-overloaded heart that is functioning normally at rest has a physiologically important impairment of endocardial flow reserve during exercise. During recovery the abnormalities may persist. (*Adapted from* Hittinger and coworkers [48].)

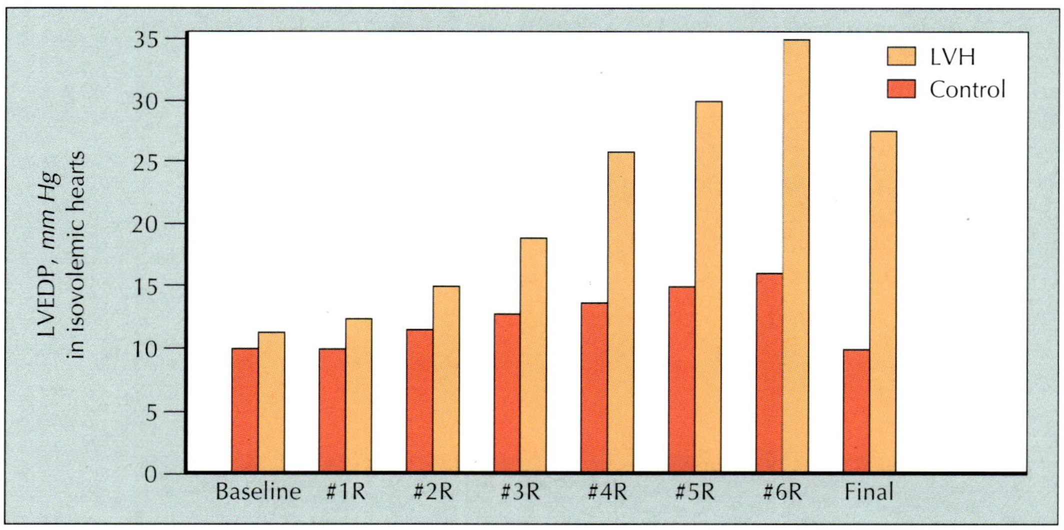

Figure 2-24. Postischemia myocardial stunning in left ventricular hypertrophy (LVH). The net effect of altered myocardial oxygen supply and demand in the hemodynamically overloaded heart makes it susceptible to the induction of ischemia [49]. In addition, alterations in cellular function may exaggerate and prolong the impact of ischemia. Repetitive bouts of ischemia were produced in rats with and without hypertrophy. Isovolumic left ventricular end-diastolic pressure (LVEDP) was measured during the reperfusion periods between the six bouts of ischemia (1R through 6R) and 25 minutes after the final reperfusion [50]. Notice that not only does ischemia produce a greater augmentation of LVEDP after each bout of ischemia but that recovery has not occurred after a prolonged period of reperfusion. This postischemic diastolic stunning of the myocardium may be related to limitations of the hypertrophied cell to maintain an ionic and metabolic environment for normal mechanical function of the sarcomere [50]. (*Adapted from* Mochizuki and coworkers [50].)

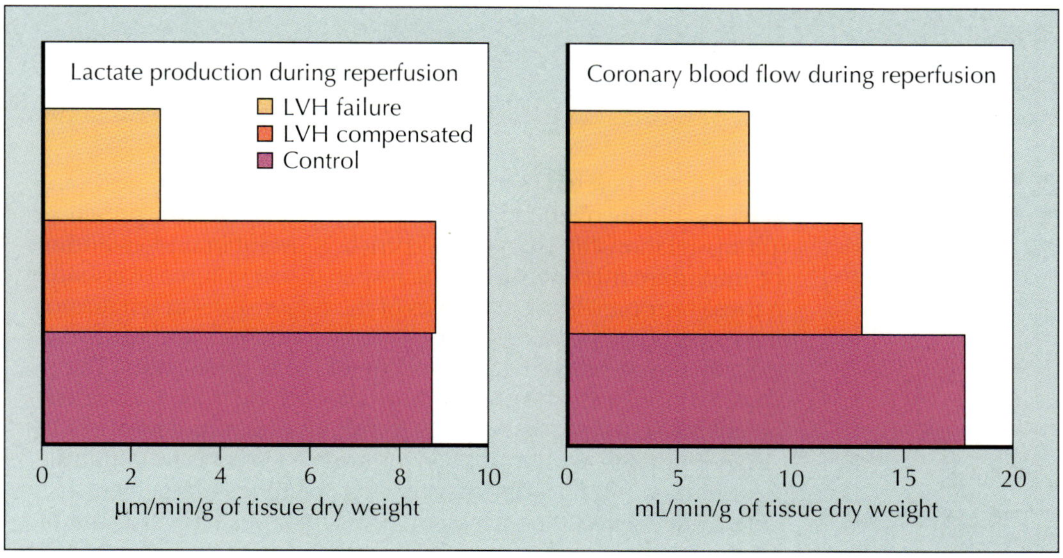

FIGURE 2-25. Reduced anaerobic glycolysis and intolerance to ischemia. Published reports have indicated a spectrum of opinion whether the hypertrophied heart has an impaired tolerance to ischemia [51]. This is an important issue because ischemia may complicate the natural history of pressure and volume overload. Ischemia has been demonstrated during exercise and atrial pacing in pressure-overload hypertrophy and is a common clinical manifestation of severe aortic stenosis even in the absence of atherosclerotic coronary artery disease.

In this series of experiments dogs with and without left ventricular hypertrophy (LVH) from aortic banding were studied to test the hypothesis that impaired tolerance to ischemia occurs in LVH with heart failure but not compensated LVH and that reduced capacity to recruit anaerobic glycolysis may explain this difference [51]. Global ischemia was produced followed by a period of reperfusion. Only dogs with LVH and decreased systolic shortening exhibited a significant impairment in lactate production (**A**). This study confirmed the blunted coronary reactive hyperemia seen in LVH (**B**). (*Adapted from* Gaasch and coworkers [51].)

NEUROHUMORAL ACTIVATION

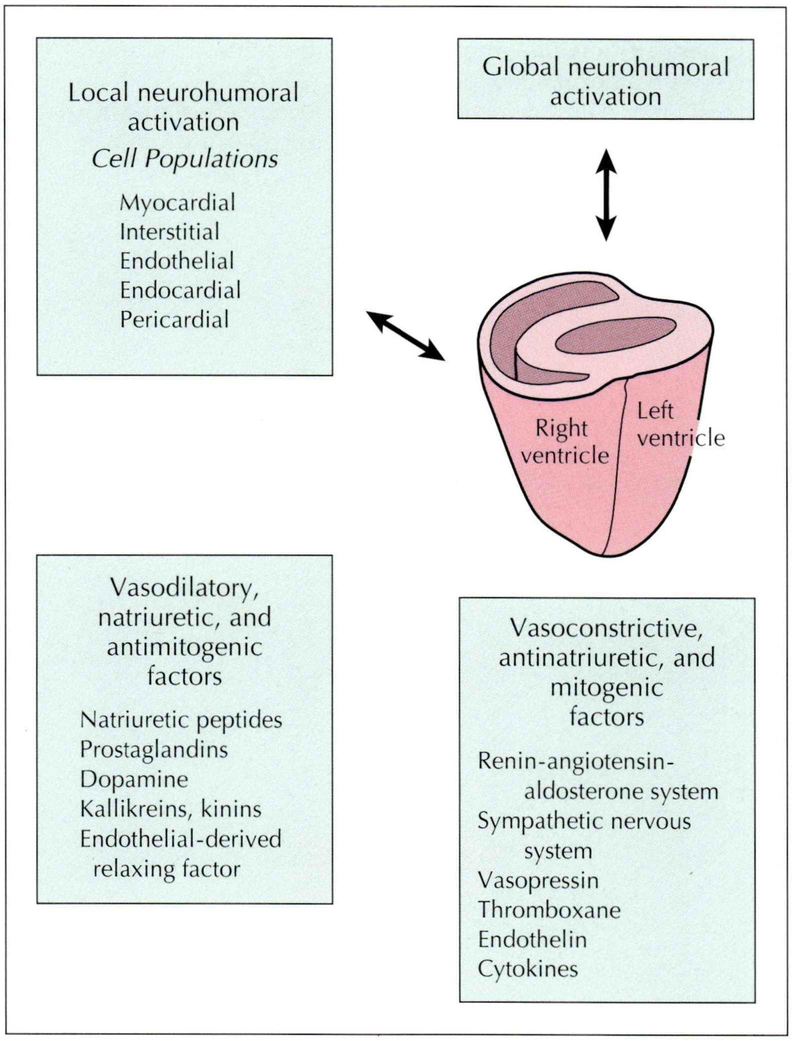

FIGURE 2-26. Sites and types of neurohumoral activation. Circulating hormones and locally synthesized and acting agents are known to exert a hemodynamic effect in congestive heart failure syndromes associated with end-stage pump failure [52]. Prognosis is adversely influenced by overt sympathetic activation [53]. At the terminal phase of pressure or volume overload, circulatory function and neurohumoral activation appear identical to those of patients with primary myocardial disease (*ie*, dilated cardiomyopathy).

In the early stage of pressure and volume overload it is not clear how important humoral mechanisms are in producing a compensated state. It is reasonable to postulate that selective activation of the neurohumoral axis may occur with certain valvular lesions. For example, the increased atrial pressures from tricuspid and mitral valve disease may preferentially activate atrial natriuretic peptides. Further work is necessary to define the role of circulating paracrine and autocrine mechanisms in valvular heart disease. The role of the endocardium as a local neurohumoral activation site is being investigated [54]. The possibilities include beneficial as well as detrimental effects on the remodeling of the myocardial, interstitial, and vascular systems. (*Adapted from* Miller and Burnett [52].)

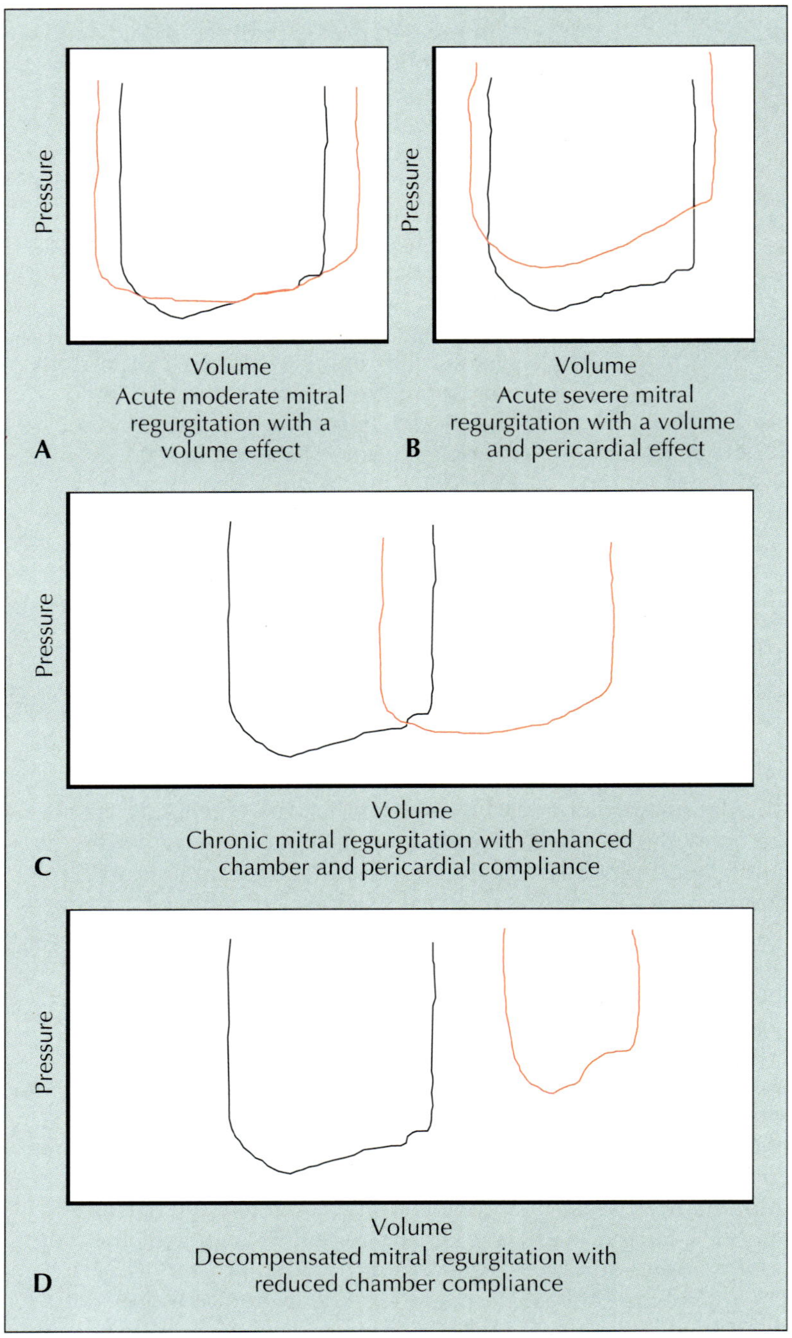

FIGURE 2-27. Left ventricular diastolic pressure-volume relationships in volume overload. The evolution of the diastolic pressure-volume relationship of the left ventricle is useful in understanding the important mechanisms in the response to a volume overload. In these four panels are examples of the major shifts in the diastolic pressure-volume relationship that are encountered, and the text presents the common mechanisms involved in these shifts. The *black line* represents the normal ventricle and the *red line* represents the volume-overloaded ventricle from mitral regurgitation.

A, A moderate acutely applied volume overload is from mitral regurgitation (*red line*). There is modest chamber enlargement at end-diastole with little increase in pressure and a leftward shift of the diastolic pressure-volume relationship due to a smaller end-systolic chamber size achieved from the hyperdynamic chamber performance.

B, A major upward shift represents a higher pressure for a wide range of chamber volumes. This is acute pericardial restraint and a right-left ventricular interaction effect [55,56]. These two mechanisms come into play when the acute mitral or aortic regurgitation is so severe that the total intrapericardial volume increases to the point of stretching the noncompliant pericardial sac (*red line*).

C, This is the classic rightward shift of compensated volume overload lesions—mitral, tricuspid, and aortic regurgitation being the most common (*red line*). With little change in wall thickness the chamber is greatly enlarged with myocardial cell slippage allowing a reduction in chamber stiffness and a growth of the pericardium allowing increased intracavitary volumes to exist with a normal low pericardial pressure.

D, Chamber stiffness increases when decompensation occurs in volume overload [57] (*red line*). Often the myocardium has become myopathic and fibrotic.

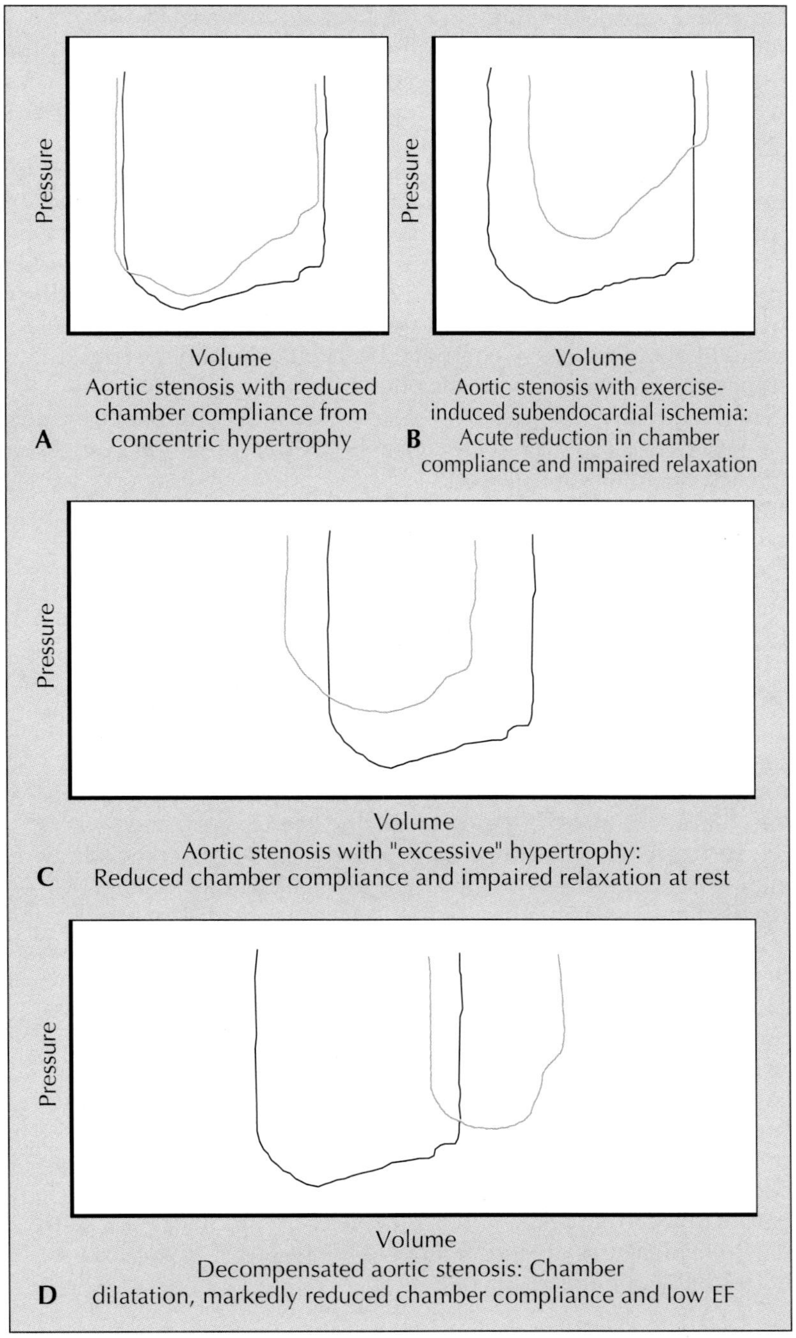

FIGURE 2-28. Left ventricular diastolic pressure-volume relationships in pressure overload. Alterations in diastolic function are common in pressure overload and are easily understood by examining the pressure-volume relationship of the left ventricle, for aortic stenosis and systemic hypertension, and of the right ventricle for pulmonic stenosis and pulmonary hypertension secondary to mitral valve disease and a variety of other etiologies. In these four panels are examples of the major shifts in the pressure-volume relationship. The text defines the common mechanisms involved in these shifts. The *black line* represents the normal ventricle and the *purple line* represents the pressure-overloaded ventricle of aortic stenosis.

A, The classic upward shift is seen for the pressure-overloaded ventricle with concentric hypertrophy (*purple line*). The thicker walled chamber is stiffer than the normal chamber such that for a given increase in volume there is a greater increase in pressure [16]. The left ventricle in compensated aortic stenosis usually has a normal end-diastolic volume with a moderately increased end-diastolic pressure.

B, The dramatic upward shift of exercise-induced ischemia is represented (*purple line*). Here the ischemia is not due to epicardial atherosclerotic coronary artery disease but to 1) the abnormalities of the coronary circulation associated with hypertrophy, 2) the increase in myocardial oxygen consumption in left ventricular hypertrophy (LVH), and 3) the more severe and prolonged manifestations seen in the setting of LVH. The major shift comes from the increased chamber stiffness from ischemia [58].

C, An upward and leftward shift is shown that is common when concentric hypertrophy actually reduces chamber size, wall stresses become lower from the smaller chamber radius with increased wall thickness, and systolic shortening is enhanced (*purple line*). This is commonly observed in elderly women with severe aortic stenosis [17]. The shift in the diastolic pressure-volume relationship is not only due to an increase in chamber stiffness from marked concentric hypertrophy but also involves an early diastolic upward shift from abnormal myocardial relaxation [59,60]. The resultant delay in left ventricular pressure decay causes increased early diastolic pressures for a given volume.

D, This pressure-volume shift is seen when the myocardium becomes myopathic from prolonged pressure overload, as in aortic stenosis with severely depressed ejection fraction (EF) (*purple line*). A marked increase in chamber stiffness is associated with chamber dilatation and increased myocardial stiffness [61].

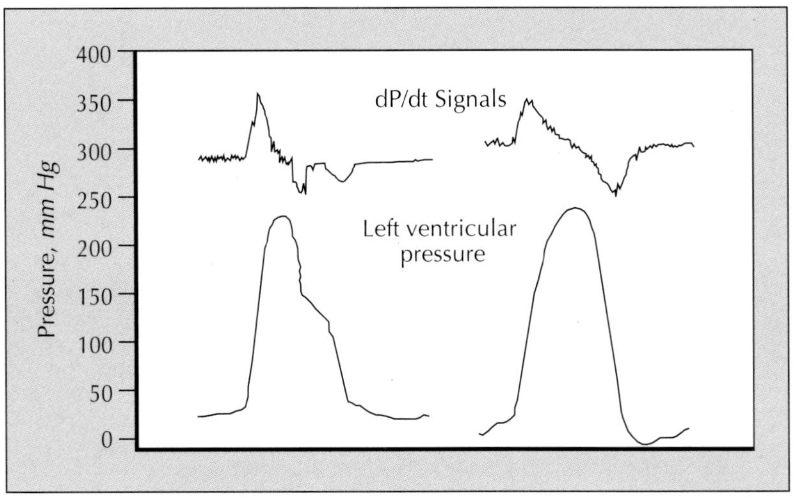

FIGURE 2-29. Abnormal left ventricular pressure decay and myocardial relaxation in the hypertrophied ventricle. Myocardial relaxation is the cellular event that is tightly linked to ventricular pressure decay, most of which occurs in the isovolumic relaxation period. In the hypertrophied myocardium there are a variety of mechanisms by which relaxation can be disrupted. Most of these lead to a reduction in the rate and extent that calcium reuptake occurs after contraction [62].

Shown here are left ventricular pressure tracings from two patients with aortic stenosis. In the *right graph*, pressure is decaying in a normal, monoexponential fashion, as indicated by the change in pressure/time (dP/dt) signal gradually returning to baseline after peak negative dP/dt. In the *left graph*, the pressure decay is markedly abnormal, taking a longer time for pressure to fall to the early diastolic nadir. In addition, the decay is not monoexponential, and the eventual minimum diastolic pressure is increased.

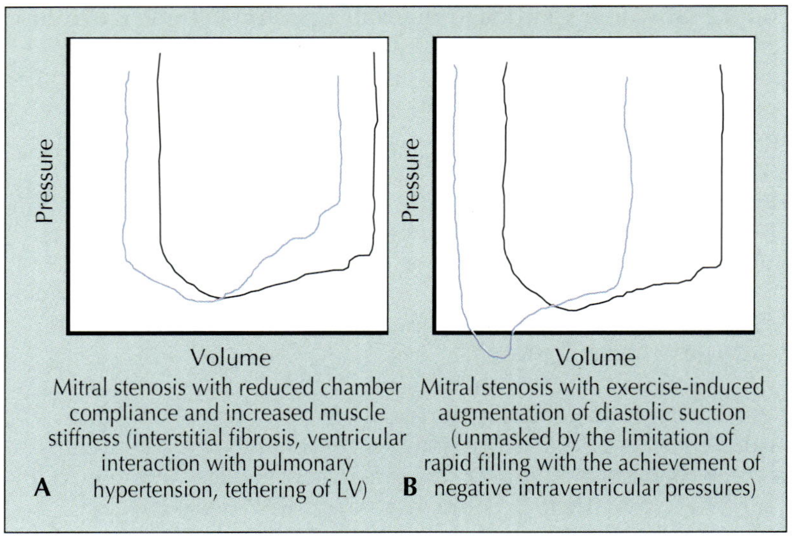

FIGURE 2-30. Left ventricular diastolic pressure-volume relationships in mitral stenosis. Mitral stenosis results in relatively unique shifts in the diastolic pressure-volume relationship. **A**, The leftward shift is seen from the smaller chamber size caused by restricted ventricular filling (*purple line*). But there is also an increase in chamber stiffness commonly seen in mitral stenosis; the potential reasons are multiple [63,64]. The associated pulmonary hypertension can cause right ventricular enlargement and hypertrophy that shifts the interventricular septum and produces a ventricular interaction. Also an increased left ventricular (LV) stiffness can be caused by interstitial fibrosis that occurred with the initial rheumatic insult. The valve and subvalvular abnormalities can effectively tether the LV, reducing its ability to enlarge without significant increase in pressure. Finally, mitral stenosis presenting in the elderly is increasingly recognized. These individuals are more likely to also have coronary artery disease and systemic hypertension—two conditions often increasing LV stiffness. A noncompliant LV coupled to a stenotic mitral valve can produce, as with exercise, markedly increased left atrial pressures compared to each condition in isolation.

B, A unique shift is seen—a downward shift in early diastole with achievement of negative interventricular pressures [64,65] (*purple line*). Mitral stenosis prevents rapid filling such that the LV contracts down to a small end-systolic volume. Elastic recoil propels pressure to negative levels until time has elapsed for filling to expand chamber size. This unique mechanism is clarified in Fig. 2-31.

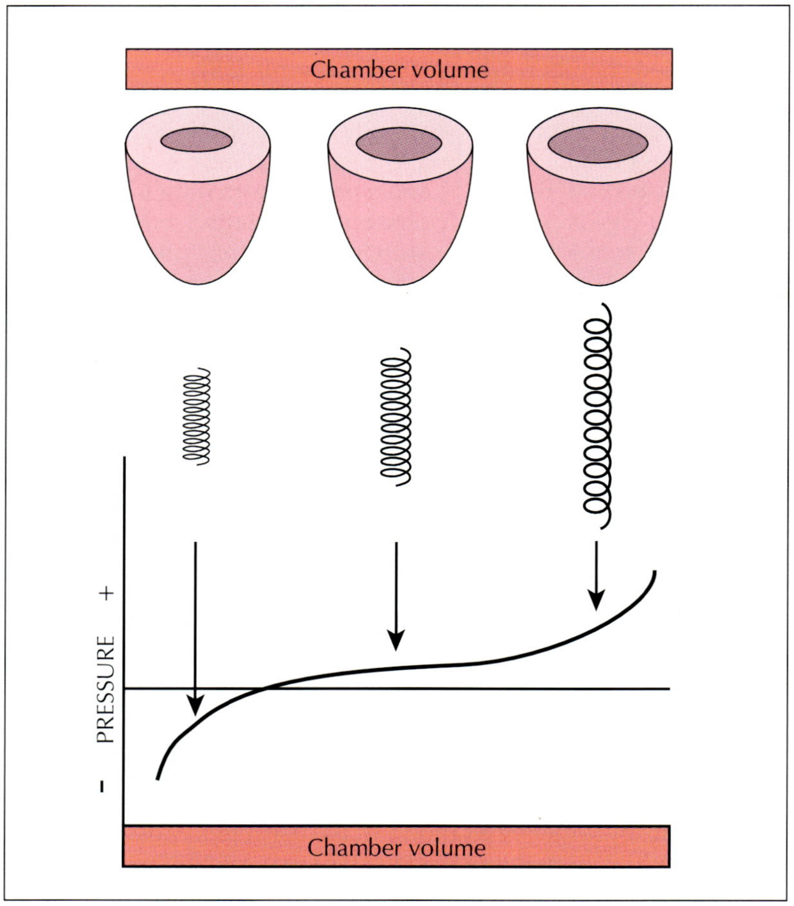

FIGURE 2-31. Diastolic suction in mitral stenosis. With more forceful contraction, especially under conditions when systemic vascular resistance decreases, as during exercise, the end-systolic left ventricle has stored energy in terms of compressed elastic elements in the wall of the left ventricle [66]. These "springs" recoil after contraction has ended. When myocardial relaxation is complete, the intracavitary pressure reaches negative values if ventricular filling does not occur or is slowed, as in mitral stenosis. Thus, mitral stenosis does not produce elastic recoil; it simply unmasks this normally occurring chamber property.

This figure schematically shows what has been demonstrated experimentally [67]. A greater reduction of end-systolic volume produces a lower pressure if no filling occurs. Normally this portion of the diastolic pressure-volume relationship is not seen because of normal, torrential early diastolic filling that occurs even before myocardial relaxation is complete. In mitral stenosis, early diastolic pressures of -5 to -8 mm Hg are recorded in approximately 60% of patients [65,68].

LEFT VENTRICULAR CHAMBER AND MYOCARDIAL STIFFNESS IN PRESSURE AND VOLUME OVERLOAD

TYPE OF OVERLOAD	CHAMBER STIFFNESS ΔP/ΔV	CHAMBER VOLUME/MASS	MYOCARDIAL STIFFNESS CONSTANT K
Acute volume overload: Acute mitral and aortic regurgitation	Increased	Increased	Normal
Chronic volume overload: *Compensated*: Chronic mitral and aortic regurgitation	Decreased	Normal	Normal
Chronic volume overload: *Decompensated*: Chronic mitral and aortic regurgitation	Increased	Increased	Increased
Chronic pressure overload: *Compensated*: Aortic stenosis	Increased	Decreased	Normal
Chronic pressure overload: *Decompensated*: Aortic stenosis	Increased	Decreased	Increased

FIGURE 2-32. Changes in chamber and myocardial passive properties in pressure and volume overload. The type and the stage of pressure and volume overload result in unique effects on chamber stiffness, geometry (volume-mass ratio), and myocardial stiffness [69]. Acute volume loads cause left ventricular dilatation, which increases operative stiffness and the volume-mass ratio. With chronic volume overload, chamber adaptation includes a decrease in chamber stiffness to accommodate the increased volume with no increase in pressure. Decompensated volume and pressure overload are frequently associated with increased myocardial stiffness as well as chamber stiffness. This occurs with eccentric hypertrophy in volume overload (increased volume-mass ratio) and concentric hypertrophy in pressure overload (decreased volume-mass ratio). (*Adapted from* Gaasch [67].)

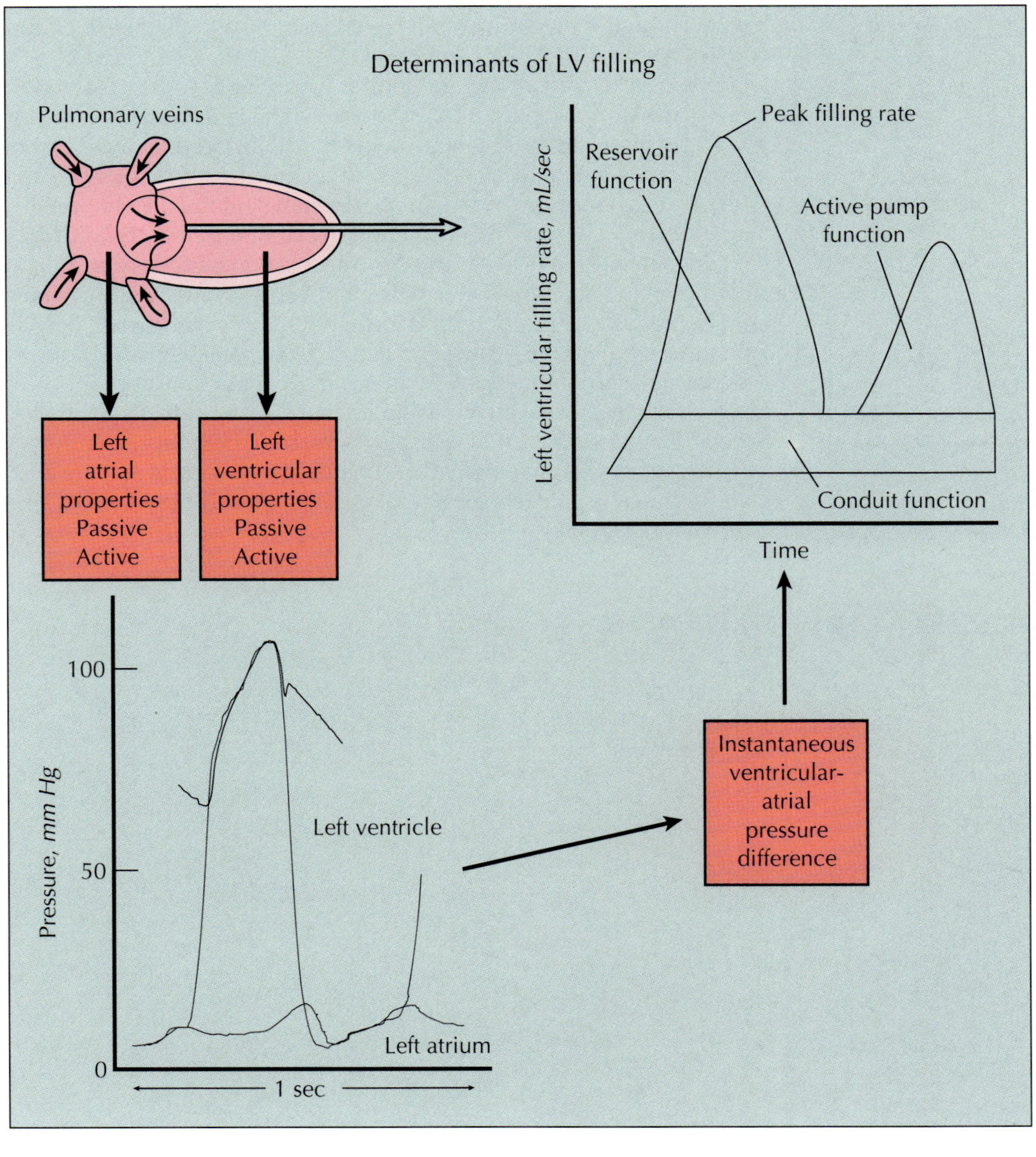

FIGURE 2-33. Determinants of ventricular filling patterns. The passive and active properties of the atria and ventricles interact to produce the transient transvalvular pressure differences causing blood to accelerate and decelerate [70,71]. These blood flow patterns are quantified in velocity terms by Doppler echocardiography or in volume terms of measuring the rate of ventricular chamber enlargement.

The filling pattern for the left ventricle shows the early diastolic rapid filling, followed by diastasis, and completed by atrial contraction giving its booster effect to left ventricular preload. The filling curve can also be viewed as representing the different functions of the left atrium [72]. It acts first as a simple conduit in allowing the passage of blood from the pulmonary veins to the left ventricle in diastole. During systole it stores blood (reservoir function), which is subsequently pushed and sucked into the left ventricle in early diastole. Finally it actively pumps blood due to atrial systole.

Left atrial and left ventricular properties are altered in pressure and volume overload; this alters the filling pattern. The valvular lesions themselves alter filling patterns. For example, aortic regurgitation gives a second pathway for left ventricular filling in diastole. Normal filling patterns are altered in a complex fashion by pressure and volume overload. Elegant experimental design and methods for data acquisition are required to dissect free the underlying determinants of a given filling pattern. Altered filling dynamics in mitral stenosis have been studied in detail in such a fashion [72].

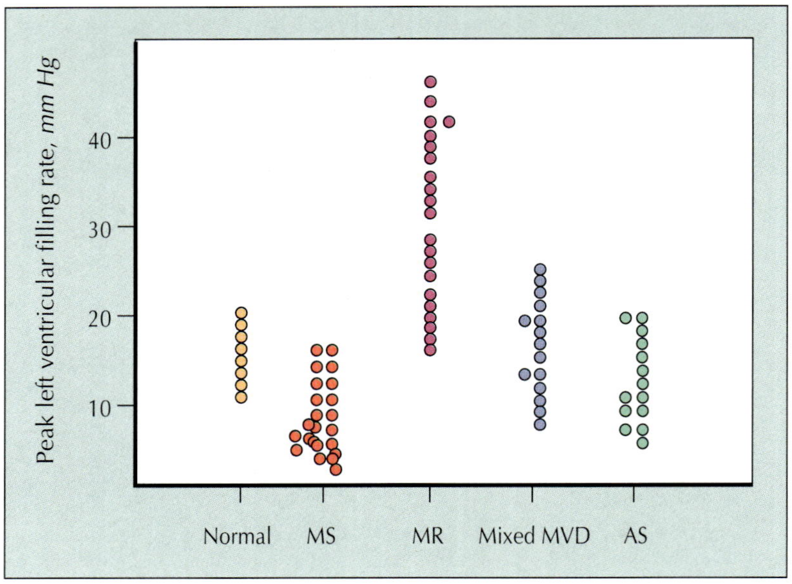

Figure 2-34. Peak left ventricular filling rates in pressure and volume overload. The rate of early diastolic filling reflects in part the diastolic properties of the ventricle, but in valvular heart disease, it also illustrates the impact of certain lesions on ventricular filling. Therefore, filling patterns are the end phenomena of multiple, interacting forces [71].

The columns show individual data points from patients with specific valve lesions [73]. In mitral stensois (MS) there is a clear impairment in diastolic filling from the valve lesion. In mitral regurgitation (MR) there is an augmentation of peak filling due to the regurgitant volume returning to the left ventricle during distole combined with the volume that proceeds forward with the next ventricular systole. In mixed mitral valve disease (MVD) the net effect on filling is a broader spectrum often in the normal range. Finally, in aortic stenosis (AS) there is a similar spectrum but with a fair proportion of the patients having a reduction in filling rate. In AS filling rates are not directly affected by the valve lesion. Rather, they reflect the interaction of the passive and active properties of the left ventricle and left atrium [74] (*Adapted from* Hall and Julian [71].)

Systolic Function

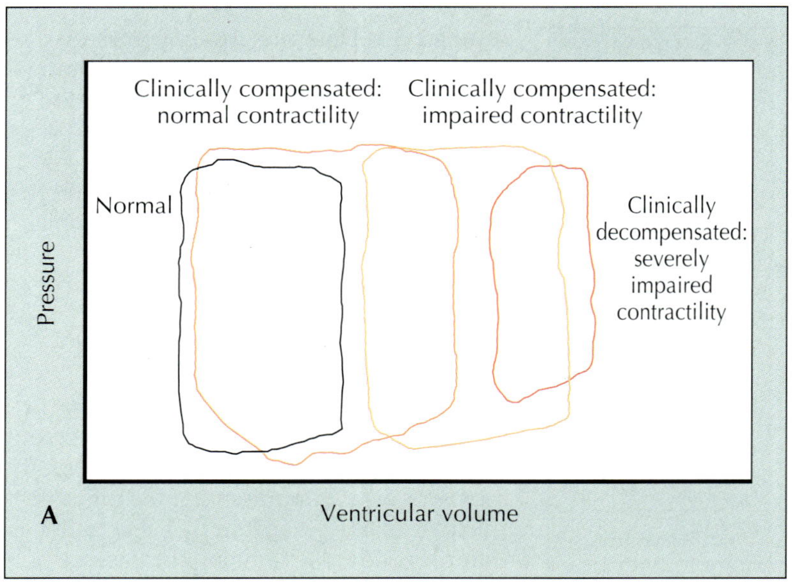

Figure 2-35. Pressure-volume relationships in mitral regurgitation (MR). The entire pressure-volume relationship is shown here, including a normal left ventricle (LV) and three LVs with MR as the cause of volume overload. In all three abnormal situations chamber dilatation pushes the loop to the right (**A**). The ejection fraction is represented by the width of the pressure-volume loop. In MR an ejection fraction in the normal range may indicate impaired myocardial performance [75,76]. These patients may be asymptomatic and have minimally abnormal hemodynamics as shown in **B** as clinically compensated, chronic MR [57]. As patients move to clinical decompensation there may be an accompanying deterioration in both chamber and myocardial performance (*panel B*). This reduced performance may be irreversible despite operative repair of the regurgitant lesion. Most patients with chronic MR are clinically compensated with normal contractility and upper limits of normal to elevated ejection fractions (as represented by the second loop from the left in *panel A*). Many become symptomatic *without* irreversible myocardial and chamber dysfunction and are effectively treated by valve repair or replacement. (Part B *adapted from* Corin and coworkers [55].)

B. PRESSURE-VOLUME RELATIONSHIPS IN MR

	CONTROLS	CLINICALLY COMPENSATED CHRONIC MR	CLINICALLY DECOMPENSATED CHRONIC MR
LV end-diastolic pressure, *mm Hg*	10±3	18±6*	18±9*
LV systolic pressue, *mm Hg*	128±14	116±15	115±18
Cardiac index, *L/min/m²*	4.3±0.7	2.7±0.5**	2.2±0.6**
End-diastolic volume index, *mL/m²*	83±19	191±44**	211±53**
Ejection fraction, %	65±3	65±5	44±8**

*P<0.05.
**P<0.01.

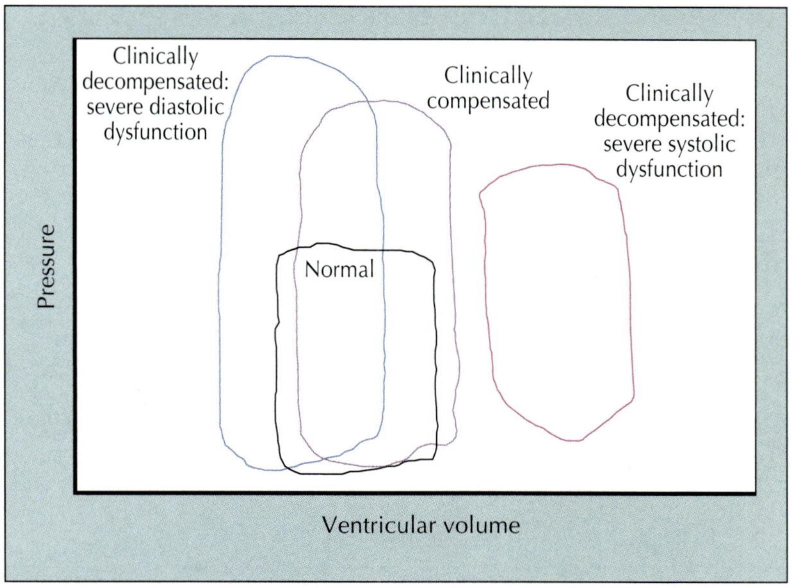

FIGURE 2-36. Pressure-volume relationship in aortic stenosis. In aortic stenosis the pressure-volume loop reveals an increased pressure generation and a fairly normal chamber size and systolic performance in the clinically compensated patient. As the obstruction progresses or an adaptive mechanism falters, the pressure-volume loop can be displaced in different directions. In some patients the chamber is actually smaller with high ejection fraction leaving a very small residual volume at end-systole. This response, common in elderly women, is still maladaptive because diastolic pressures are often markedly increased from altered chamber compliance and impaired myocardial relaxation [17]. On the other hand, some patients develop chamber dilatation with severe systolic dysfunction (rightward shift, *far right loop*), Chamber compliance is not increased and, therefore, diastolic pressures are increased.

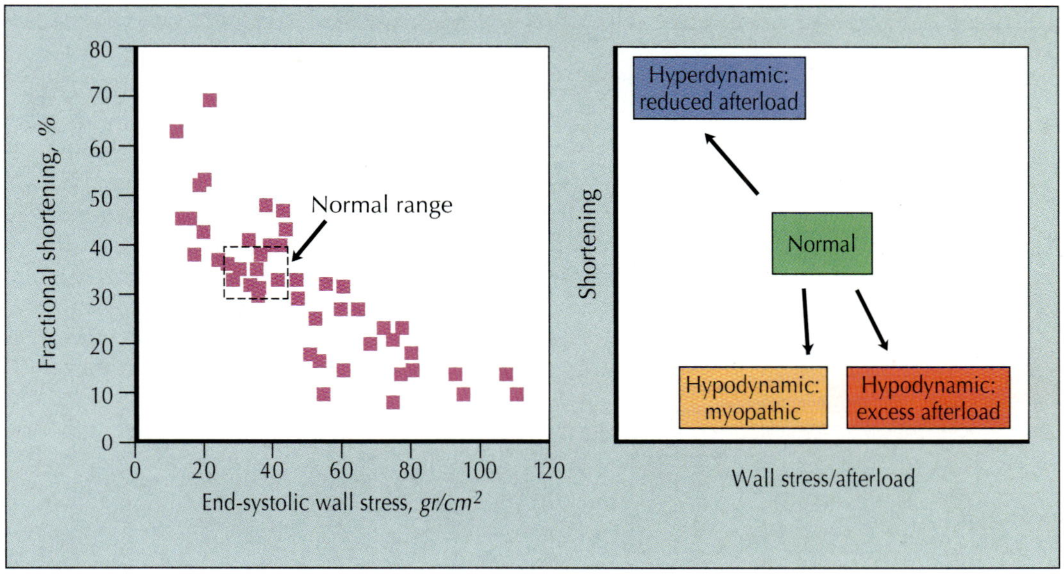

FIGURE 2-37. Stress-shortening relationship in pressure overload. Acute increases of the load against which muscle contracts reduces the speed and extent of muscle shortening. The fractional shortening versus end-systolic relation (or shortening versus afterload relation) expresses this concept and provides a framework to evaluate cardiac performance [77]. This is useful in pressure overload, such as aortic stenosis, to understand chamber mechanics and to predict clinical outcomes such as from corrective surgery. Data on the *left side* of the figure are from patients with aortic stenosis (*pink squares*) and illustrate the diversity of left ventricular adaptation. The *right side* of the figure is a schematic depiction of the data on the *left*.

Hypertrophy often normalizes wall stress because increased wall thickness neutralizes the increased pressures. Thus, those with compensated aortic stenosis have normal shortening (*ie*, ejection fraction). Some patients, particularly elderly women, have a hypertrophic process that increases wall thickness with reduced chamber size [17]. This altered geometry causes wall stress to be lower than normal and shortening is consequently greater than normal. On the other hand, some patients have reduced shortening proportional to an increase in afterload. These patients often have beneficial responses, both clinically and in terms of chamber mechanics, to aortic valve surgery. Finally, true myocardial dysfunction may develop in some patients and is indicated by reduced shortening. Shortening remains reduced even after the valve lesion has been treated.

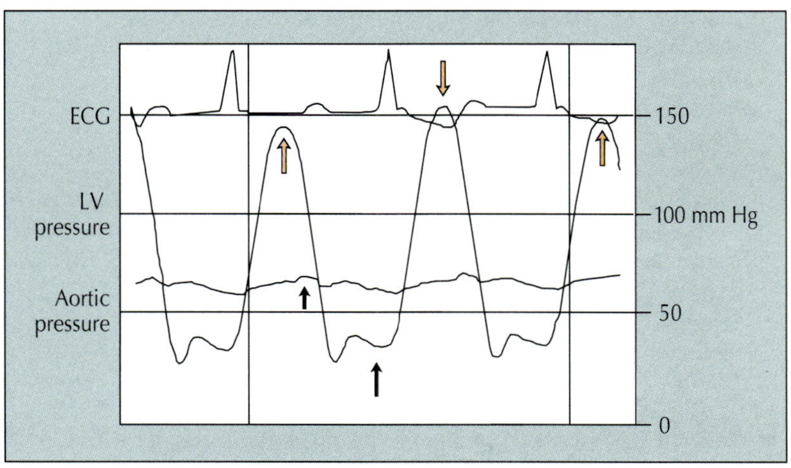

FIGURE 2-38. Cardiogenic shock as a consequence of pressure overload. Severely reduced shortening, especially with an element of myocardial depression, may occur in untreated aortic stenosis. This figure shows the pressure waveforms of cardiogenic shock with low arterial pressures (*arrowhead*) and high left ventricular diastolic pressures (*black arrow*). The *orange arrows* indicate the mechanical alternans that occurs in severe aortic stenosis with important pump dysfunction. Note the sizeable transaortic gradient. ECG—electrocardiogram; LV–left ventricle.

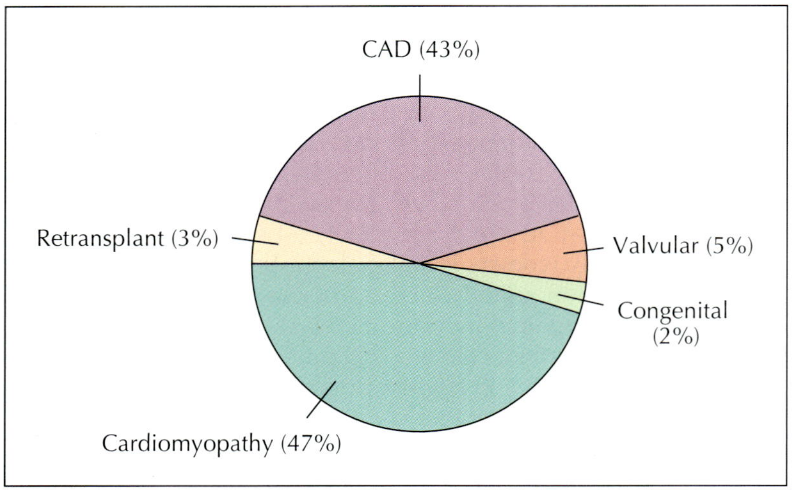

FIGURE 2-39. Severe and irreversible ventricular dysfunction leading to cardiac transplantation. Irreversible ventricular dysfunction occurs in many patients with untreated pressure and volume overload and in some patients despite corrective valve surgery. These patients may be candidates for cardiac transplantation. Shown here are data indicating the underlying heart disease of patients needing transplantation, which includes 5% with end-stage valvular disease [78]. CAD—coronary artery disease. (*Adapted from* Stevenson [78].)

SUMMARY

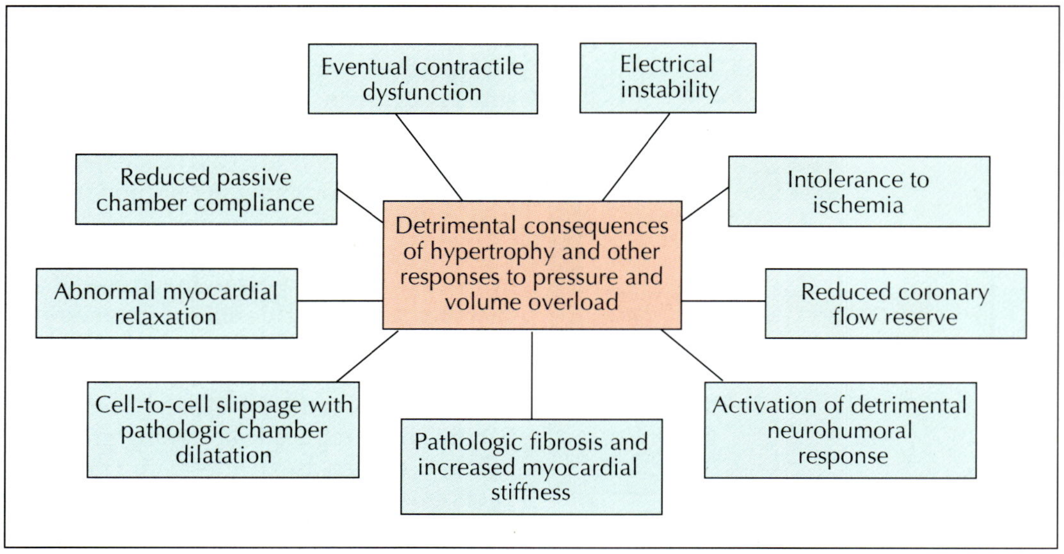

FIGURE 2-40. Summary of the detrimental consequences of hypertrophy. In this chapter the successful adaptation as well as the untoward consequences have been presented for both pressure and volume overload lesions. In this figure the detrimental consequences are summarized. Consequences occur from the adaptation and maladaptation of the myocardium as well as the interstitium, the coronary vasculature, and the neuroendocrine axis.

REFERENCES

1. Pflugfelder PW, Landzberg JS, Cassidy MM, *et al.*: Comparison of cine MR imaging with Doppler echocardiography for the evaluation of aortic regurgitation. *Am J Roentgenol* 1989, 152:729–735.
2. Katz AM: Heart failure. In *The Heart and Cardiovascular System*, 2nd edn. Edited by Fozzard HA. New York: Raven Press; 1992:333–353.
3. Ross J: Afterload mismatch in aortic and mitral valve disease: implications for surgical therapy. *J Am Coll Cardiol* 1985, 5:811–826.
4. Osler W: *The Principles and Practice of Medicine*. New York: D. Appleton; 1892.
5. Meerson FZ: On the mechanisms of compensatory hyperfunction and insufficiency of the heart. *Cor Vasa* 1961, 3:161–177.
6. Sonnenblick EH, Strobeck JE: Current concepts in cardiology: derived indexes of ventricular and myocardial function. *N Engl J Med* 1977, 296:978–982.
7. Schwartz K, Carrier L, Mercadier JJ, *et al.*: Molecular phenotype of the hypertrophied and failing myocardium. *Circulation* 1993, 87(suppl VII):VII5–VII10.
8. Le Jemtel TH, Sonnenblick EH: Heart failure: adaptive and maladaptive processes. *Circulation* 1993:87(suppl VII):VII1–VII4.
9. Schwartz K: Phenoconversion and mechanogenic transduction of the mammalian heart. *Med Sci* 1990, 6:664–673.
10. Cooper G, Kent RL, Mann DL: Load induction of cardiac hypertrophy. *J Mol Cell Cardiol* 1989, 21:(suppl V):11–30.
11. Bugaisky LB, Gupta M, Gupta MP, Zak R: Cellular and molecular mechanisms of cardiac hypertrophy. In *The Heart and Cardiovascular System*, 2nd edn. Edited by Fozzard HA, Haber E, Jennings RB, *et al*. New York: Raven Press; 1992:1621–1637.
12. Anversa P, Olivetti G, Melissari M, Loud AV: Stereological measurement of cellular and subcellular hypertrophy and hyperplasia in the papillary muscle of adult rat. *J Mol Cell Cardiol* 1980, 12:781–795.
13. Anversa P, Kajstura J, Olivetti G, *et al.*: Cellular basis of cardiac hypertrophy: myocyte cellular hypertrophy and myocyte cellular hyperplasia. *Heart Failure* 1993, 9:171–182.

14. Hess OM, Ritter M, Schneider J, *et al.*: Diastolic stiffness and myocardial structure in aortic valve disease before and after valve replacement. *Circulation* 1984, 69:855–865.
15. Linzbach AJ: Heart failure from the point of view of quantitative anatomy. *Am J Cardiol* 1960, 5:370–382.
16. Mann DL, Spann JF, Cooper G: Basic mechanisms and models in cardiac hypertrophy: part 2. Hypertrophy into failure. *Mod Concepts Cardiovasc Dis* 1988, 57:13–17.
17. Carroll JD, Carroll EP, Feldman T, *et al.*: Sex-associated differences in left ventricular function in aortic stenosis of the elderly. *Circulation* 1992, 86:1099–1107.
18. Berne RM, Levy MN: *Cardiovascular Physiology*, edn 5. St. Louis: Mosby Year Book; 1986.
19. Shroff SG, Janicki JS, Weber KT: Mechanical and energetic behavior of the intact left ventricle. In *The Heart and Cardiovascular System*, 2nd edn. Edited by Fozzard HA. New York: Raven Press; 1992:129–150.
20. Shroff SG, Motz W: Left ventricular systolic resistance in rats with hypertension and hypertrophy. *Am J Physiol* 1989, 257:H386–H394.
21. Shroff SG, Naegelen D, Clark WA: Relation between left ventricular systolic resistance and ventricular rate processes. *Am J Physiol* 1990, 258:H381–H394.
22. Hendel RD, VandeBerg JL, Shade RE, *et al.*: Cardiac beta myosin heavy chain diversity in normal and chronically hypertensive baboons. *J Clin Invest* 1989, 83:1487–1493.
23. Feldman AM, Weinberg EO, Ray PE, Lorell BH: Selective changes in cardiac gene expression during compensated hypertrophy and the transition to cardiac decompensation in rats with chronic aortic banding. *Circ Res* 1993, 73:184–192.
24. Arai M, Matsui H, Periasamy M: Review: sarcoplasmic reticulum gene expression in cardiac hypertrophy and heart failure. *Circ Res* 1994, 74:555–564.
25. Nadal-Ginard B, Mahdavi V: Molecular basis of cardiac performance: plasticity of the myocardium generated through protein isoform switches. *J Clin Invest* 1989, 84:1693–1700.
26. Alpert NR, Mulieri LA, Litten RZ: Functional significance of altered myosin adenosine triphosphatase activity in enlarged hearts. *Am J Cardiol* 1979, 44:947–953.
27. Factor SM: Role of the extracellular matrix in dilated cardiomyopathy. *Heart Failure* 1993, 9:260–268.
28. Janicki JS, Matsubara BB: Myocardial collagen and left ventricular diastolic function. In *Left Ventricular Diastolic Dysfunction and Heart Function.* Edited by Gaasch WH, LeWinter MM. Philadelphia: Lea and Febiger; 1994:125–140.
29. Weber KT: Cardiac interstitium in health and disease: the fibrillar collagen network. *J Am Coll Cardiol* 1989, 13:1637–1652.
30. Carroll EP, Janicki JS, Pick R, Weber KT: Myocardial stiffness and reparative fibrosis following coronary embolisation in the rat. *Cardiovasc Res* 1989, 23:655–661.
31. Weber KT, Pick R, Jalil JE, *et al.*: Patterns of myocardial fibrosis. *J Mol Cell Cardiol* 1989, 21(suppl V):121–131.
32. Weber KT, Janicki JS, Pick R, *et al.*: Collagen in the hypertrophied pressure-overloaded myocardium. *Circulation* 1987, 75:I–40.
33. Terracio L, Rubin K, Gullberg D, *et al.*: Expression of collagen binding integrins during cardiac development and hypertrophy. *Circ Res* 1991, 68:734–744.
34. Chapman D, Weber KT, Eghbali M: Regulation of fibrillar collagen types I and III and basement membrane type IV collagen gene expression in pressure overloaded rat myocardium. *Circ Res* 1990, 67:787–794.
35. Sadoshima J, Izumo S: Molecular characterization of angiotensin II-induced hypertrophy of cardiac myocytes and hyperplasia of cardiac fibroblasts: critical role of the AT_1 receptor subtype. *Circ Res* 1993, 73:413–423.
36. Vassalli G, Hess OM, Krogmann ON, *et al.*: Coronary artery size in mitral regurgitation and its regression after mitral valve surgery. *Am Heart J* 1993, 126:1091–1098.
37. Villari B, Hess OM, Moccetti D, *et al.*: Effect of progression of left ventricular hypertrophy on coronary artery dimension in aortic valve disease. *J Am Coll Cardiol* 1992, 20:1073–1079.
38. Dodge JT Jr, Brown BG, Bolson EL, Dodge HT: Lumen diameter of normal human coronary arteries: influence of age, sex, anatomic variation, and left ventricular hypertrophy or dilation. *Circulation* 1992, 86:232–246.
39. Bishop SP, Powell PC, Hasebe N, *et al.*: Coronary vascular morphology and reduced coronary reserve in dogs with chronic pressure overload cardiac hypertrophy [abstract]. *Circulation* 1993, 88(suppl):I–545.
40. Marcus ML: Effects of cardiac hypertrophy on the coronary circulation. In *The Coronary Circulation in Health and Disease*. Edited by Marcus ML. New York: McGraw-Hill; 1983:285.
41. Strauer BE: The coronary circulation in hypertensive heart disease. *Hypertension* 1984, 6(suppl III):III74–III80.
42. Rakusan K, Flanagan MF, Geva T, *et al.*: Morphometry of human coronary capillaries during normal growth and the effect of age in left ventricular pressure-overload hypertrophy. *Circulation* 1992, 86:38–46.
43. Olsson RA, Buenger R, Spaan JAE: Coronary circulation. In *The Heart and Cardiovascular System*, 2nd edn. Edited by Fozzard HA. New York: Raven Press; 1992:1393–1425.
44. Matsuo S, Tsuruta M, Hayano M, *et al.*: Phasic coronary artery flow velocity determined by Doppler flowmeter catheter in aortic stenosis and aortic regurgitation. *Am J Cardiol* 1988, 62:917–922.
45. Klocke FJ: Measurements of coronary flow reserve: defining pathophysiology versus making decisions about patient care. *Circulation* 1987, 76:1183–1189.
46. Nakano K, Corin WJ, Spann JF, *et al.*: Abnormal subendocardial blood flow in pressure overload hypertrophy is associated with pacing-induced subendocardial dysfunction. *Circ Res* 1989, 65:1555–1564.
47. Carabello BA, Nakano K, Ishihara K, *et al.*: Coronary blood flow in dogs with contractile dysfunction due to experimental volume overload. *Circulation* 1991, 83:1063–1075.
48. Hittinger L, Shannon RP, Kohn S, *et al.*: Exercise-induced subendocardial dysfunction in dogs with left ventricular hypertrophy. *Circ Res* 1990, 66:329–343.
49. Vatner SF, Hittinger L: Coronary vascular mechanisms involved in decompensation from hypertrophy to heart failure. *J Am Coll Cardiol* 1993, 22(suppl A):34A–40A.
50. Mochizuki T, Eberli FR, Ngoy S, *et al.*: Effects of brief repetitive ischemia on contractility, relaxation, and coronary flow: exaggerated postischemic diastolic dysfunction in pressure-overload hypertrophy. *Circ Res* 1993, 73:550–558.
51. Gaasch WH, Zile MR, Hoshino PK, *et al.*: Stress-shortening relations and myocardial blood flow in compensated and failing canine hearts with pressure-overload hypertrophy. *Circulation* 1989, 79:872–883.
52. Miller WL, Burnett JC: Circulating paracrine and autocrine mechanisms in heart failure. *Curr Opin Cardiol* 1993, 8:376–382.
53. Floras JS: Clinical aspects of sympathetic activation and parasympathetic withdrawal in heart failure. *J Am Coll Cardiol* 1993, 22(suppl A):72A.
54. Brutsaert DL: Cell communication between endocardium and myocardium: its role in cardiac overloading and failure. *Heart falilure* 1990, 6:75–80.
55. LeWinter M, Pavelec R: Influence of the pericardium on left ventricular end-diastolic pressure-segment length relations during early and later phases of experimental chronic volume overload in dogs. *Circ Res* 1982, 50:501–509.

56. Carroll JD, Lang RM, Neumann EL, *et al.*: The differential effects of positive inotropic and vasodilator therapy on diastolic properties with congestive cardiomyopathy. *Circulation* 1986, 74:815–825.
57. Corin WJ, Murakami T, Monrad ES, *et al.*: Left ventricular passive diastolic properties in chronic mitral regurgitation. *Circulation* 1991, 83:797–807.
58. Carroll JD, Carroll EP: Exercise-induced angina pectoris. In *Left Ventricular Diastolic Dysfunction and Heart failure*. Edited by Gaasch WH, LeWinter MM. Philadelphia: Lea and Febiger; 1994:259–273.
59. Carroll JD, Hess OM, Hirzel HO, Krayenbuehl HP: Exercise-induced ischemia: the influence of altered relaxation on early diastolic pressures. *Circulation* 1983, 67:521.
60. Eichhorn P, Grimm J, Koch R, *et al.*: Left ventricular relaxation in patients with left ventricular hypertrophy secondary to aortic valve disease. *Circulation* 1982, 65:1395–1404.
61. Hess OM, Schneider J, Koch R, *et al.*: Diastolic function myocardial structure in patients with myocardial hypertrophy. *Circulation* 1981, 63:360.
62. Apstein CS, Morgan JP: Cellular mechanisms underlying left ventricular diastolic dysfunction. *Left Ventricular Diastolic Dysfunction and Heart Failure*. Edited by Gaasch WH, LeWinter MM. Philadelphia: Lea and Febiger; 1994:3–24.
63. Liu CP, Ting CT, Yang TM, *et al.*: Reduced left ventricular compliance in human mitral stenosis: role of reversible internal constraint. *Circulation* 1992, 85:1447–1456.
64. Gaasch WH, Folland ED: Left ventricular function in rheumatic mitral stenosis. *Eur Heart J* 1991, 12(suppl B):66–69.
65. Sabbah HN, Anbe DT, Stein PD: Negative intraventricucular diastolic pressures in patients with mitral stenosis: evidence of left ventricular diastolic suction. *Am J Cardiol* 1980, 45:562–566.
66. Robinson TF, Factor SM, Sonnenblick EH: The heart as a suction pump. *Sci Am* 1986, 254:84–91.
67. Yellin EL, Nikolic SD: Diastolic suction and the dynamics of left ventriuclar filling. In *Left Ventricular Diastolic Dysfunction and Heart Failure*. Edited by Gaasch WH, LeWinter MM. Philadelphia: Lea and Febiger; 1994:89–102.
68. Paulus WJ, Vantrimpont PJ, Rousseau MF: Diastolic function of the nonfilling human left ventricule. *J Am Coll Cardiol* 1992, 20:1524–1532.
69. Gaasch WH: Passive elastic properties of the left ventricle. In *Left Ventricular Diastolic Dysfunction and Heart failure.* Edited by Gaasch WH, LeWinter MM. Philadelphia: Lea and Febiger; 1994:143–149.
70. Ishida Y, Meisner JS, Gallo JI, *et al.*: Left ventricular filling dynamics: influence of left ventricular relaxation and left atrial pressure. *Circulation* 1986, 74:187–196.
71. Carroll JD, Hess OM, Hirzel HO, Krayenbuehl HP: Dynamics of left ventricular filling at rest and during exercise. *Circulation* 1983, 68:59–67.
72. Meisner JS, Keren G, Pajaro OE, *et al.*: Atrial contribution to ventricular filling in mitral stenosis. *Circulation* 1991, 84:1469–1480.
73. Hall RJC, Julian DG: Ventricular function in valve disease. In *Disease of the Cardiac Valves*. Edited by Hall RJC. New York: Churchill Livingstone; 1989:285–314.
74. Murakami T, Hess OM, Gage JE, *et al.*: Diastolic filling dynamics in patients with aortic stenosis. *Circulation* 1986, 73:1162–1174.
75. Wisenbaugh T, Spann JF, Carabello BA: Differences in myocardial performance and load between patients with similar amounts of chronic aortic versus chronic mitral regurgitation. *Am Coll Cardiol* 1984, 4:916–923.
76. Starling MR, Kirsch MM, Montgomery DG, Gross MD: Impaired left ventricular contractile function in patients with long-term mitral regurgitation and normal ejection fraction. *J Am Coll Cardiol* 1993, 22:239–250.
77. Shimizu G, Hirota Y, Kita Y, *et al.*: Left ventricular midwall mechanics in systemic arterial hypertension; myocardial function is depressed in pressure-overload hypertrophy. *Circulation* 1991, 83:1676–1684.
78. Stevenson LW: Selection and management of patients for cardiac transplantation. *Curr Opin Cardiol* 1993, 8:411–418.

ROLE OF TWO-DIMENSIONAL ECHOCARDIOGRAPHY AND DOPPLER ULTRASOUND

3

CHAPTER

Peter C. Nishan and Rick A. Nishimura

The evaluation of patients with valvular heart disease has been greatly enhanced by the advent of two-dimensional echocardiography and Doppler ultrasound. Echocardiography is an ideal modality for confirming the diagnosis of a valvular lesion found on physical examination. Determination of the severity of a valvular lesion, as well as its effect on the cardiac chambers and pulmonary circulation, can be assessed by echocardiography. Because echocardiography is a noninvasive diagnostic modality, it is well suited for serial follow-up of patients with valvular lesions. The new imaging and hemodynamic laboratories not only aid physicians in the diagnosis of valvular disease but also provide valuable information to guide therapy. In experienced hands, echocardiography can provide most or all of the information necessary for a decision on timing of catheter-based and surgical intervention.

Two-dimensional echocardiography allows the cardiac structures to be imaged in multiple planes and in real time [1]. Assessment of valve morphology and valve motion can be performed for all four valves. The effect of the valvular lesion on the left and right ventricle, atria, and great vessels can be assessed. Cardiac masses related to valve disease such as thrombi, vegetations, and abscesses can now be detected reliably by two-dimensional echocardiographic imaging.

Doppler ultrasound can measure blood flow velocities in the cardiac chambers, across valves, and through the great vessels [2]. Application of the modified Bernoulli equation to high-velocity jets measured by continuous-wave Doppler ultrasound provides accurate, noninvasive measurements of valve gradients and intracardiac pressures (pressure gradient = $4 \times [\text{velocity}]^2$). Measurement of laminar flow by pulse-valve Doppler ultrasound can be used to determine volumetric flow for assessment of cardiac output, valve area, and regurgitant fractions. Color-flow imaging provides a visual display of the direction and magnitude of blood flow velocities superimposed on real-time two-dimensional imaging and is used for semiquantitative assessment of valvular regurgitation and intracardiac shunts.

In the past, one of the limitations of two-dimensional echocardiography has been inadequate image resolution in a subset of patients in which there is poor acoustic penetration (*ie*, obese patients, patients with chronic obstructive pulmonary disease, post open-heart surgery patients). Transesophageal echocardiography (TEE) has emerged as a new window on the heart, providing consistent high-resolution imaging of cardiac structures in all patients [3]. TEE is particularly useful for imaging posterior structures and has added significant information for evaluation of patients with mitral valve disease (particularly in those with mitral prostheses), suspected infective endocarditis, and diseases of the aorta.

Echocardiography is a highly operator-dependent diagnostic modality, both in its performance and in its interpretation. Careful attention to details is necessary in order to obtain consistently reliable anatomic and hemodynamic information. Correlation with the clinical findings is always necessary to derive the optimal benefit from echocardiographic data [4].

Normal Valves

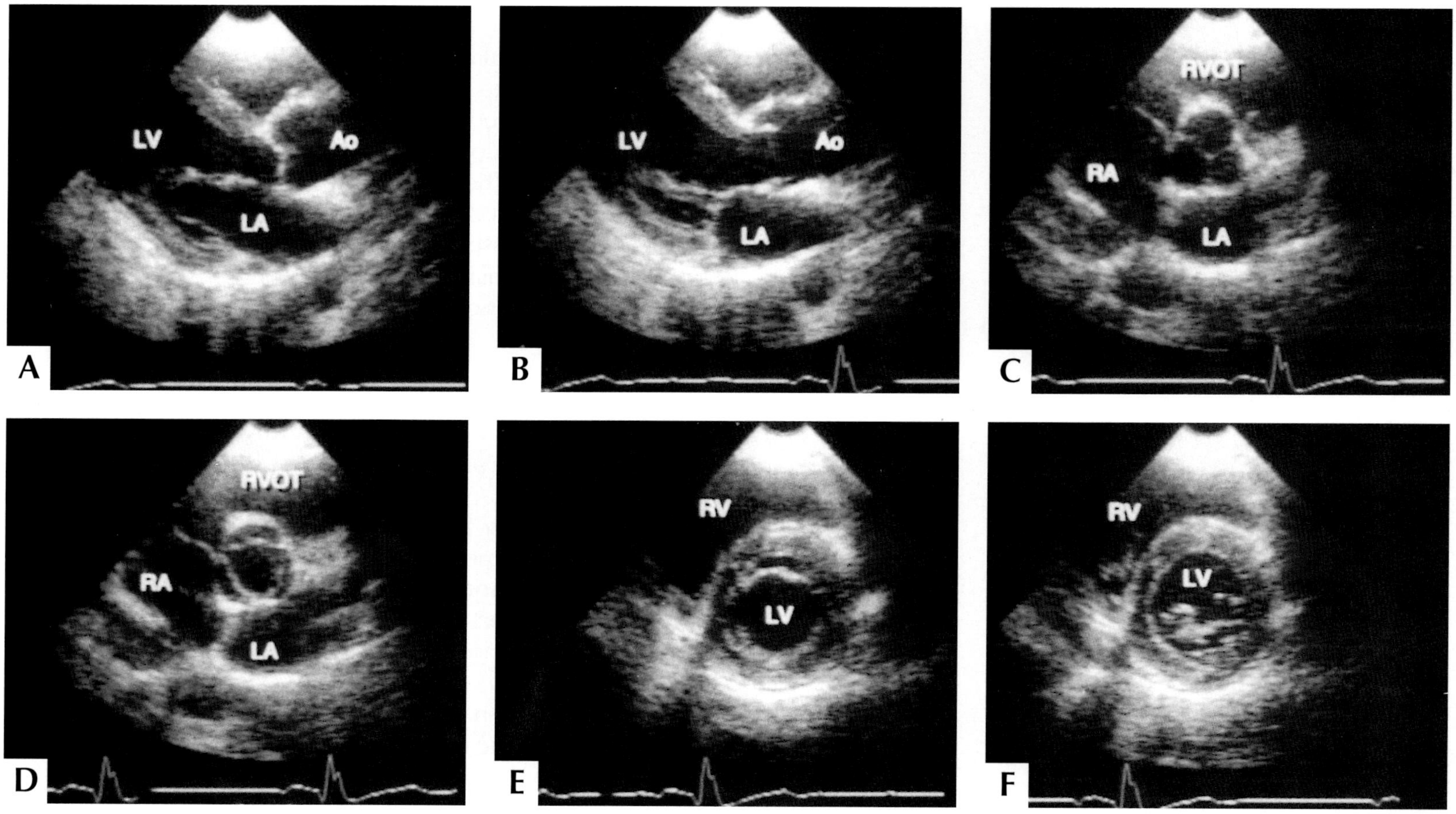

Figure 3-1. Two-dimensional echocardiography of normal heart valves. Two-dimensional echocardiography allows imaging of valve morphology and valve motion in real time. The normal valve leaflets are thin and mobile and can be seen to open widely on two-dimensional imaging. The normal parasternal long- and short-axis views of aortic and mitral valves are shown. In the long-axis view, the mitral valve opens fully during diastole (**A**) and the aortic valve opens fully during systole (**B**). The aortic valve consists of three cusps (left, right, and noncoronary), which can be seen on the short-axis view as thin, mobile, triangular structures (**C,** diastole; **D,** systole). The mitral valve consists of the large anterior leaflet and smaller posterior leaflet, which are normally thicker than the aortic valve cusps and can be seen to open into a large circular orifice on the short-axis view (**E,** diastole; **F,** systole). Ao—aorta; LA—left atrium; LV— left ventricle; RA—right atrium; RV—right ventricle; RVOT—right ventricular outflow tract.

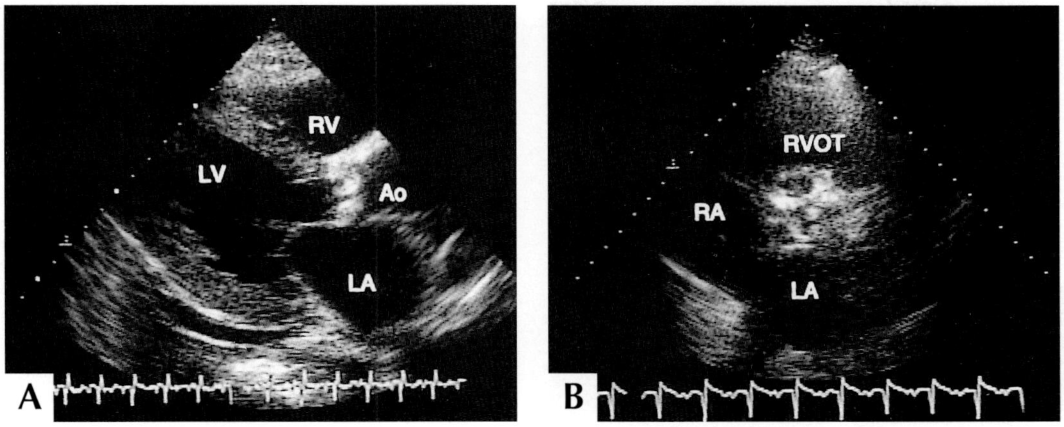

Figure 3-2. Calcific aortic stenosis (AS). In a patient with calcific AS, the aortic valve appears echo dense and immobile, as shown in the parasternal long-axis (**A**) and short-axis (**B**) views. Two-dimensional echocardiographic imaging is a highly sensitive method for determining the presence of AS. However, the severity of AS cannot be determined reliably from the two-dimensional image alone. In the presence of calcification, it is frequently difficult to visualize the number of aortic valve cusps. Other information that should be obtained from the two-dimensional echocardiogram is the response of the left ventricle (LV) to the pressure overload (chamber size, ventricular hypertrophy, and ventricular systolic function), as well as other concomitant valve disease. Ao—aorta; LA—left atrium; RA—right atrium; RV—right ventricle; RVOT—right ventricular outflow tract.

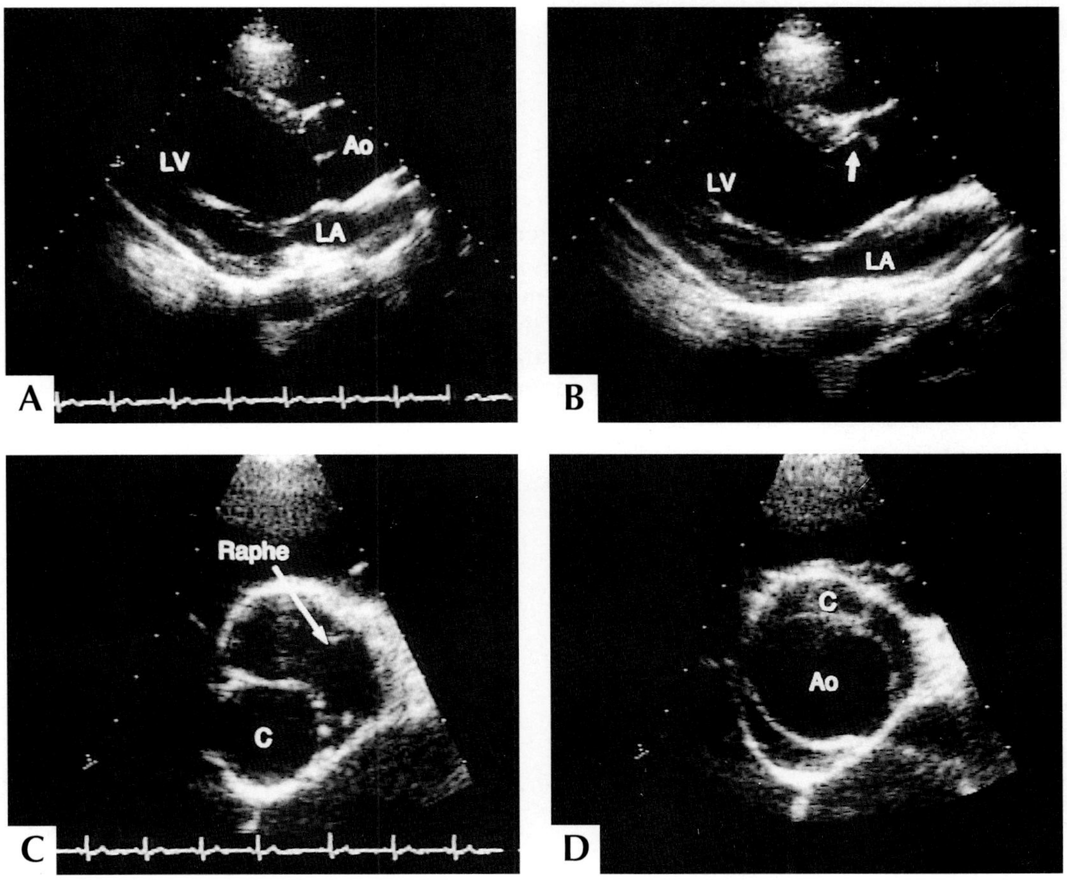

Figure 3-3. Noncalcified bicuspid aortic valve. Two-dimensional echocardiography can reliably diagnose the presence of a noncalcified bicuspid aortic valve [5]. The parasternal long-axis view may or may not show eccentric coaptation, which was the diagnostic feature on M-mode echocardiography (**A**). The diagnosis of a bicuspid aortic valve is made on the basis of systolic doming of the aortic cusps (*arrow* in **B**), as well as the direct visualization of the two cusps on the short-axis view (**C**) and (**D**). A raphe is seen at two o'clock with commissures at five and 10 o'clock in *panel C*. As with calcific aortic stenosis, the severity of the obstruction outflow cannot be determined by the two-dimensional echocardiographic appearance alone. Ao—aorta; C—cusp; LA—left atrium; LV—left ventricle.

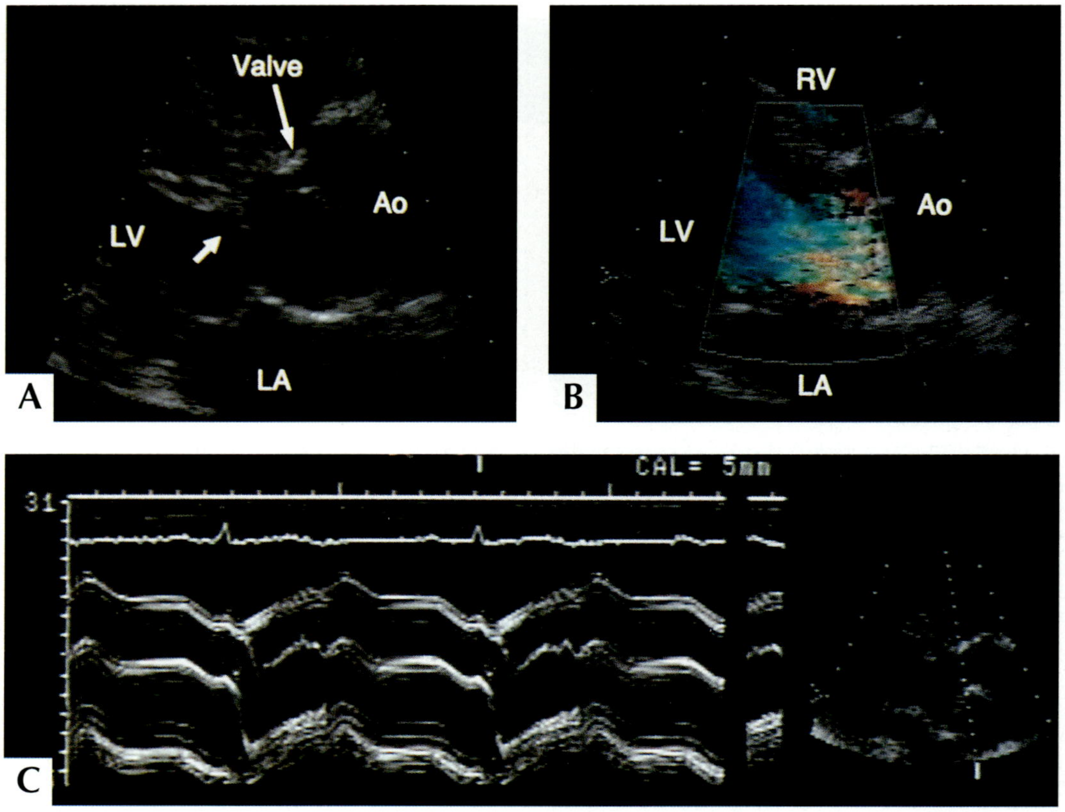

FIGURE 3-4. Left ventricular (LV) outflow obstruction. Two-dimensional echocardiography enables the determination of the different sites of LV outflow obstruction (valvular, subvalvular, and supravalvular). Discrete subvalvular obstruction is seen in approximately 9% of adolescents and adults with aortic stenosis. The three different types of subvalvular obstruction can be seen on two-dimensional echocardiography (type 1—thin,discrete membrane; type 2—thick, fibrous ring with associated subvalvular hypertrophy; type 3—subvalvular tunnel) [6]. An associated dynamic component to the obstruction may be present and is diagnosed by systolic anterior motion of the mitral valve, as well as a late-peaking Doppler velocity curve from the LV outflow tract. In instances of inadequate images, transesophageal echocardiography may be useful in further defining the presence and type of subvalvular stenosis. **A,** The long-axis view best visualizes the presence of discrete subvalvular aortic stenosis, seenas an echo-dense structure (*short arrow*) proximal to the aortic valve (*long arrow*). **B,** Color-flow imaging can be used to confirm the presence of subvalvular stenosis by demonstrating turbulence in this region, seen as a mosaic color pattern. **C,** Character-istic M-mode echocardiography shows premature systolic cusp closure followed by high-frequency fluttering, which is characteristic of this lesion. Ao—aorta; LA—left atrium; RV—right ventricle.

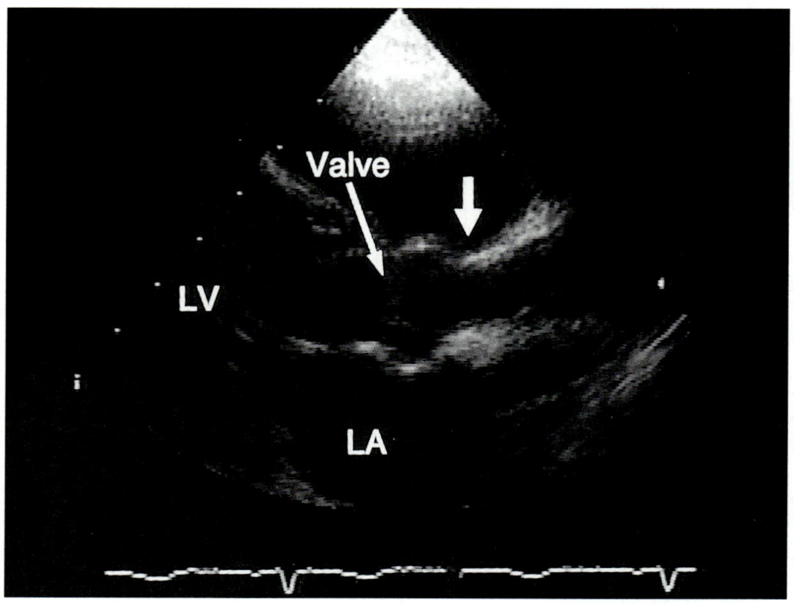

FIGURE 3-5. Supravalvular outflow obstruction. Supravalvular outflow obstruction is seen in fewer than 1% of adolescents and adults with aortic stenosis. The most common variant is an "hourglass" appearance of the ascending aorta (*thick arrow*), which can be seen best on the parasternal long-axis view. *Thin arrow* indicates aortic valve. Less commonly seen is uniform hypoplasia of the ascending aorta [7]. LA—left atrium; LV—left ventricle.

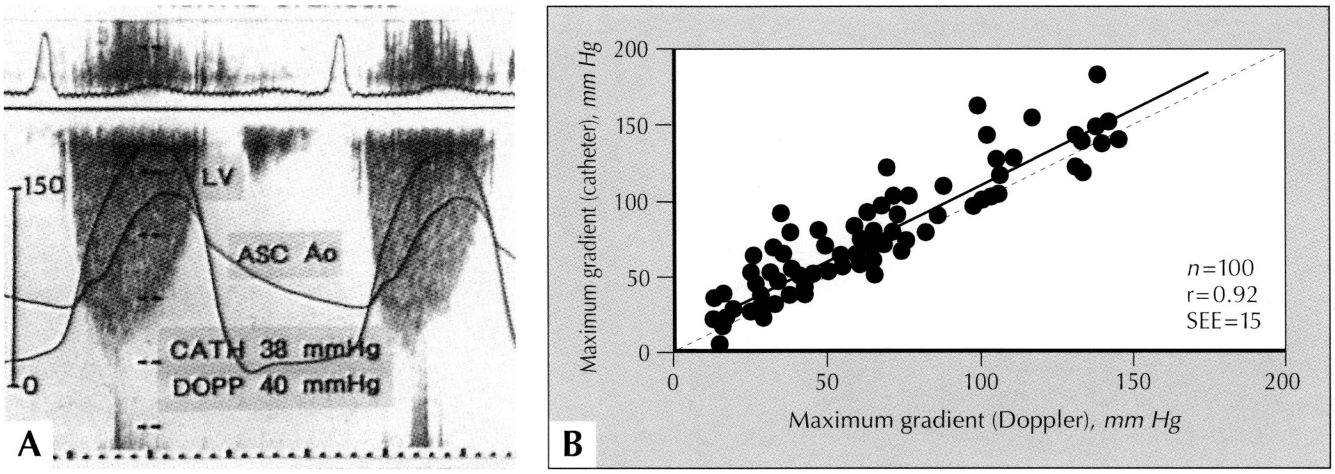

FIGURE 3-6. Aortic valve gradient in aortic stenosis (AS). Doppler ultrasound provides an accurate, noninvasive method for measurement of the aortic valve gradient in patients with AS [8]. The instantaneous pressure gradient between the left ventricle (LV) and aorta can be measured by applying the modified Bernoulli equation (pressure gradient = 4 × [velocity]^2) to the continuous-wave Doppler signal across the aortic valve. The mean aortic valve gradient, the most useful measurement of the degree of obstruction, can be obtained by averaging the instantaneous pressure gradients and can be performed on-line quickly with the calculation packages in the newer echocardiographic instruments.

In the assessment of patients with AS, it is of critical importance to interrogate the valve from multiple windows to ensure that the Doppler beam is parallel to the velocity jet [2,4,8]. A deviation of greater than 20° will result in a clinically significant underestimation of the pressure gradient. The Doppler examination can underestimate an aortic valve gradient but should not overestimate the gradient (except in the rare instances of severe anemia or coexistent LV outflow obstruction). Thus, the results should be correlated with the two-dimensional echocardiographic findings, as well as with the clinical findings. **A,** Simultaneous measurement of the aortic valve mean gradient demonstrates the excellent correlation between the gradient derived from cardiac catheterization (CATH) and continuous-wave Doppler ultrasound (DOPP). **B,** Correlation between Doppler- and catheter-derived instantaneous aortic valve pressure gradient. The regression equation, catheter gradient = 10.3 + 0.97 × Doppler gradient, is represented by the *solid line* [8]. Asc Ao—ascending aorta; SEE—standard error of the estimate. (*Adapted from* Currie and coworkers [8]; with permission.)

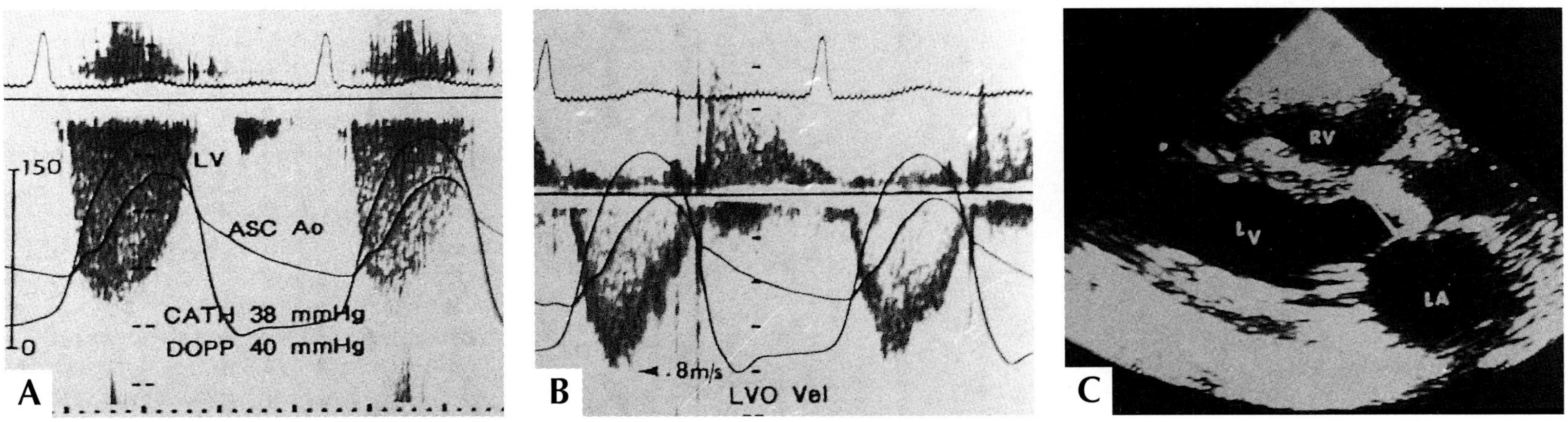

FIGURE 3-7. Determination of the aortic valve area (AVA). The pressure gradient in aortic stenosis is dependent on the flow through the aortic valve. Thus, calculation of an AVA should be performed in conjunction with measurement of the aortic valve gradient for determination of the severity of stenosis. An AVA can be calculated using the continuity principle, in which flow through the left ventricular outflow (LVO) tract is equated to flow through the aortic valve (AV). Flow is measured by the product of [area] × [velocity]. Thus, AVA = (LVO area × LVO velocity)/AV velocity. The AVA measured by Doppler continuity correlates well with that measured by cardiac catheterization [9]. The AVA calculated by Doppler ultrasound is more accurate than the AVA calculated by the Gorlin equation if there is coexistent severe aortic regurgitation or low cardiac output. The patient in Fig. 3-6 had a mean gradient of 38 mm Hg, compatible with a "moderate" degree of aortic stenosis. However, a low cardiac output was present and, thus, an AVA needed to be calculated.

A, A simultaneous catheter-Doppler tracing shows correlation between catheter-derived (CATH) and Doppler-derived (DOPP) mean gradient. The peak Doppler velocity is 3.6 m/sec. **B,** The peak LVO velocity is 0.8 ms. **C,** Parasternal long-axis view shows measurement of the LVO diameter of 2.0 cm at the insertion of the aortic valve cusps into the aortic annulus (*solid line*). The AVA is calculated by: AVA = (LVO area × LVO velocity)/AV velocity, AVA = (3.14 × 0.8)/3.6, and AVA = 0.7 cm^2. An AVA index of 0.35 cm^2/m^2 could be calculated, consistent with the clinical diagnosis of severe aortic stenosis. LA—left atrium; LV—left ventricle; RV—right ventricle.

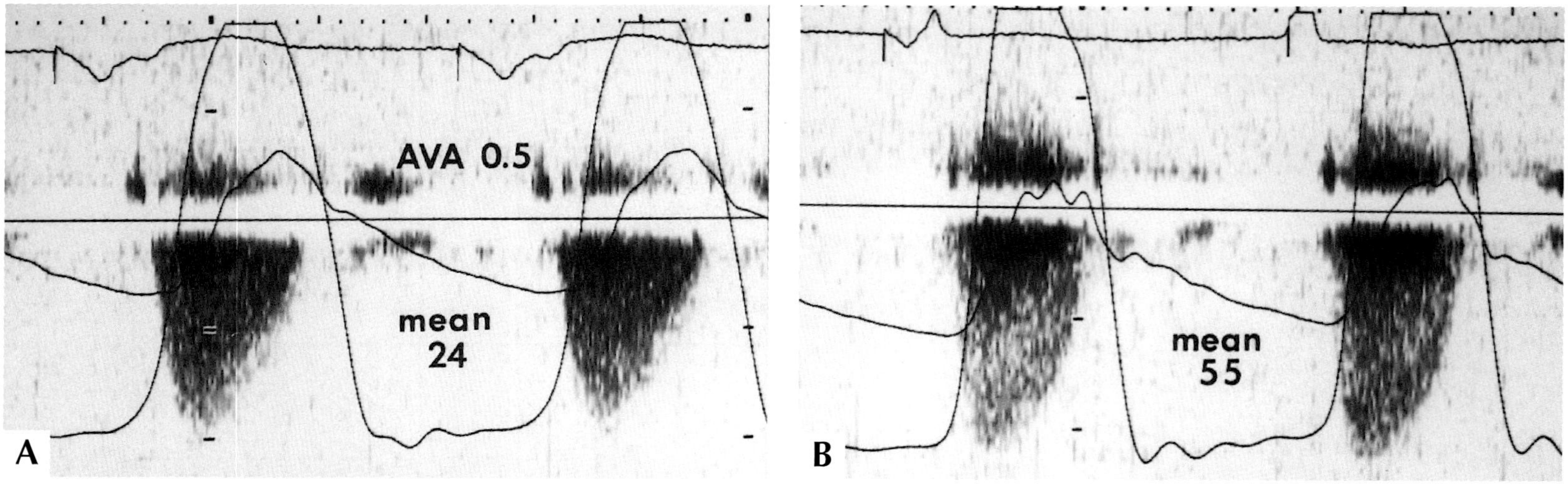

FIGURE 3-8. Dobutamine infusion in the differentiation of severe and mild aortic stenosis (AS). In patients with poor left ventricular (LV) function and AS, the combination of a low aortic valve gradient and a low aortic valve area (AVA) may be present. It may be difficult to differentiate whether these patients have 1) severe critical end-stage aortic stenosis or 2) mild AS and coexistent primary LV dysfunction [10]. In the latter circumstance, the AVA may calculate to be smaller than the true valve area because the low output may not be able to fully open the valve. This has important implications for management because surgery is indicated in the former circumstance but will not be beneficial in the latter.

Dobutamine can be used during the echocardiographic examination to differentiate these two entities. **A,** In the baseline state, this patient with AS and an ejection fraction of 20% has a calculated AVA of 0.5 cm^2 and a mean aortic valve gradient of 24 mm Hg. The simultaneous LV aortic pressures are shown. Doppler scale markers are 2.0 m/sec. **B,** At an infusion rate of 30 μg/kg/min dobutamine and normalization of cardiac output, there is an increase in the aortic valve mean gradient to 55 mm Hg, consistent with severe stenosis. In patients with a primary problem of depressed LV function and coexistent mild AS, the aortic valve velocity and mean gradient will not increase as the output is normalized by dobutamine infusion. (*Adapted from* Nishimura and Tajik [4]; with permission.)

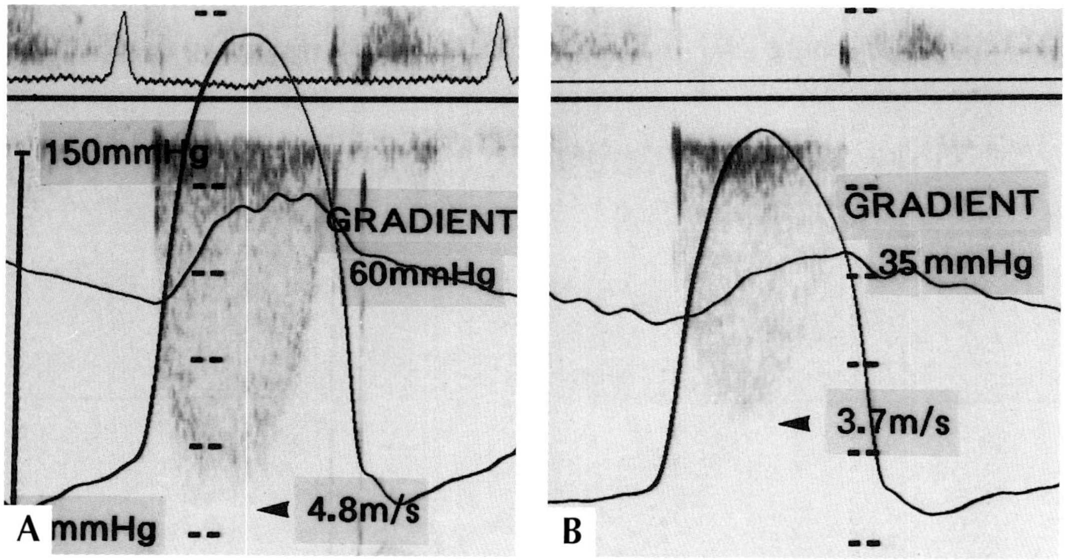

FIGURE 3-9. Percutaneous aortic balloon valvuloplasty. In selected patients with calcified aortic stenosis (AS), percutaneous aortic balloon valvuloplasty (PABV) can be used for palliation of symptoms. Inflation of one or more large balloons across the aortic valve will result in a modest improvement in hemodynamics and an improvement in symptoms of heart failure. Because of the high restenosis rate and high continued mortality, this procedure should be reserved for patients with severely symptomatic AS who are otherwise not candidates for aortic valve surgery and those who have a limited life span due to other medical problems. PABV can also be used as a "bridge" to surgery in the critically ill patient [10].

A, Simultaneous Doppler ultrasound and dual-catheter (left ventricular and aortic pressures) tracings in a patient before PABV. The mean aortic valve gradient is 60 mm Hg, and the peak Doppler velocity is 4.8 m/sec. **B,** After PABV, there has been a modest reduction in the mean gradient to 35 mm Hg and a decrease in the aortic valve velocity to 3.7 m/sec.

AORTIC REGURGITATION

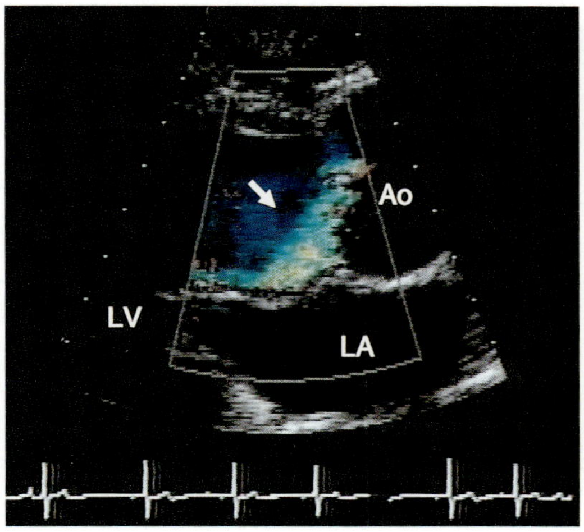

FIGURE 3-10. Aortic regurgitation (AR). Two-dimensional echocardiography and Doppler ultrasound provide valuable information for the patient with AR. The etiology of the AR can be determined. In this patient, there is AR, seen as an eccentric jet on color-flow imaging (*arrow*) due to a bicuspid aortic valve. The response of the left ventricle (LV) to the volume overload can be assessed by M-mode or quantitative two-dimensional measurements [11] and is of critical importance for timing of aortic valve operation [12]. The size of the aortic root can also be measured when considering aortic valve operation. Ao—aorta; LA—left atrium.

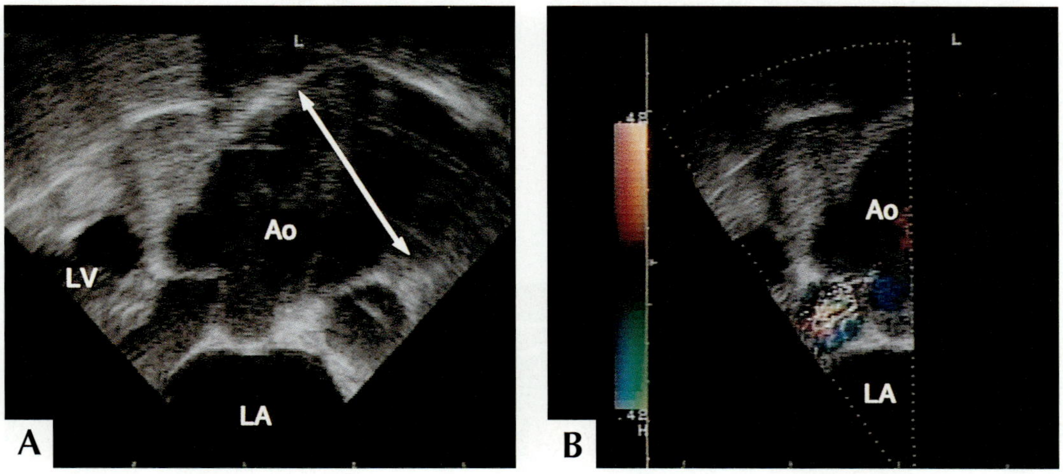

FIGURE 3-11. Transesophageal echocardiography (TEE) in diagnosis of aortic regurgitation (AR). The AR may be secondary to an abnormality of the aortic valve cusps or an abnormality of the aorta (Ao). TEE provides high-resolution images of the aortic root and ascending aorta in situations in which inadequate images are obtained by precordial echocardiography. Biplane or omniplane TEE can be used to image the entire thoracic aorta [3,13]. **A,** Transesophageal longitudinal view from a patient with a dilated aortic root (*arrow*) and severe AR, seen as a widely turbulent jet on color-flow imaging (**B**). LA—left atrium; LV—left ventricle.

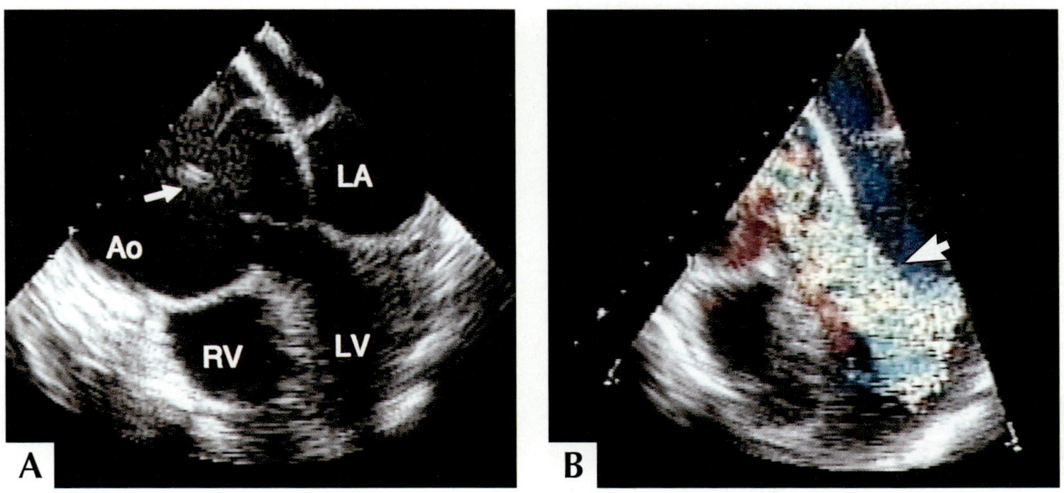

FIGURE 3-12. Transesophageal echocardiography (TEE) in the diagnosis of aortic dissection. Aortic dissection can be a cause of aortic regurgitation (AR). TEE has emerged as an ideal noninvasive method for the rapid diagnosis of aortic dissection with a 98% positive and negative predictive value [14]. **A,** The intimal flap and entry point (*arrow*) can be visualized directly on two-dimensional imaging. **B,** The complications of aortic dissection, such as AR (*arrow*), pericardial effusion, and regional wall motion abnormalities from myocardial infarction, can all be readily diagnosed by echocardiography. Ao—aorta; LA—left atrium; LV—left ventricle; RV—right ventricle.

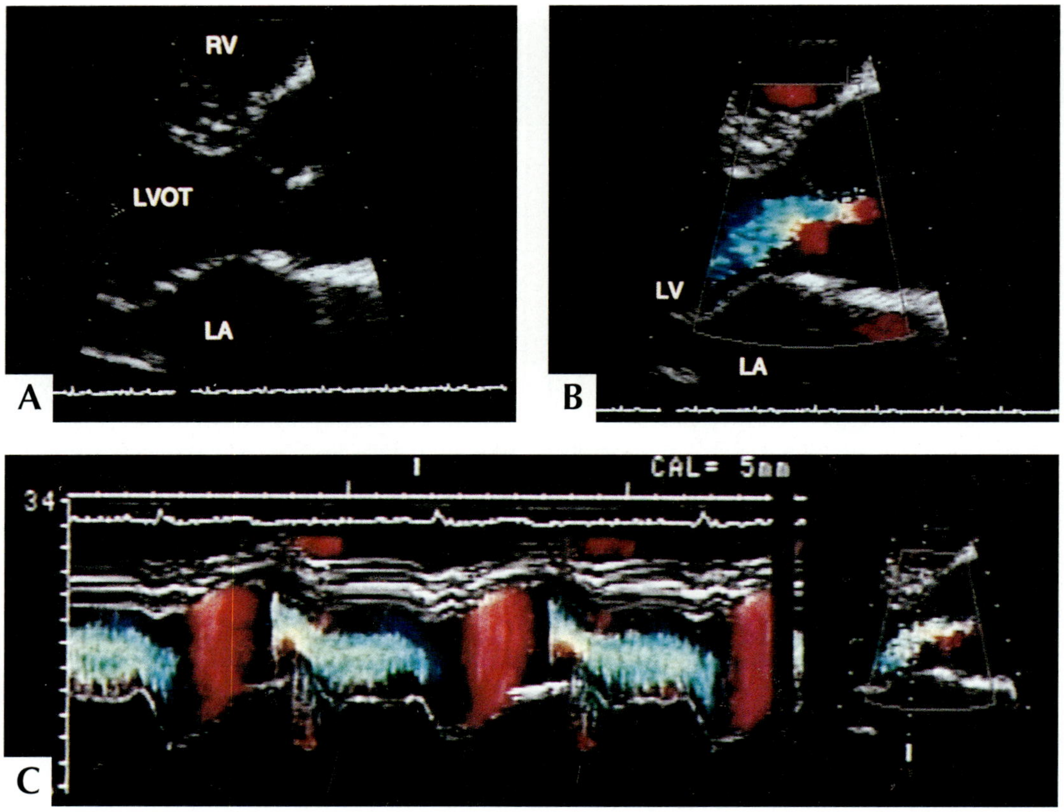

FIGURE 3-13. Doppler ultrasound imaging in the determination of the severity of aortic regurgitation (AR). The severity of AR can be assessed by several echocardiographic methods. The left ventricular (LV) size and function reflect the ventricular response to volume overload and should be considered when assessing the severity of the regurgitation. There are indirect Doppler findings, such as the diastolic half time, pulsed-wave Doppler interrogation of the descending aorta, LV outflow velocity, and mitral inflow velocity curve, which are useful in assessing the severity of regurgitation [15] and are discussed in Figs. 3–15, 3–16, and 3–17. In the absence of mitral regurgitation, quantitative Doppler ultrasound measurements of regurgitant volume and regurgitant fraction can be obtained by experienced laboratories [16]. Color-flow imaging, which superimposes a color-coded display of the intracardiac velocities directly on the real-time two-dimensional image, has been used as a semiquantitative approach for determination of the severity of regurgitation in patients with central jets [17]. For AR, it is not the extent of the jet into the LV cavity but rather the width (or area) of the jet in the LV outflow tract (LVOT) that correlates with the severity of regurgitation.

A and **B**, mild-to-moderate AR with the regurgitant jet width occupying 30% of the LVOT on the parasternal long-axis view. A color M-mode can be placed through the jet to further define the width of the jet in relation to the width of the LVOT (**C**). This method cannot be used when there is an eccentric jet of AR (*see* Fig. 3-10). LA—left atrium; RV—right ventricle.

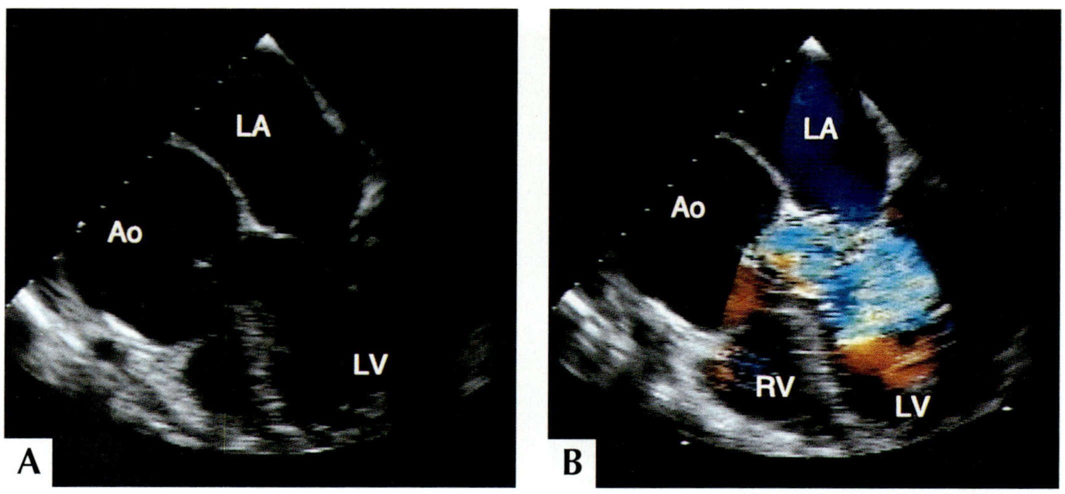

FIGURE 3-14. Transesophageal echocardiography (TEE) in the diagnosis of AR. In this patient, severe AR is seen in the apex down the long-axis view of TEE (**A**) as the regurgitant jet by color-flow imaging occupies nearly 100% of the left ventricular (LV) outflow tract (**B**). Ao— aorta; LA—left atrium; RV—right ventricle.

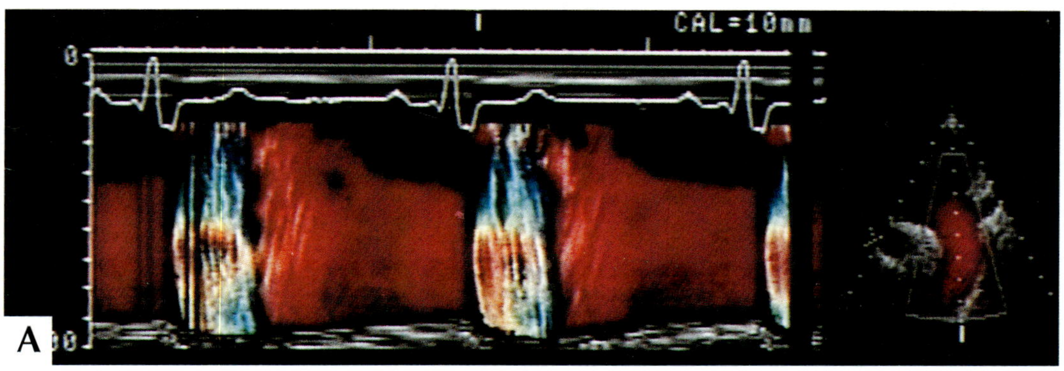

FIGURE 3-15. Diastolic flow reversal in diagnosing the severity of aortic regurgitation (AR). An indirect measure of the severity of AR is obtained by placing a pulsed-wave sample volume in the descending aorta just distal to the left subclavian artery. The degree of diastolic flow reversal correlates with the severity of AR [18]. Although other factors, such as the compliance of the aorta and force of ventricular contraction, (*continued*)

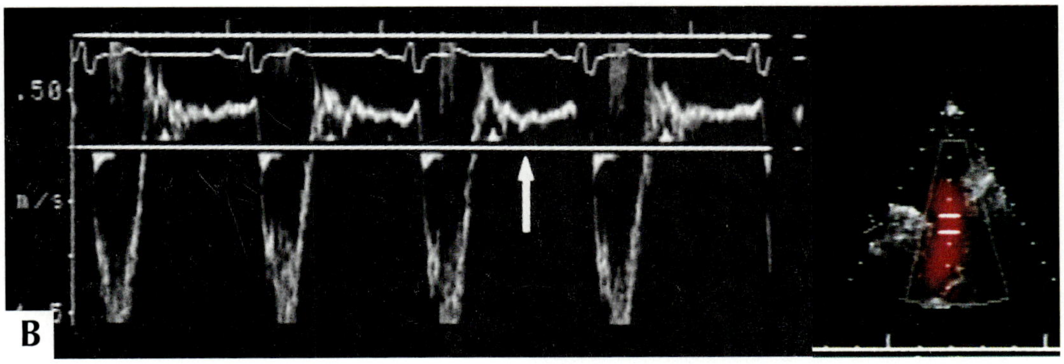

FIGURE 3-15. (*continued*) contribute to the degree of diastolic flow reversal, severe AR can be diagnosed when there is an early diastolic reversal of greater than 0.6 m/sec and a continued holodiastolic reversal greater than 0.2 m/sec [15]. **A,** Color M-mode echocardiography is used to display the velocities in the descending aorta over time in this patient with severe AR. **B,** The pulsed-Doppler tracing of the descending aorta shows a high-velocity holodiastolic flow reversal (*arrow*), indicating severe regurgitation.

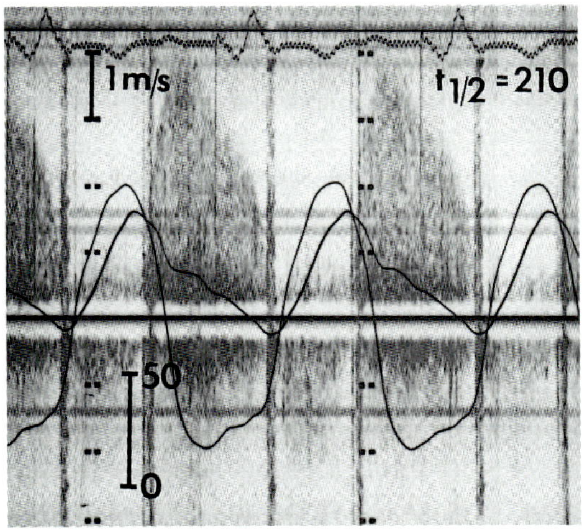

FIGURE 3-16. Continuous-wave Doppler velocity curve. The continuous-wave Doppler velocity curve of the aortic regurgitation (AR) jet is a reflection of the instantaneous gradient between the aorta and left ventricle during diastole [19]. In patients with severe AR, there is a steep decline of the AR velocity curve due to a rapid rate of rise of left ventricular diastolic pressure and rapid rate of fall of aortic pressure. The rate of fall of the velocity can be measured using a diastolic half time ($t_{1/2}$). The pressure $t_{1/2}$ is dependent on other factors such as left ventricular compliance, aortic compliance, and systolic contractility. However, a pressure ($t_{1/2}$) of less than 300 ms is indicative of severe AR [20]. Shown is an example of a patient with severe AR who has a diastolic $t_{1/2}$ of less than 300 ms. (*Adapted from* Nishimura and Tajik [4]; with permission.)

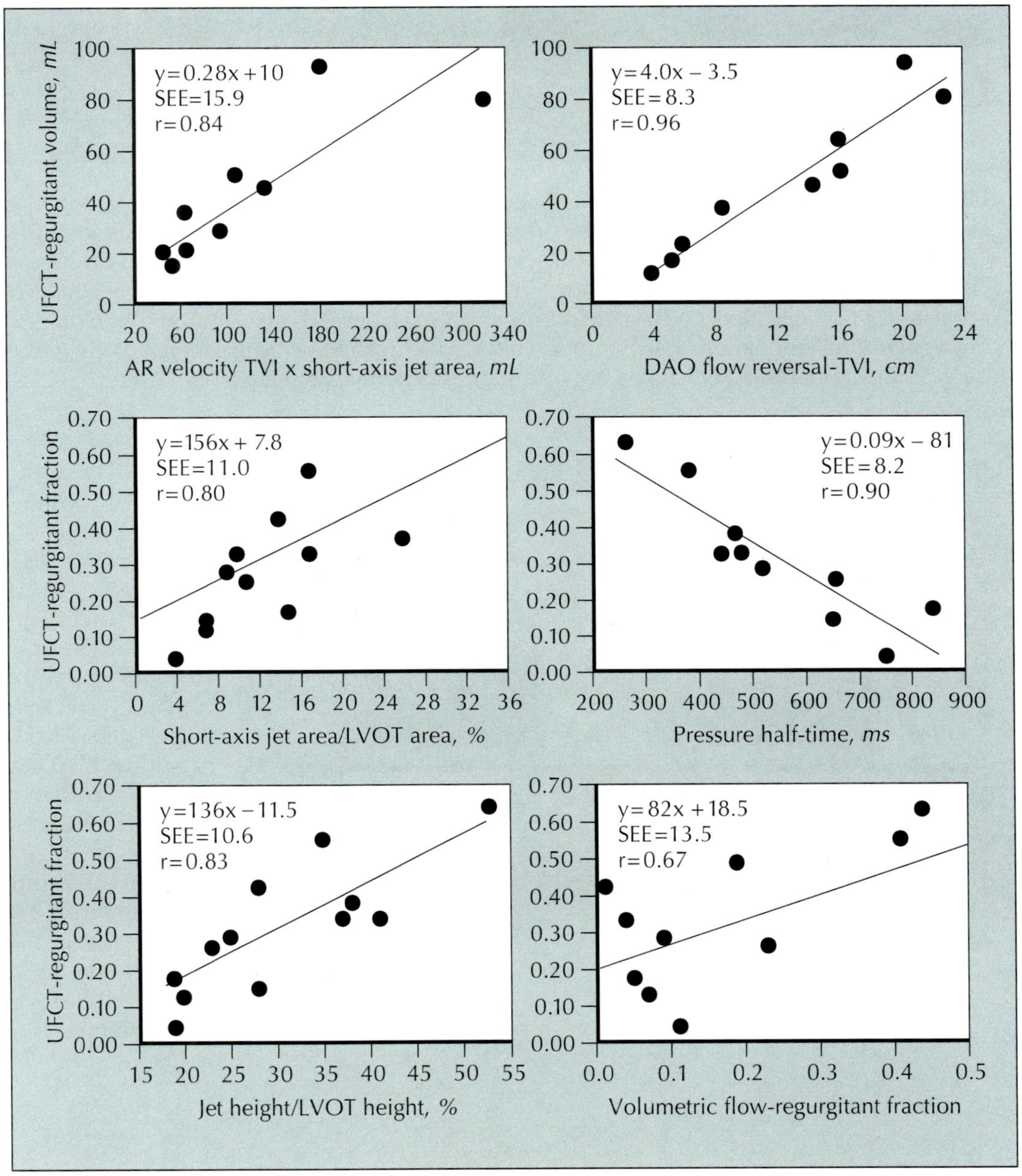

FIGURE 3-17. Ultrafast-computed tomographic regurgitant fraction/volume. In this study, several Doppler indices of the severity of aortic regurgitation (AR) were compared with ultrafast-computed tomographic (UFCT) regurgitant fraction or regurgitant volume [15]. No one Doppler method could be used as an absolute measure of AR severity. An integrated approach using multiple echocardiographic methods with the incorporation of clinical data is necessary to define fully the severity of AR in an individual patient. DAO—descending aorta; LVOT—left ventricular outflow tract; SEE—standard error of the estimate; TVI—time velocity integral. (*Adapted from* Nishimura and coworkers [15].)

Mitral Stenosis

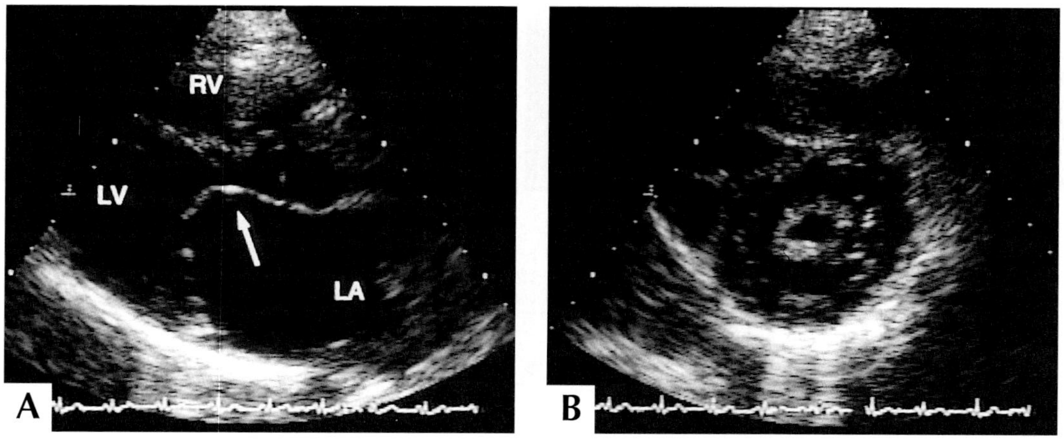

Figure 3-18. Echocardiography in the diagnosis of mitral stenosis (MS). Echocardiography is now the gold standard for the diagnosis of MS and for the determination of its severity. The diagnosis of MS is made by visualization of doming of the mitral valve leaflets in a "hockey-stick" deformity (*arrow*) on the parasternal long-axis view (**A**) and a "fish-mouth" appearance of the leaflets on the parasternal short-axis view (**B**). In addition to the diagnosis, two-dimensional echocardiography aids in the evaluation of the morphology of the mitral valve apparatus, which has important implications for therapy.

Several valve scoring systems have been devised as a method to determine whether a patient is a suitable candidate for percutaneous mitral balloon valvuloplasty [21a]. One system assigns a score of one to four for valve thickening, valve mobility, valve calcification, and subvalvular fusion, with one being the mildest and four being the most severe. The four scores are summed for a total score. A score of eight or less is predictive of excellent acute results, low risk of complications, and a low restenosis rate. This score is an objective echocardiographic measurement that indicates pliability of the mitral valve similar to the findings of a loud first heart sound and opening snap on physical examination. In this patient, the valve score is five. The degree of commissural involvement has also been shown to be predictive of the acute results of valvuloplasty [22]. LA—left atrium; LV—left ventricle; RV—right ventricle.

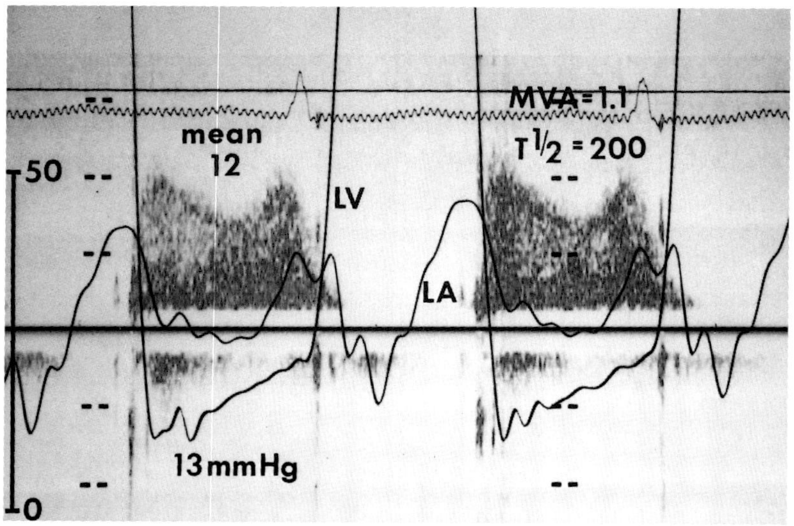

Figure 3-19. Continuous-wave velocity curve in mitral stenosis (MS). The continuous-wave velocity curve across the mitral valve provides an accurate measurement of the mean mitral gradient in patients with MS [23]. As opposed to the measurement of a mean aortic valve gradient, the measurement of the mean mitral valve gradient by Doppler ultrasound is simple to obtain from a technical standpoint. Thus a Doppler-derived mitral gradient is reliable and actually provides a more accurate measurement than conventional cardiac catheterization using pulmonary capillary wedge pressure [4]. Shown are the simultaneous pressure curves from direct left atrial (LA) and left ventricular (LV) measurements and the simultaneous mitral flow velocity curve in a patient with MS. There is an excellent correlation between the catheter-derived mean gradient of 13 mm Hg and the Doppler-derived mean gradient of 12 mm Hg. The mitral valve area (MVA) of 1.1 cm^2 is calculated from the diastolic half time ($t_{1/2}$), as described in Fig. 3-20. Doppler ultrasound can also be used to assess pulmonary pressures and the presence of coexistent mitral regurgitation in the patient with MS. (*Adapted from* Nishimura and Tajik [4]; with permission.)

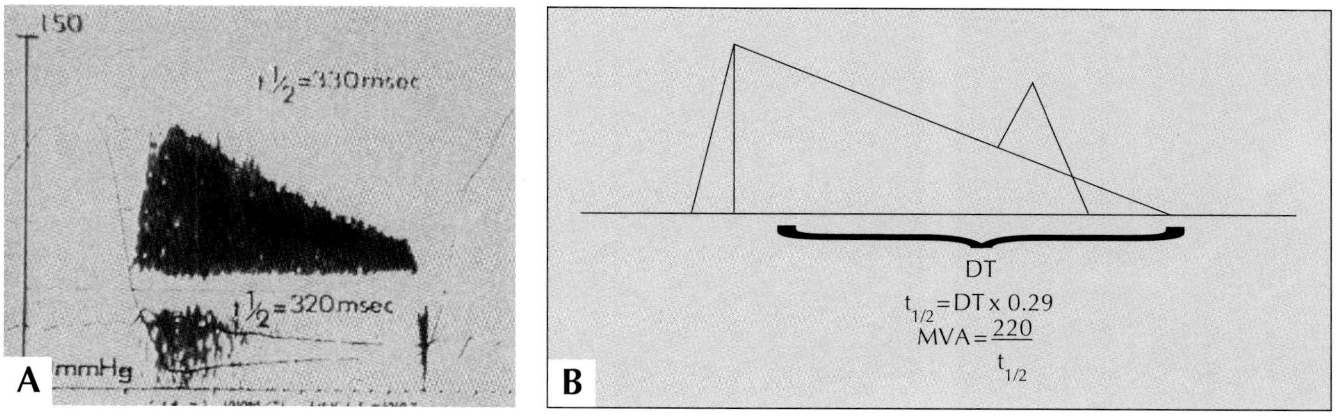

FIGURE 3-20. Diastolic half-time in estimating the severity of mitral stenosis (MS). The diastolic half time ($t_{1/2}$) is an indirect measurement of the severity of MS by reflecting the relative changes in left atrial (LA) and left ventricular (LV) pressure during diastole [24]. **A,** Simultaneous transmitral Doppler velocity curve and dual-catheter tracings (LV and pulmonary capillary wedge pressure). The diastolic $t_{1/2}$ of 330 ms measured by Doppler ultrasound correlates well with the $t_{1/2}$ of 320 ms measured by cardiac catheterization. **B,** Measurement of diastolic $t_{1/2}$ from the transmitral Doppler velocity curve can be obtained by multiplying the deceleration time (DT; time for the velocity curve to fall from its peak initial velocity to baseline) by 0.29. An independent measurement of mitral valve area (MVA) can be obtained from the Doppler-derived diastolic $t_{1/2}$ by dividing $t_{1/2}$ into a constant of 220 [25]. The diastolic $t_{1/2}$ is dependent on LV and LA compliance in addition to the severity of the obstruction and should not be used when chamber compliance changes rapidly, such as immediately after percutaneous balloon valvuloplasty or surgical commissurotomy, or when there are severe baseline abnormalities of LV compliance [26]. In these instances, the continuity principle can be applied to determination of MVA in a similar manner to that used for determination of aortic valve area [27]. (Part A *adapted from* Nishimura and Tajik [4]; with permission.)

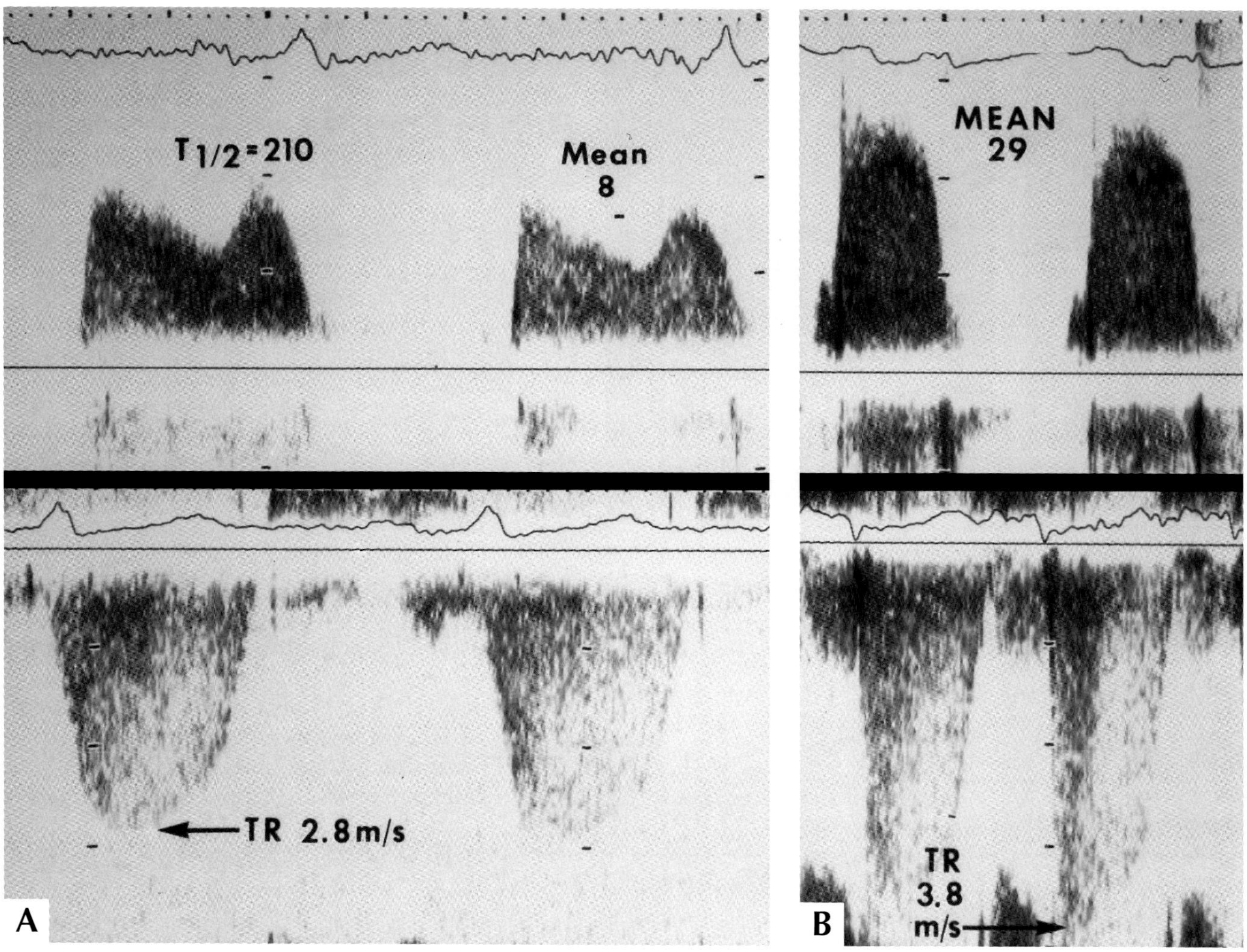

FIGURE 3-21. Doppler exercise studies. In some patients the results of the resting Doppler studies do not correlate with the symptoms. In these instances, it is useful to perform Doppler exercise studies, either with supine bicycle or upright treadmill. The change in the mean mitral gradient, as well as the pulmonary pressure (estimated from the tricuspid regurgitation [TR] peak velocity) in response to exercise, provides valuable clinical information. **A,** The resting mitral flow velocity curve (*top*) and TR signal (*bottom*) in a patient with significant limitation of activity. The mean transmitral gradient of 8 mm Hg and the mildly elevated TR velocity of 2.8 m/sec compatible with only a "moderate" degree of mitral stenosis. **B,** With graded exercise to a low workload, there is a significant increase in mean gradient to 29 mm Hg (*top*) and elevation of TR regurgitation velocity to 3.8 m/sec (*bottom*), indicating that the degree of stenosis is significant enough to produce symptoms in this patient. (*Adapted from* Nishimura and Tajik [4]; with permission.)

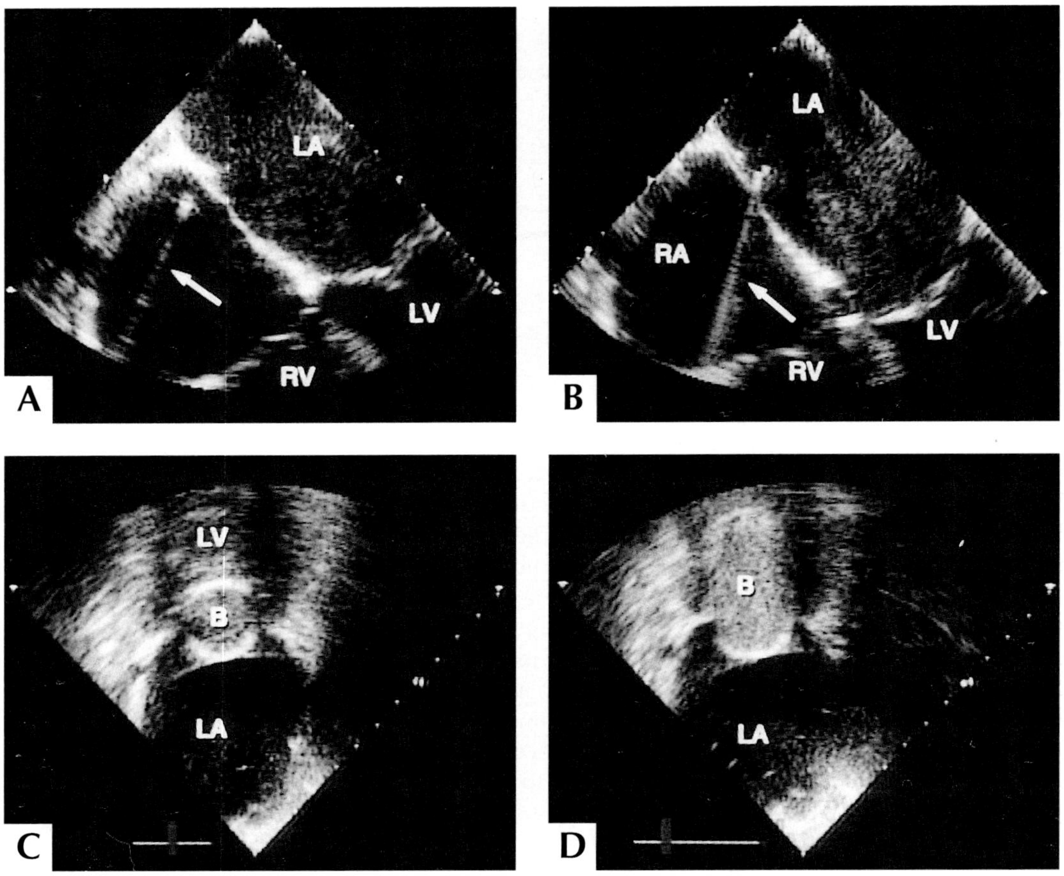

FIGURE 3-22. Transesophageal echocardiography (TEE) for percutaneous mitral balloon valvuloplasty (PMBV). TEE is useful in the patient undergoing PMBV [28]. It is performed in most patients who are deemed candidates for PMBV prior to the procedure to rule out left atrial (LA) thrombus and significant mitral regurgitation, which may not be detected by precordial echocardiography. TEE may also be used in guiding the transseptal puncture. **A,** TEE image during attempted transseptal puncture showing the needle (*arrow*) is posterior and superior to the fossa ovalis. **B,** The transseptal needle (*arrow*) has been properly positioned and now crosses the region of the fossa ovalis. TEE may also guide the position of the balloon during inflation. **C** and **D,** Sequential TEE still-frame images during inflation of an Inoue balloon (B) properly positioned across the mitral valve. LV—left ventricle; RA—right atrium; RV—right ventricle.

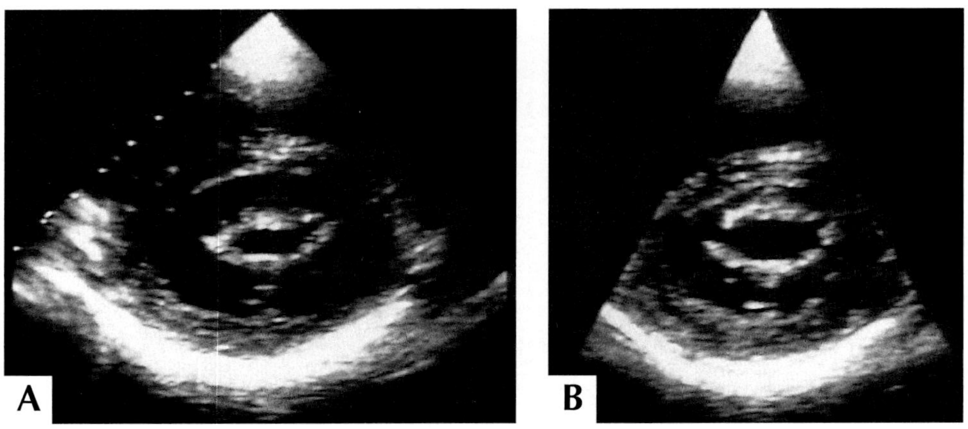

FIGURE 3-23. Effect of percutaneous mitral balloon valvuloplasty on stenotic mitral valve. The mechanism of percutaneous mitral balloon valvuloplasty (PMBV) involves splitting of fused commissures similar to the mechanism of surgical commissurotomy [29]. **A,** Parasternal short-axis view of a stenotic mitral valve before PMBV shows fusion of the posteromedial and anterolateral commissures. **B,** After the mitral valvuloplasty, both commissures have had an increase in the angle of opening, and mitral valve area (MVA) increases from 1.1 to 2.2 cm^2. (*Adapted from* Nishimura [29a]; with permission.)

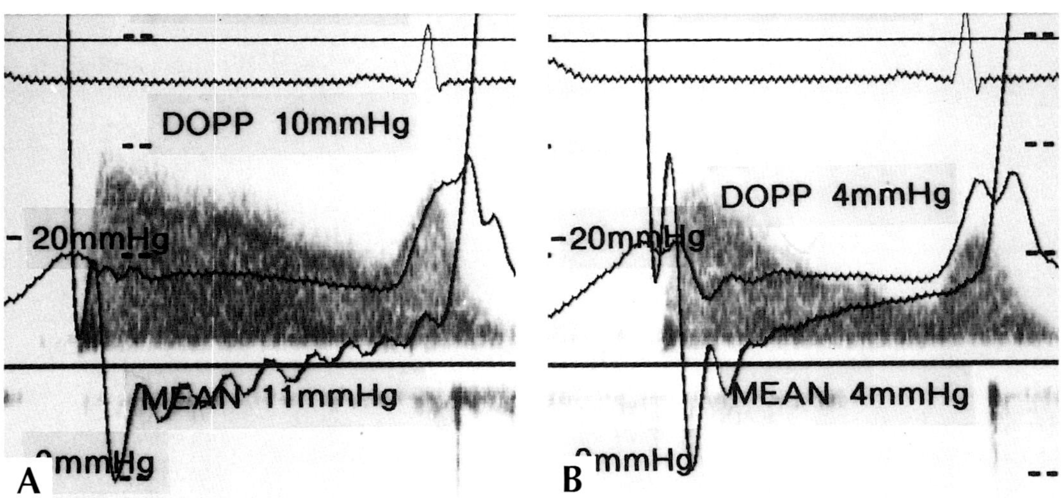

FIGURE 3-24. Percutaneous mitral balloon valvuloplasty (PMBV) can produce a decrease in gradient similar to that of surgical commissurotomy in selected patients. Simultaneous transmitral Doppler velocity curves and left ventricular/left atrial (LV/LA) pressure from an individual patient before (**A**) and after (**B**) PMBV. The mean LV/LA gradient by cardiac catheterization of 11 mm Hg before and 4 mm Hg after the PMBV matches the mean Doppler (DOPP) gradient of 10 mm Hg and 4 mm Hg.

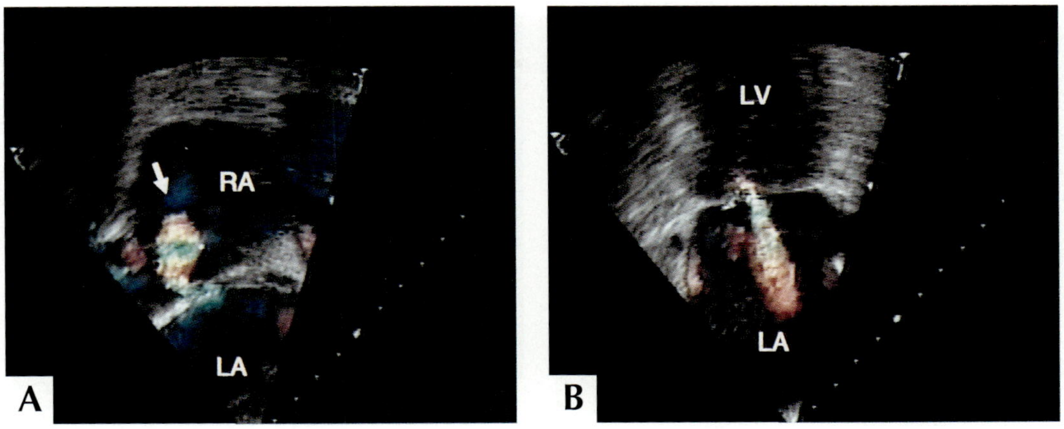

FIGURE 3-25. Transesophageal echocardiography (TEE) following percutaneous mitral balloon valvuloplasty (PMBV). Following PMBV, there is usually a small left-to-right shunt (**A**), as well as mitral regurgitation (**B**), detected by TEE. The majority of the small atrial septal defects (*arrow* in *A*) will close spontaneously over time. LA—left atrium; LV—left ventricle; RA—right atrium.

MITRAL REGURGITATION

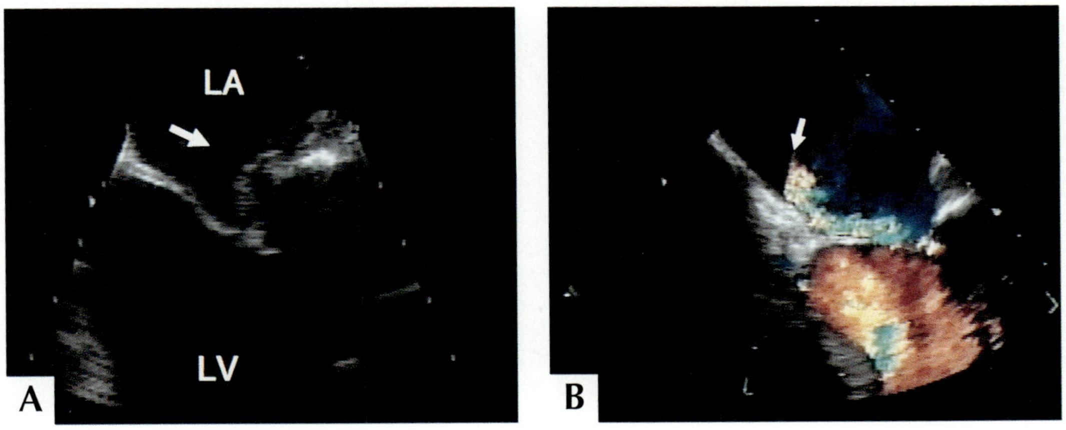

FIGURE 3-26. Evaluation of mitral regurgitation (MR). Echocardiography plays an important role in the evaluation of the patient with MR. The response of the left ventricle (LV) to the long-standing volume overload can be evaluated on serial noninvasive studies. The effect of the MR on left atrial (LA) size and the pulmonary circulation can be assessed. A semiquantitative assessment of the severity of MR can be provided by several methods (vide infra). In the era of mitral valve repair, the etiology of the MR is important for clinical decisions regarding time of valve operation.

Two-dimensional echocardiography is the diagnostic modality of choice in determining the etiology of the MR, which can be at the level of the valve, the supporting chordal apparatus, the papillary muscle, or the mitral annulus. **A,** The most common etiology of isolated MR in the 1990s is mitral valve prolapse, which can be diagnosed on two-dimensional echocardiography as thickened mitral leaflets with systolic blowing (*arrow*) into the LA. **B,** Color-flow Doppler with mitral valve prolapse demonstrates an eccentric jet. In the presence of posterior leaflet prolapse, there is an anteriorly directed regurgitant jet (*arrow*) that courses along the medial aspect of the LA. Valve repair can usually be performed in over 95% of posterior leaflet prolapses and over 80% of anterior leaflet prolapses if there is no heavy calcification of the mitral annulus [30].

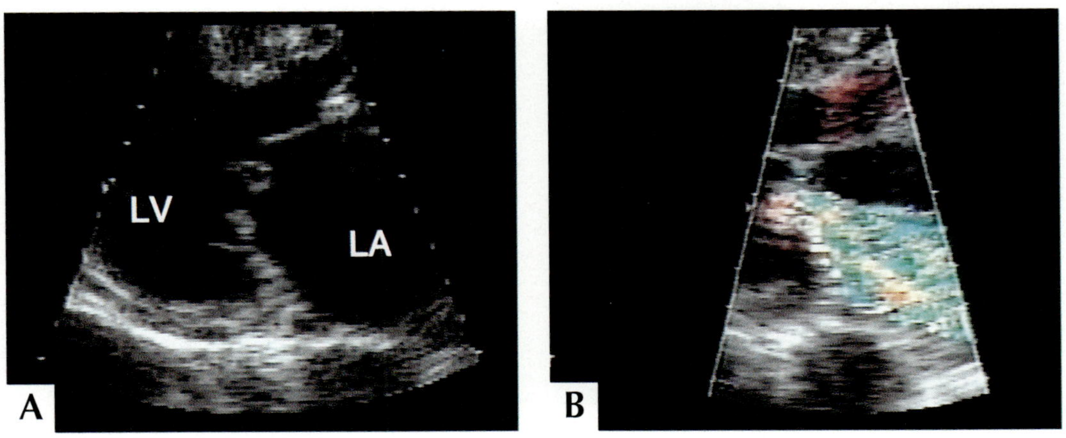

FIGURE 3-27. Rheumatic valve disease. Rheumatic valve disease is another etiology of mitral regurgitation and will appear as calcified, poorly mobile mitral valve leaflets on two-dimensional echocardiography (**A**). A central regurgitant jet will be present on color-flow imaging (**B**). LA—left atrium; LV—left ventricle.

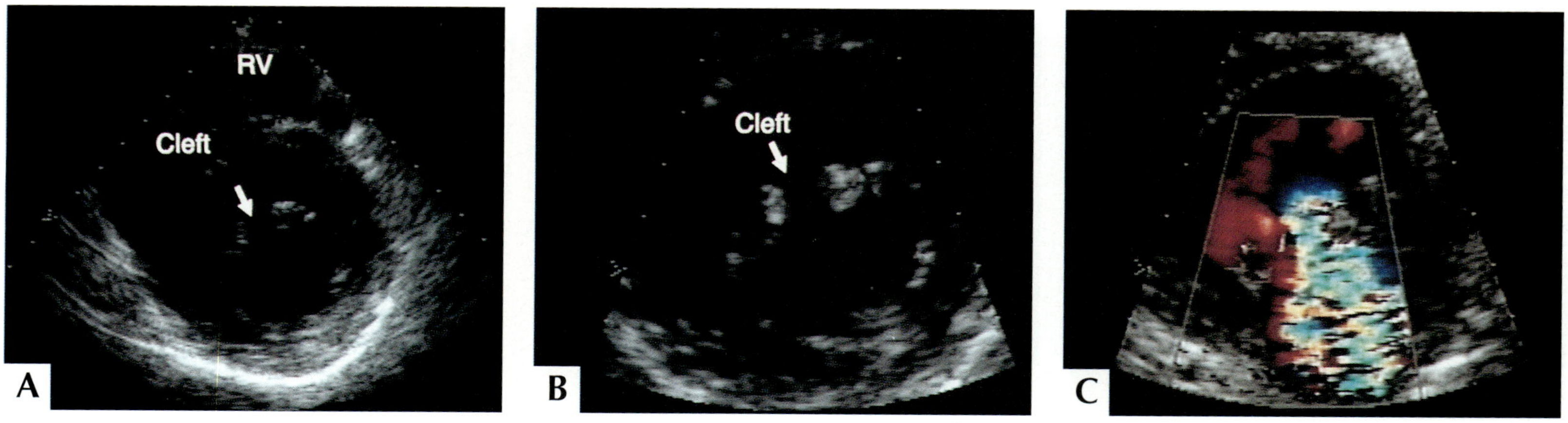

FIGURE 3-28. Cleft mitral valve. A cleft mitral valve is an unusual form of regurgitation in the adult. The cleft of an anterior leaflet can be seen on two-dimensional echocardiography (*arrows*) in the parasternal short-axis view (**A** and **B**). **C,** On color-flow imaging, the regurgitant jet can be seen to emanate from the area of the cleft itself. A cleft mitral valve leaflet is part of an atrioventricular canal defect and is associated frequently with a primum atrial septal defect and an inflow ventricular septal defect. RV—right ventricle.

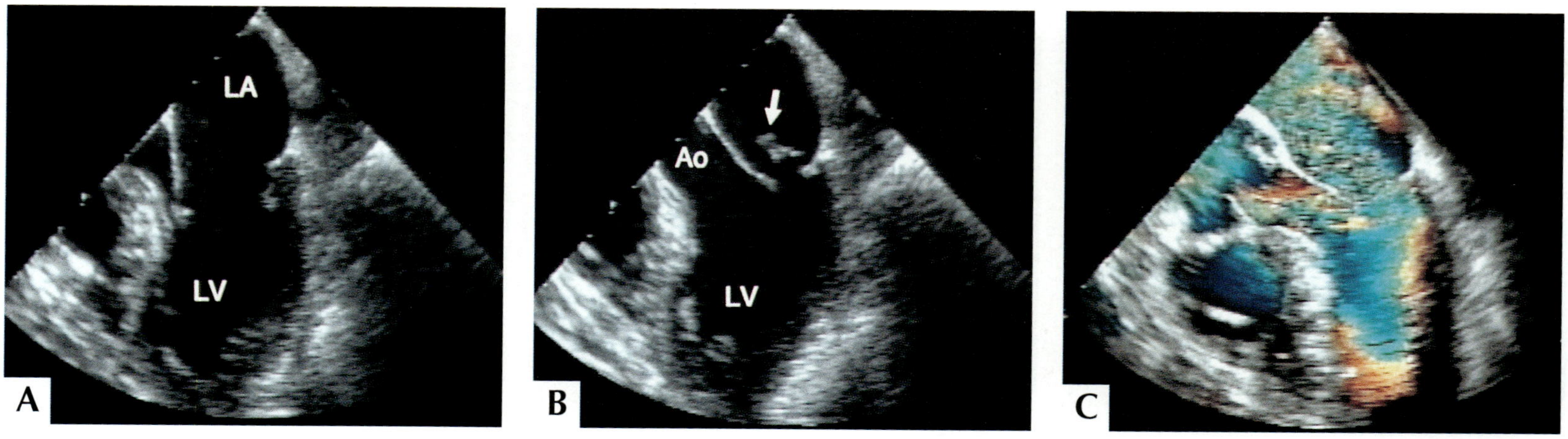

FIGURE 3-29. Rupture of the mitral chords. Severe acute mitral regurgitation can occur secondary to loss of the supporting mitral valve apparatus. In the setting of a myocardial infarction, this is usually due to a rupture of the posteromedial papillary muscle. A rupture of the mitral chord(s) may occur spontaneously but is usually associated with the redundant chords seen with a floppy mitral valve. On two-dimensional echocardiography, the mitral valve leaflet motion opens normally in diastole (**A**), but in systole, there is loss of coaptation and severe prolapse of the mitral valve leaflets into the left atrium (LA) (**B**). Frequently, the ruptured chord can be seen (*arrow*). On color-flow imaging, there is turbulence in the entire LA during systole (**C**). Ao—aorta; LV—left ventricle.

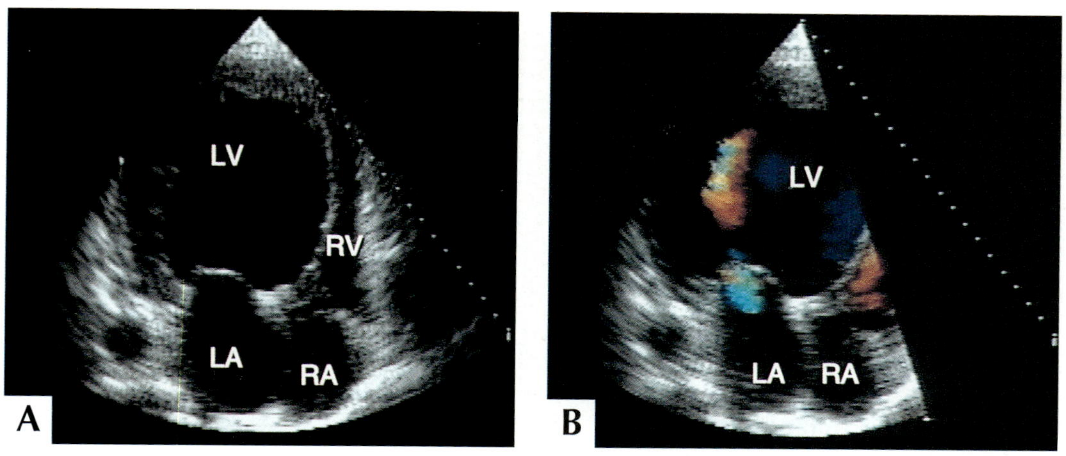

FIGURE 3-30. Mitral regurgitation (MR) due to annular dilatation. A common etiology of MR is annular dilatation, usually from an ischemic or idiopathic dilated cardiomyopathy. This form of MR will appear on echocardiography as structurally normal mitral valve leaflets (**A**) and a central jet of regurgitation on color-flow imaging (**B**). LA—left atrium; LV—left ventricle; RA—right atrium; RV—right ventricle.

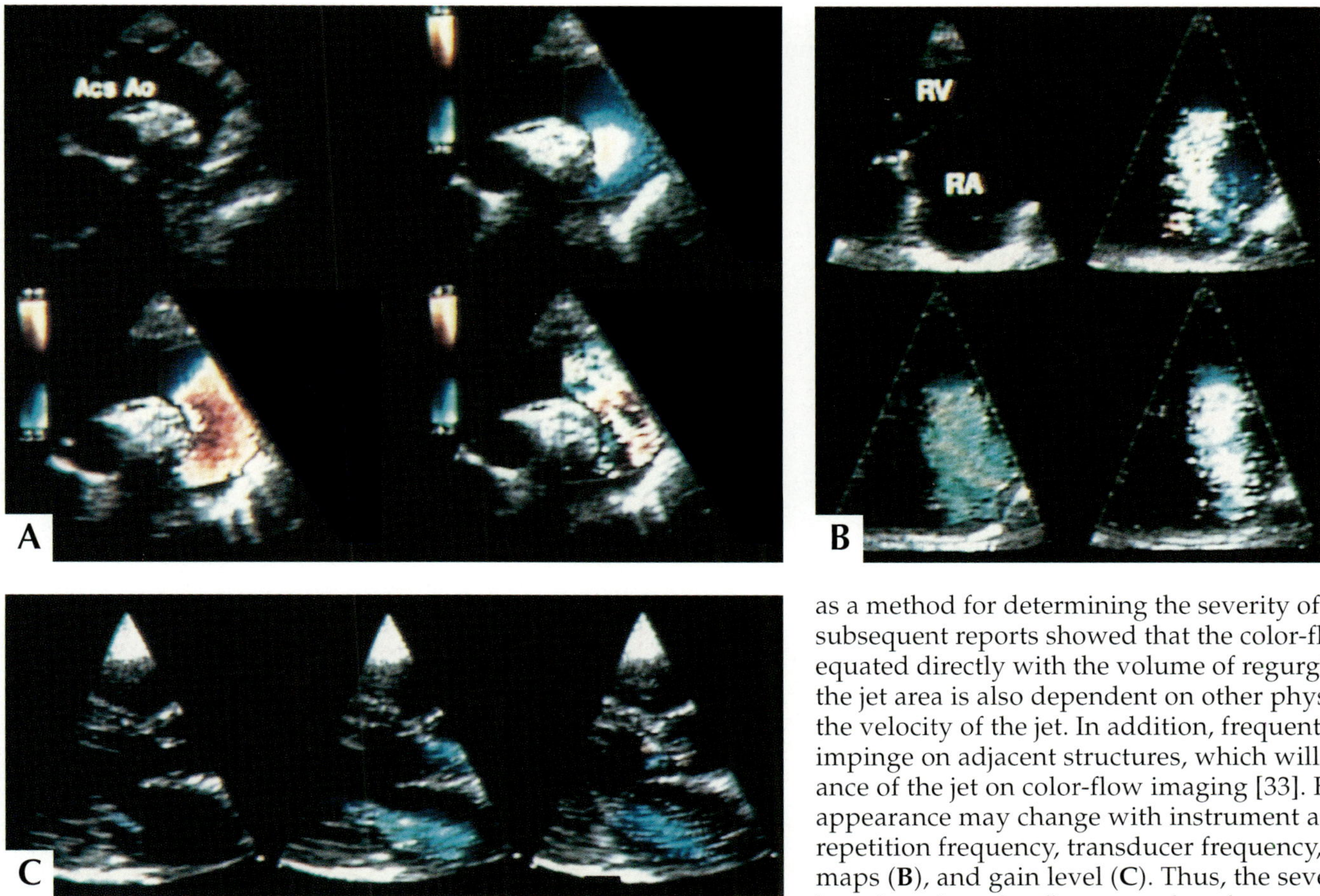

FIGURE 3-31. Determination of severity of mitral regurgitation (MR). It is difficult to determine the exact severity of MR on echocardiography. Two-dimensional echocardiographic findings that suggest severe MR include a dilated hyperdynamic left ventricle or a flail mitral valve leaflet. Indirect clues to the severity of MR include the continuous-wave Doppler mitral regurgitation jet intensity, the initial mitral inflow velocity, the contour of the continuous-wave Doppler MR velocity curve, and interruption of pulmonary venous flow (vide infra). The area or extent of the jet into the left atrium on color-flow imaging was initially proposed as a method for determining the severity of MR [31]. However, subsequent reports showed that the color-flow jet area cannot be equated directly with the volume of regurgitation [32], because the jet area is also dependent on other physical factors such as the velocity of the jet. In addition, frequently eccentric jets impinge on adjacent structures, which will decrease the appearance of the jet on color-flow imaging [33]. Finally, the jet area appearance may change with instrument adjustments in pulse repetition frequency, transducer frequency, filter setting (**A**), color maps (**B**), and gain level (**C**). Thus, the severity of MR cannot be based on the color-flow area alone but must be a culmination of all information provided by the clinical setting, two-dimensional echocardiographic findings, the color-flow jet, and the indirect Doppler findings, which are discussed in Figs. 3-32 through 3-36. In experienced laboratories, a regurgitant fraction or volume can be calculated from volumetric flow rates [16]. Newer techniques such as amplitude-weighted continuous-wave signal intensity [34] and proximal isovelocity surface areas [35] show promise as future methods of further quantitating the severity of MR. Asc Ao—ascending aorta; RA—right atrium; RV—right ventricle.

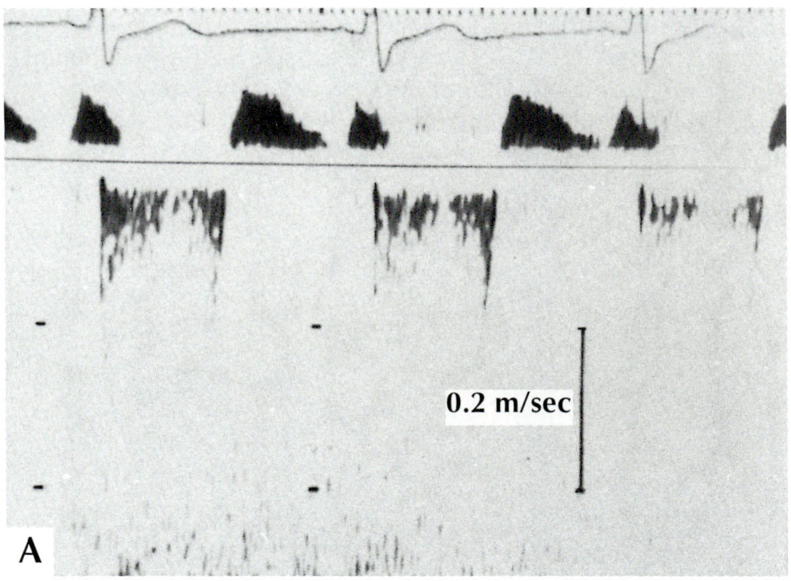

FIGURE 3-32. Doppler signal in the determination of severity of mitral regurgitation (MR). The signal strength of the continuous-wave MR Doppler signal is proportional to the number of erythrocytes in the regurgitant jet [36]. Although certain investigational instruments can perform objective measurements of the continuous-wave intensity [34], a subjective estimation of the regurgitation severity can be made from the MR spectral display. Mild MR will produce a faint continuous-wave regurgitant signal (**A**). *(continued)*

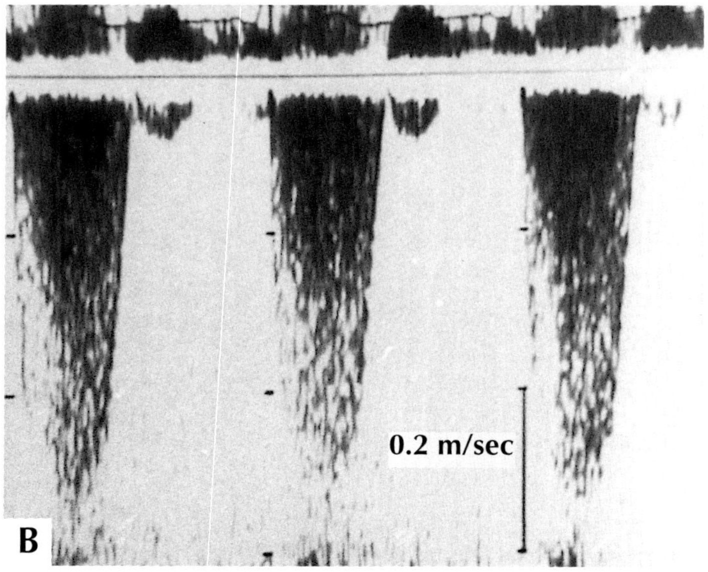

FIGURE 3-32. (*continued*) This is in contrast with the dense continuous-wave signal of severe MR (**B**).

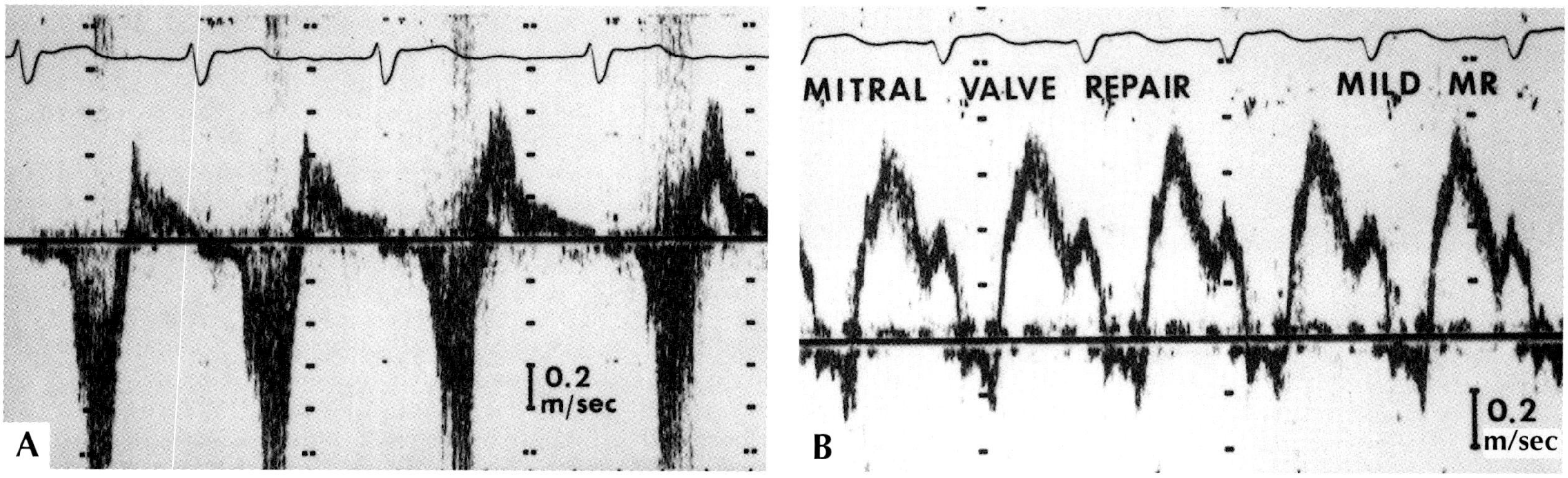

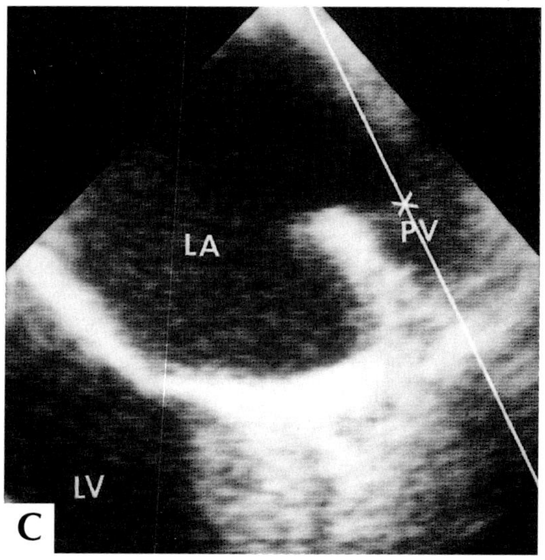

FIGURE 3-33. Pulsed-wave sampling for mitral regurgitation (MR). An indirect measure of the severity of MR can be made from pulsed-wave sampling of the pulmonary venous inflow [37]. The normal pulmonary vein velocity curve consists of a systolic and a diastolic forward flow velocity. **A,** In the presence of severe MR, there is reversal of the systolic forward flow. **B,** After valve repair, the systolic forward flow returns. Although pulmonary venous flow velocities can be obtained in nearly 80% of patients by the transthoracic approach, transesophageal echocardiography (TEE) allows interrogation of pulmonary venous flow in 99% of patients. **C,** The left upper pulmonary vein is the easiest site to sample using TEE. The systolic forward flow is dependent on other factors than just the severity of MR, such as jet direction, left atrial (LA) size, LA compliance, ventricular function, and LA systolic function. LV—left ventricle; PV—pulmonary vein. (*Adapted from* Freeman and coworkers [30]; with permission.)

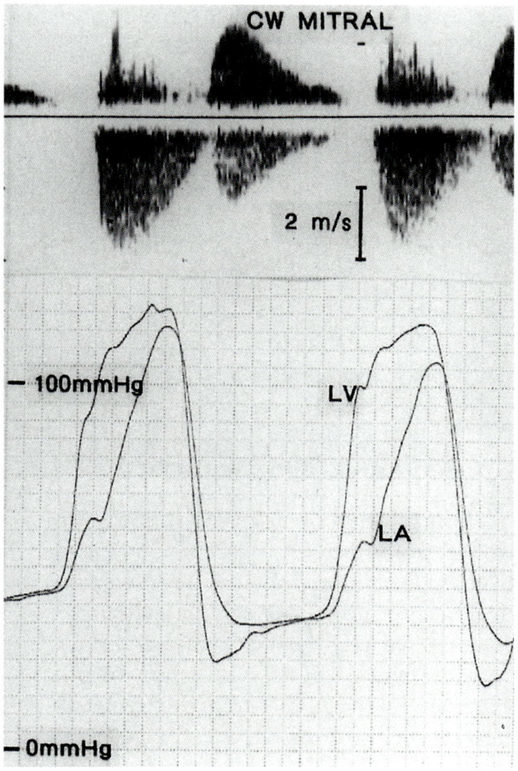

Figure 3-34. Doppler velocity in severe acute mitral regurgitation (MR). The continuous-wave (CW) Doppler velocity curve reflects the instantaneous pressure gradient between the left atrium (LA) and left ventricle (LV) during systole. Shown is the simultaneous MR Doppler velocity curve and LA/LV pressure curves in a patient with severe acute MR. There is a large *v* wave on the LA pressure, which is seen as a "cutoff" sign on the downslope of the continuous-wave Doppler velocity curve. There is also a relatively low peak velocity (<4 m/sec), indicating the combination of a high LA pressure and a low systemic pressure. (*Adapted from* Nishimura [37a]; with permission.)

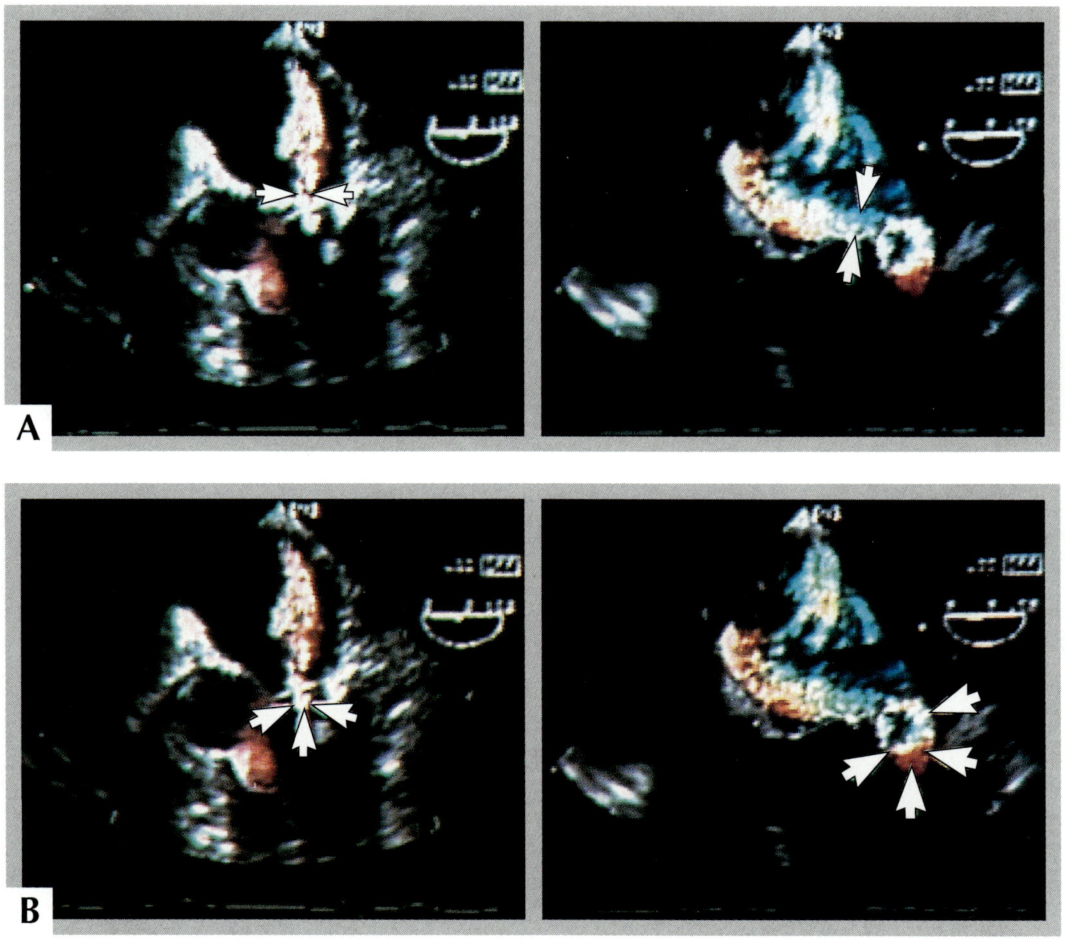

Figure 3-35. Transesophageal echocardiography (TEE) in mitral regurgitation (MR). TEE from two patients with MR and similar color-flow MR jet areas. **A,** The patient in the *left panel* has mild MR, and the patient in the *right panel* has severe MR. The jet width at its origin (*arrows*) may help in further determining the severity of regurgitation [38]. **B,** These panels outline the proximal isovelocity surface area (PISA), a promising new method of quantitating the severity of MR. The volume of blood that passes through the regurgitant orifice is proportional to the hemispheric area of the flow acceleration proximal to the mitral valve, as seen on color-flow imaging at any given Nyquist limit [35]. The flow acceleration area can be subjectively assessed visually (*arrows*). The *left panel* shows a small flow acceleration area with mild MR, and the *right panel* shows a large flow acceleration area with severe MR.

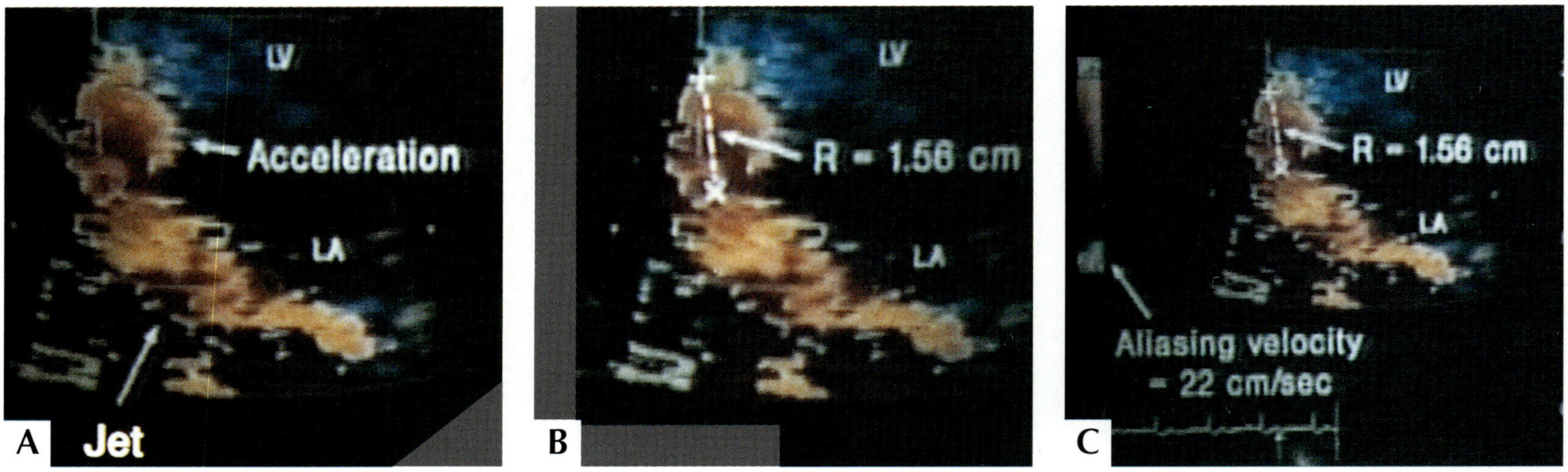

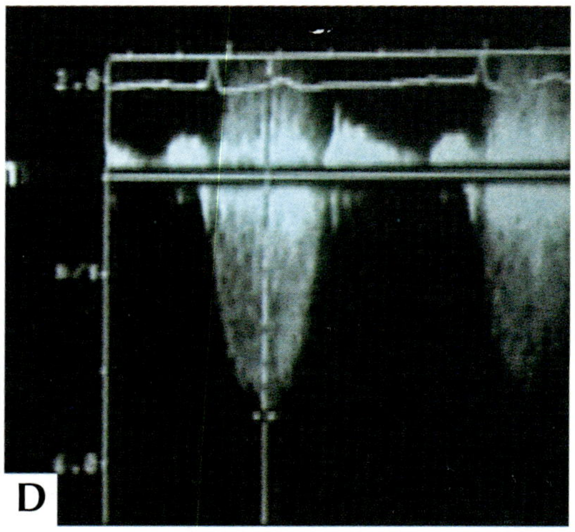

FIGURE 3-36. Proximal isovelocity surface area. A quantitative measurement of regurgitant flow and regurgitant orifice can be calculated from the proximal isovelocity surface area (PISA). **A**, After optimization of the two-dimensional image, the color-flow baseline is shifted downward to decrease the Nyquist limit on the color-flow imaging display. The aliasing velocity = 22 cm/sec. There will be an isovelocity surface area proximal to the regurgitant orifice formed by color aliasing at the Nyquist limit, which has the shape of a hemisphere. **B** and **C**, The radius (R) of the isovelocity hemisphere is measured to be 1.56 cm. Instantaneous flow rate is then calculated by multiplying the calculated area of the hemisphere ($2 \times \pi \times r^2$) by the Nyquist limit velocity (Vr): Flow $_{MR}$(mL/sec) = $6.28\ r^2 \times V_r$ (cm/sec). **D**, An effective regurgitant orifice area (ERO) can be calculated by dividing the peak velocity of the mitral regurgitation (MR) continuous-wave signal (V_{MR}) of 500 cm/sec (or 5 m/sec) into the flow of 336 mL/sec: ERO_{MR}(cm^2) = low_{MR} (mL/sec)/ V_{MR}(m/sec). The ERO_{ME}= 67 mm^2. Although standards are still evolving, severe MR is present with an ERO of greater than 40 mm^2. LA—left atrium; LV—left ventricle.

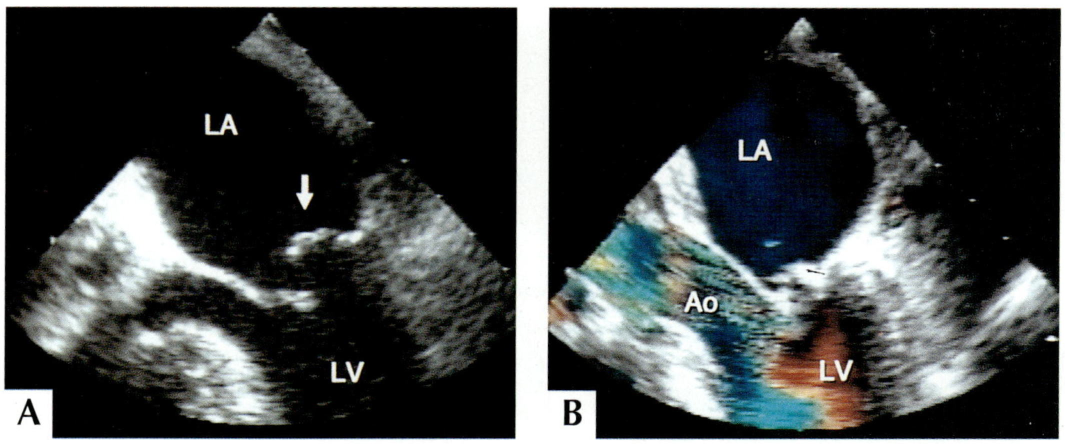

FIGURE 3-37. Transesophageal echocardiography (TEE). TEE is now becoming an integral part of the cardiac operating room. The TEE probe can be inserted before sternotomy, and images can be obtained throughout the operation without disturbing the operative field. The major value of intraoperatic echocardiography is during mitral valve repair [30]. TEE can identify the etiology of the (MR) before the operation (**A**—flail posterior leaflet [*arrow*]) and can assess the adequacy of the repair after the operation (**B**—plicated posterior leaflet with no MR seen on color-flow imaging). Complications such as residual MR, systolic anterior motion of the mitral valve, poor left ventricular (LV) function, and right ventricular failure can be identified [30]. Intraoperative TEE is also used for evaluation of the results of myectomy in patients with hypertrophic cardiomyopathy following LV function and regional wall abnormalities in high-risk coronary artery disease patients, aiding in surgical removal of intracardiac masses, and guiding surgical therapy in aortic dissection. Ao—aorta; LA—left atrium.

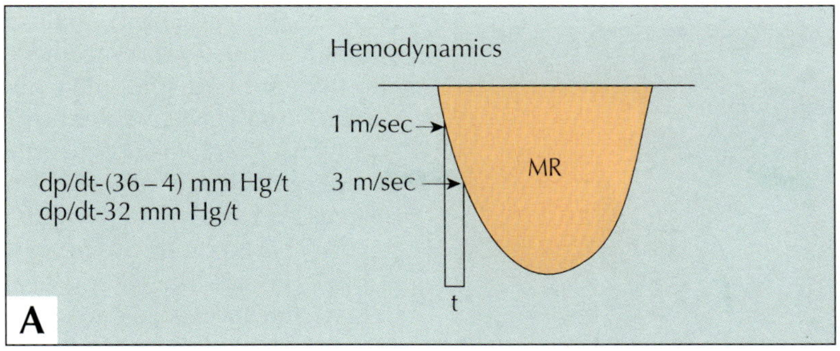

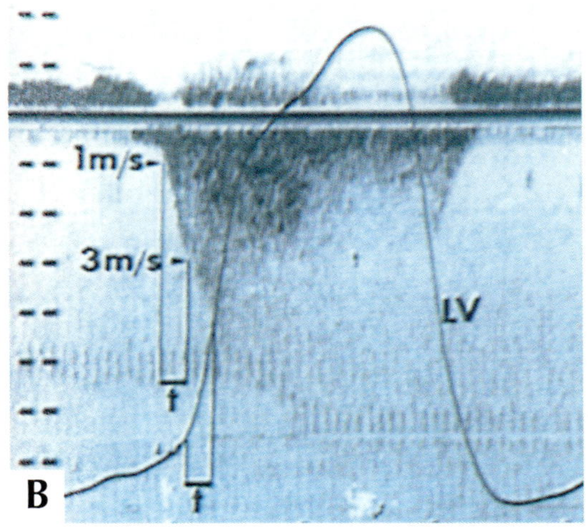

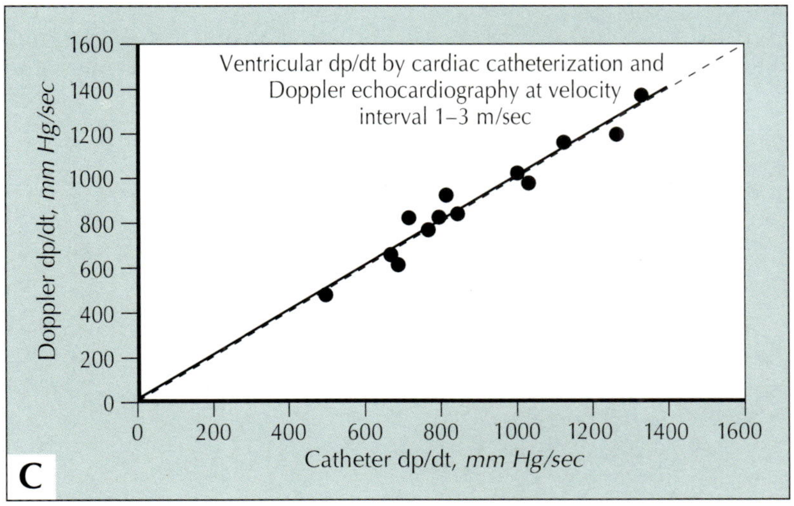

FIGURE 3-38. Doppler velocity curve for mitral regurgitation (MR). The MR continuous-wave Doppler velocity curve contains valuable information about left ventricular (LV) function. The Doppler velocity represents the instantaneous gradient between the LV and left atrium [19]. If left atrial pressure is assumed to be constant during systole, a reconstruction of the LV pressure curve can be derived by application of the modified Bernoulli equation. The peak positive LV dp/dt can be derived from the ascending limb of the mitral regurgitation velocity curve (**A**), by measuring the time interval between 1 and 3 m/sec. This time interval (t) is divided into the pressure difference between 1 and 3 m/sec (32 mm Hg) to obtain the rate of pressure rise. The measured "t" by Doppler ultrasound correlates well with that obtained by high-fidelity measurements of LV pressure (**B**). **C,** There is an excellent correlation between the ratio of change of ventricular pressure to change in time (dp/dt) between the two methods [39]. The dp/dt calculated from Doppler velocity curves in patients with severe MR has been shown to be predictive of postoperative LV function following mitral valve operation independent of LV size and function [40]. The same concept can also be applied to the descending limb of the MR curve for calculation of the time constant of relaxation in assessment of diastolic function [41]. (*Adapted from* Chung and coworkers [39]; with permission.)

TRICUSPID AND PULMONARY VALVE DISEASE

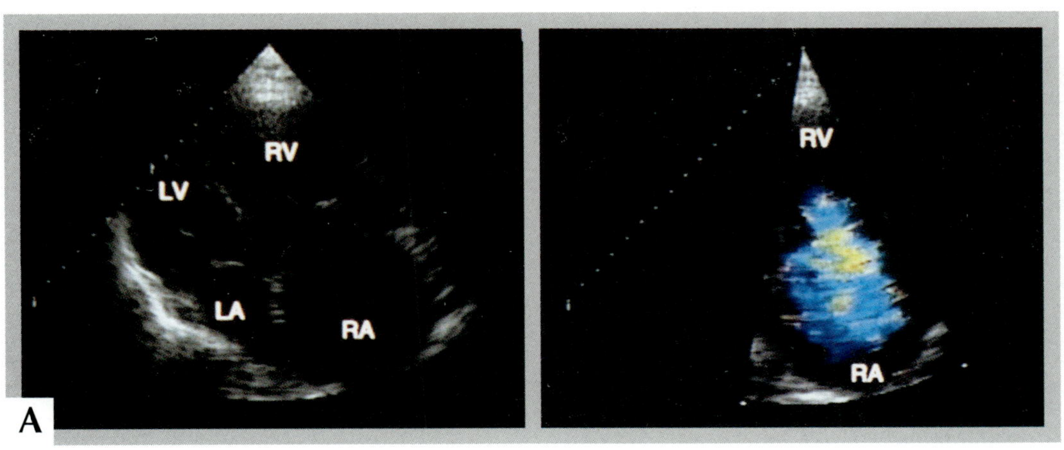

FIGURE 3-39. Doppler ultrasound of tricuspid regurgitation (TR). TR is a common valvular lesion. Mild degrees of TR as assessed by Doppler ultrasound are present in over 70% of normal subjects. Pathologic TR can be seen in the presence of elevated pulmonary artery pressures of intrinsic disease of the tricuspid valve or annulus. **A,** Apical four-chamber view showing TR from rheumatic involvement of the valve. (*continued*)

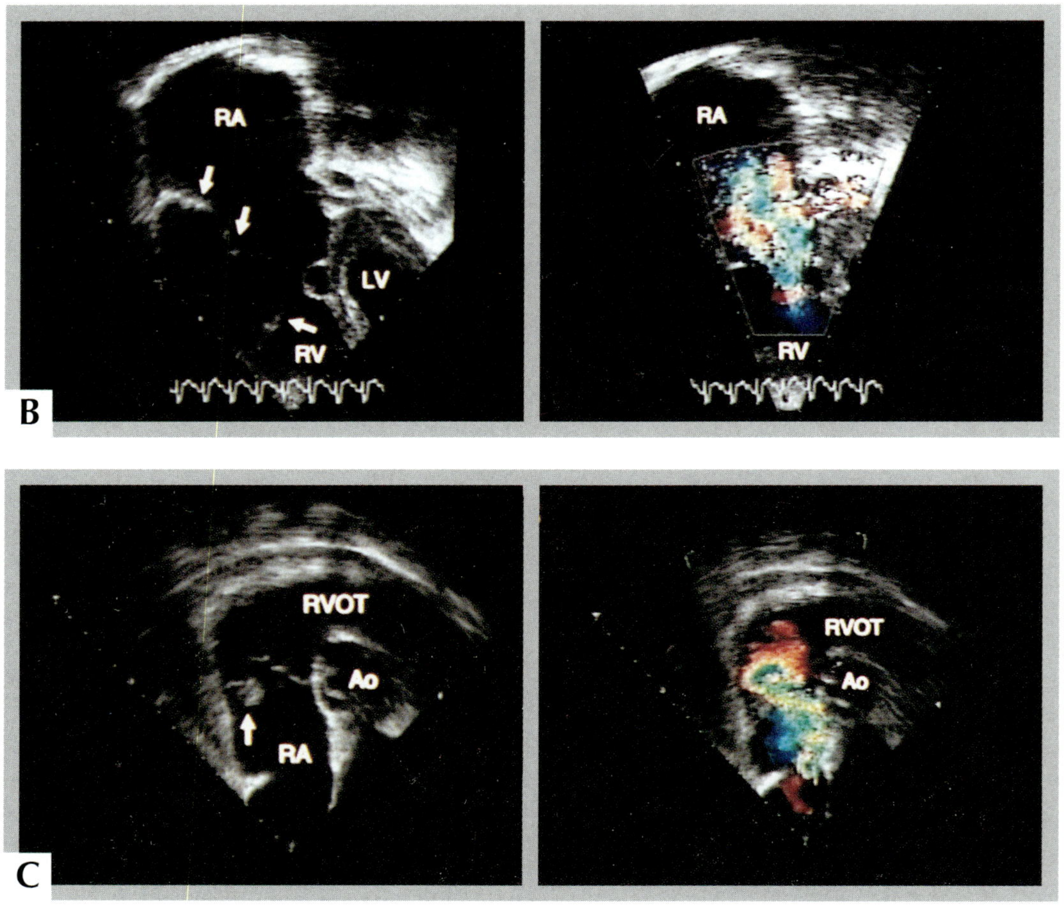

FIGURE 3-39. (*continued*) **B,** Ebstein's anomaly is due to displacement of a large and tethered tricuspid valve into the right ventricle (RV) (*arrows*). Two-dimensional echocardiography is the diagnostic modality of choice for the diagnosis of Ebstein's anomaly. The suitability for valve repair is based on the degree of tethering of the large sail-like anterior leaflet. **C,** Parasternal short-axis view shows severe TR from right-sided endocarditis with valvular vegetations (*arrow*). Ao–aorta; LA—left atrium; LV—left ventricle; RA—right atrium; RVOT—right ventricular outflow tract.

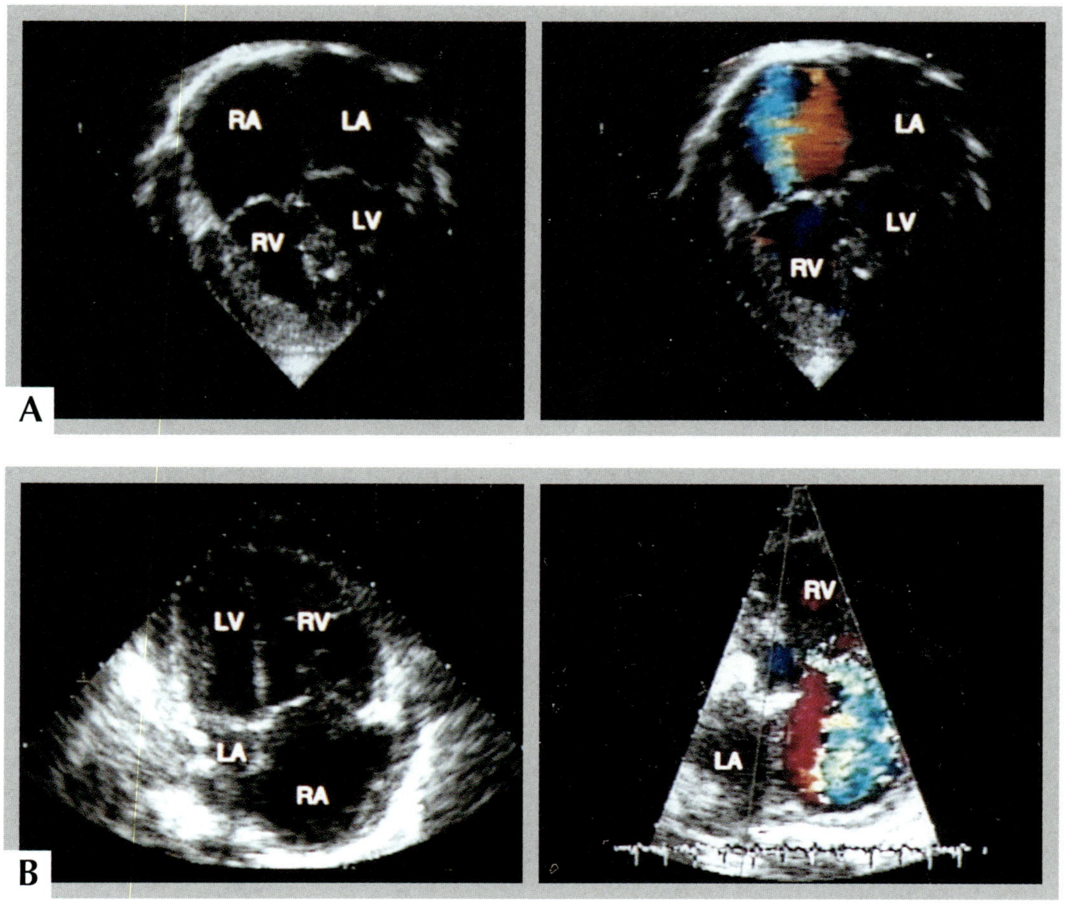

FIGURE 3-40. Doppler ultrasound tricuspid regurgitation (TR). **A,** Apex down four-chamber view demonstrates TR due to primary pulmonary hypertension. Severe right ventricular (RV) hypertrophy is present. **B,** Apex down four-chamber view demonstrates TR secondary to RV infarction. There is severe enlargement of both the RV and right atrium (RA). (*continued*)

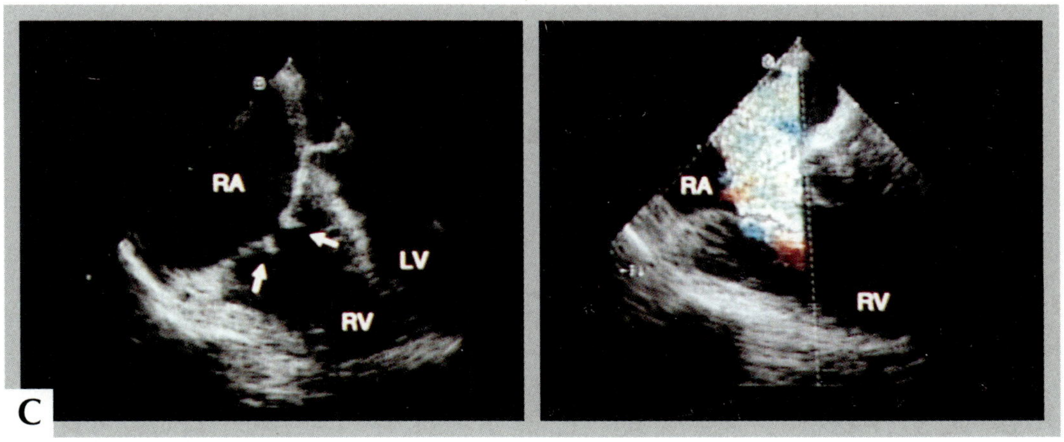

FIGURE 3-40. *(continued)* **C,** Systemic carcinoid syndrome will primarily affect the right-sided valves. The characteristic valve appearance is that of thickened, immobile leaflets with severe regurgitation of both the tricuspid and pulmonic valves (*arrows*) [42]. LA—left atrium; LV—left ventricle.

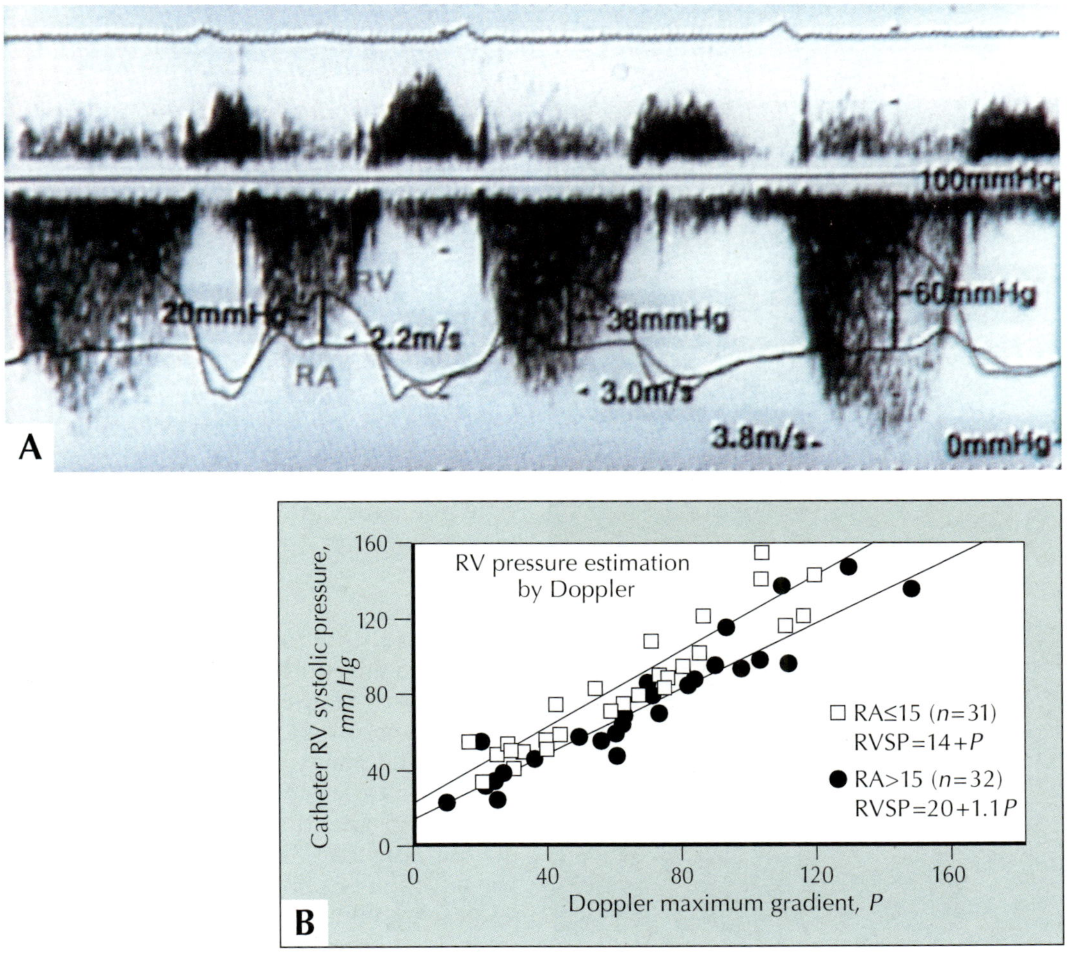

FIGURE 3-41. Right ventricular/right atrial pressure gradient. The tricuspid regurgitation (TR) peak systolic velocity can be used to calculate right ventricular (RV) systolic pressure (RVSP; and pulmonary artery systolic pressure in the absence of RV outflow obstruction) [43]. The modified Bernoulli equation can be applied to the peak TR peak velocity to obtain the peak gradient between the RV and right atrium (RA). **A,** Simultaneous continuous-wave TR velocity curves and RA and RV pressures. The peak velocities (in m/sec) can be converted to the simultaneous RV/RA pressure gradient (in mm Hg) on a beat-to-beat basis. **B,** An accurate, noninvasive estimate of the RVSP can be obtained from the Doppler-derived RV/RA gradient. Assumed RA pressures can be based on regression equations [43] but are best determined for an individual patient by examination of the inferior vena cava dynamics. P—mm Hg. (*Adapted from* Currie and coworkers [43]; with permission.)

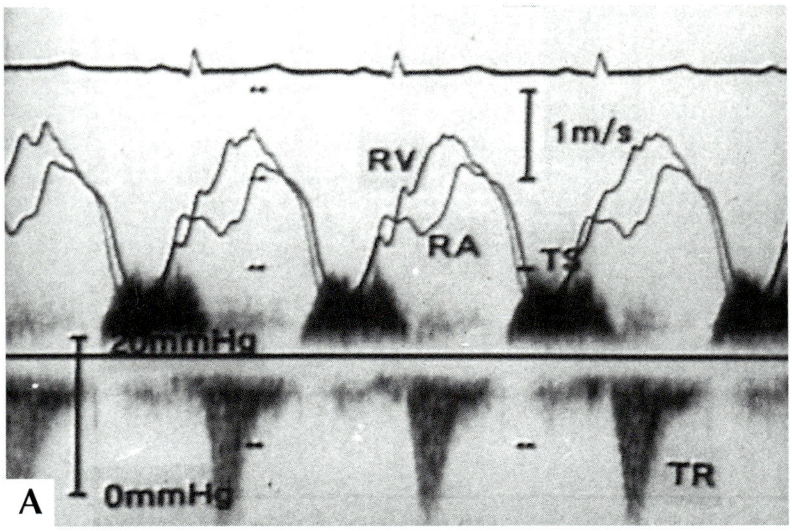

FIGURE 3-42. Severe tricuspid regurgitation (TR) in carcinoid heart disease. Simultaneous catheter-Doppler traces in the presence of severe TR, such as in this patient with carcinoid heart disease. **A,** Right ventricular (RV) and right atrial (RA) pressure tracings show large *v* waves with rapid systolic equalization of pressure. This is reflected in the continuous-wave Doppler velocity curves by a low velocity TR signal with an early systolic peak and rapid decline of velocity in mid-to-late systole. Tricuspid stenosis (TS) is also present. *(continued)*

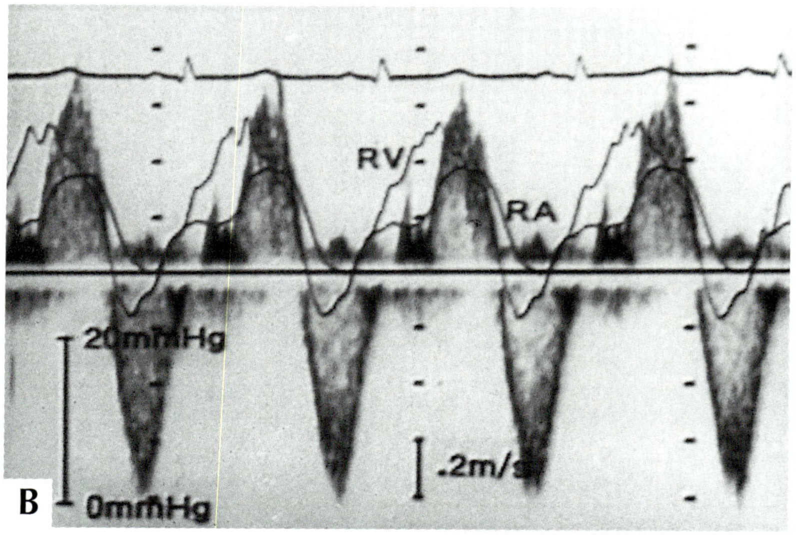

FIGURE 3-42. (*continued*) **B,** Pulsed-Doppler examination of the hepatic veins in the same patient shows prominent systolic reversals, indicating severe insufficiency. The simultaneous RV and RA pressures are shown. (*Adapted from* Nishimura and Tajik [4]; with permission.)

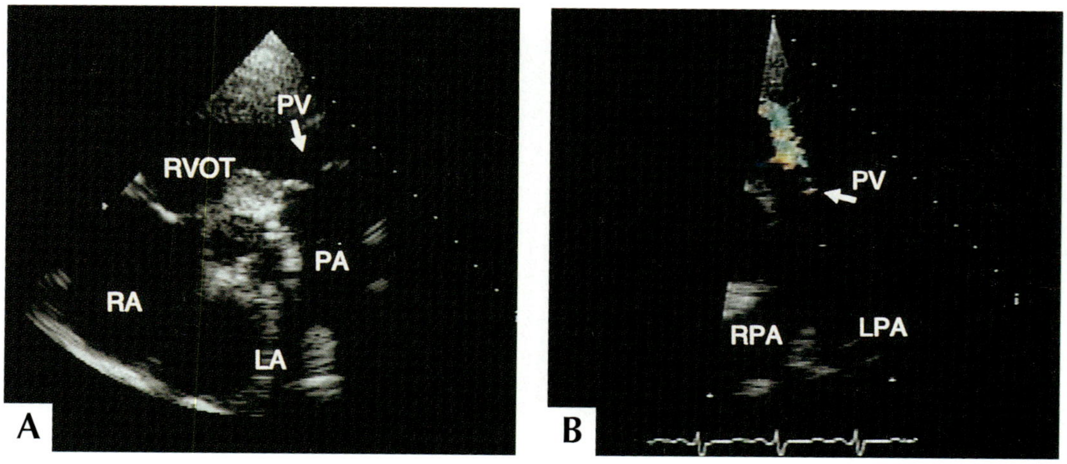

FIGURE 3-43. Pulmonary valve (PV) echocardiography. The examination of the pulmonary valve by echocardiography is technically more difficult than the other valves due to the limited acoustic windows that can be used. **A,** Parasternal short-axis view of a thickened PV in a patient with primary pulmonary hypertension. **B,** Color-flow imaging shows a characteristic pulmonary regurgitant jet during diastole. Doppler analysis of this jet can be used to estimate pulmonary artery (PA) pressure [44]. LA—left atrium; LPA—left pulmonary artery; RA—right atrium; RPA—right pulmonary artery; RVOT—right ventricular outflow tract.

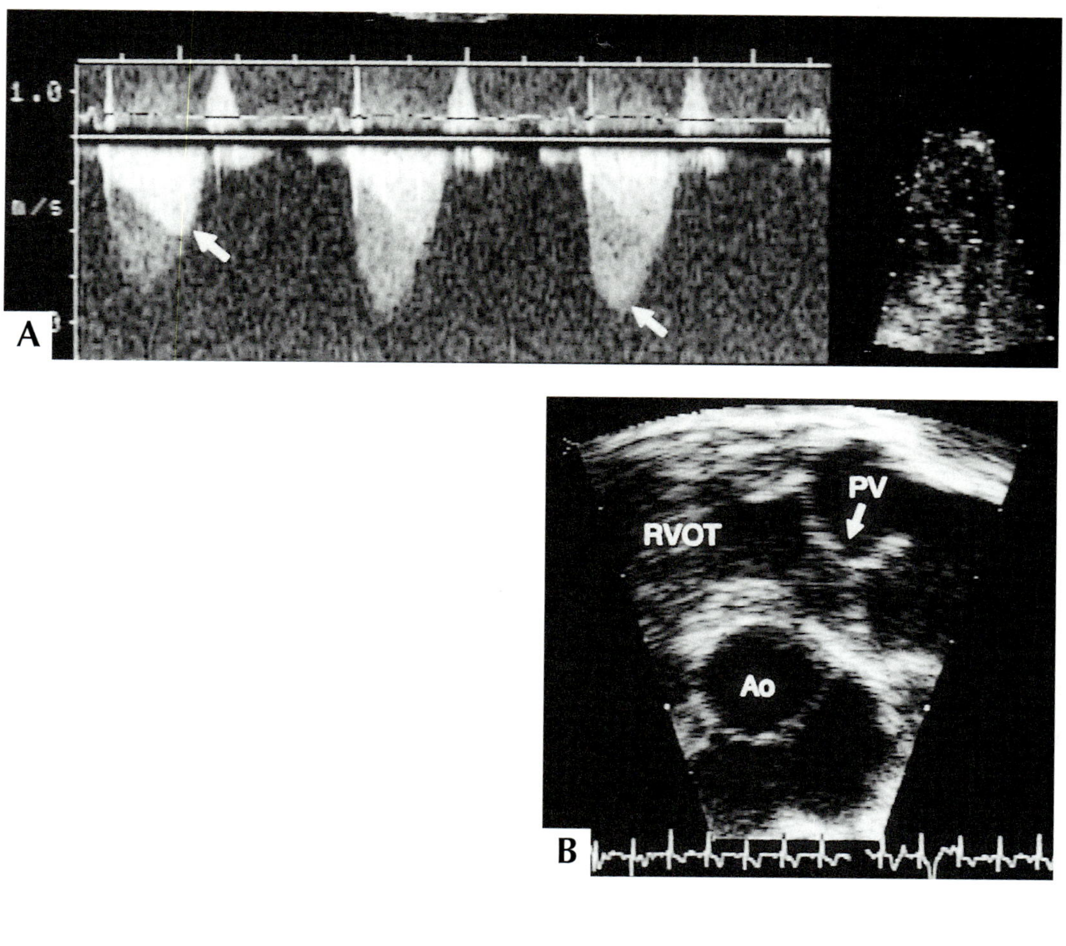

FIGURE 3-44. Pulmonic stenosis. Pulmonic stenosis in the adult is rare but is one of the causes of a loud murmur, in which a routine echocardiographic examination may not detect any obvious etiology. It may be necessary to repeat the examination with special attention to the right ventricular outflow tract (RVOT). **A,** Continuous-wave Doppler examination of a young adult with pulmonary valve (PV) stenosis. There is a high velocity jet of 3.8 m/sec (*arrow on the third beat*), indicating the presence of valvular stenosis. The Doppler profile also shows a late-peaking subvalvular velocity of 2 m/sec (*arrow on the first beat*). **B,** Horizontal transesophageal echocardiographic image of the RVOT shows subvalvular hypertrophy secondary to the calcified and stenotic PV. Ao—aorta.

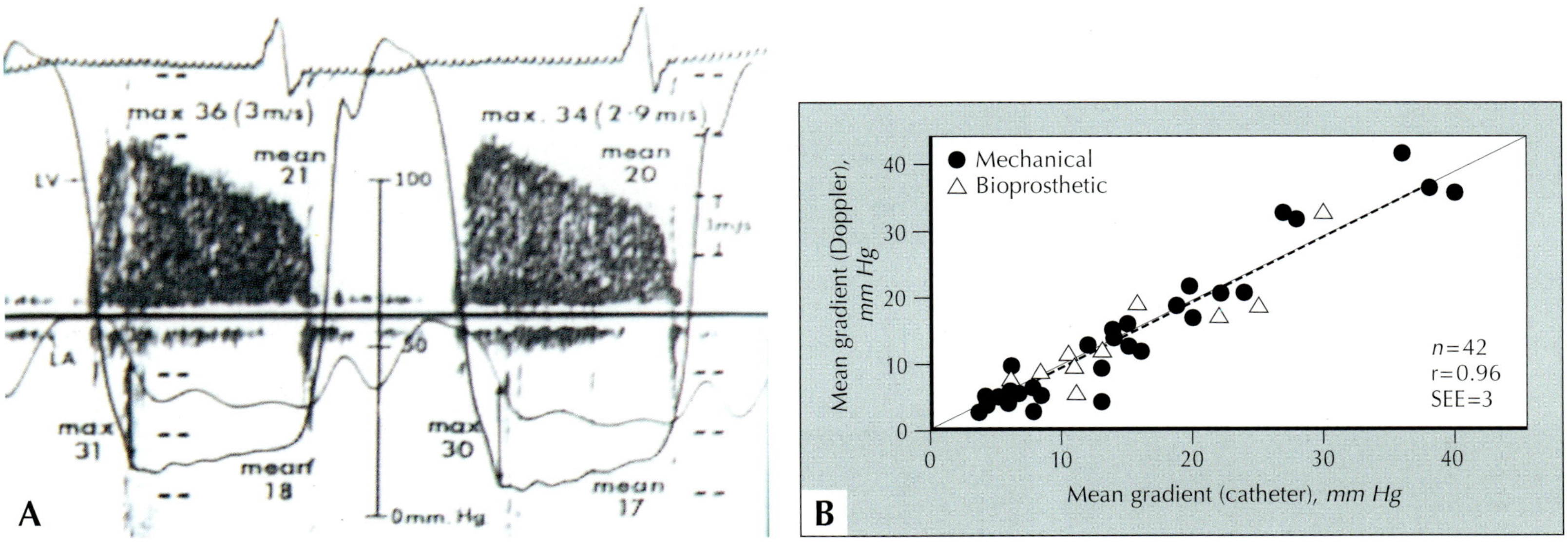

FIGURE 3-45. Assessment of prosthetic valves. Two-dimensional echocardiography and Doppler ultrasound are useful in the assessment of the patient with a prosthetic valve. All prosthetic valves have an inherent degree of stenosis, which must be considered when interpreting the echocardiographic studies. Continuous-wave Doppler examination can be used to accurately measure the mean gradient across a prosthesis [45] and is a valuable modality for the diagnosis of prosthetic valve obstruction. **A,** Simultaneous left atrial (LA)/left ventricular (LV) pressures and transmitral Doppler velocity of a stenotic Hancock bioprosthesis showing the excellent correlation between the maximum (max) and mean catheter and Doppler gradients. **B,** Correlation between catheter and Doppler mean gradients in a group of patients with mechanical and bioprosthetic valves. Because each prosthesis has its own inherent degree of obstruction, the mean gradient from a Doppler examination should be compared with the normal values that have been established in the literature for the individual size and type of prosthesis. Ideally, a Doppler examination should be performed postoperatively so that each patient can serve as his or her own control. The continuity equation (and pressure half time for mitral prosthesis) can also be used to estimate an effective prosthetic orifice area. SEE—standard error of the estimate. (*Adapted from* Burstow and coworkers [45]; with permission.)

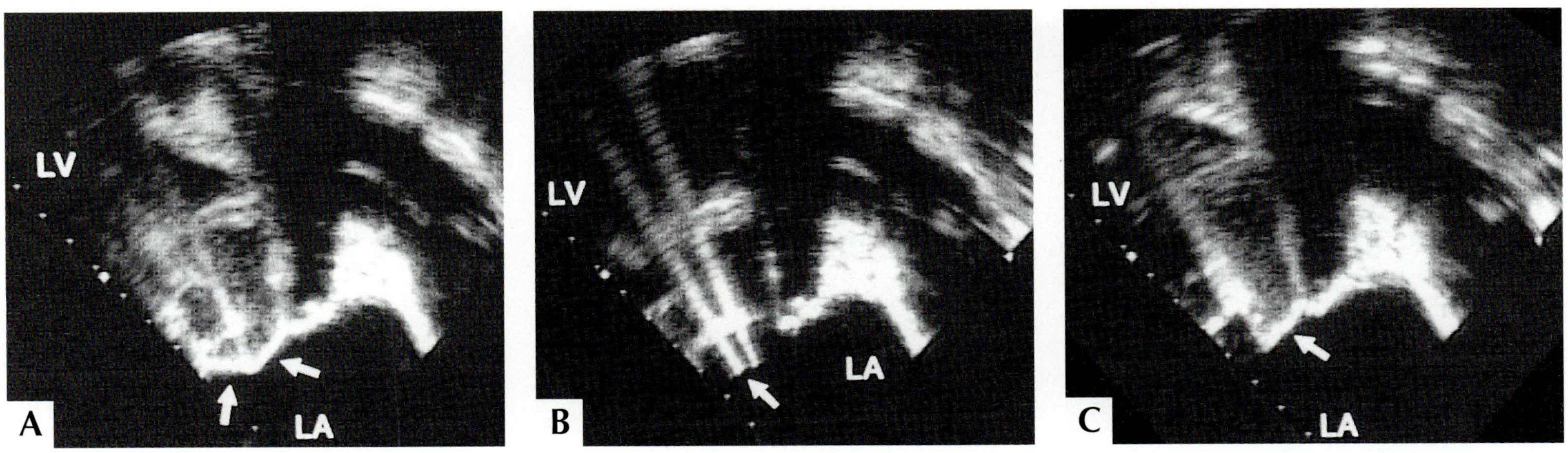

FIGURE 3-46. Prosthetic valve dysfunction. Prosthetic valve dysfunction can include stenosis, regurgitation (perivalvular or central), thrombosis, hemolysis, ball variance, and vegetations. Transthoracic echocardiography (TTE) examination is frequently suboptimal in assessing morphologic abnormalities due to acoustic shadowing, especially with mitral prostheses. Transesophageal echocardiography (TEE) complements TTE and can frequently elucidate the anatomic mechanism of valve dysfunction. In a large prospective series, overall sensitivity and specificity were 57% and 63%, respectively, for TTE and 86% and 88% for TEE in detecting morphologic valve abnormalities [46]. **A,** TEE longitudinal two-chamber view of a bileaflet St. Jude prosthetic valve. In systole, both leaflets are seen closed (*arrows*). **B,** Diastolic frame shows wide opening of both disc leaflets (*arrow*). **C,** Diastolic frame shows the sporadic occurrence of reduced opening of the right leaflet (*arrow*) causing intermittent stenosis. At operation, a small pannus of fibrous tissue was excised from the disc leaflet restoring normal function. LA—left atrium; LV—left ventricle.

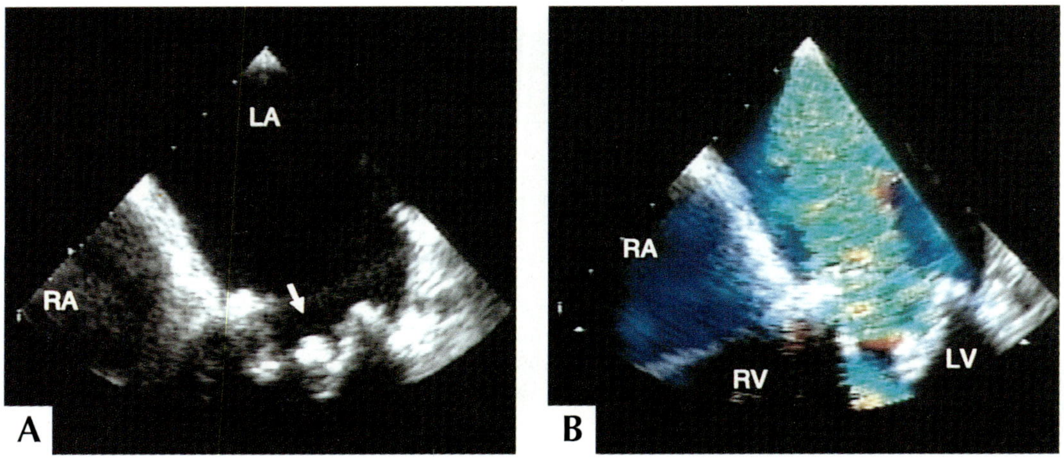

FIGURE 3-47. Prosthetic valve regurgitation. Transesophageal echocardiography (TEE) is the diagnostic modality of choice for the evaluation of prosthetic valve regurgitation, particularly in the mitral position. The posterior approach and high-frequency transducer are ideal for examining prosthetic valve structure, motion, and the color-flow velocities in the left atrium (LA). Each prosthesis does have an intrinsic degree of prosthetic valve regurgitation with a "closing volume," and the echocardiographer needs to be familiar with the color-flow velocities associated with the normal prostheses. Pathologic regurgitation can easily be identified on TEE and can be seen to be either perivalvular or through an abnormally functioning prosthesis. **A,** TEE horizontal four-chamber view of a bioprosthesis in the mitral position with a large vegetation (*arrow*) on one of the leaflets. **B,** Severe regurgitation through the prosthesis is seen on color-flow imaging. LV—left ventricle; RA—right atrium; RV—right ventricle.

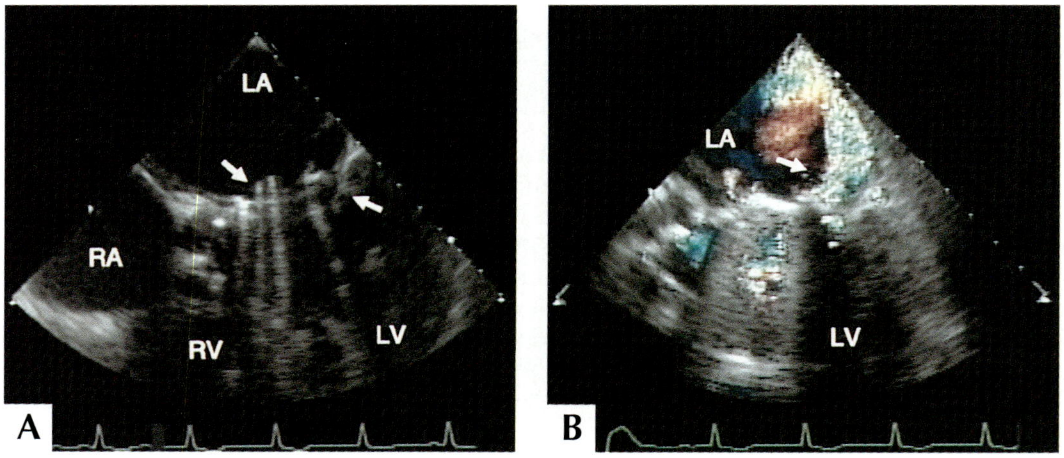

FIGURE 3-48. Perivalvular defects. Unlike the central regurgitation seen in Fig. 3-47, perivalvular defects can produce eccentric wall jets. **A,** Transesophageal echocardiographic horizontal diastolic frame shows a bileaflet St. Jude prosthesis in an open position. The *arrows* indicate dehisced sewing ring at the junction of the lateral left atrial (LA) wall from infective endocarditis. **B,** Color-flow imaging shows a large eccentric perivalvular regurgitant jet (*arrow*). LV—left ventricle; RA—right atrium; RV—right ventricle.

INFECTIVE ENDOCARDITIS

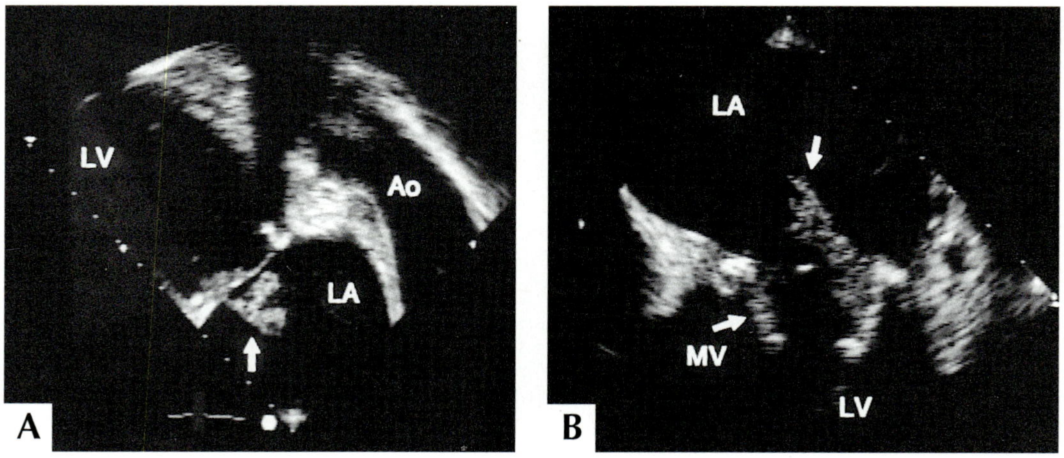

FIGURE 3-49. Lesions of infective endocarditis. The enhanced image resolution afforded by high-frequency transesophageal echocardiographic (TEE) transducers allows for better identification of vegetations in patients with infective endocarditis as compared with transthoracic echocardiography [47]. **A,** TEE long-axis view of a large vegetation (*arrow*) on a Carpentier-Edwards bioprosthesis. **B,** TEE horizontal image of the same vegetation (*arrow*). Vegetation size, extent, mobility, and texture have all been shown to be univariate predictors of complications in endocarditis. Ao—aorta; LA—left atrium; LV—left ventricle; MV—mitral valve.

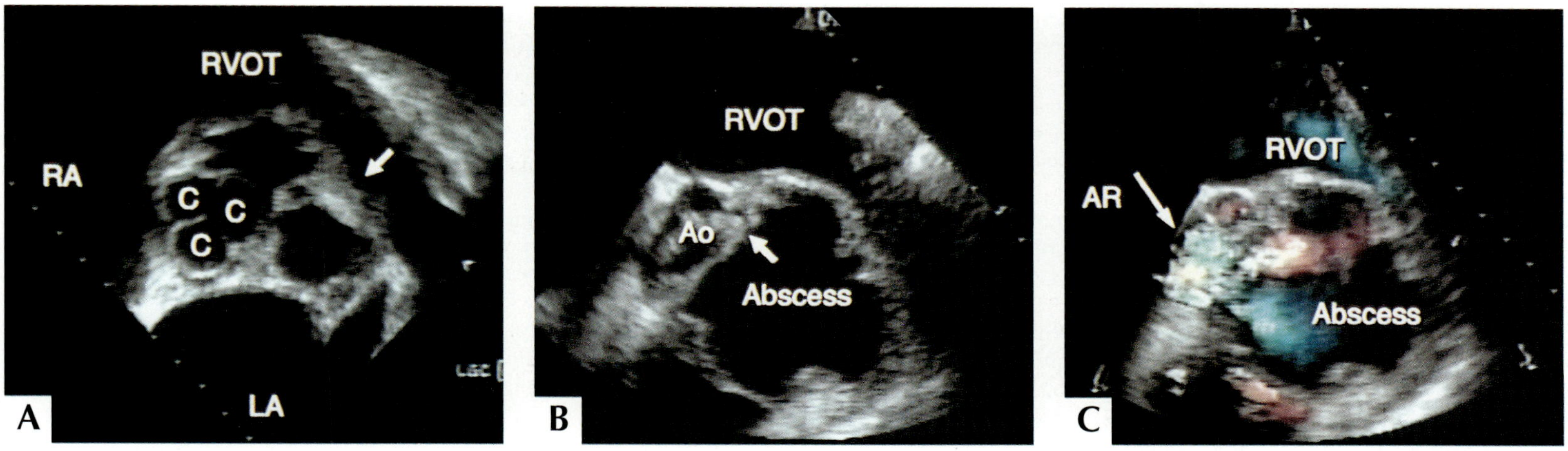

FIGURE 3-50. Complications of infective endocarditis. Patients with persistent fever, positive blood cultures, congestive heart failure, and heart block may have complications of endocarditis such as perivalvular extension and abscess formation. Transesophageal echocardiography is now one of the imaging modalities of choice in diagnosing these complications [48]. **A,** Short-axis diastolic omniplane view of a large aortic root abscess (*arrow*) visualized as echolucent structures between the aortic valve cusps (C) and right ventricular outflow tract (RVOT). **B,** Systolic frame shows expansion of the cavity and compression of the outflow tract. **C,** Diastolic frame shows regurgitation through the native aortic valve (*arrow*) and flow into the abscess. As many as 40% of patients with aortic valve endocarditis will have complications such as formation of sinus of Valsalva aneurysms, fistulous tracts through the intervalvular fibrosa, and "kissing" lesions on the anterior leaflet of the mitral leaflet. Ao—aorta; AR—aortic regurgitation; LA—left atrium; RA—right atrium.

REFERENCES

1. Tajik AJ, *et al.*: Two-dimensional real-time ultrasonic imaging of the heart and great vessels: technique, image orientation, structure identification, and validation. *Mayo Clin Proc* 1978, 53:271–303.
2. Nishimura RA, Miller FA, Callahan MJ, *et al.*: Doppler echocardiography: theory, instrumentation, technique, and applications. *Mayo Clin Proc* 1985, 60:321–343.
3. Seward JB, Khandhheria BK, Oh JK: Transesophageal echocardiography: technique, anatomic correlations, implementation, and clinical applications. *Mayo Clin Proc* 1988, 63:649–680.
4. Nishimura RA, Tajik AJ: Quantitative hemodynamics by Doppler echocardiography: a noninvasive alternative to cardiac catheterization. *Prog Cardiovasc Dis* 1994, 36:309–342.
5. Brandenburg RO, Tajik AJ, Edwards WD, *et al.*: Accuracy of two-dimensional echocardiographic diagnosis of congenitally bicuspid aortic valve. *Am J Cardiol* 1983, 51:1469–1473.
6. Wilcox W, Seward JB, Hagler DJ, *et al.*: Discrete subaortic stenosis: two-dimensional echocardiographic features with angiographic and surgical correlation. *Mayo Clin Proc* 1980, 55:425–433.
7. Weyman A, Caldwell R, Hurwitz R, *et al.*: Cross-sectional echocardiographic characterization of aortic obstruction. I. Supravalvular aortic stenosis and hypoplasia. *Circulation* 1982, 57:491–497.
8. Currie PJ, Seward JB, Reeder GS, *et al.*: Continuous-wave Doppler echocardiographic assessment of severity of calcific aortic stenosis: a simultaneous Doppler-catheter correlative study in 100 adult patients. *Circulation* 1985, 711:1162–1169.
9. Oh JK, Taliercio CP, Holmes DR Jr, *et al.*: Prediction of the severity of aortic stenosis by Doppler aortic valve area determination: prospective Doppler-catheterization correlation in 100 patients. *J Am Coll Cardiol* 1988, 11:1227–1234.
10. Nishimura RA, Holmes DR Jr, Michela M, *et al.*: Follow-up of patients with low-output, low-gradient hemodynamics after percutaneous balloon aortic valvuloplasty: the Mansfield Scientific Aortic Valvuloplasty Registry. *J Am Coll Cardiol* 1991, 17:828–833.
11. Schiller N, Shah P, Crawford M, *et al.*: Recommendations for quantitation of the left ventricle by two-dimensional echocardiography. *J Am Soc Echocardiogr* 1989, 2:358–367.
12. Bonow R, Dodd J, Maron BJ, *et al.*: Long-term serial changes in left ventricular function and reversal of ventricular dilatation after valve replacement for chronic aortic regurgitation. *Circulation* 1988, 77:1345–1355.
13. Seward JB, Khandheria BK, Freeman WK, *et al.*: Multiplane transesophageal echocardiography: image orientation, examination technique, anatomic correlations, and clinical applications. *Mayo Clin Proc* 1993, 68:523–551.
14. Erbel R, Daniel W, Visser C, *et al.*: Echocardiography in diagnosis of aortic dissection. *Lancet* 1989, 1:457–460.
15. Nishimura RA, Vonk GD, Rumberger JA, *et al.*: Semiquantitation of aortic regurgitation by different Doppler echocardiographic techniques and comparison with ultrafast-computed tomography. *Am Heart J* 1992, 124:995–1001.
16. Enriquez-Sarano M, Bailey KR, Seward JB, *et al.*: Quantitative Doppler assessment of valvular regurgitation. *Circulation* 1993, 87:841–848.
17. Perry G, Helmcke F, Nanda N, *et al.*: Evaluation of aortic insufficiency by Doppler color-flow mapping. *J Am Coll Cardiol* 1987, 9:952–959.
18. Touche T, Prasquier R, Nittenberg A, *et al.*: Assessment and follow-up of patients with aortic regurgitation by an updated Doppler echocardiographic measurement of the regurgitant fraction in the aortic arch. *Circulation* 1985, 72:819–824.
19. Nishimura RA, Tajik AJ: Determination of left-sided pressure gradients by utilizing Doppler aortic and mitral regurgitant signal: validation by simultaneous dual-catheter and Doppler studies. *J Am Coll Cardiol* 1988, 11:317–321.
20. Teague S, Heinsimer J, Anderson J, *et al.*: Quantification of aortic regurgitation utilizing continuous-wave Doppler ultrasound. *J Am Coll Cardiol* 1986, 8:592–599.

21. Abascal V, Wilkins G, O'Shea J, *et al.*: Prediction of successful outcome in 130 patients undergoing percutaneous balloon mitral valvotomy. *Circulation* 1990, 82:448–456.

21a. Reid CL, Chandratna PA, Kawanishi DT, *et al.*: Influence of mitral valve morphology in double balloon catheter balloon valvuloplasm in patients with mitral stenosis. *Circulation* 1989, 80(3):515–524.

22. Fatkin D, Paul R, Morgan J, *et al.*: Percutaneous balloon mitral valvotomy with the Inoue single-balloon catheter: commissural morphology as a determinant of outcome. *J Am Coll Cardiol* 1993, 21:319–397.

23. Holen J, Aaslid R, Landmark K, *et al.*: Determination of pressure gradient in mitral stenosis with a noninvasive ultrasound Doppler technique. *Acta Med Scand* 1976, 199:455–460.

24. Libanoff A, Rodbard S, *et al.*: Atrioventricular pressure halftime: measurement of mitral valve orifice area. *Circulation* 1968, 38:144–150.

25. Hatle LK, Angelson B, Romsdal T, *et al.*: Noninvasive assessment of the atrioventricular halftime by Doppler ultrasound. *Circulation* 1979, 60:1096–1104.

26. Thomas J, Wilkins G, Choong C, *et al.*: Inaccuracy of the mitral pressure halftime immediately following percutaneous mitral valvotomy: dependence of transmitral gradient on left atrial and ventricular compliance. *Circulation* 1988, 78:980–993.

27. Nakatani S, Masuyama Y, Kodoma K, *et al.*: Value and limitations of Doppler echocardiography in the quantification of stenotic mitral valve area: comparison of the pressure halftime and the continuity equation methods. *Circulation* 1988, 77:78–85.

28. Goldstein S, Cambell A: Mitral stenosis: evaluation and guidance of valvuloplasty by transesophageal echocardiography. *Cardiol Clin* 1993, 11:409–425.

29. Reid C, McKay C, Chandraratna P, *et al.*: Mechanisms of increase in mitral valve area and influence of anatomic features in double-balloon valvuloplasty in adults with rheumatic mitral stenosis: a Doppler and two-dimensional echocardiographic study. *Circulation* 1987, 76:628–636.

29a. Nishimura RA: Mitral Stenosis. In *Mayo Clinic Practical Cardiology, edn 3.* Edited by Guiliani ER, *et al.*: Mosby-Yearbook, 1995 .

30. Freeman WK, Schaff HV, Khandheria BK, *et al.*: Intraoperative evaluation of mitral valve regurgitation and repair by transesophageal echocardiography: incidence and significance of systolic anterior motion. *J Am Coll Cardiol* 1992, 20:599–609.

31. Helmcke F, Nanda N, Ming H, *et al.*: Color Doppler assessment of mitral regurgitation with orthogonal planes. *Circulation* 1987, 75:175–183.

32. Spain M, Smith M, Grayburn P, *et al.*: Quantitative assessment of mitral regurgitation by Doppler color-flow imaging: angiographic and hemodynamic correlations. *J Am Coll Cardiol* 1989, 13:585–590.

33. Cape E, Yoganathan P, Weyman A, *et al.*: Adjacent solid boundaries alter the size of regurgitant jets on Doppler color-flow maps. *J Am Coll Cardiol* 1991, 17:1094–1102.

34. Jenni R, Ritter M, Eberli F, *et al.*: Quantification of mitral regurgitation with amplitude-weighted mean velocity. *Circulation* 1989, 79:1294–1299.

35. Bargiggia G, Tronconi L, Sahn D, *et al.*: A new method for quantification of mitral regurgitation based on color-flow Doppler imaging of flow convergence proximal to regurgitant orifice. *Circulation* 1991, 84:1481–1489.

36. Utsunomiya T, Patel D, Doshi R, *et al.*: Can signal intensity of the continuous-wave Doppler regurgitant jet estimate severity of mitral regurgitation? *Am Heart J* 1992, 123:166–171.

37. Castello R, Pearson A, Lenzen P, *et al.*: Effect of mitral regurgitation on pulmonary venous flow velocities derived from transesophageal echocardiographic color-guided pulsed-Doppler imaging. *J Am Coll Cardiol* 1991, 17:1499–1506.

37a. Nishimura RA: The role of echocardiography. In *Atherosclerosis and Coronary Artery Disease.* Edited by Foster V, Ross R, Topol EJ. Philadelphia: Lippincott-Raven; 1996.

38. Tribouilloy C, Shen W, Quere J, *et al.*: Assessment of severity of mitral regurgitation by measuring regurgitant jet width at its origin with transesophageal Doppler color-flow imaging. *Circulation* 1992, 85:1248–1253.

39. Chung N, Nishimura RA, Holmes DR Jr, *et al.*: Measurement of left ventricular dp/dt by simultaneous Doppler echocardiography and cardiac catheterization. *J Am Soc Echocardiogr* 1992, 5:147–152.

40. Pai R, Bansal R, Shah P: Doppler-derived rate of left ventricular pressure rise: its correlation with the postoperative left ventricular function in mitral regurgitation. *Circulation* 1990, 82:514–520.

41. Nishimura RA, Schwartz RS, Tajik AJ, *et al.*: Noninvasive measurement of rat of left ventricular relaxation by Doppler echocardiography. Validation with simultaneous cardiac catheterization. *Circulation* 1993, 88:146–155.

42. Pellikka PA, Tajik AJ, Khandheria BK, *et al.*: Carcinoid heart disease: clinical and echocardiographic spectrum in 74 patients. *Circulation* 1993, 87:1188–1196.

43. Currie PJ, Seward JB, Chan K, *et al.*: Continuous-wave Doppler determination of right ventricular pressure: a simultaneous Doppler-catheterization study in 127 patients. *J Am Coll Cardiol* 1985, 6:750–756.

44. Masuyama T, Kodama K, Kitabatake A, *et al.*: Continuous-wave Doppler echocardiographic detection of pulmonary regurgitation and its application to noninvasive estimation of pulmonary artery pressure. *J Am Coll Cardiol* 1986, 74:484–492.

45. Burstow DJ, Nishimura RA, Bailey KR, *et al.*: Continuous-wave Doppler echocardiographic measurement of prosthetic valve gradients: a simultaneous Doppler-catheter correlative study. *Circulation* 1989, 80:504–514.

46. Daniel W, Mugge A, Grote J, *et al.*: Comparison of transthoracic and transesophageal echocardiography for detection of abnormalities of prosthetic and bioprosthetic valves in the mitral and aortic positions. *Am J Cardiol* 1993, 71:210–215.

47. Erbel R, Rohmann M, Drexler S, *et al.*: Improved diagnostic value of echocardiography in patients with infective endocarditis by transesophageal approach: a prospective study. *Eur Heart J* 1988, 9:43–53.

48. Daniel W, Mugge A, Martin R, *et al.*: Improvements in the diagnosis of abscesses associated with endocarditis by transesophageal echocardiography. *N Engl J Med* 1991, 324:795–800.

Magnetic Resonance Imaging and Radionuclide Angiography in Assessment

4

CHAPTER

Gerald G. Blackwell and
Gerald M. Pohost

Transthoracic echocardiography is the initial noninvasive imaging test used in the evaluation of most patients with known or suspected valvular heart disease and endocarditis. In selected cases, transesophageal echocardiography provides valuable diagnostic information, especially in patients with poor thoracic acoustic windows. The excellent temporal and spatial resolution of ultrasound-based techniques allows real-time, high-resolution evaluation of the normal and abnormal heart valve. Further, Doppler echocardiographic methods provide important physiologic information about both regurgitant and stenotic valves and estimates of their effects on chamber sizes and dynamics. Recently, magnetic resonance imaging (MRI) has emerged as a useful tool for the evaluation of patients with valvular heart disease. MRI uses a strong external magnetic field, transiently applied magnetic gradients, and radiowaves to interact with hydrogen atoms in the intact organism. Inherently, three-dimensional tomograms are acquired without the need for vascular intrusion or contrast administration and without using ionizing radiation. Cine MRI allows recognition of regurgitant valvular lesions with an accuracy comparable to Doppler ultrasound. Serial assessment of ventricular volumes and function can also be accomplished using MRI in these patients. Finally, quantitative flow information can be obtained using an MRI technique known as phase velocity mapping. A discussion of the details of magnetic resonance physics and the modifications of standard MRI required for successful cardiovascular applications are beyond the scope of this chapter and the interested reader is referred to several reviews of the topic [1–4].

The usefulness of MRI for cardiovascular applications is being increasingly recognized, and this chapter focuses on its role in the evaluation of patients with valvular heart disease and endocarditis. Although infrequently used in this specific patient population, radionuclide methods are also briefly mentioned.

NONINVASIVE IMAGING MODALITIES IN THE ASSESSMENT OF PATIENTS WITH VALVULAR HEART DISEASE AND ENDOCARDITIS

- Transthoracic echocardiography
- Transesophageal echocardiography
- MRI
- Radionuclide angiography

FIGURE 4-1. Noninvasive imaging modalities in the assessment of patients with valvular heart disease and endocarditis. Ultrasound-based techniques are the cornerstone for the initial noninvasive imaging evaluation of patients with known or suspected valvular heart disease and endocarditis. Magnetic resonance imaging (MRI) can detect regurgitant and stenotic lesions with a diagnostic accuracy comparable to that of echocardiography. However, fine valvular detail is not routinely seen on MRI and, hence, its role in the diagnosis of patients with endocarditis is more limited. Radionuclide angiography can assess the effects of valvular lesions on right and left ventricular systolic function. Regurgitant fractions can also be estimated by radionuclide-based techniques although these are seldom applied clinically. The role of single photon emission computed tomography (SPECT) blood pool imaging for the assessment of ventricular volumes remains to be defined.

MAGNETIC RESONANCE IMAGING

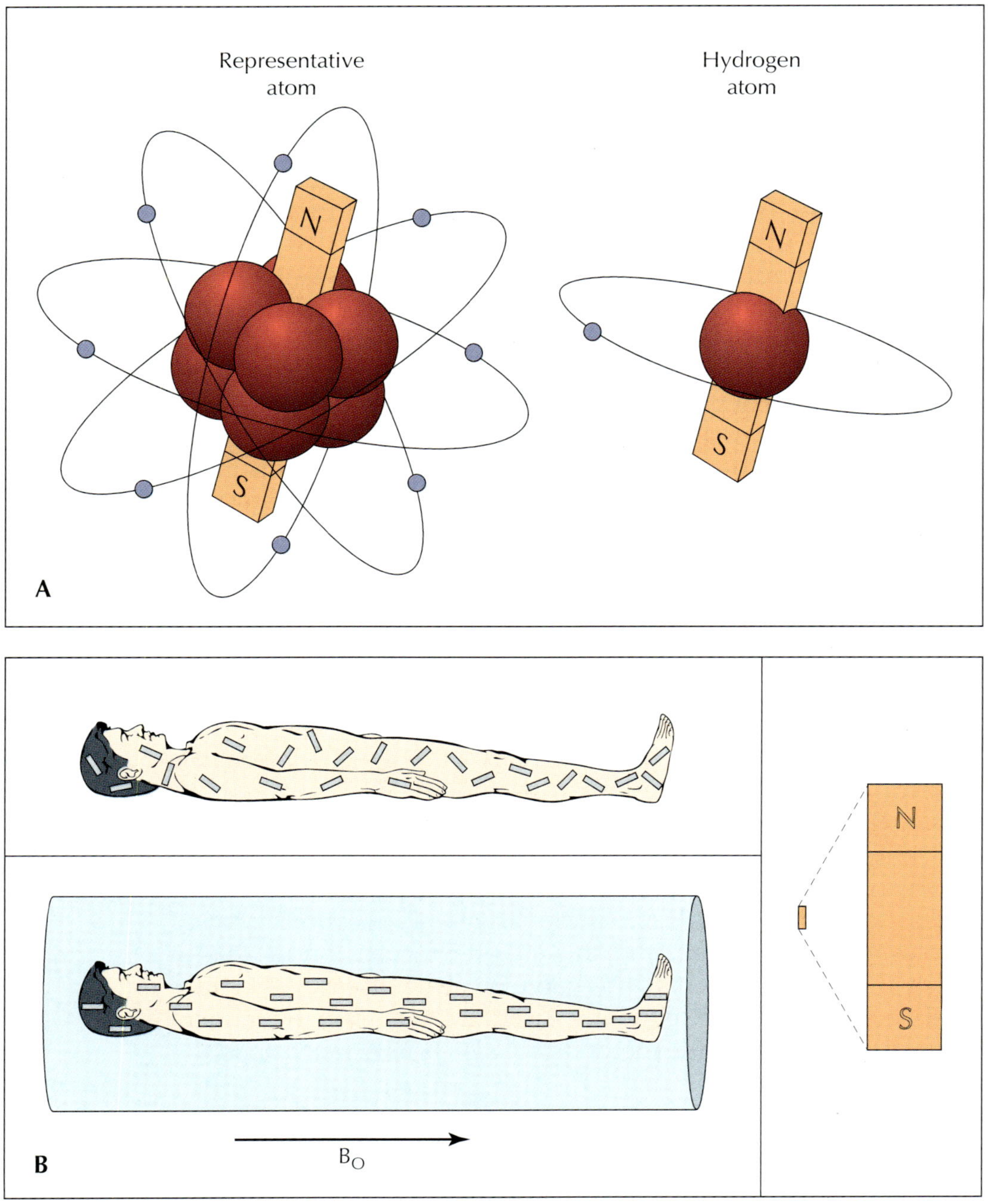

FIGURE 4-2. Basic principles of MRI. Magnetism arises as a result of the motion of a charged particle within the atomic nucleus, and MRI generally exploits the magnetic properties of the hydrogen nucleus [2]. Medical MR images depict the distribution of hydrogen nuclei, primarily in water and fat, throughout the body. **A**, the hydrogen nucleus as a tiny bar magnet. The hydrogen nucleus has a microscopic magnetic field associated with its nuclear spin. **B**, The *top panel* represents the distribution of these tiny bar magnetics (hydrogen nuclei) in the human body. In the absence of an external magnetic field, the nuclei are randomly oriented in space and no magnetic moment is produced. The *lower panel* represents the effect of an external magnetic field (cylinder) on nuclear alignment. In the presence of an external magnetic field, many of the nuclei align themselves in a specific orientation. This orderly arrangement produces a measurable magnetic moment (B_O). (*continued*)

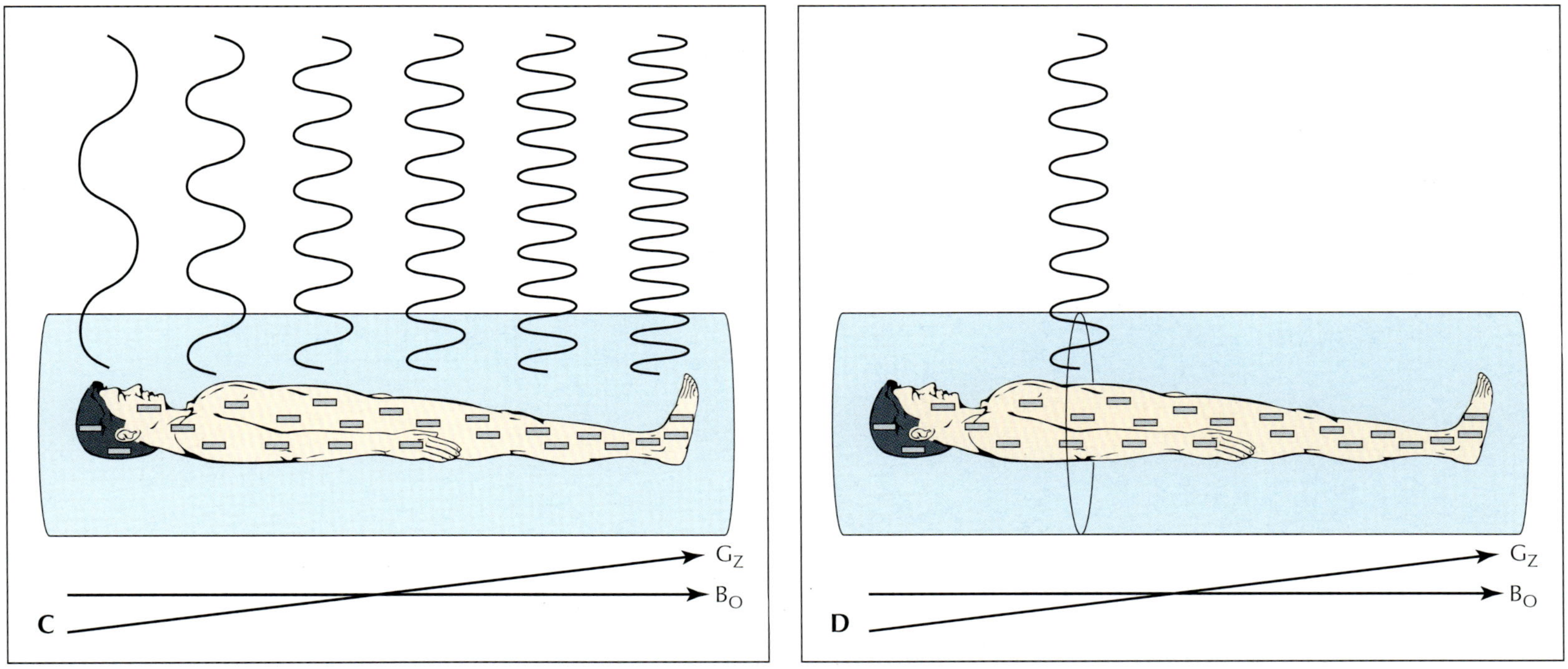

FIGURE 4-2. *(continued)* **C**, The effect of a magnetic field gradient on the homogeneous external magnetic field. A small magnetic field gradient is applied, which leads to a progressively increasing magnetic field strength from the patient's head to foot. Because hydrogen nuclei spin at a specific frequency depending on the strength of the external magnetic field, nuclei located in a weaker magnetic field spin slowly in relation to the rotational frequency of hydrogen nuclei exposed to a stronger magnetic field. Using magnetic field gradients in three dimensions, radiofrequency energy, and powerful computers, specific regions of the body can be selected for imaging. **D**, A slice taken at the level of the heart. High-resolution three-dimensional data sets may be acquired with excellent temporal and spatial resolution using MRI techniques. These data sets can be acquired to highlight morphologic information (spin echo, black blood), functional information (gradient echo, cine MRI), or flow data (phase velocity mapping). G_z— the magnetic gradient (G) in the z direction along the long axis of the body.

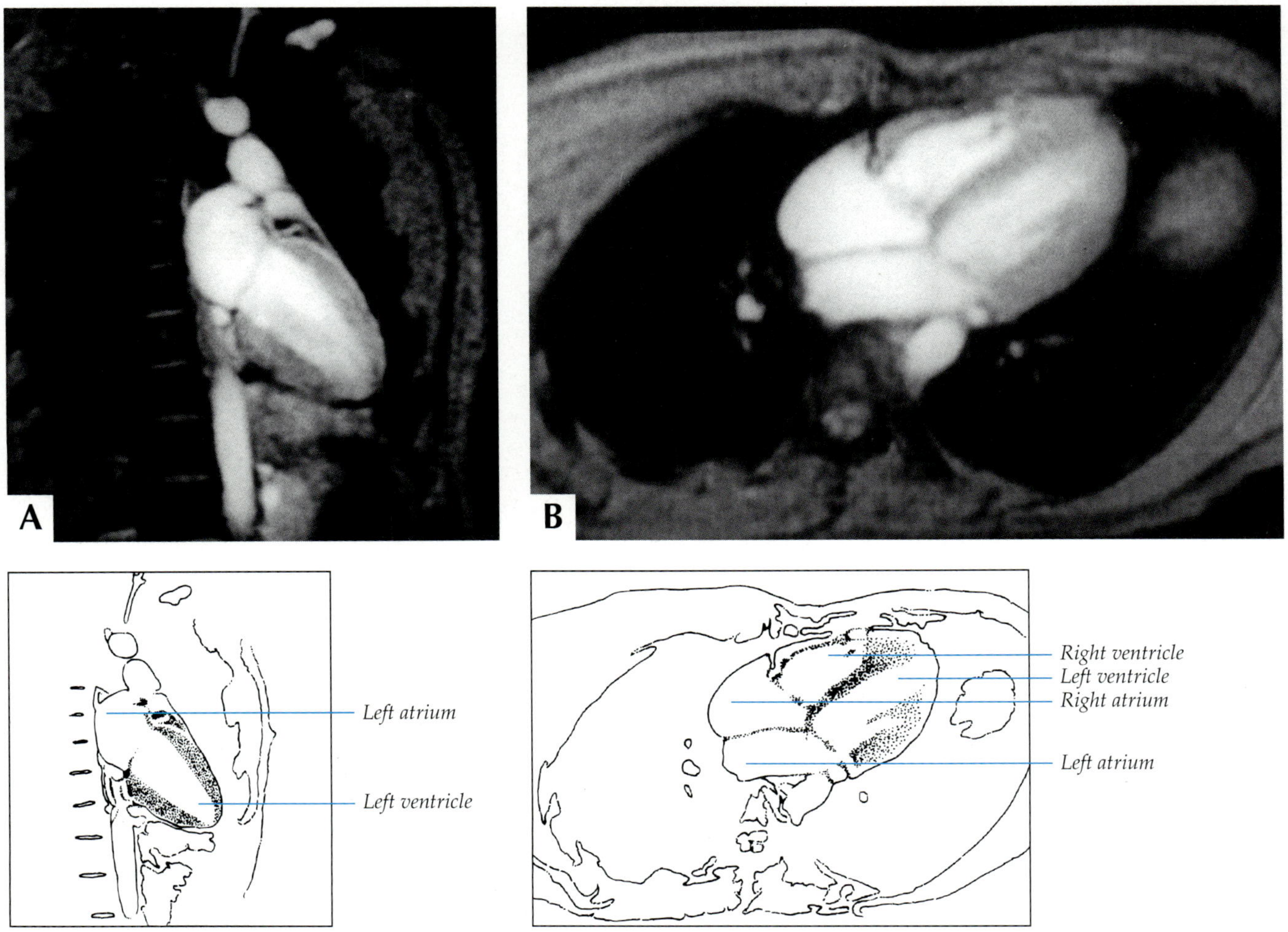

FIGURE 4-3. Tomographic planes. A major advantage of MRI is the ability to acquire images in any desired tomographic plane. This figure demonstrates several tomographic planes that are useful in the evaluation of patients with known or suspected valvular heart disease.

A, In the right anterior oblique (RAO) plane, left ventricular function and mitral regurgitation can be assessed. **B**, In the four-chamber plane, biventricular systolic function can be assessed, as well as mitral and tricuspid valve disease. *(continued)*

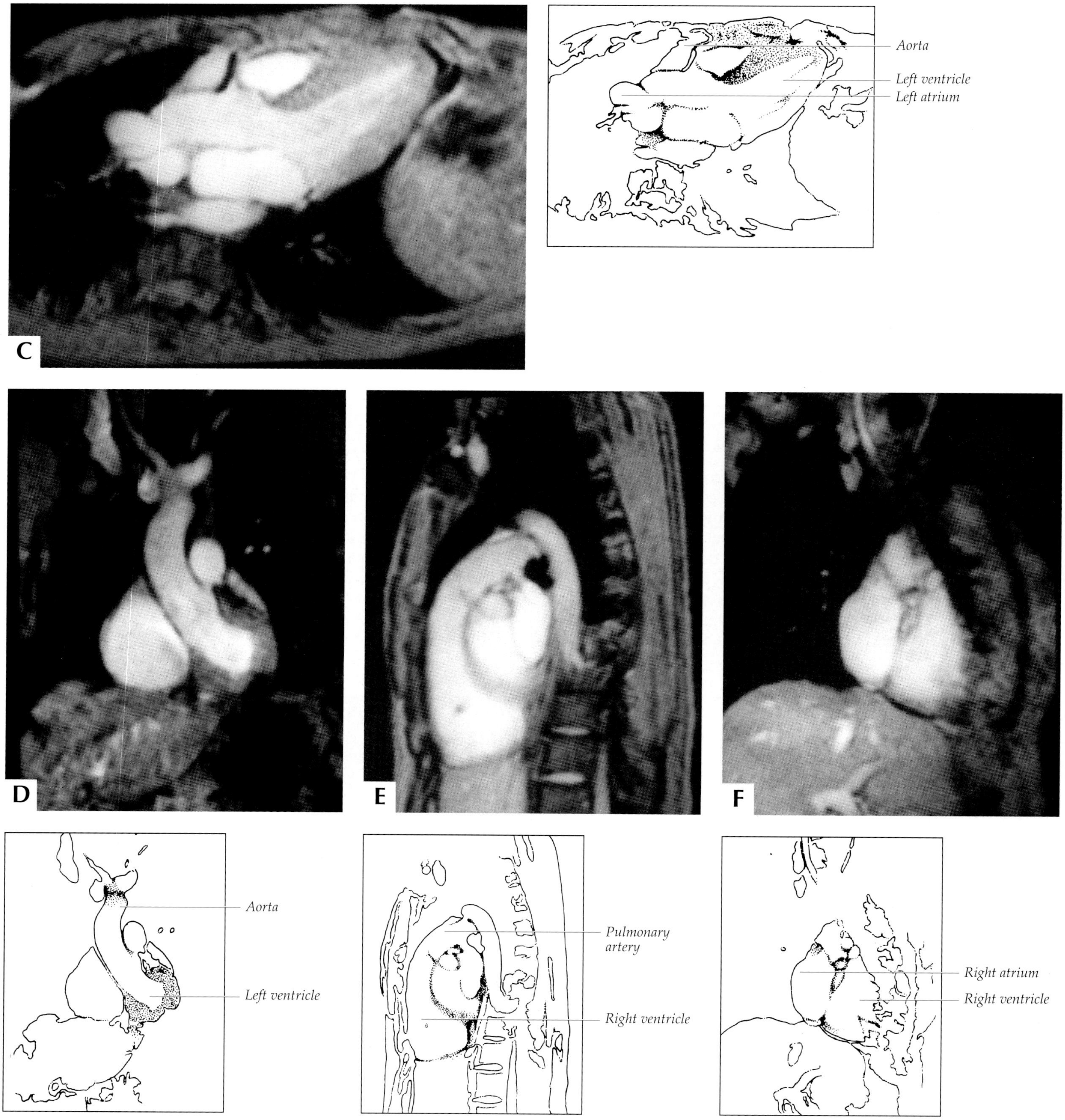

FIGURE 4-3. (*continued*) **C**, The left ventricular outflow tract plane allows assessment of ventricular function as well as mitral and aortic valve disease. **D**, The coronal ascending aortic plane facilitates assessment of the aortic valve. **E**, The right ventricular outflow tract plane is well suited for the assessment of right ventricular (RV) function as well as pulmonic valve disease. **F**, The RAO plane through the RV facilitates assessment of RV function as well as tricuspid and pulmonic valve disease. (*continued*)

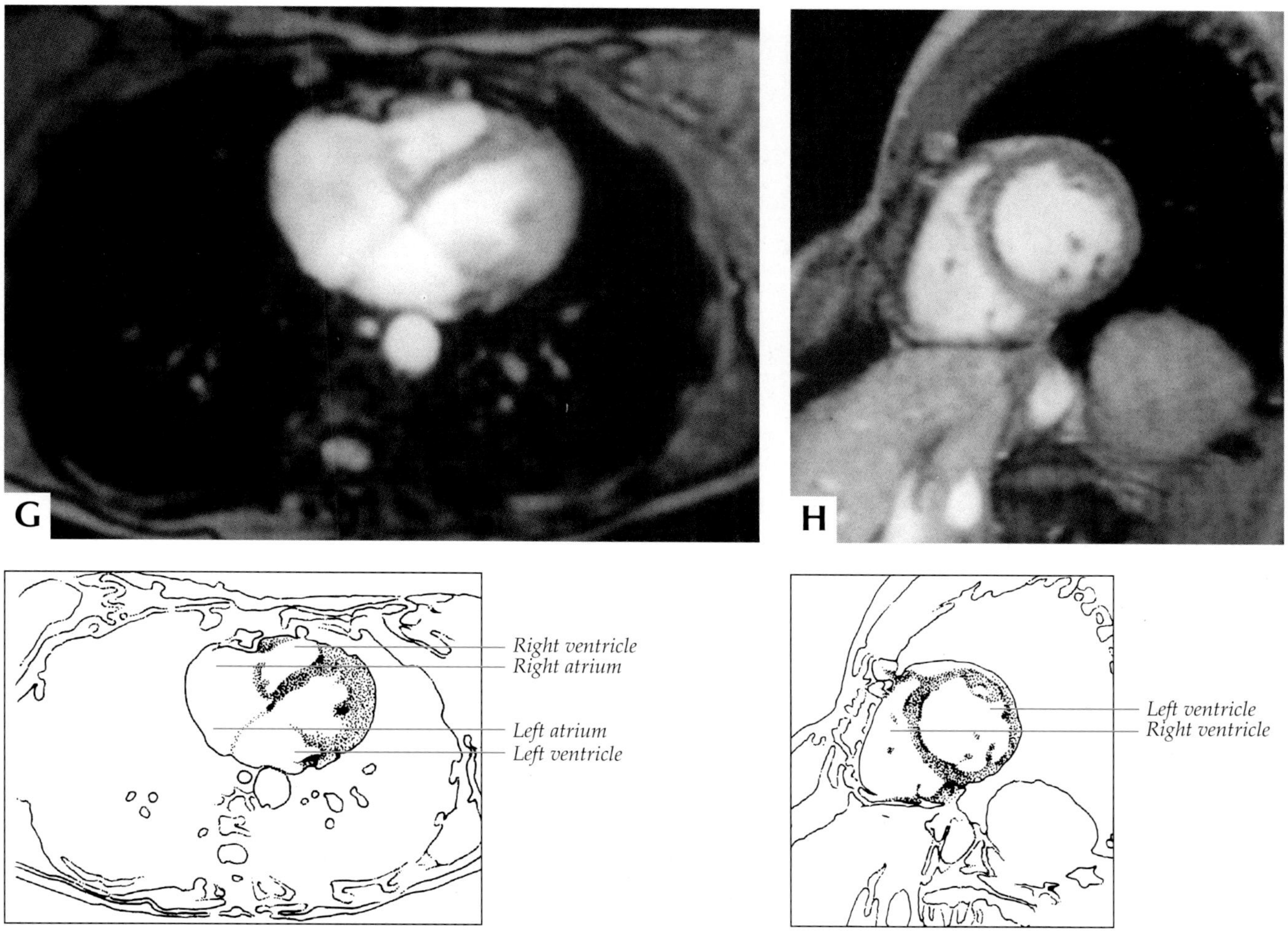

FIGURE 4-3. (*continued*) In addition to the above planes, stacked tomographic sets, which encompass the heart, can be acquired in either the straight axial projection (**G**), or aligned with the true cardiac short axis (**H**).

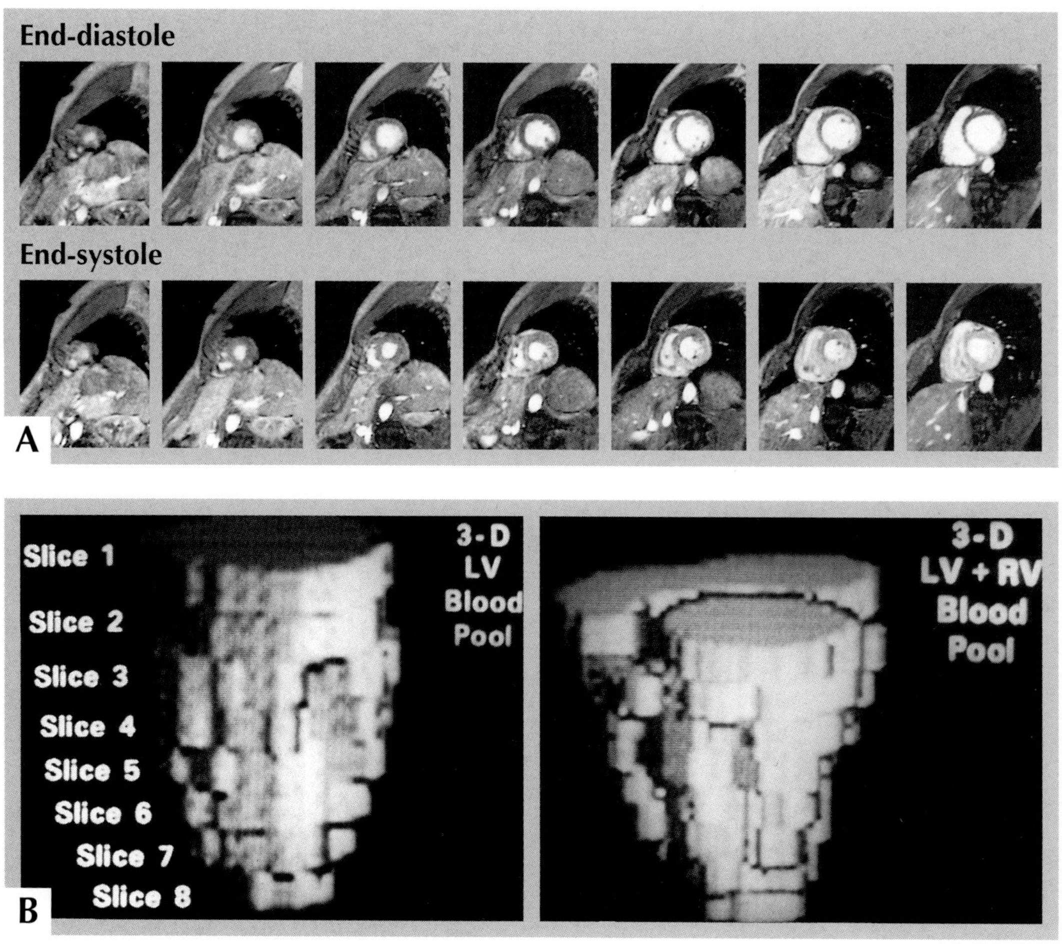

FIGURE 4-4. Serial short-axis tomograms. Cine MRIs can provide accurate and reproducible measurements of ventricular volume and mass [5–8]. Both right ventricular (RV) and left ventricular (LV) volumes can be accurately assessed using axial tomographs aligned with the axes of the body. However, in many situations it is useful to acquire images that are aligned with the cardiac axes. Cranney *et al.* [6] have provided validation of LV volumes using cardiac axial MRI in comparison with calibrated invasive ventriculography. **A**, A stacked set of short-axis tomograms that encompass the entire heart. End-diastolic and end-systolic frames are shown from the apex to the cardiac base. **B**, A three-dimensional reconstruction of the LV blood pool (*left*) and of the combined LV and RV blood pool (*right*). Unprecedented insight into ventricular shape and function can be obtained using MRI. These data are particularly useful in the serial follow-up of patients with chronic valvular heart disease.

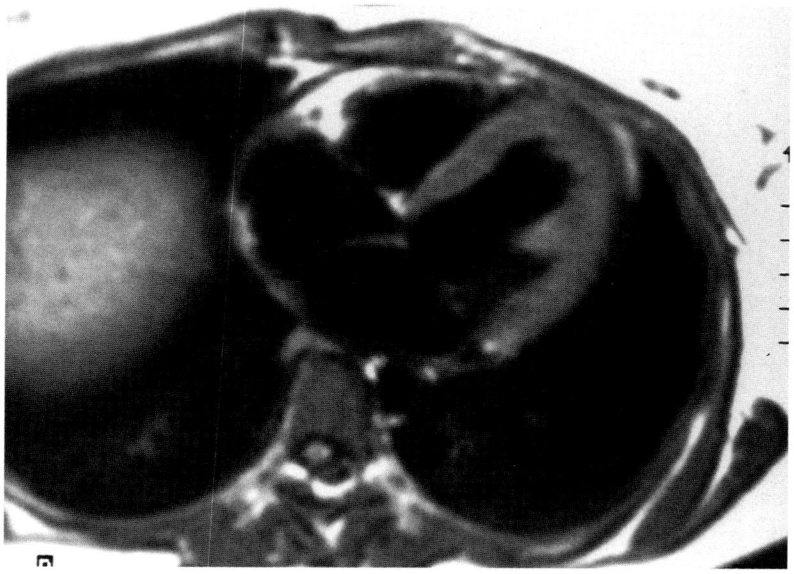

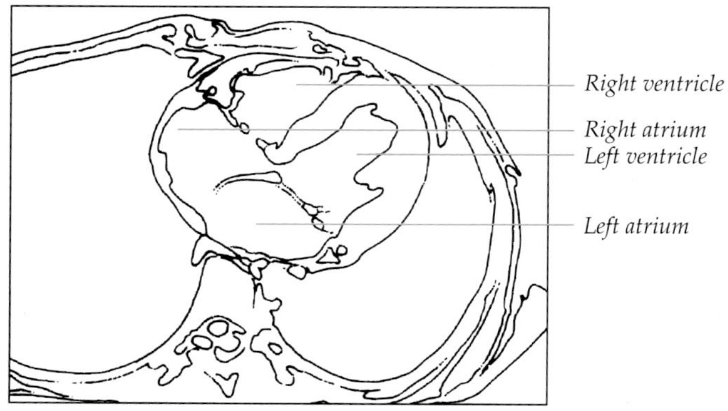

FIGURE 4-5. Spin echo imaging. Spin echo (black blood) image is from a patient with surgically documented bacterial endocarditis involving the mitral valve. Although large vegetations can often be appreciated using MRI, in general, echocardiography provides much better resolution of fine valvular detail and vegetations.

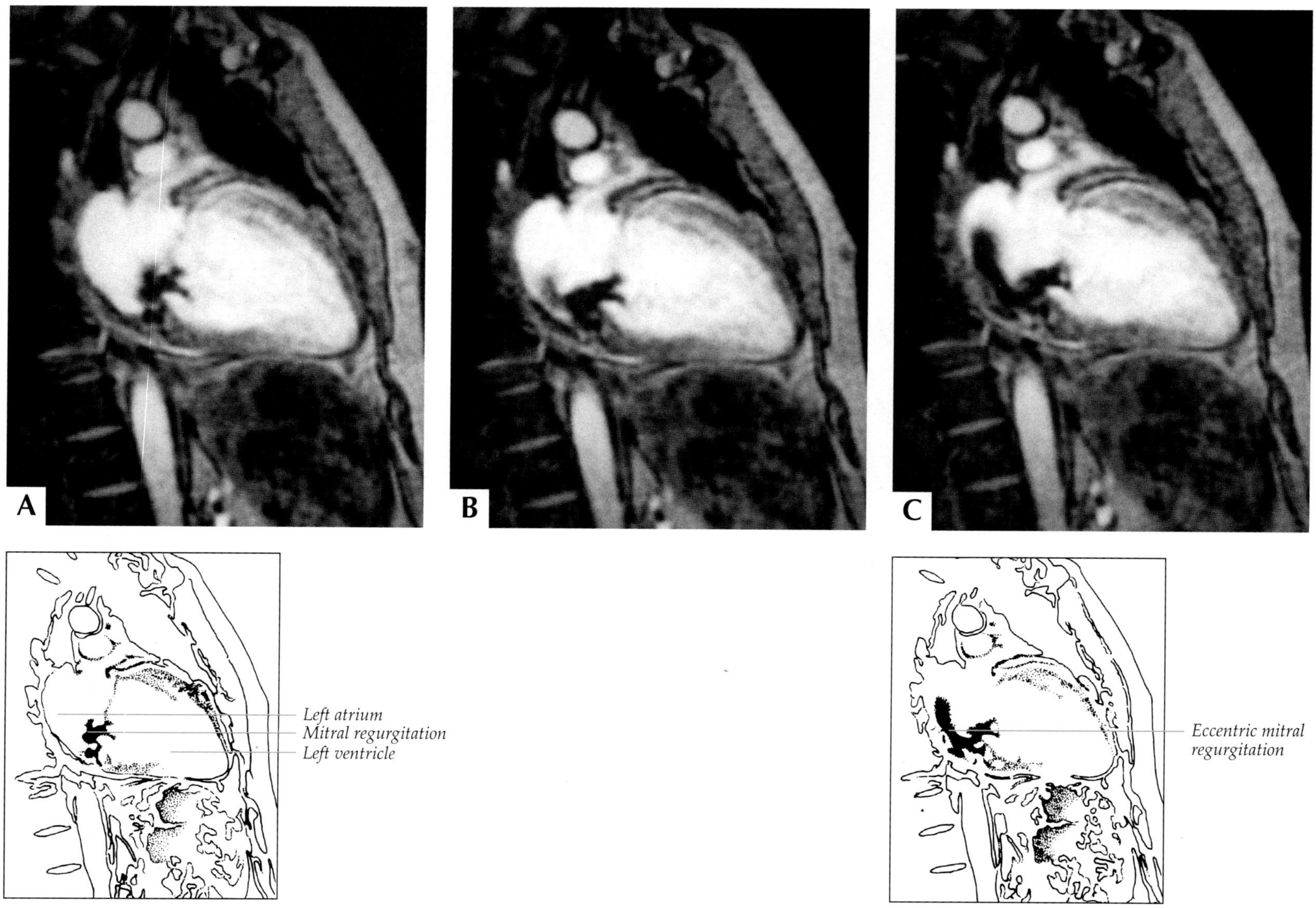

FIGURE 4-6. Cine MRI. Cine MRI is well suited to assessing the presence and severity of valvular regurgitation [9]. Turbulent blood flow appears as a region of decreased MRI signal intensity on cine MRI. The signal loss appears as a black void within the normally white blood pool. Signal void patterns are associated with opening and closing of normal cardiac valves. However, these voids are small and have been well characterized by Mirowitz *et al.* [10]. Many studies have demonstrated the sensitivity and specificity of cine MRI for detecting valvular regurgitation [11–15]. However, as with Doppler ultrasound, display and imaging parameters can affect the appearance of regurgitant jets on cine MRI [16].

This figure represents sequential frames (**A** through **F**) from a cine loop in a patient with bacterial endocarditis affecting the mitral valve. Right anterior oblique (RAO) and four-chamber planes are shown. (*continued*)

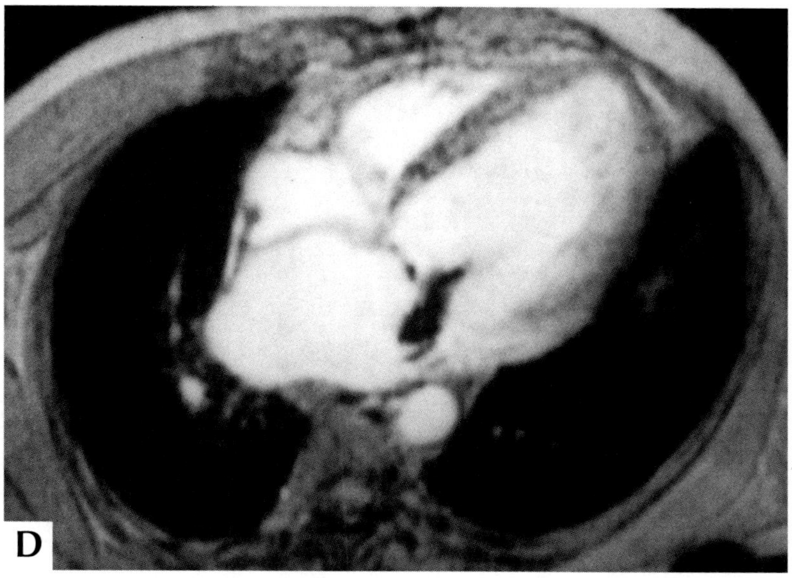

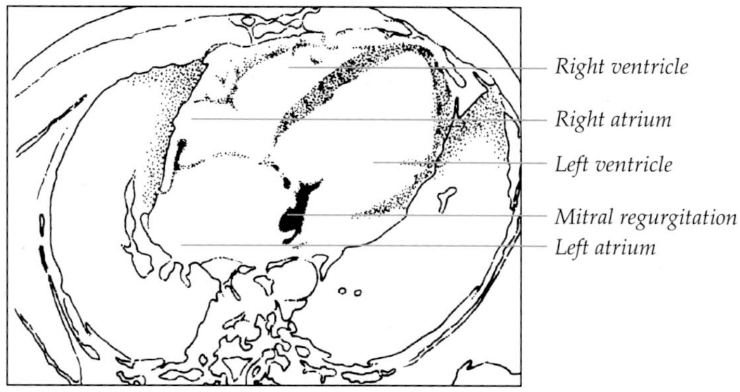

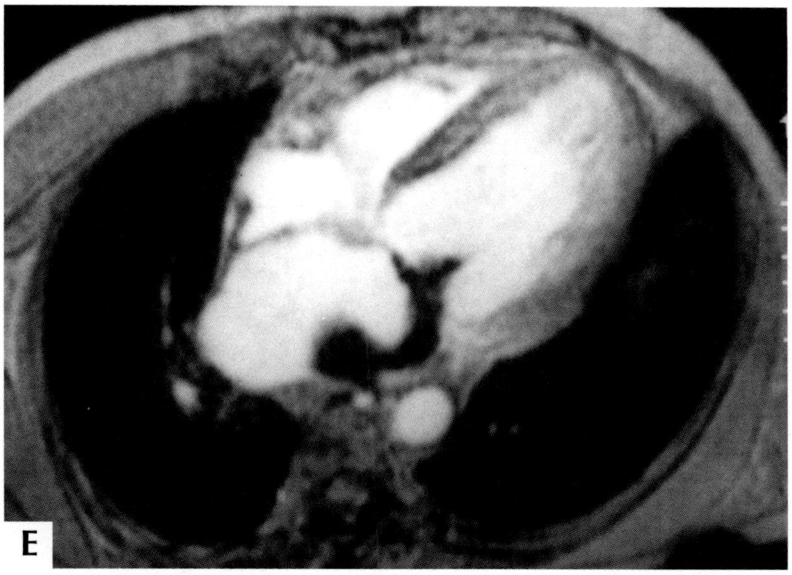

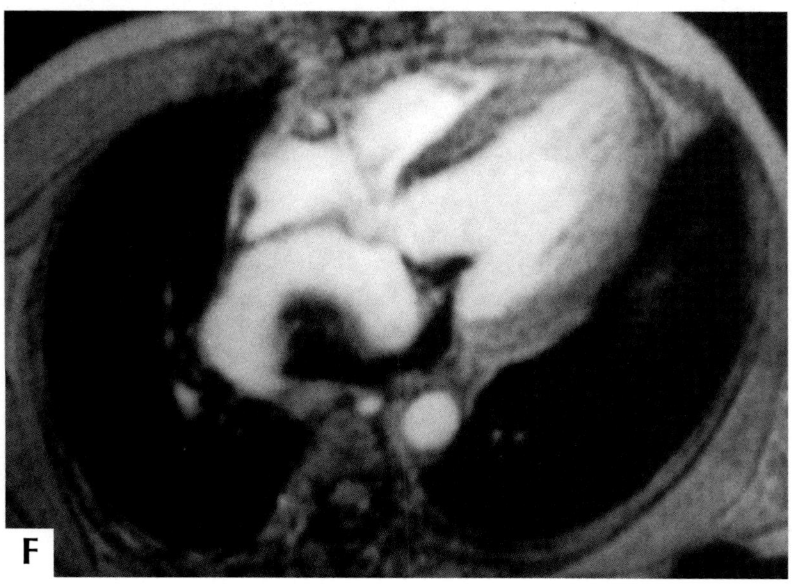

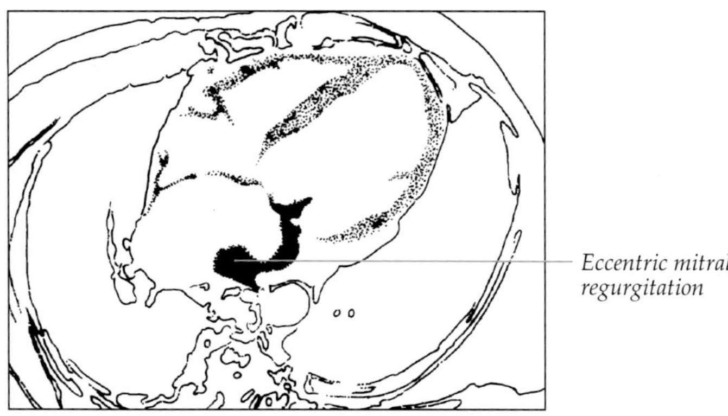

FIGURE 4-6. (*continued*) Early in systole a small signal void can be seen originating at the level of the mitral valve. As systole progresses, a much larger jet is visualized directed toward the posterolateral wall of the left atrium. The jet is eccentric and occupies a large portion of the atrium. In patients with endocarditis the regurgitant jet is often eccentric and occasionally multiple jets can be visualized due to perforations of the valve leaflets.

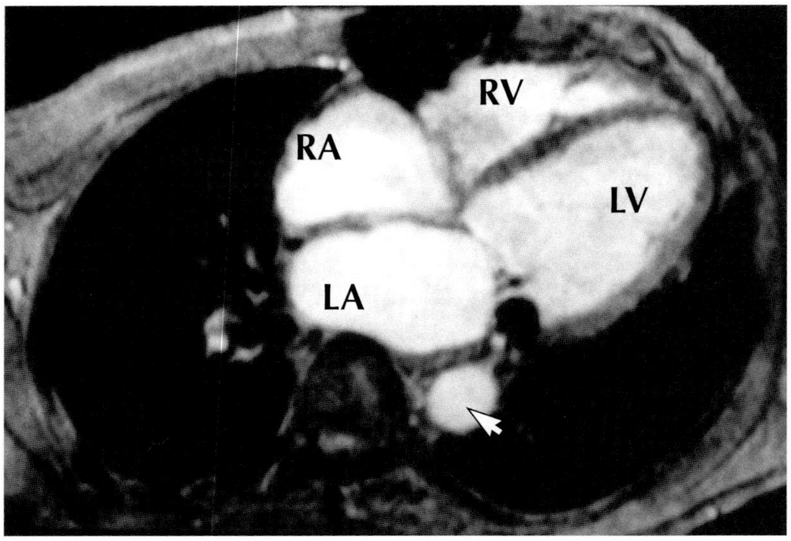

FIGURE 4-7. Mitral annular calcification. This four-chamber cine MRI frame shows mitral annular calcification (*arrow*). MRIs visualize only hydrogen nuclei; therefore, calcification appears as a region of signal dropout. Mitral annular calcium is frequently associated with mitral regurgitation. LA—left atrium; LV—left ventricle; RA—right atrium; RV—right ventricle.

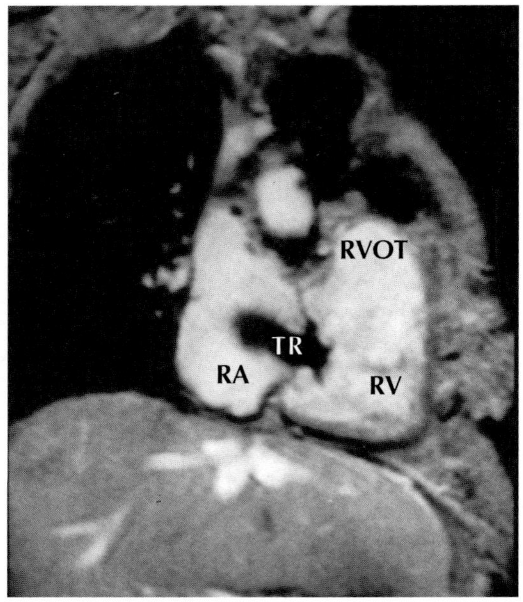

FIGURE 4-8. Severe tricuspid regurgitation (TR). In this mid-systolic frame from a right anterior oblique view of the right ventricle (RV), a large signal void originates at the level of the tricuspid valve and extends well into the body of the right atrium (RA). TR is most often functional secondary to RV chamber enlargement from a variety of causes. In this patient there was a contribution from rheumatic disease because she had previously undergone replacement of both her mitral and aortic valves. In this imaging plane her two prostheses are not visualized. RVOT—right ventricular outflow tract.

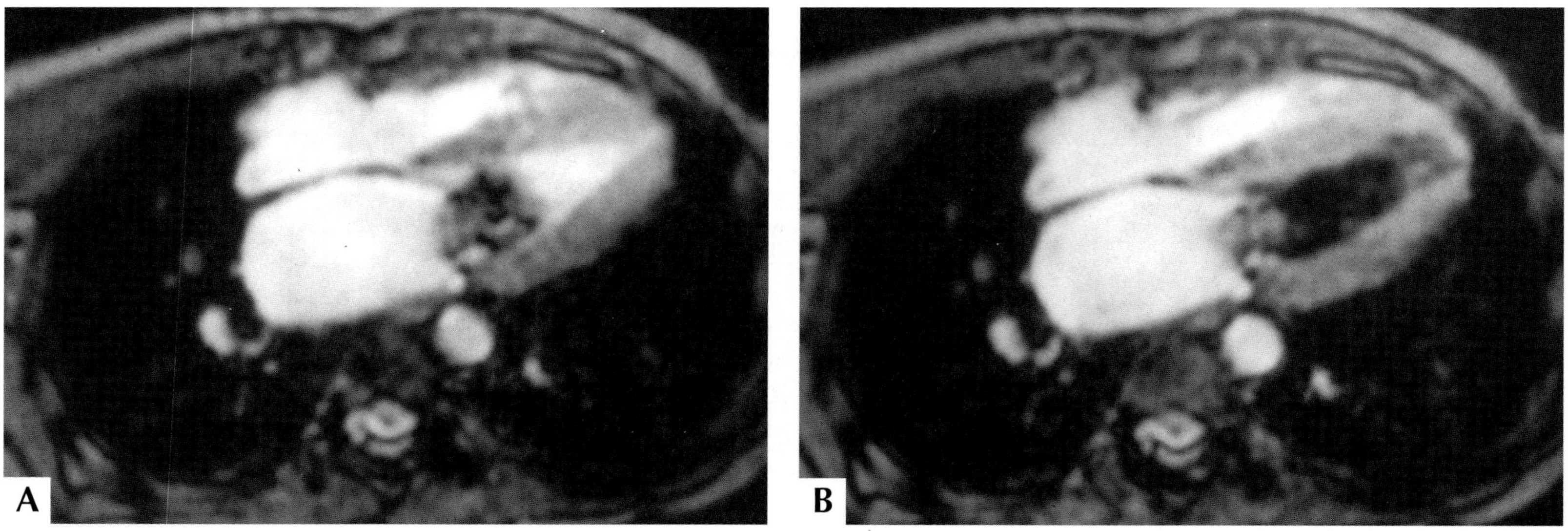

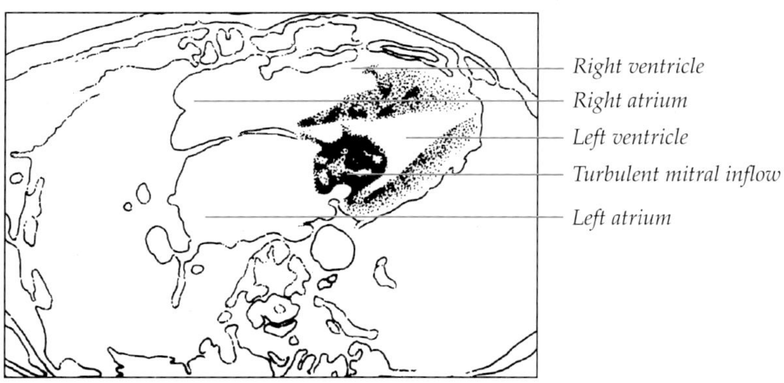

FIGURE 4-9. Mitral stenosis (MS). Sequential diastolic frames are from a four-chamber cine MRI (**A–D**, early to end diastole). In this patient mitral valve opening is associated with turbulent left ventricle (LV) inflow (*panel A*) as identified by the region of signal loss (*panel B*). As diastole progresses, the signal void encompasses the entire body of the LV consistent with significant MS. (*continued*)

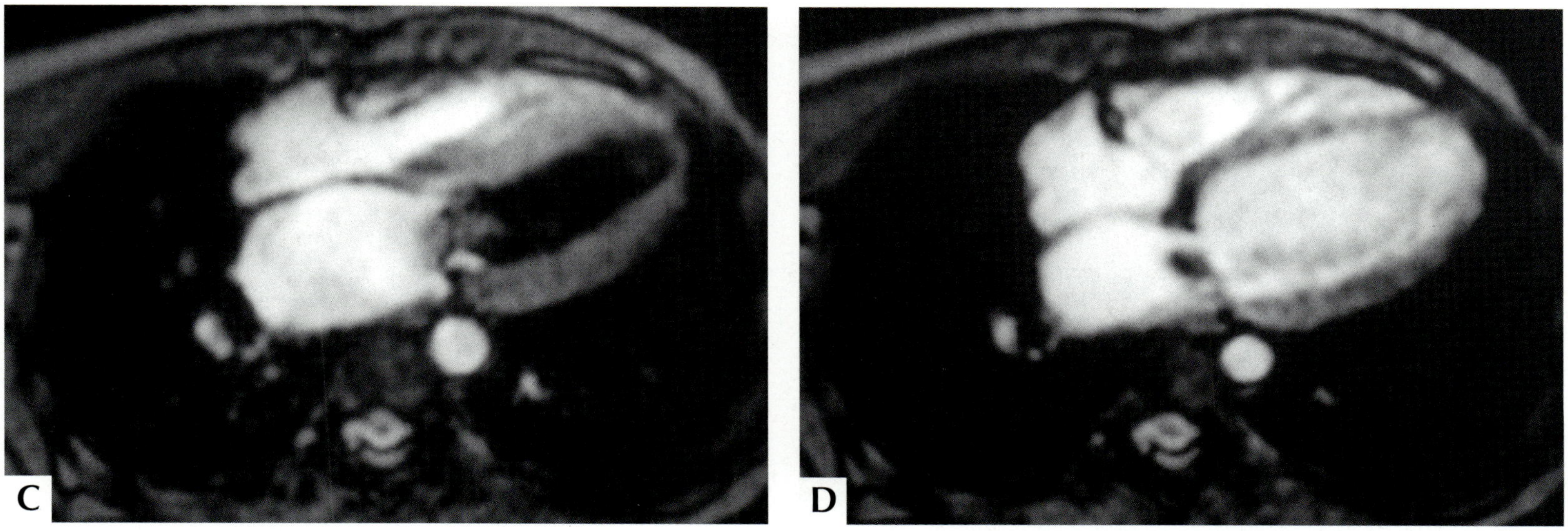

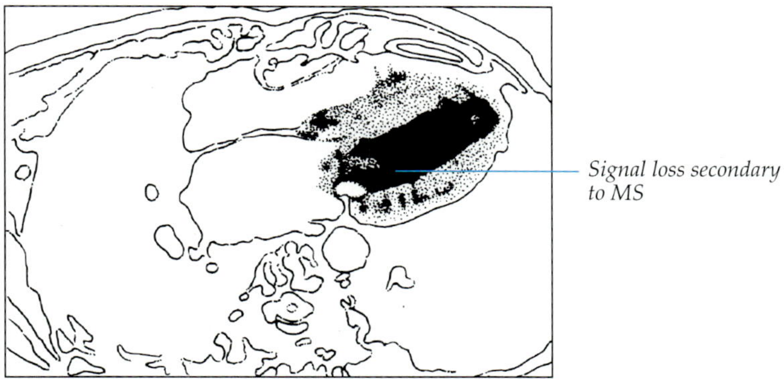

FIGURE 4-9. *(continued)* The end-diastolic frame demonstrates the restoration of MRI signal within the LV cavity. Conventional cine MRI has been correlated with Doppler ultrasound estimates of MS [17]. It is anticipated that phase velocity mapping techniques will increase the utility of cine MRI for detecting stenotic valve gradients [18].

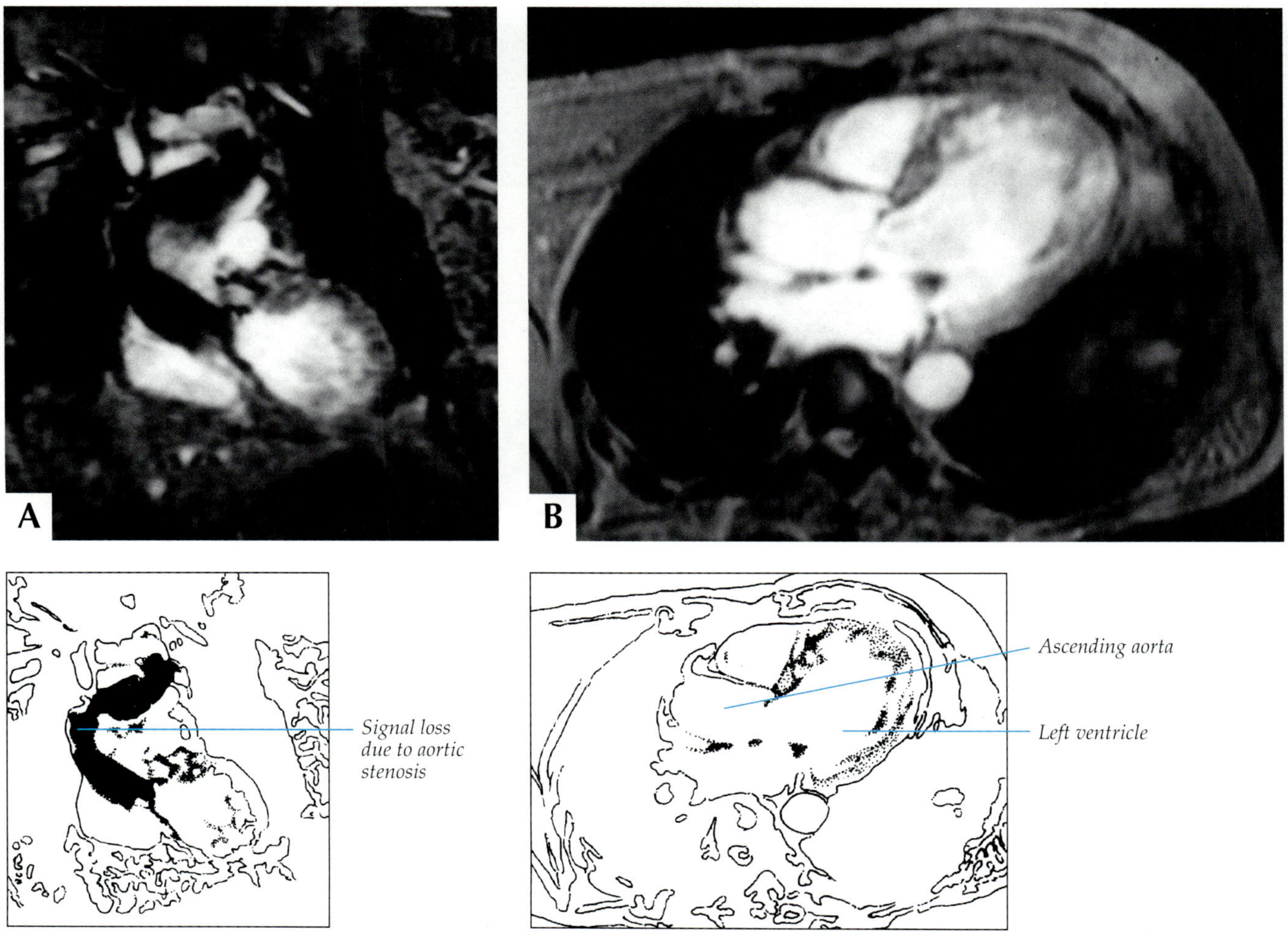

FIGURE 4-10. Valvular aortic stenosis (AS). Coronal ascending aorta and left ventricular outflow tract (LVOT) images, seen in a patient with severe valvular AS. As systole progresses (**A**), there is extensive signal loss extending to the level of the aortic arch. The extent of signal loss in the ascending aorta has been correlated with the degree of obstruction [19]. However, phase velocity mapping techniques allow precise quantitative assessment of the stenotic valvular gradients [20]. *(continued)*

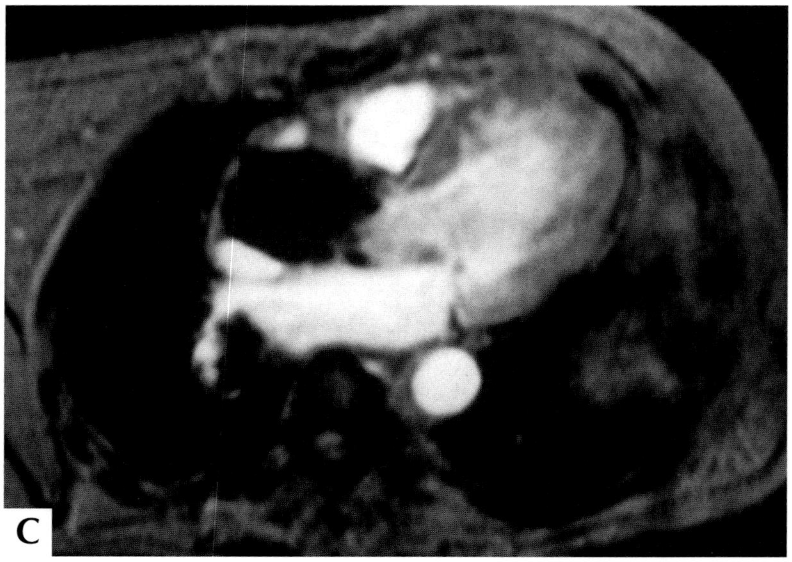

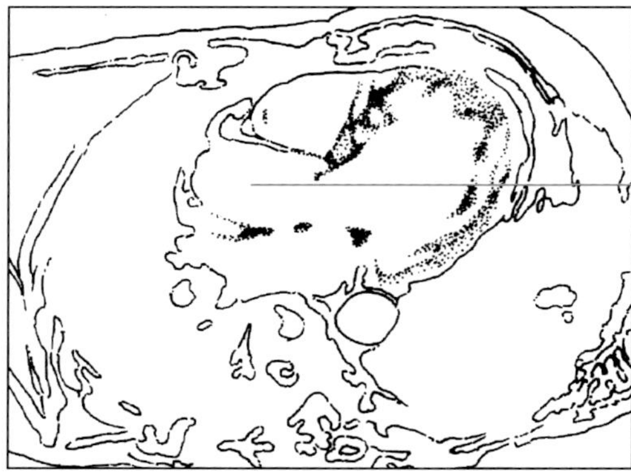

FIGURE 4-10. (*continued*) On the LVOT images (**B** and **C**) chamber function and hypertrophy can be assessed.

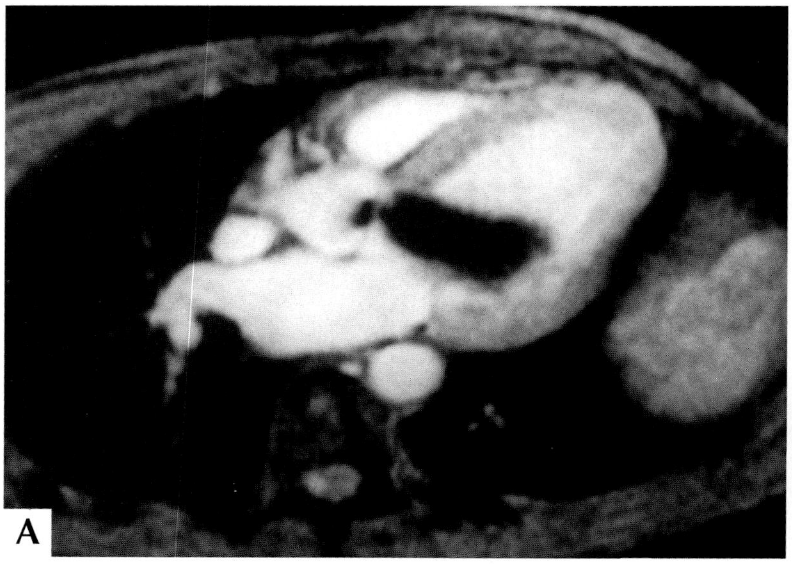

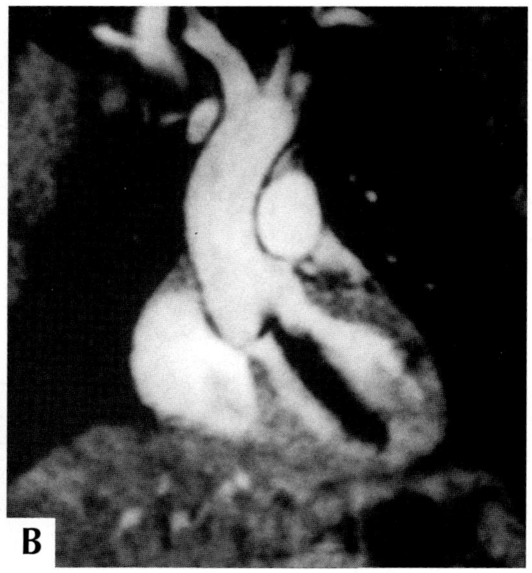

FIGURE 4-11. Severe aortic regurgitation (AR) .Shown are left ventricular outflow tract (**A**), coronal, ascending aorta (**B**), and serial short axis images (*continued*)

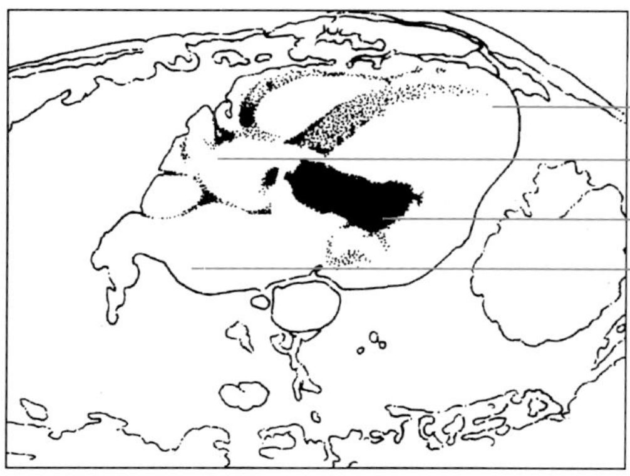

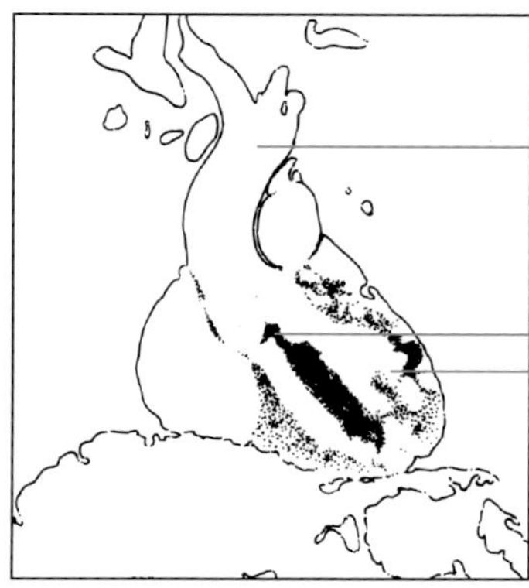

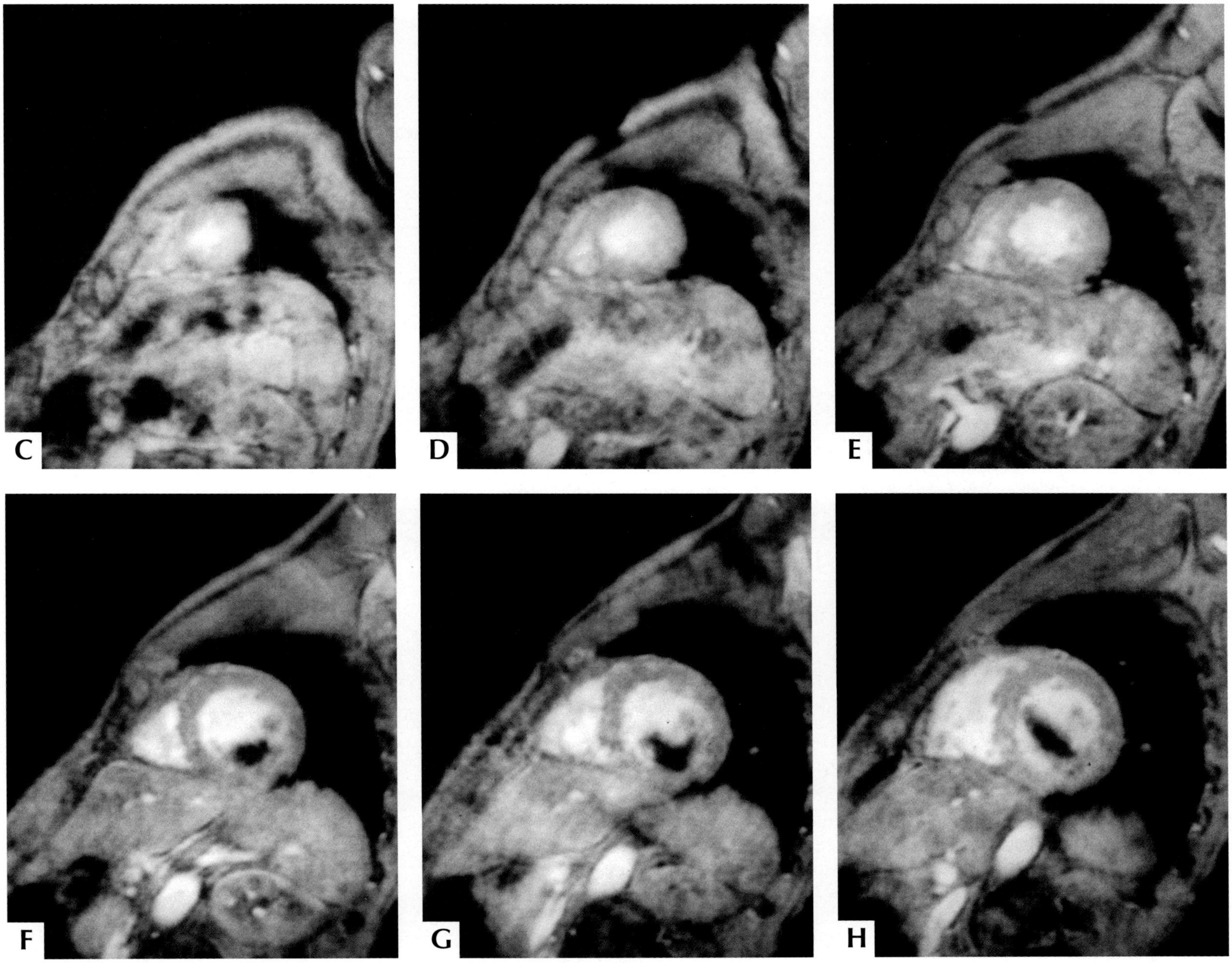

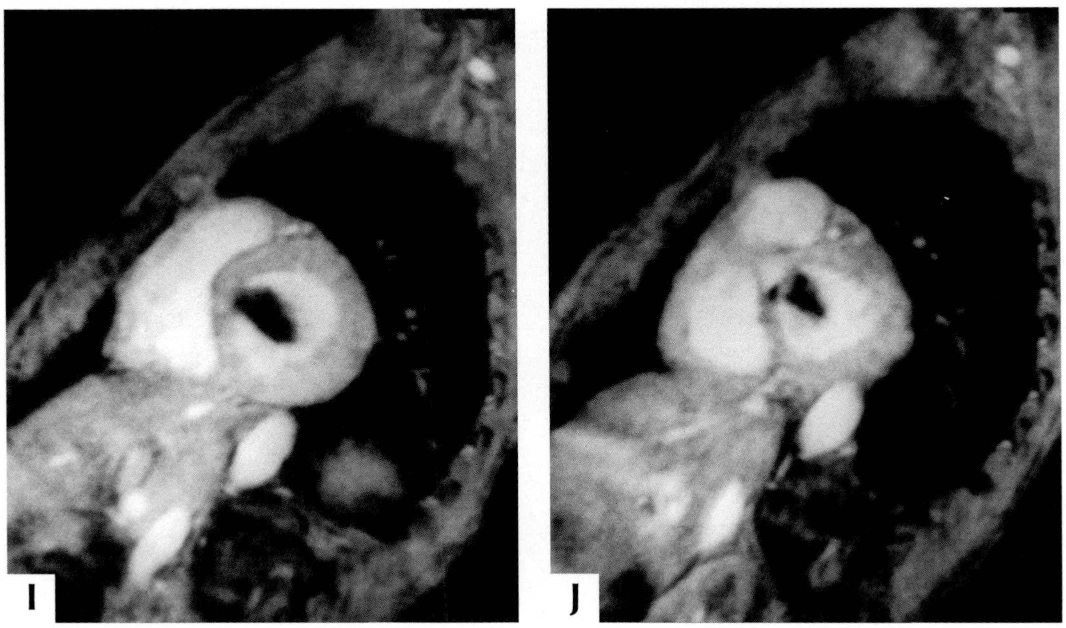

FIGURE 4-11. (*continued*) (**C–J**, apex to base) from a patient with severe AR. The regurgitant jet extends far into the left ventriclular cavity and there is significant chamber enlargement. Several studies have demonstrated the accuracy of MRI for assessing aortic regurgitation [21–23]. MRI is ideally suited for providing serial follow-up of chamber dimensions, ventricular volumes and ventricular systolic function in patients with chronic valvular regurgitation.

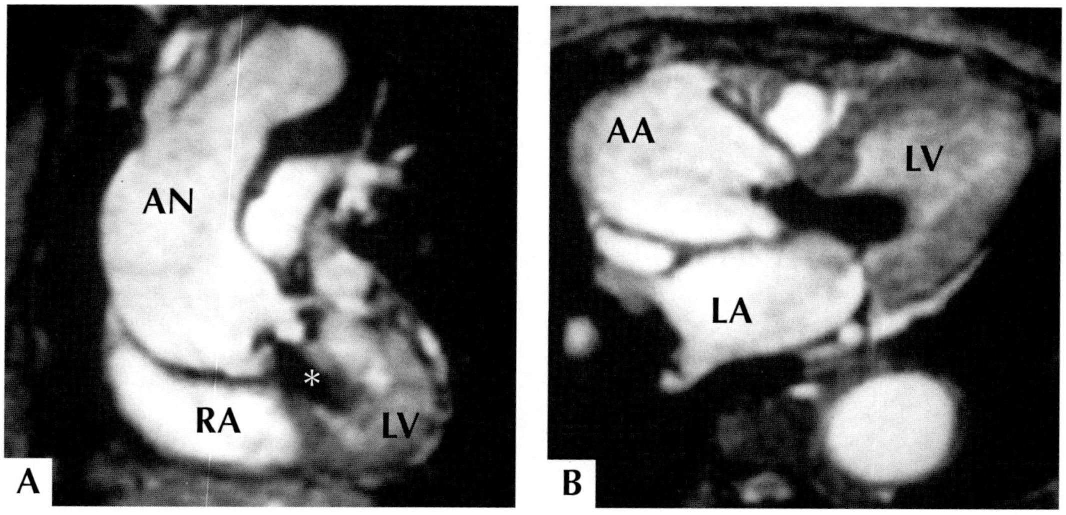

FIGURE 4-12. Aortic regurgitation (AR) secondary to a dilated aortic root. Cine MRI is the noninvasive imaging modality of choice for assessing thoracic aortic disease in stable patients. In the coronal ascending aortic view (**A**), aortic size and morphology are well demonstrated, as is an aortic aneurysm (AN) andAR (*asterisk*). The left ventricular outflow tract view (**B**) can be used to assess left ventricular (LV) wall thickness, systolic function, and the severity of AR. AA—ascending aorta; LA—left atrium; RA—right atrium.

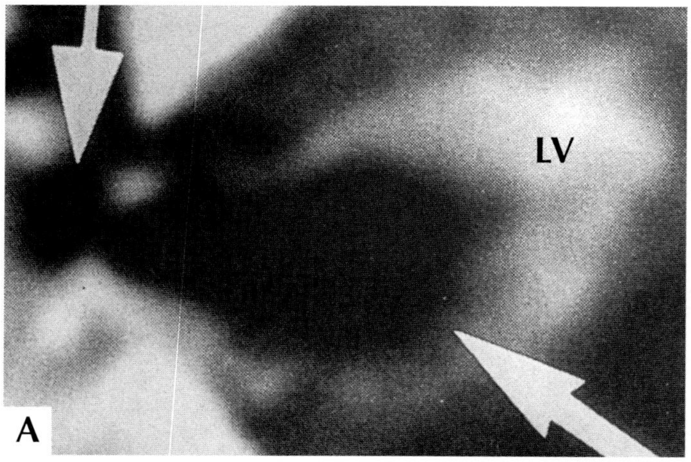

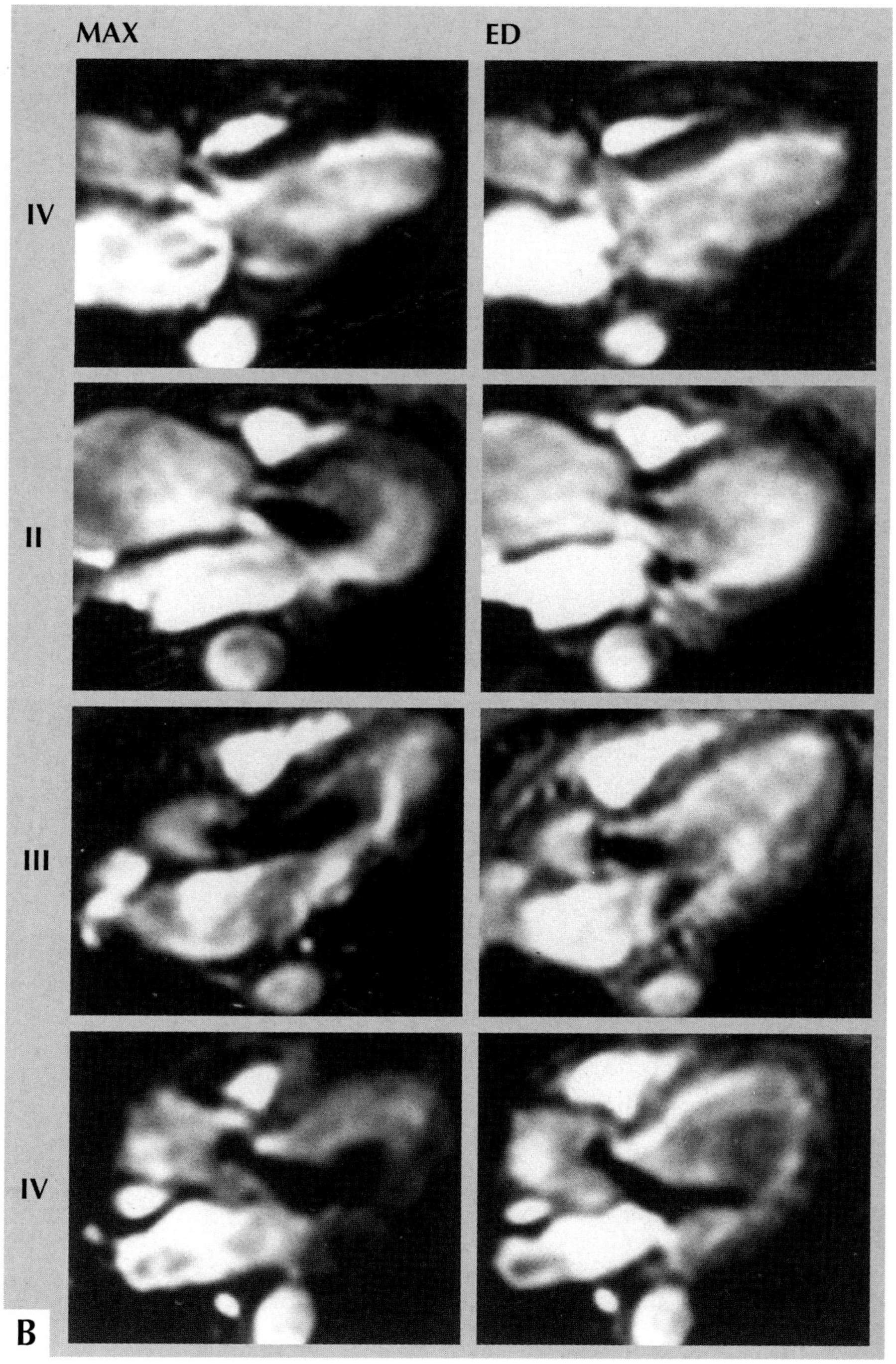

FIGURE 4-13. Aortic regurgitation (AR). A technique for the rapid assessment of AR and left ventricular (LV) function using cine MRI and the proximal convergence zone has been validated by Cranney *et al.* [24]. The LV outflow tract plane is used to calculate a single plane area-length ejection fraction. AR is assessed using the presence, size, and persistence of not only the regurgitant jet but also the zone of proximal signal loss. As fluid approaches an orifice, there is an acceleration of flow. The isovelocity surfaces proximal to the regurgitant orifice can be described by a series of hemispheres centered around the orifice. The greater the flow rate, the larger the hemisphere that is described. Using the size and persistence of this proximal convergence zone and the regurgitant jet, MRI determination of the severity of AR correlates very closely with Doppler and invasive aortography. **A**, A zoomed image of an aortic regurgitant jet. The *lower arrow* identifies the main body of the AR jet. The hemispheric proximal convergence zone is identified by the *upper arrow*. **B**, Four grades of AR are distinguished by MRI. The *left column* represents the phase during which the jet is of maximal size. The *right column* represents end diastole. Image window settings are standardized to enhance contrast between the regurgitant jet and surrounding blood. In grade I AR there is a small regurgitant jet that is not seen at end diastole. Grade IV AR is characterized by a large maximal jet and proximal convergence zone that persists to end-diastole and remains large. Grades II and III are intermediate between these two extremes. (*Adapted from* Cranney and coworkers [24]; with permission.)

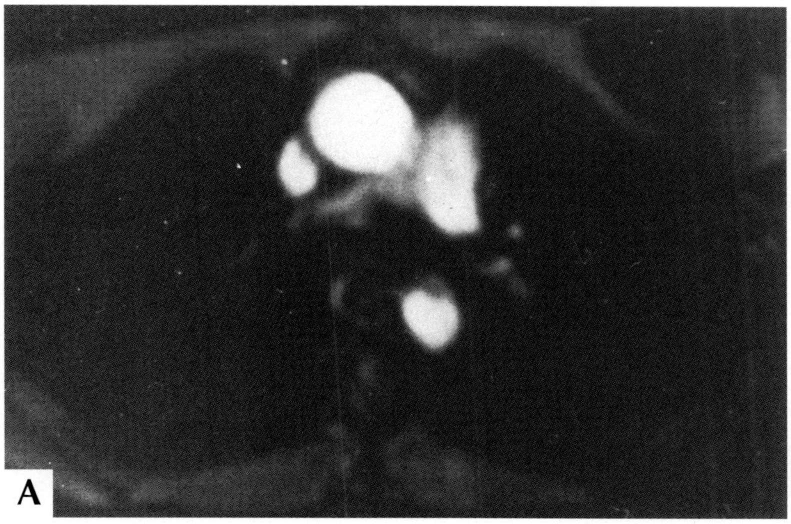

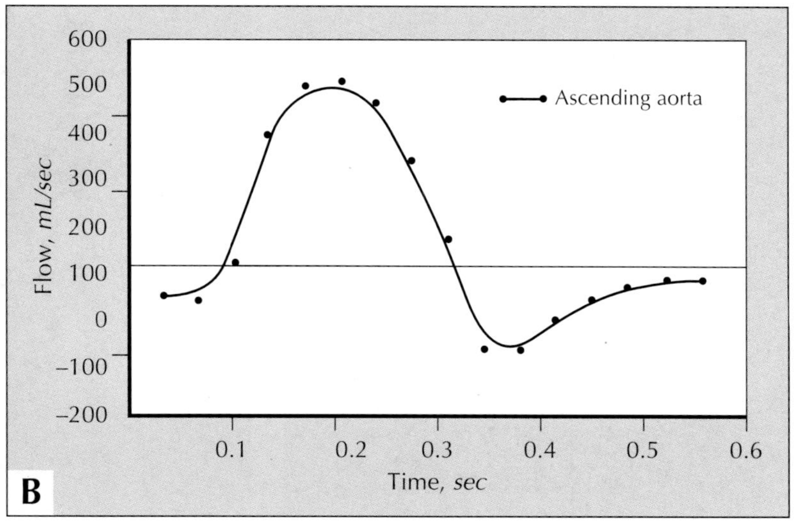

FIGURE 4-14. Phase velocity mapping. Conventional MRI techniques produce an amplitude (modulus) image based on the magnitude of radiofrequency signal. Encoded within the raw data of MR signal, however, is information regarding the radiofrequency phase angle, and phase angle can be made proportional to velocity in any direction. Using this phase velocity mapping technique, precise measurements of vascular flow can be obtained. **A**, The standard amplitude image is shown on top and the corresponding phase image on the bottom. Flow directed caphalad in the ascending aorta appears black, whereas caudal flow in the descending aorta appears white. Stationary tissue acquires no phase, and thereby, appears gray in this image [18,25].

B, This is a flow curve from a patient with aortic regurgitation . The data were obtained by integrating cross-sectional velocities in the aortic root throughout the cardiac cycle. Integration of this curve during systole represents forward stroke volume; regurgitant volume can be determined by integration of the curve during diastole. This approach may lead to more precise quantitation of regurgitation severity [23,26]. (*Adapted from* Cranney and coworkers [9]; with permission.)

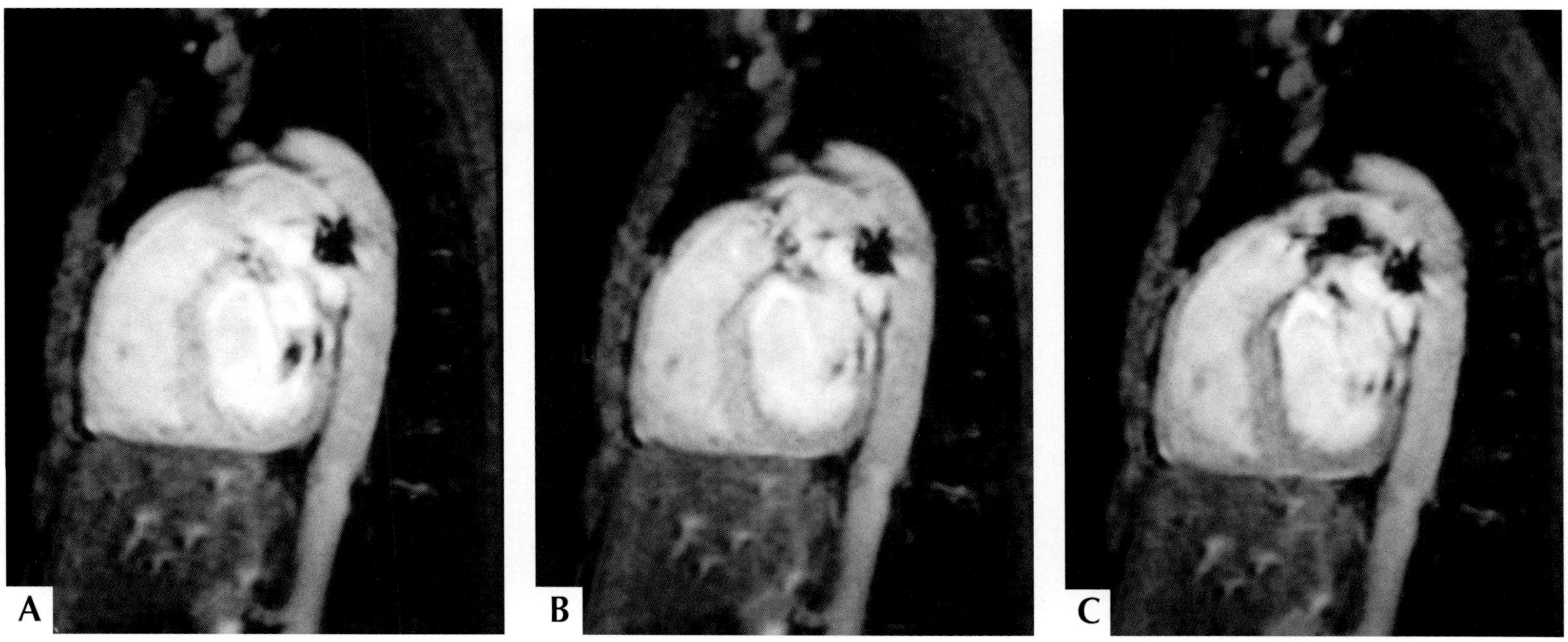

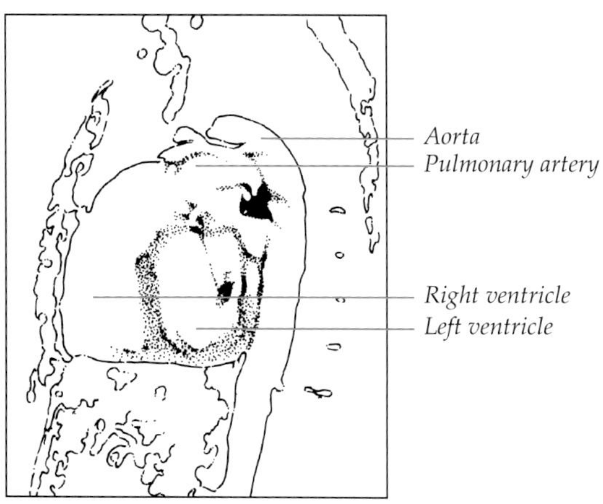

FIGURE 4-15. Valvular pulmonic stenosis (PS). Cine MRI in the right ventricular outflow tract plane is from a patient with valvular PS, the etiology of which is congenital in almost all cases. As shown in these images, from diastole through late systole (**A–F**), patients with valvular PS develop concentric right ventricular hypertrophy. Occasionally, right heart failure may develop if the transvalvular gradient is severe and the lesion is left untreated. (*continued*)

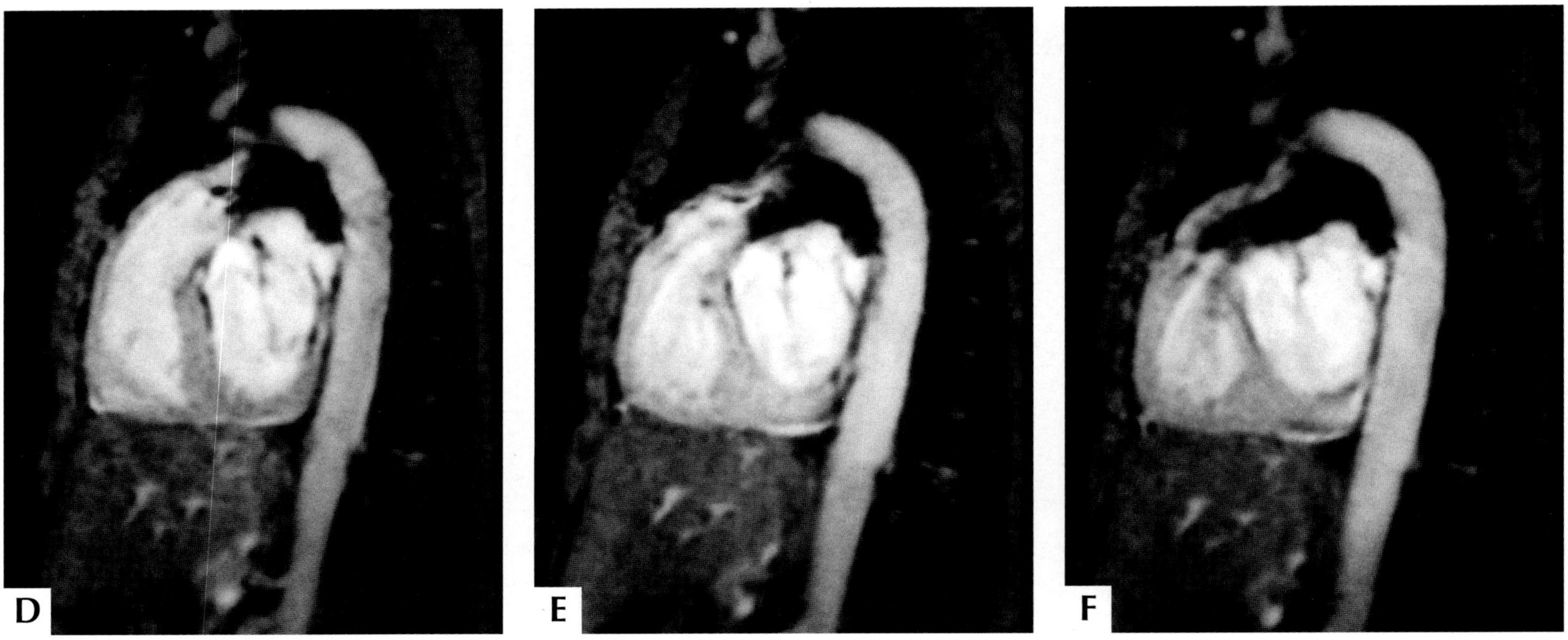

FIGURE 4-15. (*continued*) Most patients with hemodynamically important valvular PS have undergone correction as children, often with balloon valvuloplasty. This lesion is unique in that adult patients with mild to moderate PS seldom progress to a hemodynamically important gradient. MRI is useful in assessing right heart structures, which are often inadequately visualized with echocardiography [27,28].

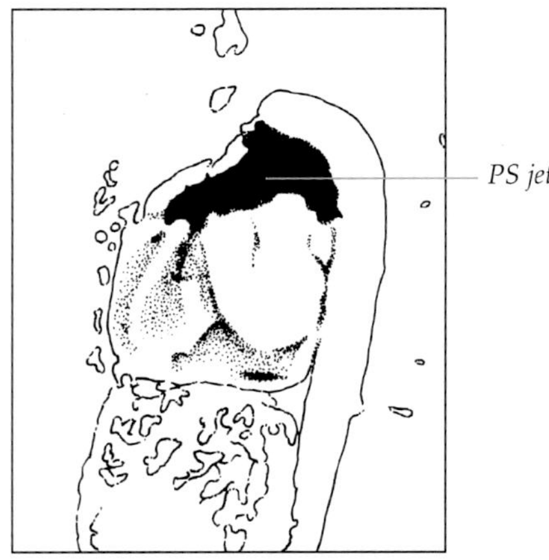

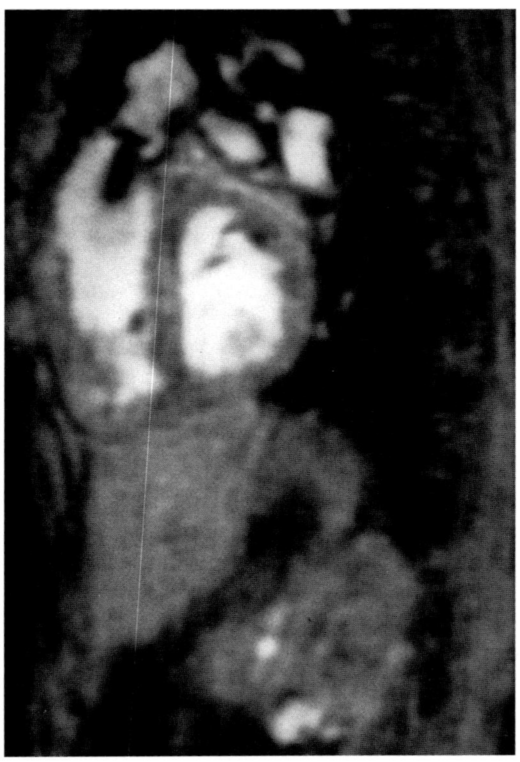

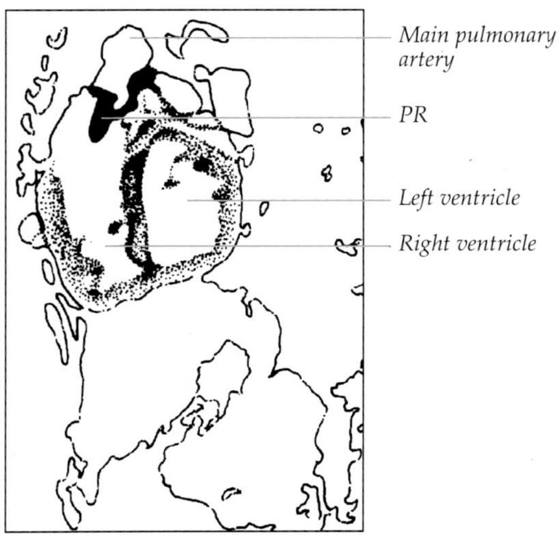

FIGURE 4-16. Pulmonary regurgitation (PR). Early diastolic cine MRI is from a patient with PR. Small jets of PR are frequently identified in normal patients but are seldom of hemodynamic importance. However, severe PR can be a late sequela in some patients after surgical repair of congenital heart disease. Cine MRI with phase velocity mapping is well suited for follow-up of patients with severe PR [29].

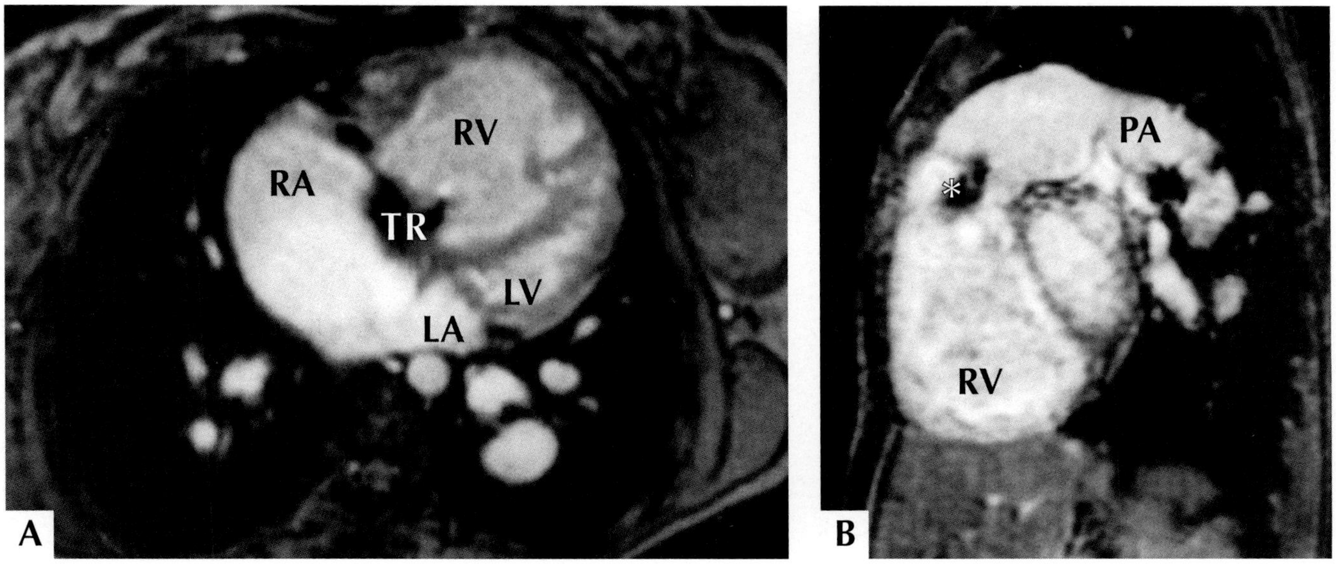

FIGURE 4-17. Combined tricuspid regurgitation (TR) and pulmonic regurgitation in a patient with pulmonary hypertension. There is marked dilatation of the right atrium (RA), right ventricle (RV), and main pulmonary artery (PA). TR is identified on the systolic axial image (**A**). Pulmonic regurgitation (PR) is identified in the early diastolic RV outflow tract (RVOT) image (*asterisk* in **B**). MRI techniques have been used to assess right and left lung perfusion in normal patients [30]. In addition, pulmonary flow has been quantified in patients with pulmonary hypertension using phase velocity mapping techniques [31]. LA—left atrium; LV—left ventricle.

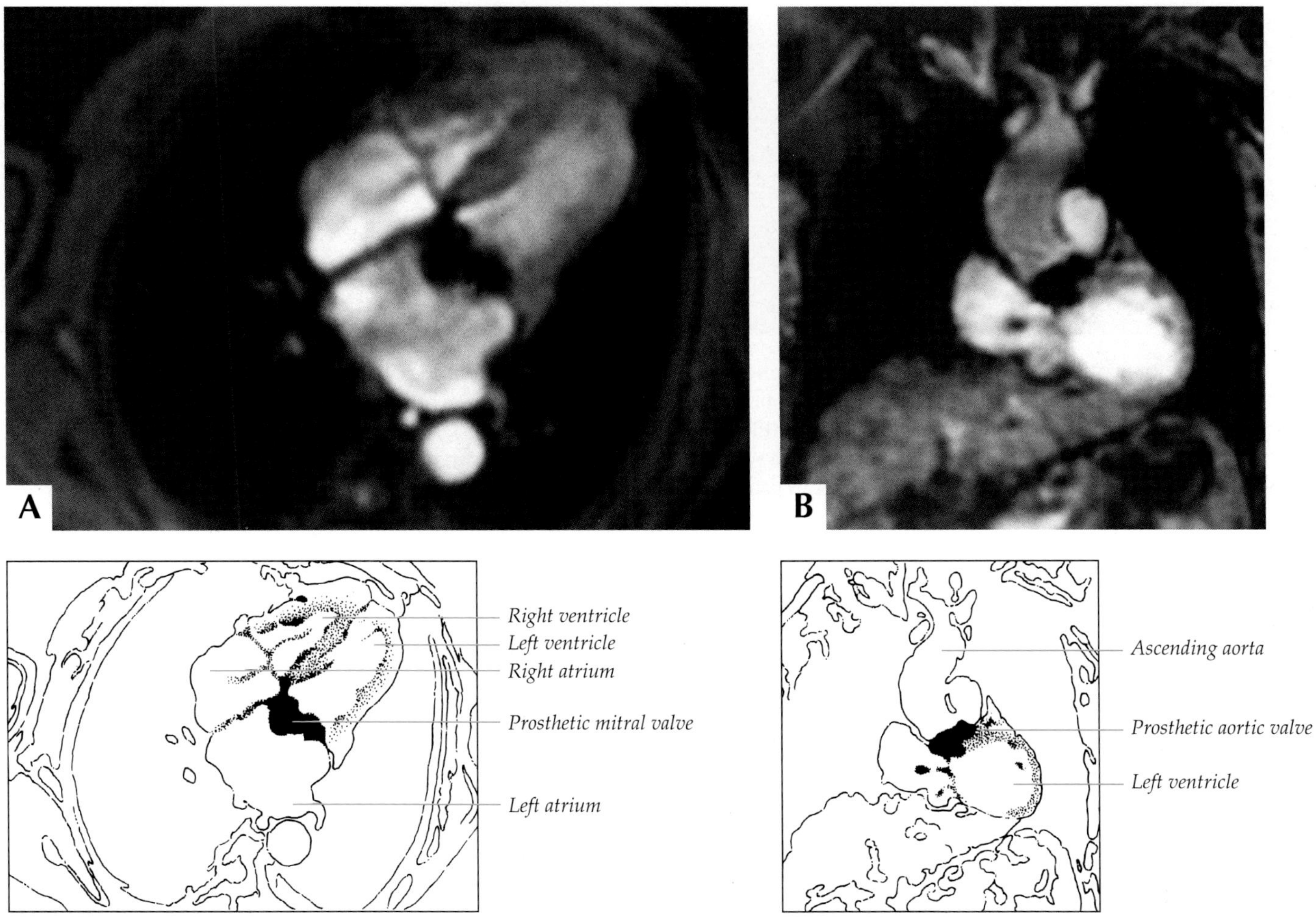

FIGURE 4-18. MRI of prosthetic valves. **A**, This four-chamber cine MRI frame is from a patient with a prosthetic mitral valve. Note the extensive signal loss in the region of the prosthesis and the markedly enlarged left atrium. **B**, The coronal ascending aortic image is from a patient with an aortic prosthesis. Virtually all prosthetic cardiac valves can be imaged safely using MRI [32]. The signal loss precludes assessment of the paravalvular region, but significant valvular and paravalvular regurgitation can be identified.

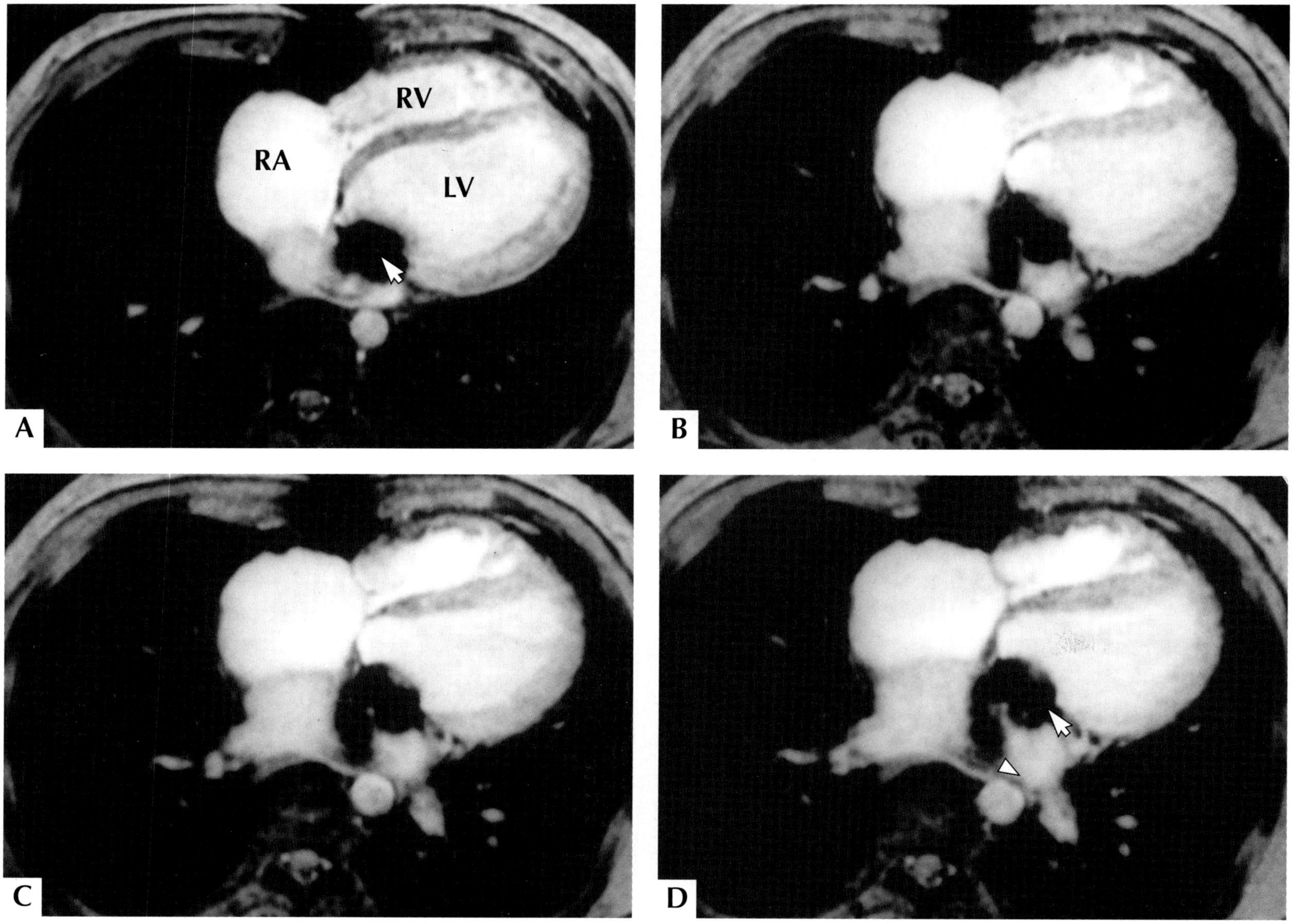

FIGURE 4-19. Perivalvular mitral regurgitation (MR) in a patient after St. Jude's mitral valve (MV) replacement. On the end-diastolic image (**A**) the normal signal void induced by the prosthesis is identified (*arrow*). **B** through **D**, An eccentric jet of MR can be easily identified on subsequent frames ending with systole and arises from the perivalvular region. Perivalvular regurgitation can be well demonstrated on transesophageal echocardiography; however, cine MRI can also be useful in these selected patients [33]. The *arrow* in *panel D* indicates the MV prosthesis; the *arrowhead* shows the area of periprosthetic MR. LV—left ventricle; RA—right atrium; RV—right ventricle.

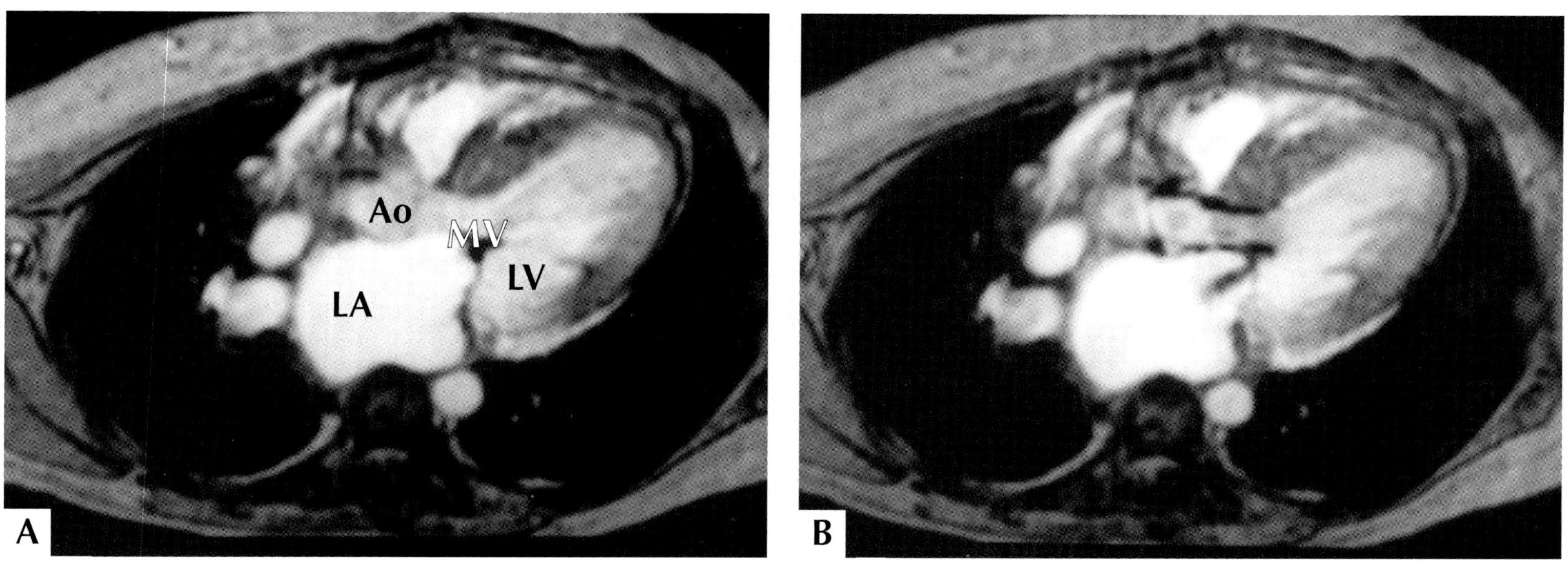

FIGURE 4-20. Left ventricular outflow tract (LVOT) cine MRIs in a patient with hypertrophic obstructive cardiomyopathy. LV hypertrophy with asymmetric septal thickening is identified in the end-diastolic image (**A**). (*continued*)

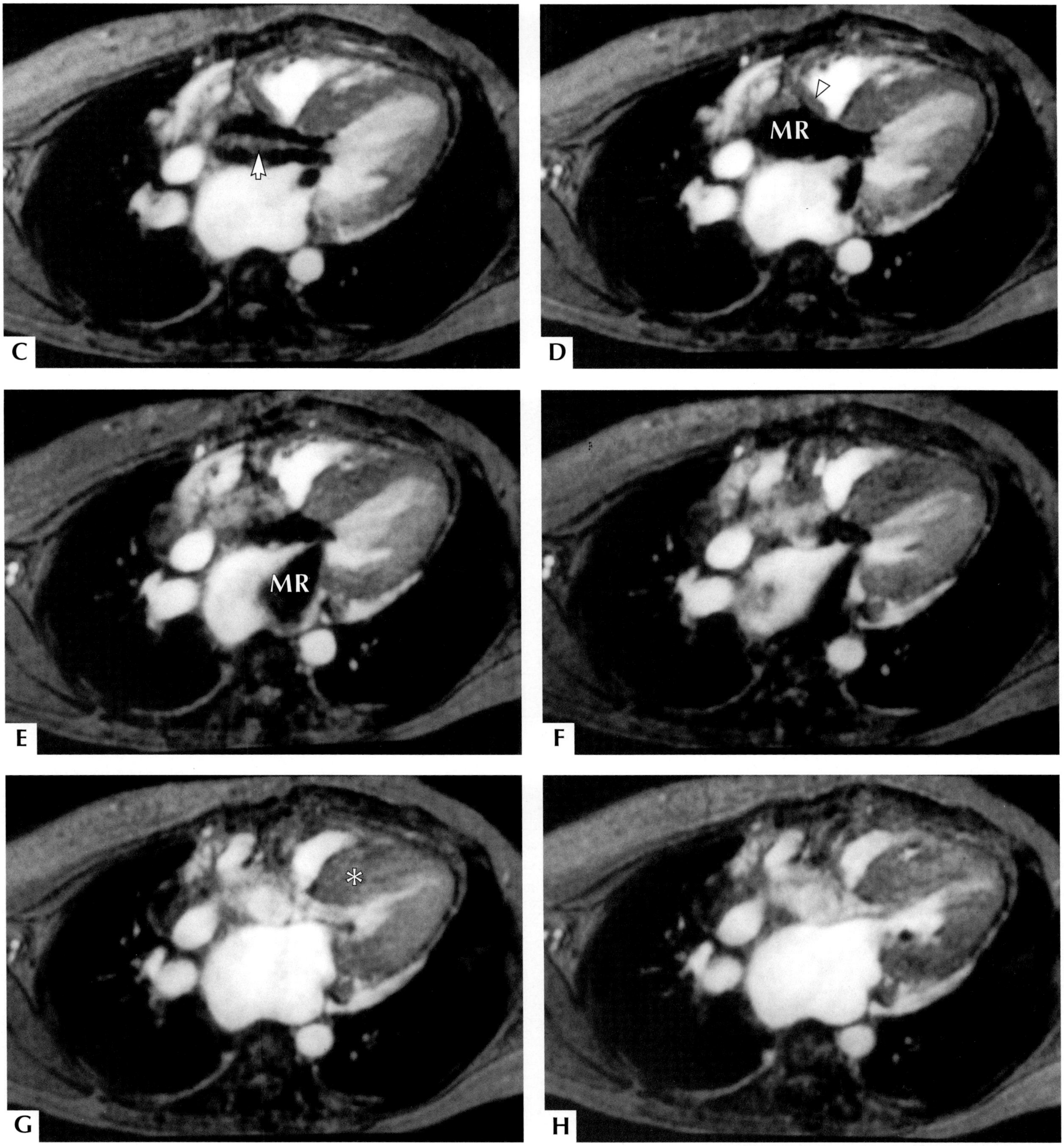

FIGURE 4-20. *(continued)* As systole progresses (**B** through **G**), signal loss is noted in the subvalvular LVOT region (*arrow* in *C*) secondary to intracavity obstruction (*arrowhead* in *D*). A large jet of mitral regurgitation (MR) is also identified and is quite common in patients with hypertrophic cardiomyopathy. Near total cavity obliteration can be seen on the late systolic images (*asterisk* in *G*). Ao—aorta; LA—left atrium; MV—mitral valve.

Radionuclide Angiography

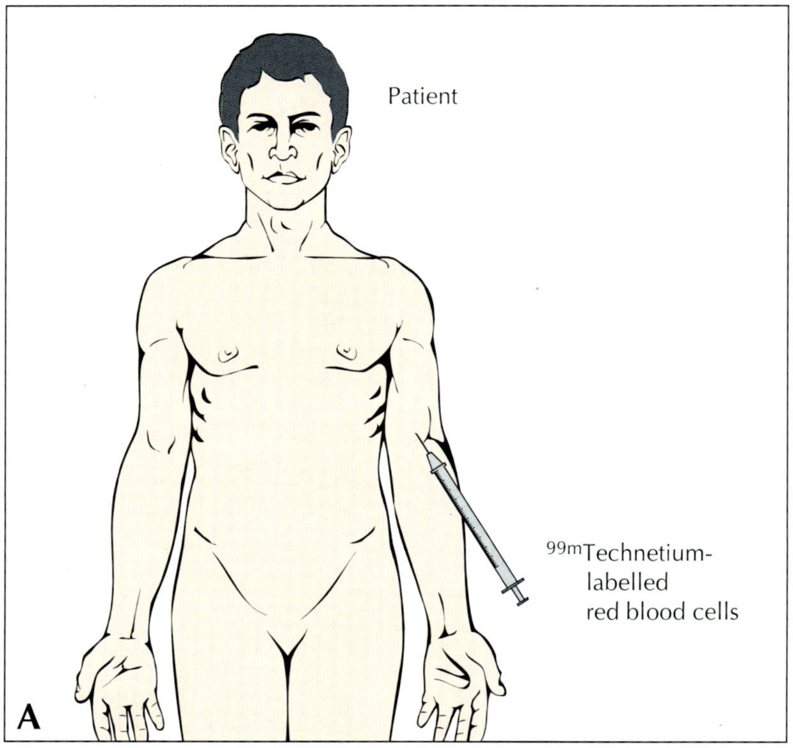

Figure 4-21. Basic principles of radionuclide angiography. Technetium-labeled red blood cells are injected intravenously and circulate throughout the blood pool (**A**). Electrocardiographic (ECG) electrodes are attached to the patient and a scintillation camera is positioned over the chest (**B**). Gamma emissions over the region of interest (heart) are detected by the camera and the acquisition gated to the R wave of the ECG. Data from many cardiac cycles are obtained and averaged. An endless loop cine of an "average" cardiac cycle is then displayed for interpretation. A region of interest is drawn around the left ventricle (LV) (or right ventricle) and radioactive counts recorded throughout the cardiac cycle. End-diastolic (**C**) and end-systolic (**D**) frames from a patient with normal LV function. Left anterior oblique or best septal separation views are shown here, but data can be acquired in different imaging projections depending on the clinical indication. This technique allows accurate and reproducible assessment of LV function and also can be used to determine regional wall motion. Special techniques facilitate quantitation of ventricular volumes, detection of intracardiac shunts, and regurgitant fraction [34–36].

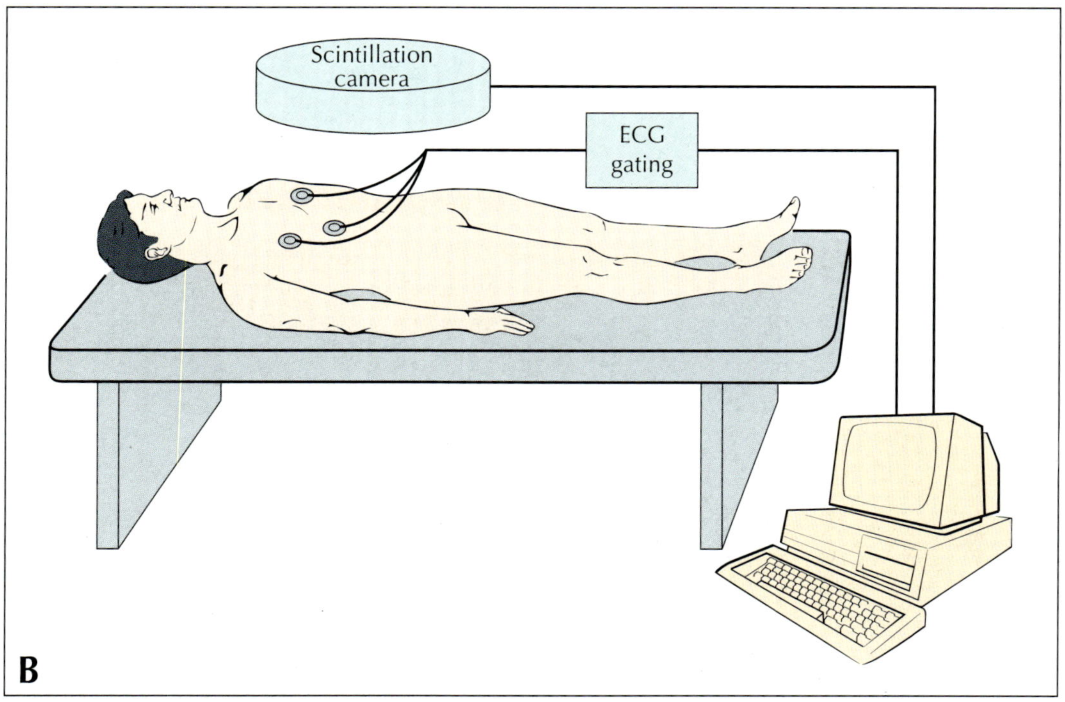

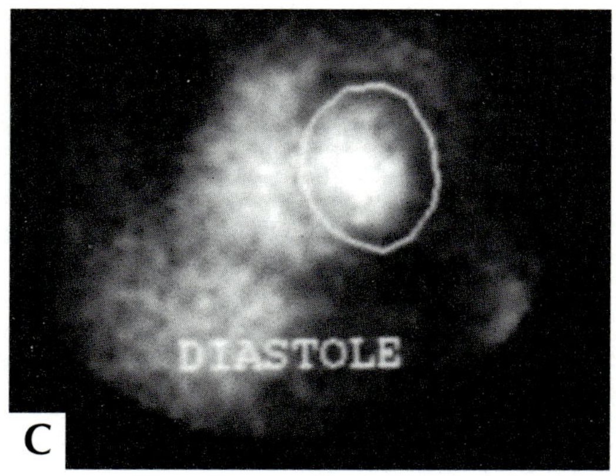

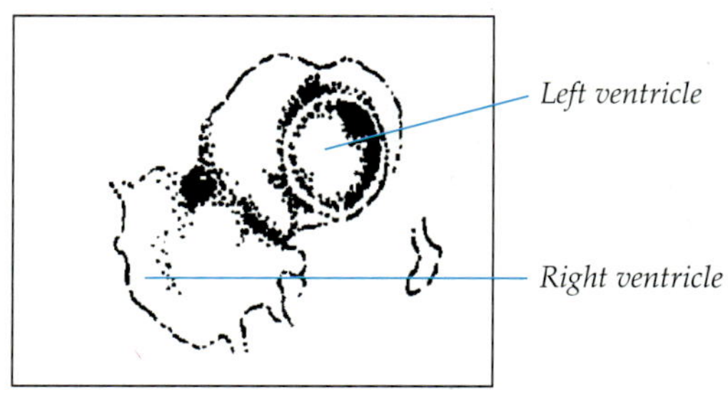

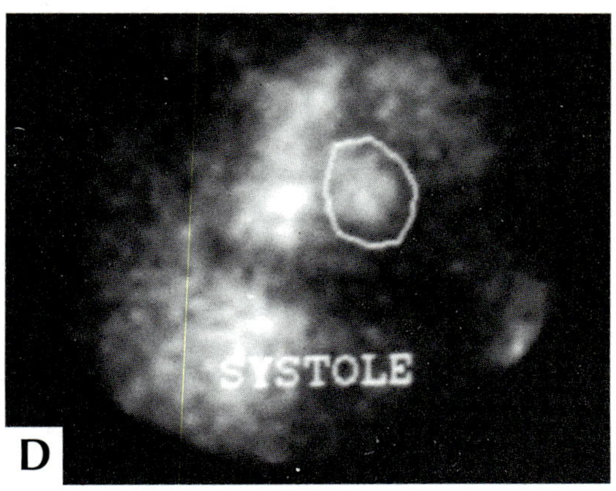

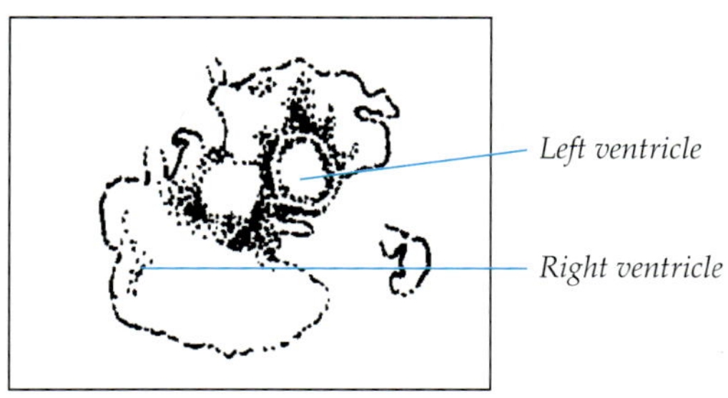

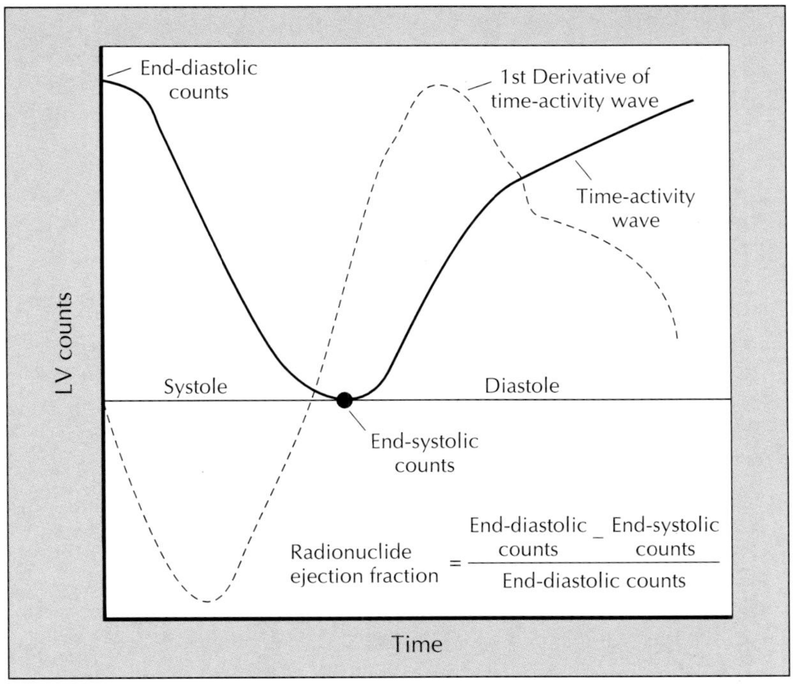

FIGURE 4-22. Left ventricular (LV) time-activity curve. End diastole is defined as the point with maximal radioactive counts and end systole the point of minimum counts. All points throughout the acquisition can be quantitated and a smooth curve constructed. Radionuclide ejection fraction (EF) is given by the equation shown. The time-activity curve and its first derivative provide important information relative to both systolic and diastolic performance of the LV.

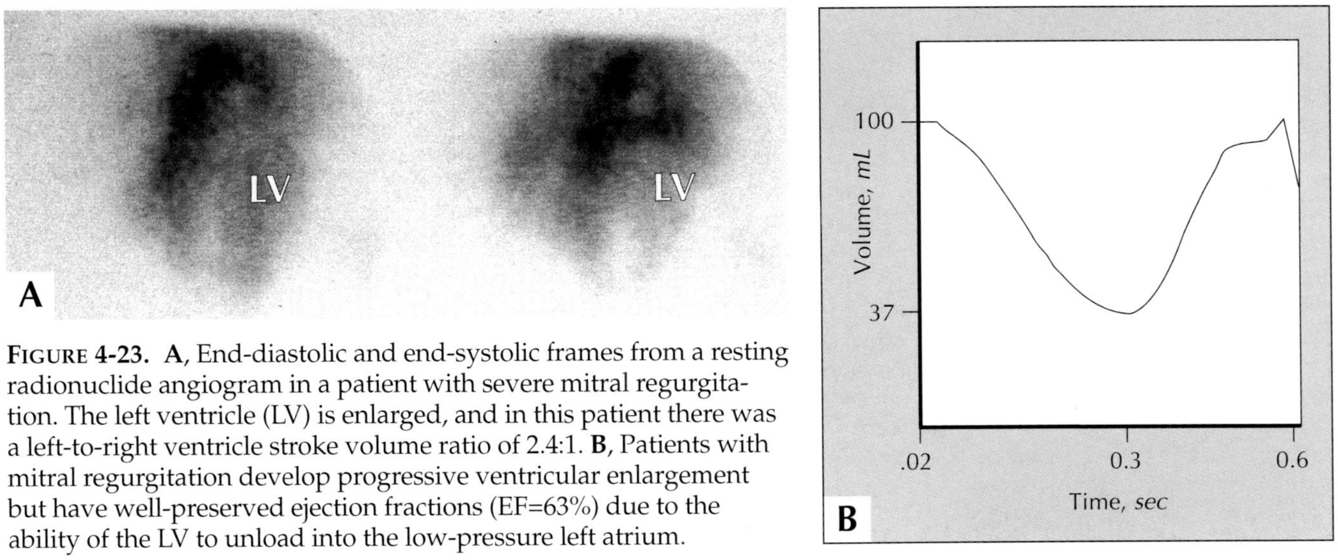

FIGURE 4-23. A, End-diastolic and end-systolic frames from a resting radionuclide angiogram in a patient with severe mitral regurgitation. The left ventricle (LV) is enlarged, and in this patient there was a left-to-right ventricle stroke volume ratio of 2.4:1. **B**, Patients with mitral regurgitation develop progressive ventricular enlargement but have well-preserved ejection fractions (EF=63%) due to the ability of the LV to unload into the low-pressure left atrium.

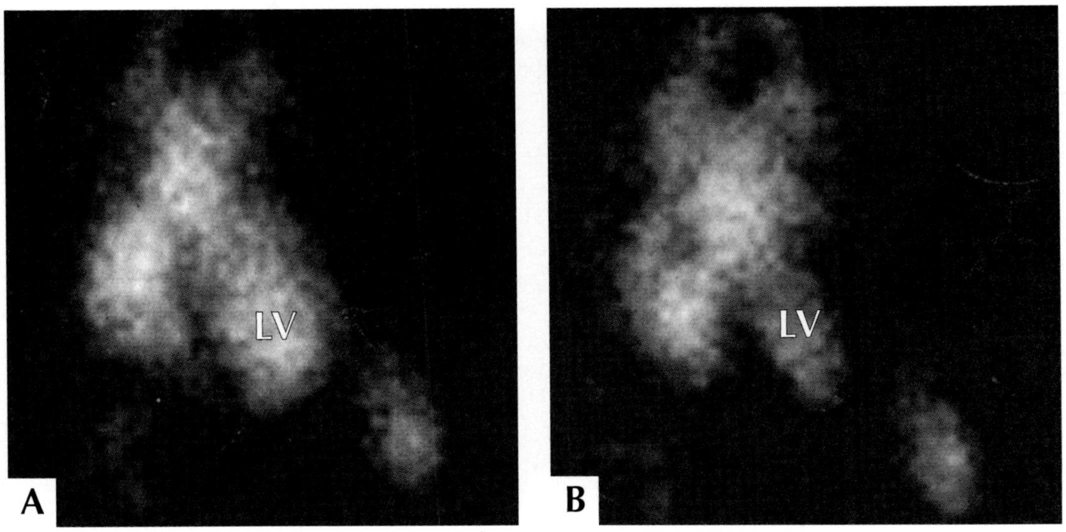

FIGURE 4-24. Radionuclide angiography plus exercise. In addition to resting studies, radionuclide angiography combined with exercise may provide an objective assessment of functional status. This figure represents rest (**A**) and exercise (**B**) radionuclide angiograms, of end-diastole in a patient with chronic aortic insufficiency,[37]. LV–left ventricle.

References

1. Doyle M, Blackwell G: Basic principles of MRI. In *MRI: Cardiovascular System*. Edited by Blackwell G, Cranney G, Pohost G. New York: Gower Medical Publishing; 1992: 1.1–1.11.
2. Saini S, Frankel RB, Stark DD, Ferrucci JT: Magnetism: a primer and review. *Am J Roentgenol AJR* 1988, 150:735–744.
3. Blackwell GG, Pohost GM: The usefulness of cardiovascular magnetic resonance imaging. *Curr Probl Cardiol* 1994, 19:117–176.
4. Blackwell G, Doyle M, Cranney G: *Cardiovascular MRI techniques.* In MRI: Cardiovascular System. Edited by Blackwell G, Cranney G, Pohost G. New York; Gower Medical Publishing; 1992: .
5. Blackwell G, Cranney G, Lotan C: Ventricular volume, function, and mass. In *MRI: Cardiovascular System*. Edited by Blackwell G, Cranney G, Pohost G. New York; Gower Medical Publishing; 1992:
6. Cranney GB, Lotan CS, Dean L, *et al.*: Left ventricular volume measurement using cardiac axis NMR imaging—validation by calibrated ventricular angiography. *Circulation* 1990; 82:154–163.
7. Sechtem U, Pflugfelder PW, Gould RG, *et al.*: Measurement of right and left ventricular volumes in healthy individuals with cine MR imaging. *Radiology* 1987, 163:697–702.
8. Weiss JL, Shapiro EP, Buchalter MB, *et al.*: Magnetic resonance imaging as a noninvasive standard for the quantitative evaluation of left ventricular mass, ischemia, and infarction. *Ann N Y Acad Sci* 1990, 601:95–106.
9. Cranney GB, Lotan CS, Pohost GM: Nuclear magnetic resonance imaging for assessment and follow-up of patients with valve disease. *Circulation* 1991, 84:216–227.
10. Mirowitz SA, Lee JKT, Gutierrez FR, *et al.*: Normal signal-void patterns in cardiac cine MR images. *Radiology*: 1990, 176:49–55.
11. Wagner S, Auffermann W, Buser P, *et al.*: Diagnostic accuracy and estimation of the severity of valvular regurgitation from the signal void on cine magnetic resonance imaging. *Am Heart J* 1989, 118:760–767.
12. Pflugfelder PW, Sechtem UP, White RD, *et al.*: Noninvasive evaluation of mitral regurgitation by analysis of left atrial signal loss in cine magnetic resonance. *Am Heart J* 1989, 117:1113–1119.
13. Nishimura T, Yamada N, Itoh A, Miyatake K: Cine MR imaging in mitral regurgitation: comparison with color Doppler flow imaging. *Am J Roentgenol* 1989, 153:721–724.
14. Higgins CB, Wagner S, Kondo C, *et al.*: Evaluation of valvular heart disease with cine gradient echo magnetic resonance imaging. *Circulation* 1991, 84:198–207.
15. Aurigemma G, Reichek N, Schieber M, Axel L: Evaluation of mitral regurgitation by cine magnetic resonance imaging. *Am J Cardiol* 1990, 66:621–625.
16. Suzuki J, Caputo GR, Kondo C, Higgins CB: Cine MR imaging of valvular heart disease: display, and imaging parameters affect the size of the signal void caused by valvular regurgitation. *Am J Roentgenol* 1990, 155:723–717.
17. Casolo GC, Zampa V, Rega L, *et al.*: Evaluation of mitral stenosis by cine magnetic resonance imaging. *Am Heart J* 1992, 123:1252–1260.
18. Mohiaddin RH, Longmore DB: Functional aspects of cardiovascular nuclear magnetic resonance imaging: techniques and application. *Circulation* 1993, 88:264–281.
19. Mitchell L, Jenkins JPR, Watson Y, *et al.*: Diagnosis and assessment of mitral and aortic valve disease by cine-flow magnetic resonance imaging. *Magn Reson Med* 1989, 12:181–197.
20. Søodergaard L, Hildebrandt P, Lindvig K, *et al.*: Valve area andcardiac output in aortic stenosis: quantification by magnetic resonance velocity mapping. *Am Heart J* 1993, 126:1156–1164.
21. Sechtem U, Pflugfelder PW, Cassidy MM, *et al.*: Mitral or aortic regurgitation: quantification of regurgitant volumes with cine MR imaging. *Radiology* 1988, 167:425–430.
22. Pflugfelder PW, Landzberg JS, Cassidy MM, *et al.*: Comparison of cine MR imaging with Doppler echocardiography for the evaluation of aortic regurgitation. *Am J Roentgenol* 1989, 152:729–735.
23. Cranney GB, Lotan CS, Pohost GM: Evaluation of aortic regurgitation by magnetic resonance imaging. *Curr Probl Cardiol* 1990, 15:87–114.
24. Cranney GB, Benjelloun H, Perry GJ, *et al.*: Rapid assessment of aortic regurgitation and left ventricular function using cine nuclear magnetic resonance imaging and the proximal convergence zone. *Am J Cardiol* 1993, 71:1074–1081.
25. Mostbeck GH, Caputo GR, Higgins CB: MR measurement of blood flow in the cardiovascular system. *Am J Roentgenol* 1992, 159:453–461.
26. Dulce MC, Mostbeck GH, O'Sullivan M, *et al.*: Severity of aortic regurgitation: interstudy reproducibility of measurements with velocity-encoded cine MR imaging. *Radiology* 1992, 185:235–240.
27. Kilner PJ, Firmin DN, Reese RSO, *et al.*: Valve and great vessel stenosis: assessment with MR jet velocity mapping. *Radiology* 1991, 178:229–235.
28. Martinez JE, Mohiaddin RH, Kilner PJ, *et al.*: Obstruction in extracardiac ventriculopulmonary conduits: value of nuclear magnetic resonance imaging with velocity mapping and Doppler echocardiography. *J Am Coll Cardiol* 1992, 20:338–344.
29. Rebergen SA, Chin JGJ, Oeenkamp J, *et al.*: Pulmonary regurgitation in the late postoperative follow-up of tetralogy of Fallot. *Circulation* 1993, 88:2257–2266.
30. Caputo GR, Kondo C, Masui T, *et al.*: Right and left lung perfusion: in vitro and in vivo validation with oblique-angle, velocity-endcoded cine MR imaging. *Radiology* 1991, 180:693–698.
31. Kondo C, Caputo GR, Masui T, *et al.*: Pulmonary hypertension: pulmonary flow quantification and flow profile analysis with velocity-encoded cine MR imaging. *Radiology* 1992, 183:751–758.
32. Pohost GM, Blackwell GG, Shellock F: Safety of patients with medical devices during application of magnetic resonance methods. *Ann N Y Acad Sci* 1992, 649:302–312.
33. Deutsch HJ, Bachmann R, Sechtem U, *et al.*: Regurgitant flow in cardiac valve prostheses: diagnostic value of gradient echo nuclear magnetic resonance imaging in reference to transesophageal two-dimensional color Doppler echocardiography. *J Am Coll Cardiol* 1992, 19:1500–1507.
34. Rozanski A, Rodrigues E, Nichols K, Berman D: Equilibrium and first-pass radionuclide cineangiography. *The Technology of Cardiovascular Imaging*. Boston: Little, Brown; 1991:221–260.
35. Blackwell G, Pohost GM: Radionuclides in the assessment of impaired ventricular function. *Nuclear Medicine in Clinical Diagnosis and Treatment*. Edited by Murray IPC, Ell, PJ. New York: Churchill Livingstone; 1994: 1181–1197.
36. Rigo P, Alderson PO, Robertson RM, *et al.*: Measurement of aortic and mitral regurgitation by gated cardiac blood pool scans. *Circulation* 1979, 60:306–312.
37. Boucher CA, Wilson RA, Kanarck DJ, *et al.*: Exercise testing in asymptomatic or minimally symptomatic aortic regurgitation. *Circulation* 1983, 67:1091–1100.

Role of Cardiac Catheterization and Angiography in Assessment

5

CHAPTER

Morton J. Kern

In the identification and treatment of valvular heart disease, the cardiac catheterization laboratory has been the longest standing arena in which diagnostic and, most recently, therapeutic procedures have been performed. Data obtained from the catheterization laboratory provide clinicians with confirmatory hemodynamic and angiographic information regarding the presence, severity, and associated conditions complicating valvular heart disease. The cardiac catheterization laboratory historically grew out of the work of physiologists studying hemodynamics in experimental animal models. It was not until the early 1950s that cardiac catheterization became a routine laboratory procedure around the world. Hemodynamic data elucidated the physiology of atrial septal defects, ventricular septal defects, stenotic and insufficient mitral and aortic valves, and left ventricular function in a consistent and widely available manner. The cardiac catheterization laboratory was then established as a physiologic laboratory to evaluate valvular and nonvalvular heart disease of all types. Coronary angiography was not added, however, until the early 1960s. Cineangiography and ventriculography permitted investigation of previously unapproachable anatomic sites, clinical conditions, and unique disease entities.

In the past decade, significant advances in both surgical and nonsurgical reparative techniques for valvular heart disease have been established, in large part due to innovation both within and outside the cardiac catheterization laboratory. With the enhancement of two-dimensional echocardiogram and Doppler ultrasound techniques, valvular heart disease can now be readily confirmed and, in some cases, echocardiography may obviate the exacting hemodynamic measurements of the past. In addition, although the valvular lesions may be precisely identified by noninvasive techniques, the presence of coexisting conditions, such as coronary artery disease, myocardial infarction, or peripheral vascular disease cannot be established without direct angiographic data. With this approach in mind, the role of cardiac catheterization and angiography [1–4] in the assessment of valvular heart disease is reviewed in this chapter.

INDICATIONS FOR CARDIAC CATHETERIZATION

INDICATIONS	PROCEDURES
Myocardial infarction	
Unstable angina postinfarction	Left ventriculography, coronary arteriography
Failed thrombolysis	Left ventriculography, coronary arteriography, right heart catheterization
Shock	Left ventriculography, coronary arteriography, right heart catheterization
Mechanical complications (ventricular septal defect, rupture of wall or papillary muscle)	Left ventriculography, coronary arteriography, right heart catheterization
Sudden cardiovascular death	Right and left catheterization, left ventriculography, coronary arteriography
Valvular heart disease	Right and left catheterization, left ventriculography, coronary arteriography, aortography
Congenital heart disease (before anticipated corrective surgery)	Right and left catheterization, left ventriculography, coronary arteriography, aortography
Aortic dissection	Aortography, coronary arteriography
Pericardial constriction or tamponade	Right and left catheterization, left ventriculography, coronary arteriography
Cardiomyopathy	Right and left catheterization, left ventriculography, coronary arteriography, biopsy
Initial and follow-up assessment for heart transplant	Right and left catheterization, left ventriculography, coronary arteriography, biopsy

Figure 5-1. Indications for cardiac catheterization. In most circumstances, a clinical evaluation and noninvasive testing, including electrocardiography, chest roentgenography, and echocardiography, have narrowed the differential diagnosis to include a valvular lesion as a contributing etiology. Among the most important indications is the evaluation of a patient with dyspnea of uncertain etiology, especially when noninvasive testing is inconclusive. (*Adapted from* Kern [4].)

CONTRAINDICATIONS AND COMPLICATIONS OF CARDIAC CATHETERIZATION

CONTRAINDICATIONS	COMPLICATIONS
Absolute contraindications	Death
Inadequate equipment or catheterization facility	Myocardial infarction
Relative contraindications	Cerebral vascular accident
Uncontrolled congestive heart failure, high blood pressure, arrhythmias	Serious arrhythmia
Recent cerebral vascular accident (<1 mo)	Ventricular tachycardia
Infection	Fibrillation
Electrolyte imbalance	Atrial fibrillation
Acute gastrointestinal bleeding or anemia	Supraventricular tachyarrhythmia
Pregnancy	Heart block, asystole
Anticoagulation (or known, uncontrolled bleeding diathesis)	Vascular injury
Uncooperative patient	Hemorrhage (local, retroperitoneal, pelvic)
Medication intoxication (*eg*, digitalis, phenothiazine)	Pseudoaneurysm
	Thrombosis/embolus/air embolus
	Aortic dissection
	Cardiac perforation, tamponade
	Contrast reaction/anaphylaxis/nephrotoxicity
	Protamine reaction
	Infection
	Congestive heart failure
	Vasovagal reaction

FIGURE 5-2. Contraindications to cardiac catheterization and potential complications of cardiac catheterization. Most catheterizations are elective procedures with a number of correctable conditions that should be considered before proceeding. Serious complications are related to arrhythmias, allergic reactions to radiographic contrast material, and trauma due to vascular access [5]. Medications used to reverse the anticoagulation, such as protamine, may also rarely be involved with hypotension and subsequent complications of the procedure. The safety of cardiac catheterization to date remains excellent with morbidity (stroke, vascular injury, serious arrhythmias) and mortality less than 0.1% for the majority of patients. The risks of stroke, myocardial infarction, and death have been reduced over the decades by increased operator experience, better radiography equipment, improved catheter materials and contrast media, and careful patient management during high-risk procedures. (*Adapted from* Kern [4].)

SPECIALIZED CATHETERIZATION TECHNIQUES FOR VALVULAR HEART DISEASE ASSESSMENT

- Transseptal puncture
- Direct left ventricular puncture
- Dual high-fidelity micromanometer catheters
- Multiple arterial access
- Long sheaths/double-lumen catheters
- Endomyocardial biopsy
- Pericardial pressure/drainage
- Transcoronary pressure/flow velocity
- Intra-arterial/intracardiac ultrasound imaging
- Indication dilution curves

FIGURE 5-3. Special catheterization techniques. In addition to routine catheter access from the femoral artery and vein, a variety of special techniques may be required for assessment of valvular heart disease. The technique of transseptal access to the left atrium or ventricle is most often used when prosthetic valves are located either in the aortic or mitral positions. In conditions (such as mitral stenosis) in which an accurate pulmonary capillary wedge pressure is required but the measurements are considered unreliable, direct left atrial pressure measurement via the transseptal approach is highly desirable, if not critical to accurate decision making.

In the assessment of aortic stenosis, high-fidelity manometer-tipped pressure catheters are available to record small differences between left ventricular and aortic pressures. This technique can identify aortic gradients with greater precision than fluid-filled transducer systems. Another method using a double-lumen micromanometer catheter system is also available, but it has not provided sufficient fidelity required for routine hemodynamic assessment. In patients with prosthetic aortic and mitral valves, direct left ventricular puncture can be attempted. This uncommonly used technique employs echo-guided needle positioning through the fifth intercostal space at the apex if necessary. Direct left ventricular puncture is used for assessment of mitral regurgitation and left ventricular function in patients with two mechanical prosthetic tilting disc valves in the mitral and aortic positions or in patients in whom access to the left ventricle cannot be achieved via the transseptal route. In rare circumstances, the assessment of pericardial pressure may be an adjunctive technique required for the assessment of valvular lesions.

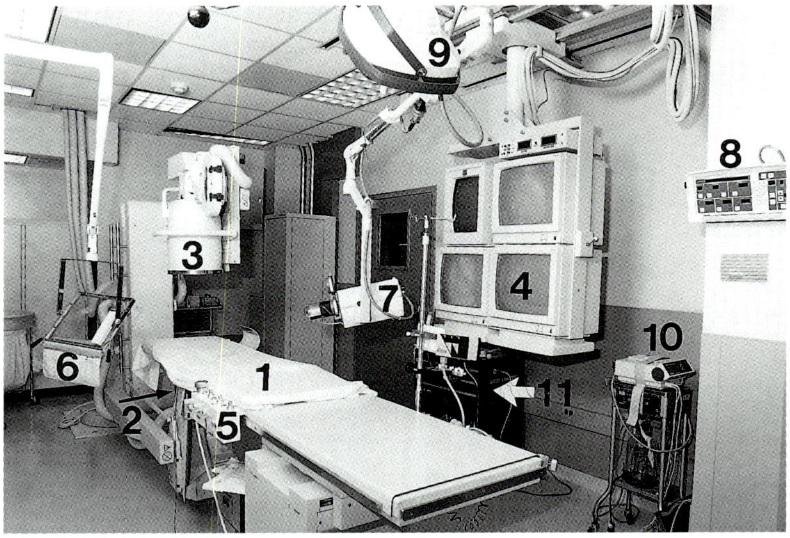

FIGURE 5-4. The cardiac catheterization laboratory. A cardiac catheterization laboratory may have several angiographic and hemodynamic suites. The patient lies supine on a table under a C-arm fluoroscopic unit. The fluoroscopic images are displayed on video monitors. Hemodynamic data obtained through catheters and transducers are transmitted to another video monitor next to the fluoroscopic images [6].

The numerous components and equipment of the cardiac catheterization laboratory are an integral part of the procedure and safety system for the patient. The patient table (*1*) is mounted so that it can be moved over the radiography tube (*2*). The radiographic beam is projected upward through the patient to the image intensifier (*3*) and then after appropriate digital signal processing, transmitted to the video monitor screens (*4*). Two of the three video monitors for fluoroscopic images are able to contain a static image and are able to recall other stored digital images for future review. The cardiac catheterization operators stand to the right side of the patient in front of the table control mechanisms (*5*) and are protected by lead aprons, thyroid guards, eyeglasses, and table/ceiling-mounted lead shields (*6*). Radiographic contrast media injections are made through a specially designed, ceiling-mounted power injector (*7*) that is controlled remotely from a wall-mounted panel (*8*). This unit provides instruction for exact delivery of the quantity, pressure, and flow rate through preset parameters of contrast delivery. The patient's vascular access site is visualized directly, assisted by an overhead operative light (*9*). After catheters are positioned using fluoroscopic guidance, cardiac output can be measured with an indicator dilution technique using the thermodilution computer (*10*) at the side of the patient. In case of emergency, a cardiac "crash" cart (*11*) is always available and fully supplied with emergency equipment and drugs.

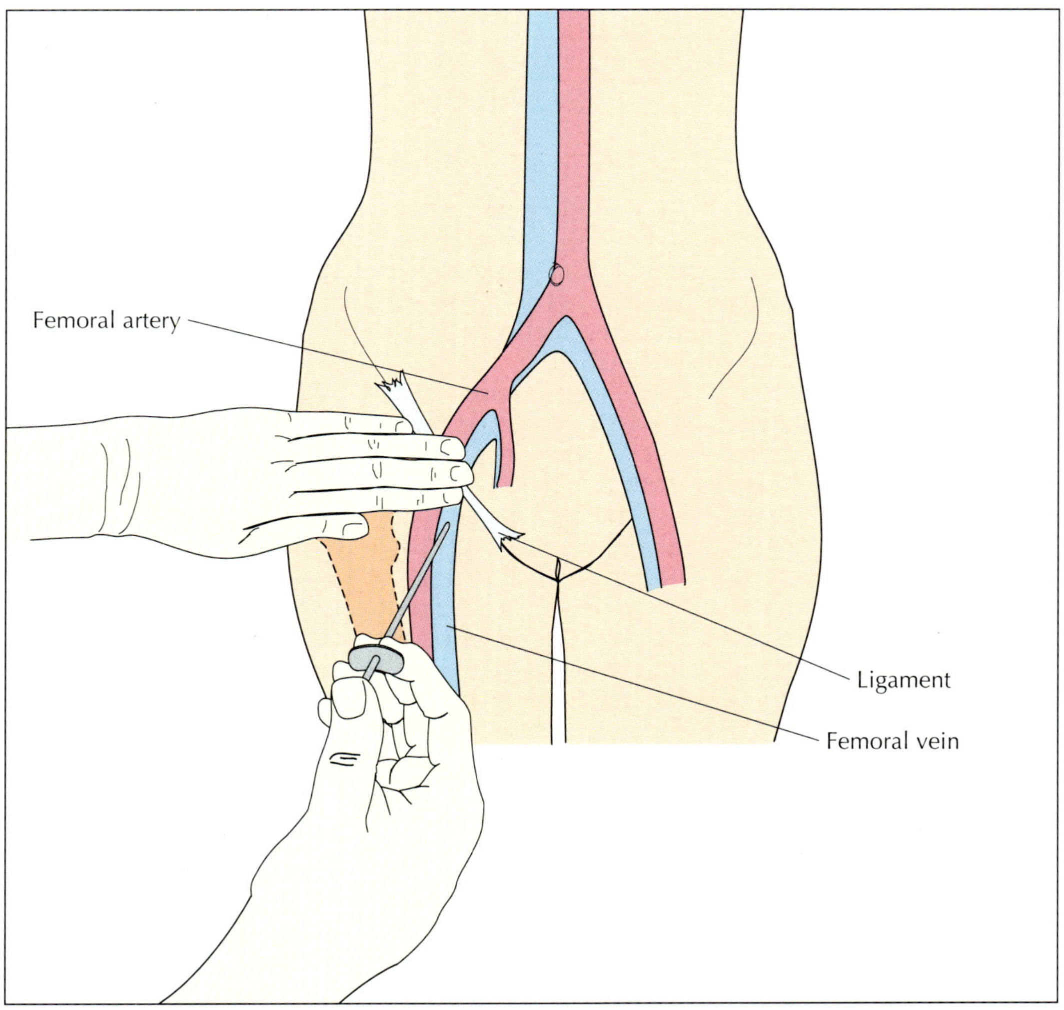

FIGURE 5-5. Vascular access. The vascular system can be approached through a femoral artery and vein using a modified Seldinger technique with sheath introducers. The operator palpates the femoral artery after establishing its course below the inguinal ligament. The inguinal (groin) skin crease is located. The inguinal ligament, which lies directly beneath the inguinal skin crease from the iliac crest to the pubis, is palpated. In obese patients, the inguinal skin crease may be lower than the inguinal ligament. There may be additional skin folds above and below the inguinal ligament, which can confuse the proper positioning for needle insertion. The femoral artery is approximately 1 cm in diameter running across the inguinal ligament. In most patients, the femoral artery crosses the inguinal ligament at a point dividing the ligament into one-third and two-thirds lateral portions. The femoral artery pulse is located with the middle and index fingers with the fingers placed parallel to the long axis of the femoral artery. The index finger palpates the artery 1 to 2 cm below the inguinal ligament where the site of actual arterial entry with the needle will be. The Seldinger or Cook-type needle is introduced into the femoral artery at its medial aspect. Once within the vascular lumen, a flexible spring guidewire (diameter 0.035 or 0.038 in) is advanced. The needle is withdrawn from the wire, the wire wiped clean, and the introducer sheath advanced over the wire into the artery or vein. The sheath introducer and guidewire are then removed; the sheath is flushed, and the system is ready to accept catheters.

The femoral vein is found medially to the femoral artery, running parallel within 1 to 2 cm, and can be cannulated in the same manner as the femoral artery. The drawing shows correct hand positioning for the arterial puncture using the Seldinger technique. Five steps are used: 1) The vessel is punctured with the needle at an angle of 30° to 40°. 2) Free blood flow return is observed. 3) The guidewire is then passed through the needle into the vessel. 4) The needle is removed over the wire while firm pressure is applied at the site. 5) The sheath is passed over the wire and advanced into the vessel with a rotating motion [7]. (*Adapted from* Tilkian and Daily [7].)

INDICATIONS FOR ALTERNATIVE ROUTES TO FEMORAL ARTERIAL CATHETERIZATION

- Claudication
- Absent dorsalis pedis and posterior tibialis pulses
- Absent popliteal pulses
- Femoral bruits
- Absent femoral pulses
- Prior femoral artery graft surgery
- Extensive inguinal scarring from radiation therapy, surgery, or prior catheterization
- Excessively tortuous or diseased iliac arteries
- Severe back pain, inability to lie flat
- Patient request

FIGURE 5-6. The indications for using alternative routes to femoral artery catheterization. Femoral artery access may not always be available due to peripheral arterial disease or prior surgery. Alternative arterial access sites should be considered. (*Adapted from* Kern [4].)

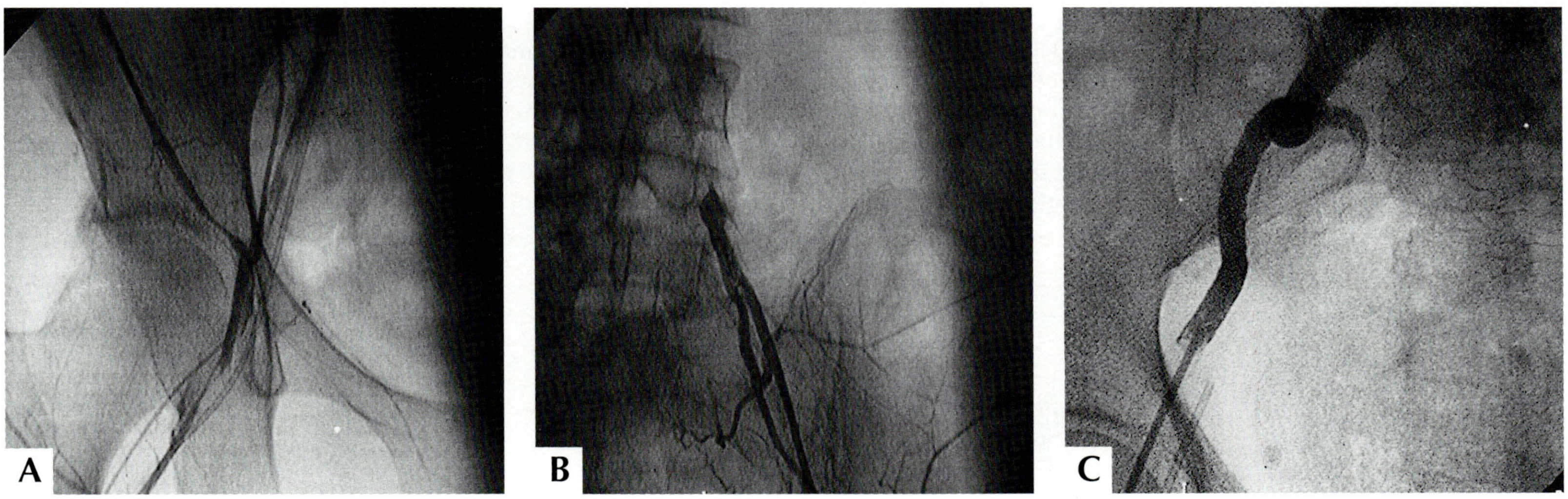

FIGURE 5-7. Identification of peripheral vascular disease. Although the femoral approach for catheterization is the most widely used method and is associated with minimal complications, the presence of significant peripheral vascular disease may complicate diagnostic catheterization for patients with valvular heart disease. The Seldinger technique can achieve vascular access in patients with peripheral arterial disease using modified or specialized guidewires. Peripheral angiography may be required at the time of diagnostic catheterization to identify the route best suited for arterial catheter advancement. **A,** An occluded right common femoral artery with collateral filling of the hypogastric artery in a patient in whom diminished femoral pulses were noted but who had no symptoms of claudication. Although venous access was obtained and a right heart catheter could be advanced without difficulty, no arterial access through the right femoral artery could be accomplished.

B, Cannulation of the contralateral femoral artery was performed, but complete left iliac occlusion was also identified. Thus, a brachial approach was required. This finding has important clinical implications for exercise studies, placement of intra-aortic balloon pump support, and future surgical outcome. This patient had successful catheterization from the right brachial artery approach. **C,** Normal femoral artery access through a mildly tortuous right femoral artery.

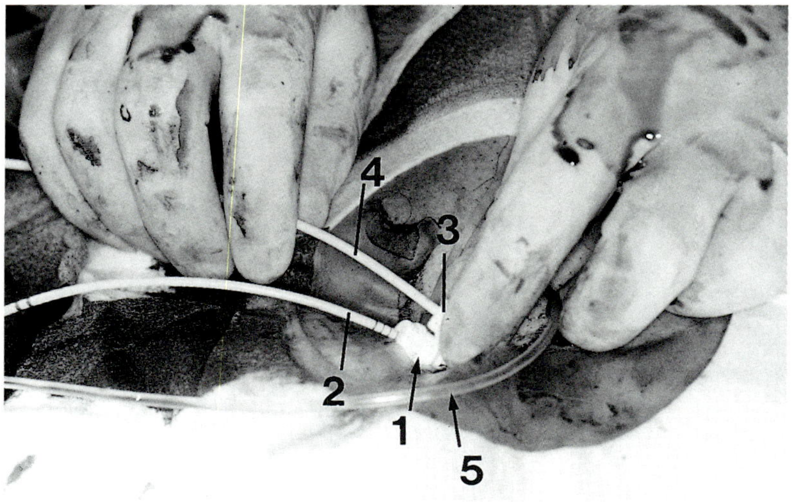

FIGURE 5-8. Catheter placement. After using the appropriate Seldinger needle and guidewire technique, catheter placement in the femoral artery and vein is straightforward. Through the 8-F venous sheath (*1*), an 8-F balloon-tipped flotation pulmonary artery catheter is advanced (*2*). Through the 7-F arterial sheath (*3*), the 6-F arterial, diagnostic coronary angiographic, or ventriculographic catheter (*4*) is advanced. By using an arterial sheath one French size larger than the arterial catheter, the side arm of the arterial sheath (*5*) can measure peripheral arterial pressure throughout the procedure. This method uses three pressure transducers and a systematic data collection methodology to provide complete hemodynamic and angiographic data in 95% of all cardiac catheterization studies in a rapid and comprehensive manner.

Collection of hemodynamic data in an organized manner should be an integral part of every catheterization protocol, especially for studies evaluating valvular heart disease. Complex hemodynamic data recording can be accomplished accurately and rapidly if a consistent method is established. The routine collection of right and left heart hemodynamic data with appropriate blood oxygen saturations and cardiac output measurements can usually be accomplished safely in less than 30 minutes. Cardiac output determinations by thermodilution technique is routine, although the Fick (oxygen consumption method) cardiac output method is preferred for valvular lesions. Indicator (indocyanine) green dye curves are reserved for suspected intracardiac shunt studies. Multiple blood samples for oxygen saturation are also obtained throughout the right and left heart for intracardiac shunt identification. Simultaneous pressure measurements across the heart, concentrating on the aortic and mitral valves, facilitate accurate evaluation of those valves that are affected most commonly. Different and unique hemodynamic measurements, such as simultaneous pulmonary artery and right ventricular pressures for pulmonary stenosis, are, at times, necessary.

The most common complication of right heart catheterization (*catheter 2*) is stimulation of the right ventricular outflow tract, which may result in ventricular arrhythmias, rarely,advanced atrioventricular block, or right bundle branch block. Significant but transient ventricular arrhythmias occur in patients undergoing right heart catheterization, are self-limited, and do not require treatment. The arrhythmia is terminated when the catheter is removed. Sustained ventricular arrhythmias have been reported, especially in unstable patients or those with electrolyte imbalance, acidosis, or concurrent myocardial ischemia. The prophylactic use of lidocaine is generally not necessary.

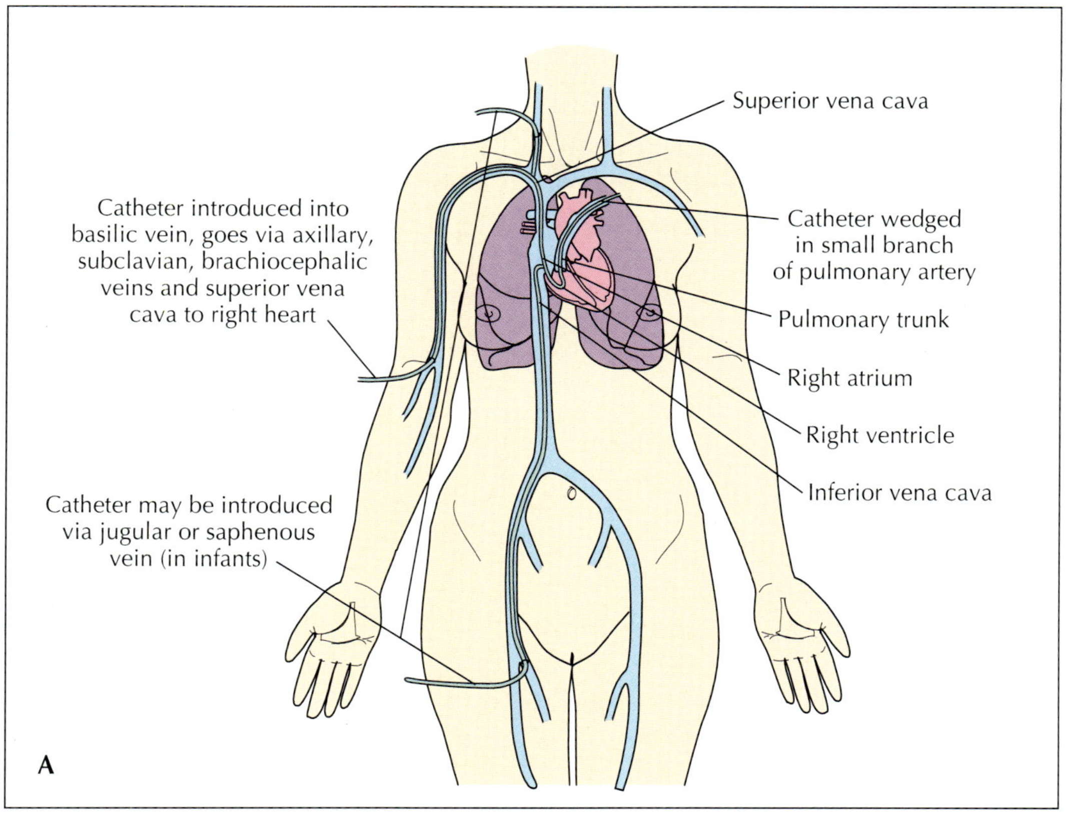

FIGURE 5-9. A, Right-heart catheterization. Catheter routes for assessment of hemodynamic and angiographic data are shown from the right femoral and right brachial vein through the right atrium, right ventricle, pulmonary artery, and to the pulmonary capillary wedge position. (*continued*)

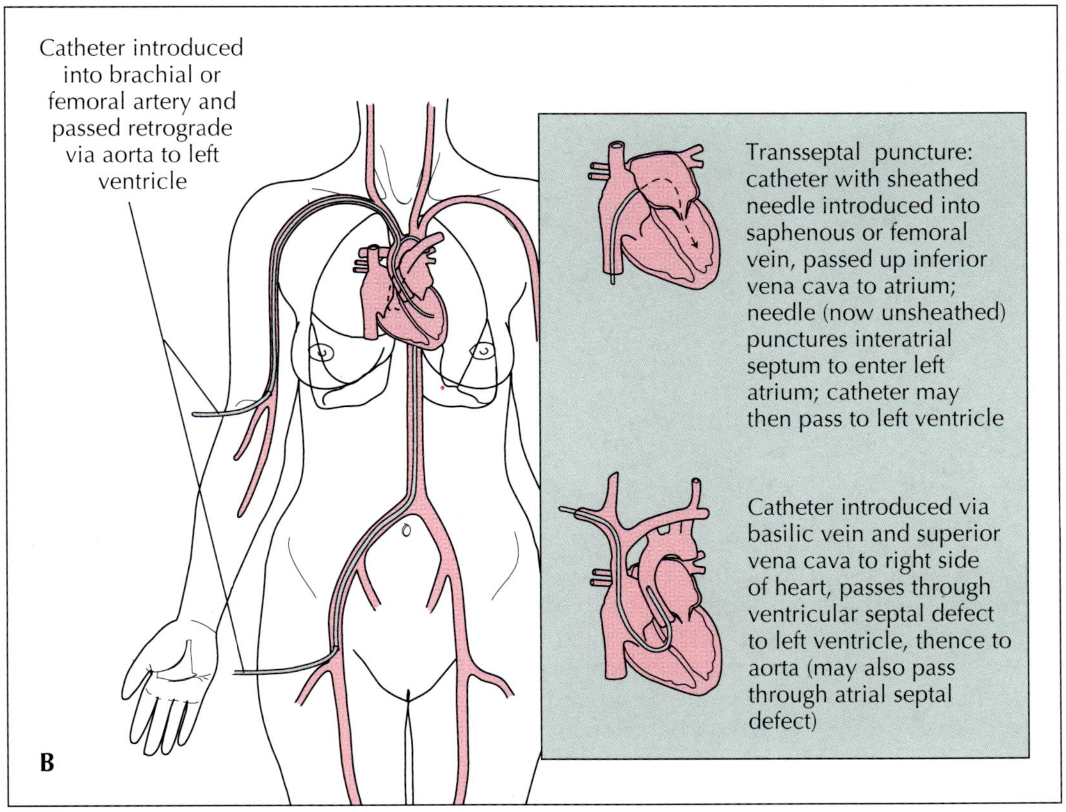

FIGURE 5-9. *(continued)* **B,** Left heart catheterization. Access to the left ventricle is obtained through either a retrograde femoral artery route to the central aortic position or via an antegrade approach through a transseptal puncture with a catheter passing from the right to the left atrium and left ventricular locations [4]. (*Adapted from* Kern [4].)

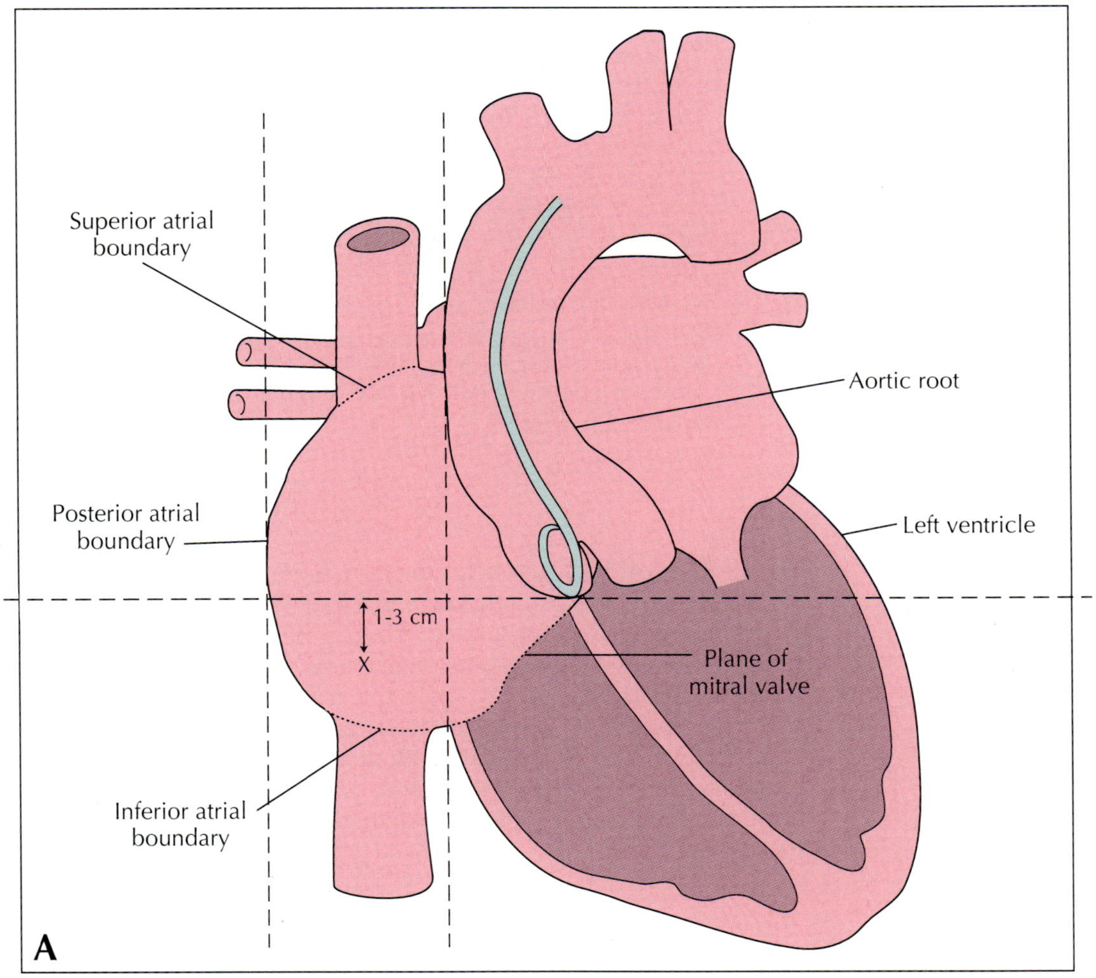

FIGURE 5-10. The transseptal approach. Transseptal catheterization is often required for precise assessment of left atrial or left ventricular pressures in the presence of mitral and aortic prosthetic valve surgery. **A,** The transseptal catheter crosses the intra-atrial septum at a level of the aortic valve in the anteroposterior projection. The correct positioning of the transseptal puncture requires localization through a technique identifying the mid-point of the interatrial septum demarcated by the inferior aortic cusp (by a pigtail catheter), posterior atrial wall border in the right anterior oblique projection. The operator centers the transseptal needle and catheter prior to puncture according to the description of Croft and Lipscomb [8]. Once the catheter has crossed the atrial septum, contrast can be injected (as shown in **B**) to identify the location within the left atrium before entry through the mitral valve into the left ventricle [4]. The pressure wave form and an arterialized blood oxygen sample confirms that the catheter is within the left atrium. *(continued)*

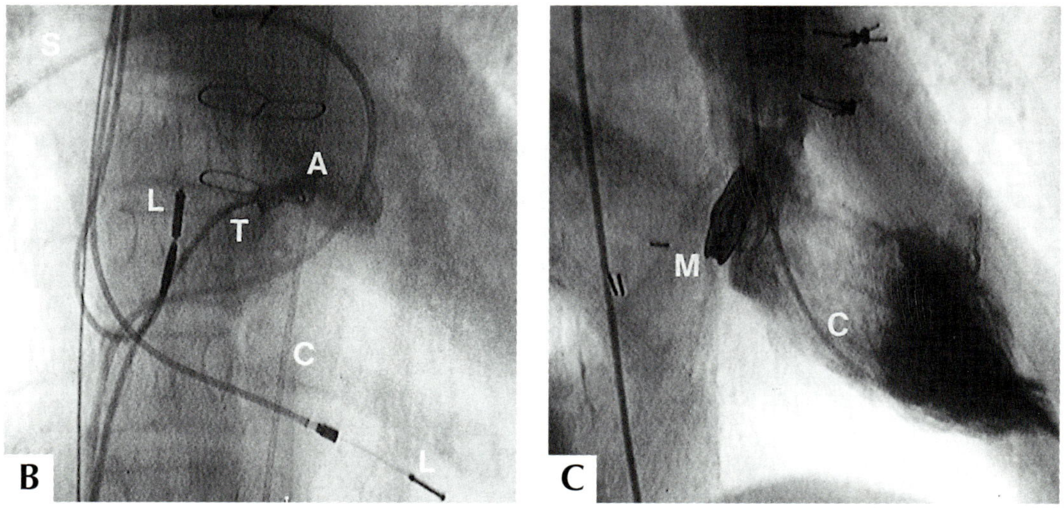

FIGURE 5-10. (*continued*) **B,** A cineangiographic frame from a study in a patient with a prosthetic aortic tilting disc valve (A) requiring transseptal evaluation for valvular malfunction. This patient had atrial and ventricular pacing wires which can be seen with the heavy electrode marks (L). The transseptal catheter is identified by the letter T. The Swan-Ganz catheter (S) is positioned in the pulmonary artery, and the ascending portion of the pigtail catheter (C) is adjacent to the spine. Radiographic contrast media was injected through the transseptal catheter identifying the left atrial appendage and indicated catheter repositioning before crossing into the left ventricle.

C, For comparison, this panel shows a tilting-disc prosthesis (M) in the mitral position with a catheter (C) across the aortic valve during ventriculography. Note the angle of the mitral valve and the difference in the large prosthetic valve size of the mitral prosthesis ring relative to that of the aortic prosthesis. (Part A *adapted from* Croft and Lipscomb [8].)

A. INDICATIONS FOR TRANSSEPTAL LEFT HEART CATHETERIZATION

MEASUREMENT OF HEMODYNAMICS FOR VALVE AREA CALCULATION

Mitral valve
- Pulmonary capillary wedge pressure in question
- Doppler mitral valve gradient in question
- Prosthetic mitral valve
- Previous mitral valve surgery

Aortic valve
- Retrograde catheterization not possible
- Mechanical prosthetic valve, especially the tilting disk
- Echocardiographic data inconclusive

LEFT VENTRICULAR ANGIOGRAPHY

To assess mitral regurgitation when retrograde catheterization not possible

VALVULOPLASTY

Mitral

Antegrade aortic

ASCERTAINMENT OF PULMONARY VENO-OCCLUSIVE DISEASE

B. CONTRAINDICATIONS TO THE TRANSSEPTAL APPROACH

Patient cannot lie flat or fully cooperate

Anticoagulant therapy or other hemostatic abnormality (coumadin should be discontinued several days before transseptal puncture so that the prothrombin time is ≤ 14 sec)

Left atrial thrombus

Atrial myxoma

FIGURE 5-11. A, Indications for the transseptal approach. Crossing a tilting disc-type prosthetic valve in the aortic position has been performed with varying success using a retrograde catheter technique, although death in some patients from a lodged catheter has been reported.

B, The risks of transseptal left heart catheterization should be carefully evaluated in patients with distorted cardiac anatomy secondary to congenital heart disease, dilated aortic root, marked atrial enlargement, or thoracic skeletal deformity. (Part A *adapted from* Kern [4].)

RISKS RELATED TO TRANSSEPTAL CATHETERIZATION

Cardiac perforation of:
- Right atrium
- Posterior left atrium
- Left atrial appendage
- Pulmonary vein
- Left ventricle

Puncture into the aortic root
Pericardial tamponade*
Embolus from the left atrium

*Almost all deaths related to transseptal catheterization are secondary to tamponade.

FIGURE 5-12. Risks of transseptal catheterization. Transseptal needle puncture of the aortic root, coronary sinus, or the posterior free wall of the atrium are potentially lethal complications. In patients who have not been given anticoagulants, the needle puncture alone rarely causes a problem. However, if the transseptal catheter is advanced into these spaces, cardiac tamponade may occur. If the operator is not satisfied with the position of the Brockenbrough catheter in the right atrium, the catheter/needle combination should not be advanced, and if the equipment is not in the correct position, the procedure must start over again with removal of the transseptal needle, reinsertion of the guidewire to the superior vena cava, and repositioning of the catheter/needle assembly. (*Adapted from* Kern [4].)

ANGIOGRAPHY

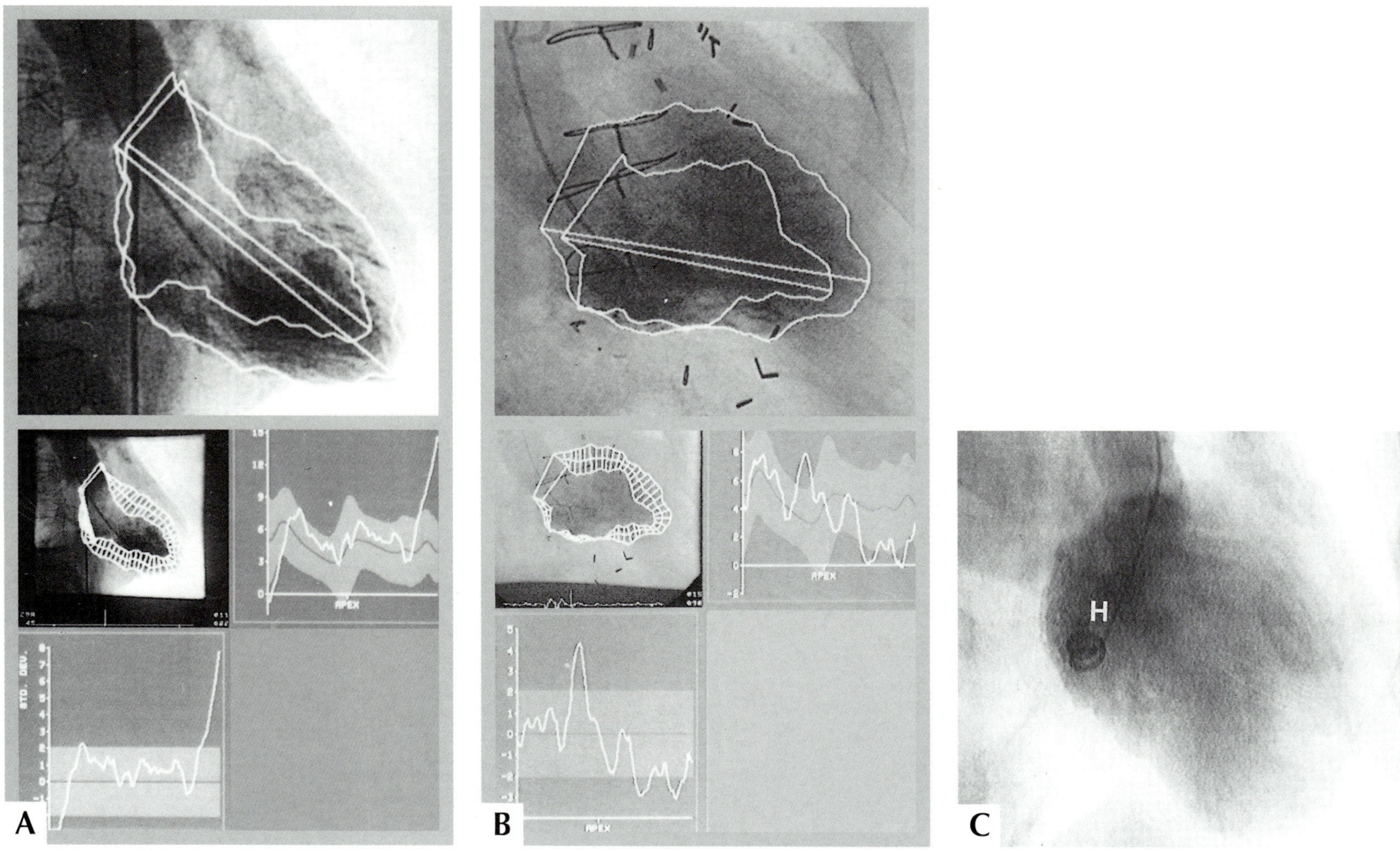

FIGURE 5-13. Role of contrast ventriculography. Ventriculography is performed by rapid injection of radiographic contrast medium through a specially designed catheter into the ventricular chamber. A predetermined contrast volume is injected at a given maximal injection pressure and over a selected period of time. The radiographic contrast opacifies the ventricular chamber over several cardiac cycles. Changes in the dimensional configuration ascribed to abnormal regional myocardial contractility are identified and quantitated. The end-systolic (ES) and end-diastolic (ED) dimensions are planimetered and an ejection fraction [(ED-ES)/ED] for stroke volume is computed.

A, Normal left ventricular contractility with ventriculography performed in a 30° right anterior oblique projection. The end-diastolic volume is 96 mL; the end-systolic volume is 31 mL, with an ejection fraction calculated at 67% and stroke volume at 65 mL. The *lower panel* shows quantification of regional wall motion using the centerline method, wherein end-diastolic and end-systolic left ventricular endocardial contours are established and a centerline constructed by the computer midway between the two contours. Wall motion is measured along 100 chords constructed perpendicular to the centerline. Motion at each chord is normalized by the end-diastolic perimeter to yield a shortening fraction. (*continued*)

D. COMPLICATIONS OF VENTRICULOGRAPHY

Cardiac arrhythmias, especially ventricular tachycardia and ventricular fibrilliation, require immediate cardioversion. All arrhythmias are more common with end-hole catheters.

Intramyocardial "staining" or injection of contrast into the myocardium is generally transient and not clinically important unless it is deep or perforating (emergency pericardiocentesis may be required).

Embolism from thrombi or air may occur. These events are minimized with careful catheter preparation, flushing, and systemic heparinization.

Contrast-related complications noted previously may occur during this procedure.

Transient hypotension (<15–30 sec) is common with ionic contrast media.

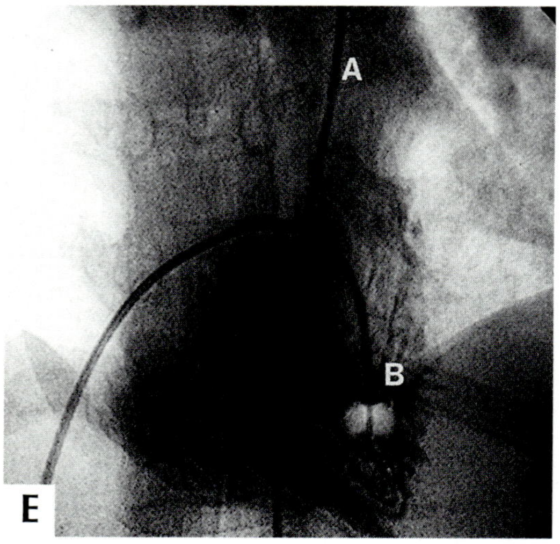

FIGURE 5-13. (*continued*) Motion along each chord is plotted (*dark line*). The mean motion in the normal ventriculogram group (*white line*) and 1 SD above and below the mean (*gray zone*) are shown for reference comparison. Wall motion is also plotted as the difference, in units of SDs, from the normal mean. The normal ventriculogram group mean is represented by the *horizontal zero line*.

B, The SD for wall motion from apex is plotted for normal reference group with 1 SD as the light zones. The patient's wall motion index is plotted over the normal zones. Variance from the 2 SD line marks abnormal contractility for this patient. Compare the normal contractile function in patient A to that of patient B who has an ejection fraction of 63% with a marked inferior akinetic zone. Although the ejection fractions are similar with similar volumetric calculations, wall motion abnormality is apparent using the centerline method (*lower panel*). The *lower panel* thus shows a marked 3 SD variance in wall motion from the apex to the base of the heart, indicating significant contractile dysfunction. These findings have critical importance to the immediate outcome and long-term prognosis following valve replacement.

C, An end-systolic frame of a left ventriculogram performed in the 30° right anterior oblique projection with a new helical design ventriculographic catheter (H) that produces minimal ectopy. The ejection fraction in this patient was only 10% with global hypokinesis, a finding not related to abnormalities of the coronary arteries. The cardiomyopathic ventricle may alter decisions for surgical intervention in patients with valvular heart disease.

D, Complications of ventriculography. Serious complications can occur during ventriculography. Meticulous attention to detail is useful in prevention.

E, Right ventriculography performed in the anteroposterior projection using a Berman-type balloon-tipped catheter (B) positioned across the tricuspid valve. Right ventriculography is used to quantitate tricuspid regurgitation, Ebstein's anomaly, right ventricular outflow tract dysplasia, anomalies of the pulmonary valve, and right-to-left shunts at the ventricular level. The Berman catheter crosses the tricuspid valve to the right ventricular apex. An aortic catheter (A) ascends beyond the cardiac silhouette along the left side of the spine. No tricuspid regurgitation can be seen in this study.

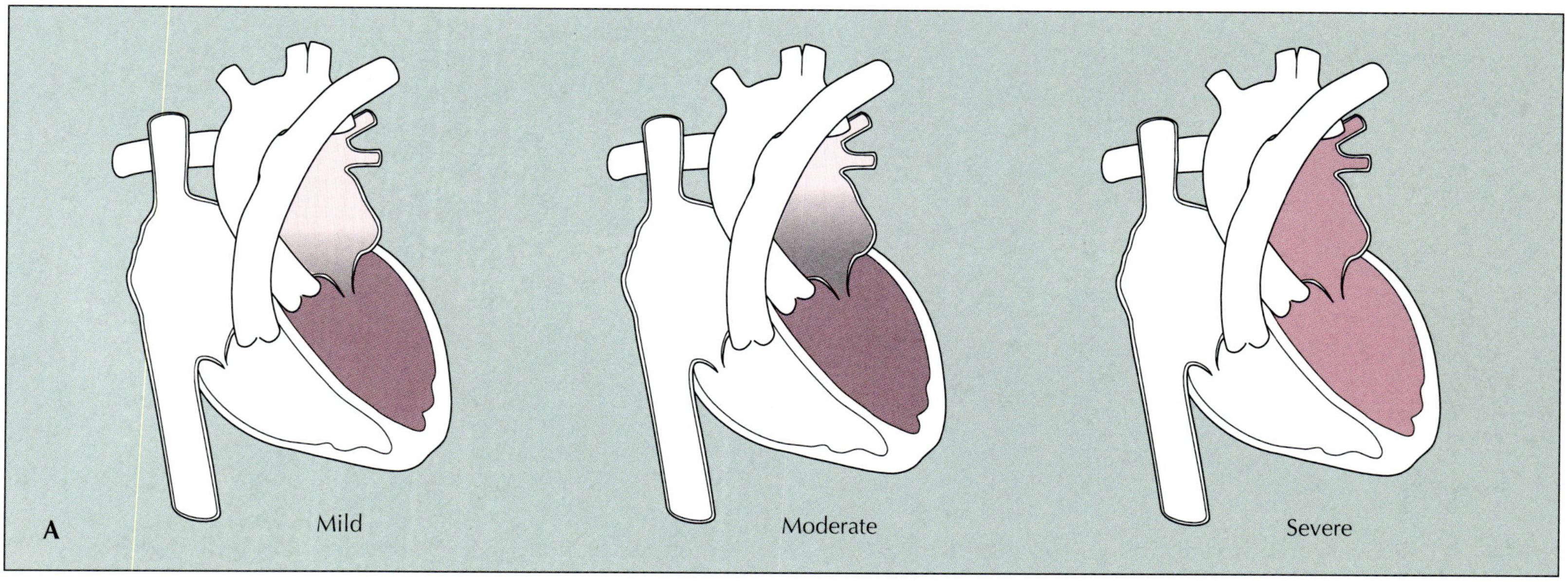

FIGURE 5-14. A, Valvular regurgitation. Regurgitation through the mitral or tricuspid valve can easily be recognized during ventriculography. The quantitation of regurgitation by angiography uses a qualitative grading scale related to the degree and rate of atrial opacification. Mild mitral regurgitation is characterized by a well-localized, brisk systolic jet of contrast filling the left atrium through at least one to two cardiac cycles. Moderate mitral regurgitation is a larger, more diffuse jet opacifying the left atrial chamber and the chamber opacification is maintained through three cardiac cycles. Severe mitral regurgitation is characterized by a rapid, brisk filling of the entire left ventricle, often with opacification of the pulmonary veins or left atrial appendage. The contrast medium remains as dense as the contrast within the left ventricular chamber. Catheter interference with the valve apparatus, however, may induce artifactual regurgitation. The degree of catheter-induced regurgitation is related to stiffness and calcification of the valve leaflets. (*continued*)

$$RF = \frac{\text{Regurgitant flow}}{\text{Total flow}}$$

$$= \frac{\text{CO from angiogram} - \text{CO from Fick/thermodilution}}{\text{CO from angiogram}}$$

B

RF<40%	Mild
RF=40% to 60%	Moderate
RF>60%	Severe

C

FIGURE 5-14. *(continued)* At times, noninvasive Doppler echocardiographic confirmation of this finding is important. In addition, although a semiquantitative method has been proposed, the precise quantitation based on angiographic data is variable among operators and among the conditions that influence contrast appearance in the left atrium.

B, Computation of the regurgitant fraction (RF). **C,** Semiquantitation of severity of regurgitation can be determined [4]. CO—cardiac output. (Part A *adapted from* Pujadas [9]; parts B and C *adapted from* Kern [4].)

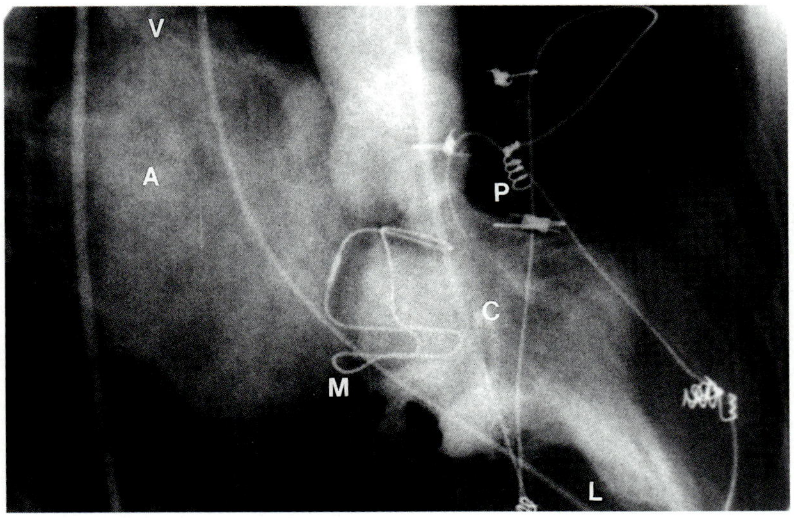

FIGURE 5-15. Severe mitral regurgitation through failing bioprosthetic mitral valve. A cineangiographic frame of a 59-year-old woman with congestive heart failure 10 years after implantation of a mitral bioprosthetic valve for mitral regurgitation. The systolic frame of the cineangiogram demonstrates satisfactory contraction of the left ventricle with extensive opacification of the atrium (A) filling the superior pulmonary vein (V). Epicardial pacing wires (P) from prior multiple procedures implanted into the myocardium are seen. Endomyocardial pacing leads (L) are also evident. The metal struts (M) supporting the bioprosthetic valve are well localized within the mitral valve ring and the pigtail catheter (C) can be seen within the left ventricle. The severity of angiographic mitral regurgitation is often associated with characteristic hemodynamic findings to be described later [10]. (*Adapted from* Kern [10].)

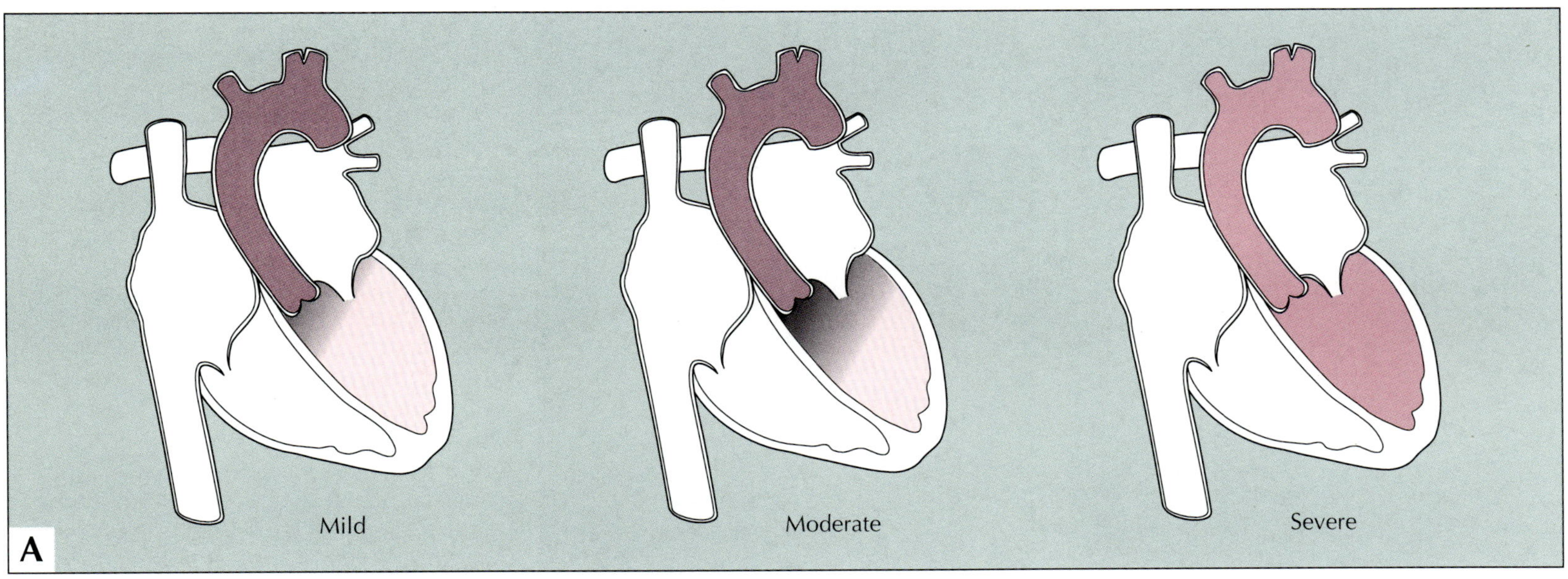

FIGURE 5-16. Role of aortography in aortic valve disease. Aortography opacifies the ascending aorta using techniques similar to ventriculography. The angiographic evaluation of aortic regurgitation uses a large-volume contrast injection through a catheter in the ascending aorta. The semiquantitative nature of angiographic data precludes more precise quantitative determination of the contribution of aortic regurgitation to the clinical status. **A,** The semiqualitative method, using the degree of opacification within the first several beats, provides a grading scale of aortic regurgitation that correlates with that seen by Doppler *(continued)*

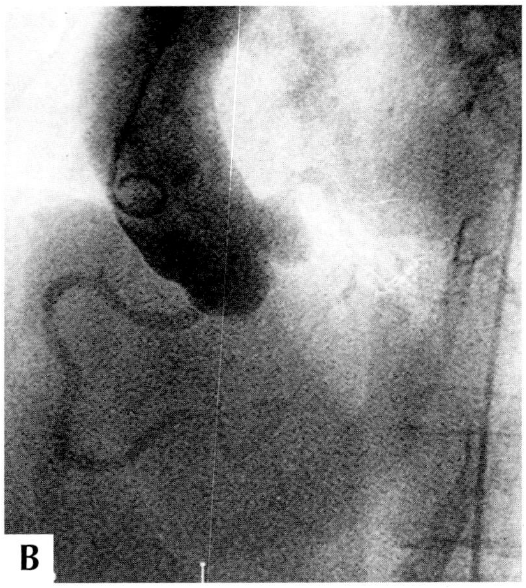

FIGURE 5-16. (*continued*) ultrasound and carries valuable prognostic implications. The angiographic characteristic of mild aortic regurgitation is a faint retrograde contrast opacification of the left ventricle during diastole during the aortic root injection. Moderate aortic insufficiency is characterized by immediate chamber opacification covering one half to two thirds of the left ventricular chamber, but contrast opacification is not maintained more than two beats. Severe aortic regurgitation is identified as immediate filling of the left ventricular chamber with contrast opacification equal to that of the aortic root.

The indications for ascending aortography include 1) defining the presence of aortic aneurysm or aortic dissection, 2) quantification of aortic insufficiency, 3) nonselective coronary artery bypass graft aortography, 4) supravalvular aortic stenosis, 5) disease of the brachiocephalic or arch vessels, 6) documentation of coarctation of the aorta, 7) opacification of aortic to pulmonary artery communications, 8) aortic or periaortic neoplastic diseases, arterial thromboembolic disease, and arterial inflammatory diseases, all of which may accompany valvular heart disease to one degree or another. **B,** Aortogram of a patient with mild aortic stenosis and trivial aortic insufficiency. The bicuspid valve is clearly seen with the right and left coronary origins well opacified. The aorta is only mildly dilated. A pigtail catheter was used for this study and is positioned 1 to 2 cm above the aortic valve cusps to prevent catheter interference with valve leaflet motion and artifactual aortic insufficiency [4]. (Part A *adapted from* Pujadas [9].)

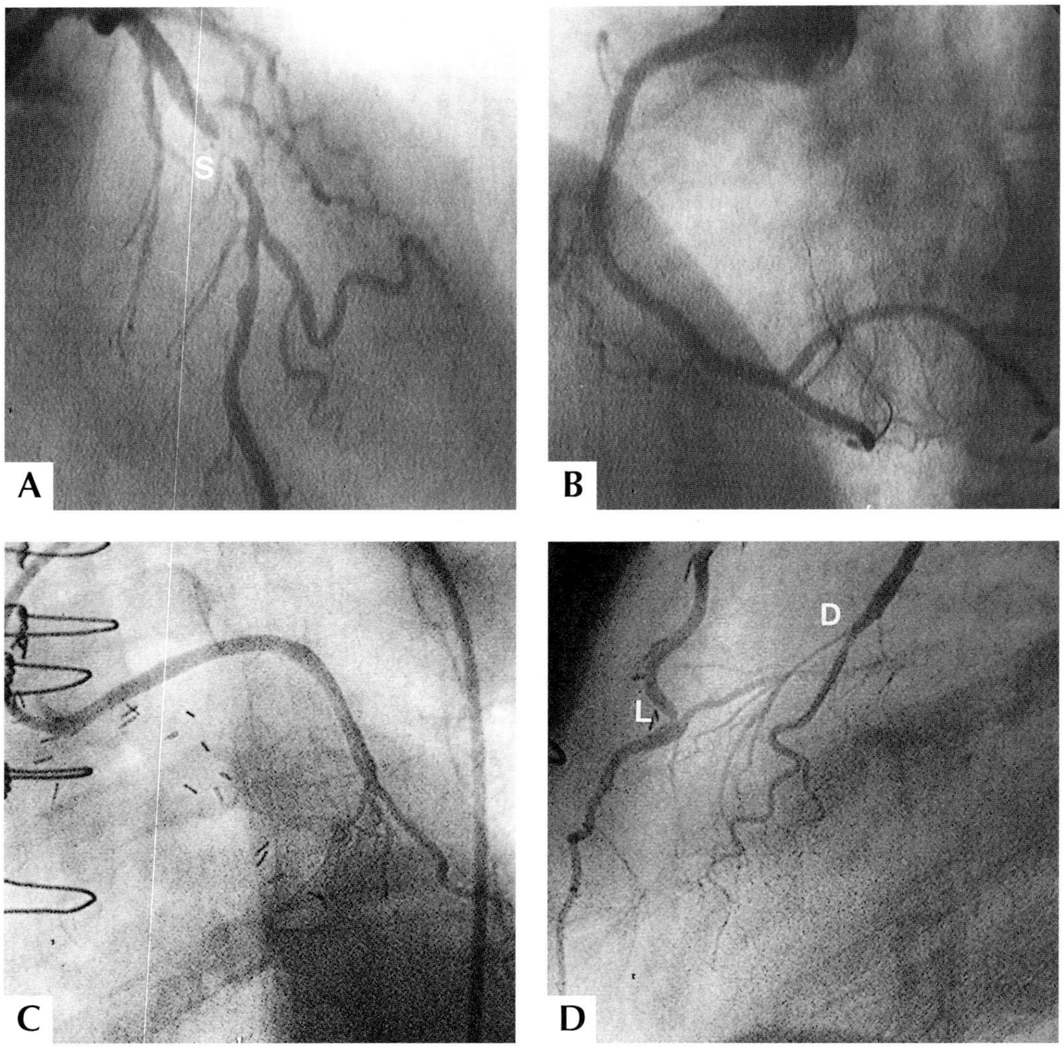

FIGURE 5-17. Coronary arteriography defines the associated atherosclerotic coronary artery narrowings, the course and supply regions of the coronary arteries, and the presence of anomalous coronary arteries, which may complicate valvular surgery. The outcome of valve surgery is directly related to the extent and severity of coexisting coronary artery disease.

A, Left anterior descending coronary artery with a 95% stenosis (S) in the mid-vessel. In the presence of significant valvular disease, this lesion would complicate the valve replacement procedure. If this lesion is not addressed, surgery may be associated with acute myocardial infarction in the perioperative period. Coronary artery bypass graft surgery or angioplasty are considerations in the decisions for valve lesion management.

B, Left anterior oblique (LAO) projection shows the right coronary artery well opacified and free of atherosclerotic narrowing with arterial dominance of the posterior descending and large posterolateral branches. Defining the contribution of coronary artery disease to the immediate intervention and future events is critical to management of such patients.

C and **D**, Course of a reversed saphenous vein coronary artery bypass graft to the left anterior descending and diagonal branch artery. The LAO projection (*panel C*) is supplemented with other angiographic views. The left lateral (LAT) view (*panel D*) is particularly helpful in delineating the left anterior descending (L) and diagonal (D) anastomotic sites more clearly. The identification of disease in the saphenous vein grafts in patients with valvular heart disease after previous surgery is also important to the surgical approach and clinical outcome. Coronary arteriography is required in many patients at risk for coronary artery disease with chest pain syndromes. The coronary angiogram obtained in a patient with aortic stenosis before aortic valve replacement has obvious implications in that many patients with aortic valve stenosis may have concomitant chest pain syndromes due to impaired coronary vasodilatory reserve and not to atherosclerotic coronary disease limiting epicardial blood flow.

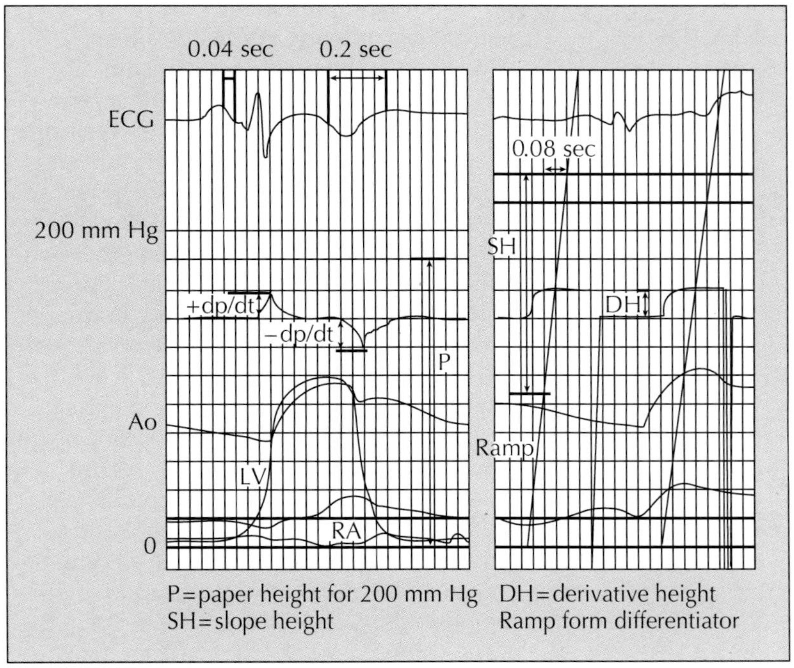

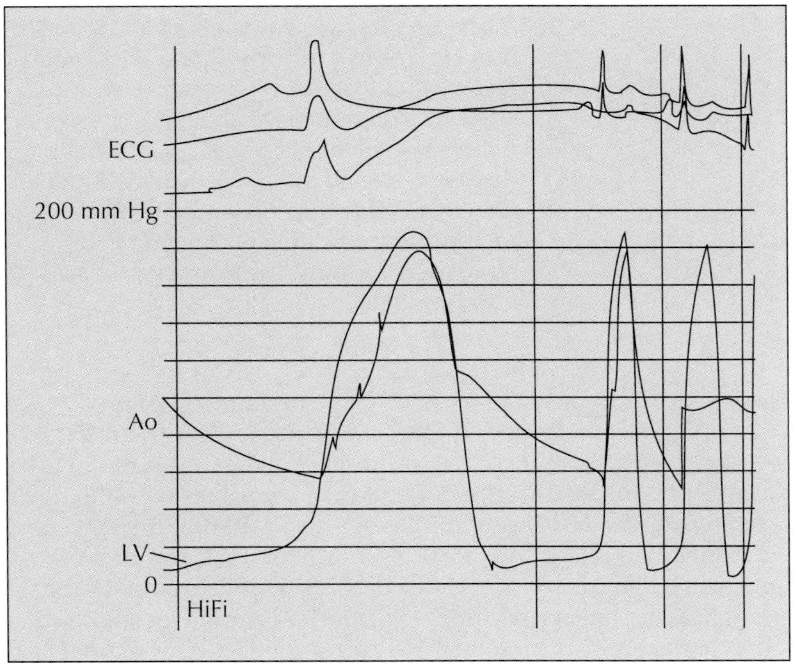

FIGURE 5-18. Hemodynamic data can be precisely obtained using high-fidelity micromanometer-tipped transducer catheter systems in addition to those obtained with fluid-filled systems. When using high-fidelity pressure catheters, the timing sequence of cardiac events can be exactly delineated. **A,** Hemodynamic tracing of simultaneous aortic (Ao) and left ventricular (LV) pressures and right atrial (RA) and pulmonary artery pressures in a patient with a chest pain syndrome. Using high-fidelity signals, the change in pressure/time relationship (dP/dt) of LV pressure (the first derivative of pressure) will indicate the level of contractility. For routine hemodynamic studies, simultaneous pressure measurements across the valve in question are preferable to that of a single transducer technique. It is not necessary to use high-fidelity pressure catheters for every valve lesion, but with the improved ease of use of these catheters this technique has gained widespread interest. The pulmonary artery pressure is not labeled but appears immediately above the RA pressure. The +dP/dt is equal to 200/p x (12.5 SH)/DH [14].

B, Simultaneous LV and aortic pressures measured with high-fidelity (HiFi) dual micromanometer-tipped transducer catheter with one transducer positioned within the LV body and the other transducer positioned immediately above the aortic valve demonstrate a small transvalvular gradient. Note the minimal differences in the timing of the upstroke of pressure transmitted to the aorta and the sawtooth pattern of the aortic pressure wave as the jet vibrates the catheter. The aortic pressure rises as LV pressure exceeds aortic diastolic pressure. In this patient with minimal aortic stenosis, an early transvalvular gradient can be demonstrated. The peak-to-peak pressure gradient is less than 10 mm Hg. High-fidelity assessment of small gradients is more precise than that obtained with fluid-filled systems [4]. DH—derivative height; ECG—electrocardiogram; P—paper height for 200 mm Hg; Ramp—electrontic input signal of 2000 mm Hg/sec; SH—slope height. (*Adapted from* Kern [4].)

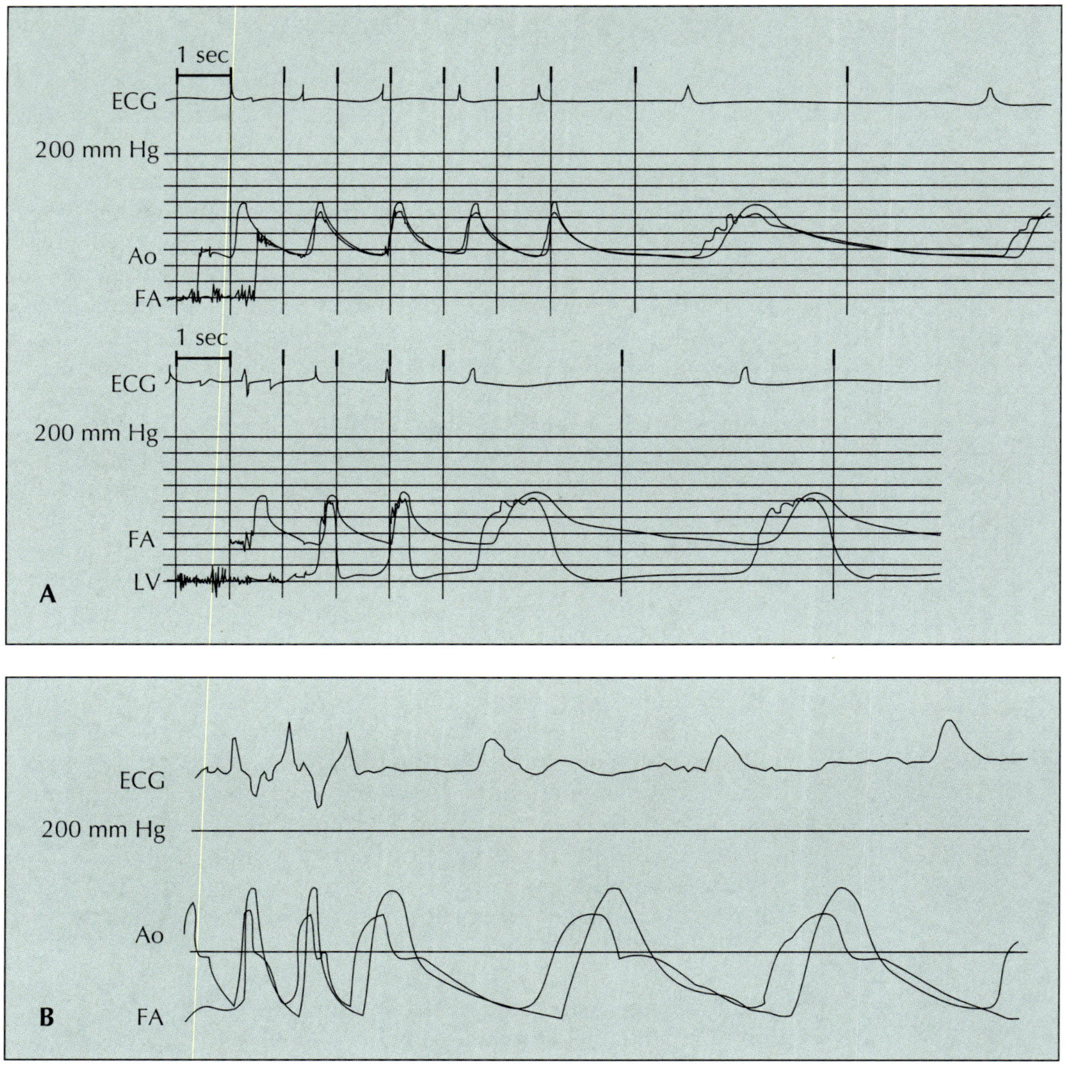

Figure 5-19. **A**, Simultaneous femoral artery (FA) and central aortic (Ao) pressures measured with fluid-filled sheath side arm and an angiographic pigtail catheter, respectively. These pressures can be used for accurate assessment of transvalvular and transventricular pressure gradients. The *top panel* shows a hemodynamic tracing of the aortic pressure measured with a 7-F pigtail catheter and femoral artery pressure measured through the 8-F sheath side arm using fluid-filled transducers. The pressure scale is 0 to 200 mm Hg. Vertical time lines are 1 second apart. Before crossing the aortic valve, both pressures are recorded. The sheath pressure demonstrates the normal features of a delay in the peripheral arterial pressure upstroke, overshoot of the femoral artery systolic pressure, and the matching of diastolic pressures after the dicrotic notch.

Left ventricular (LV) and FA pressure measurements (*bottom panel*) demonstrate the consistent relationship of central and peripheral arterial systolic pressures with no change in the pressure amplification of the femoral artery. Thus, the gradient across the aortic valve is zero. Aortic stenosis is not present in this patient.

The FA pressure overshoot of less than 20 mm Hg, relative to aortic pressure, is satisfactory for most clinical decisions for aortic stenosis. When this overshoot is excessive or if there is evidence of peripheral vascular disease, a second arterial catheter positioned above the valve may be required [4]. **B,** FA pressure amplification by 20 mm Hg or more over the aortic pressure. (Part A *adapted from* Kern [4].)

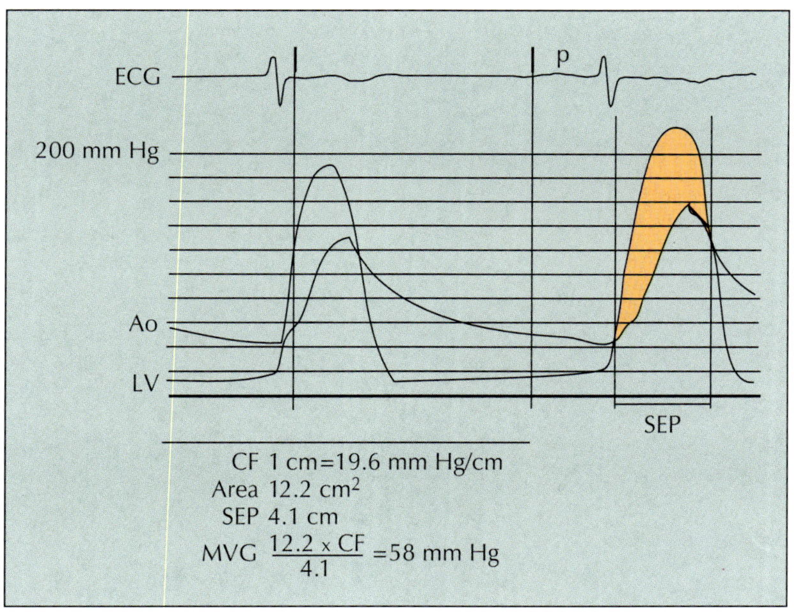

FIGURE 5-20. Aortic (Ao) stenosis. Aortic pressure, measured with a pigtail catheter above aortic valve and left ventricular (LV) pressure, using the transseptal technique demonstrates the simultaneous pressures with a precise gradient (*orange area*). In this case, in contrast to using a peripheral artery pressure, there is no requirement to phase shift aortic pressure for the transmission time delay. Planimetry of the area of this pressure gradient is classically used in the application of the Gorlin formula for the calculation of the aortic orifice. [4]. CF—correction factor for planimetry calculation to aortic valve area; ECG—electrocardiogram; MVG—mitral valve gradient; SEP—systolic ejection period. (*Adapted from* Kern [4].)

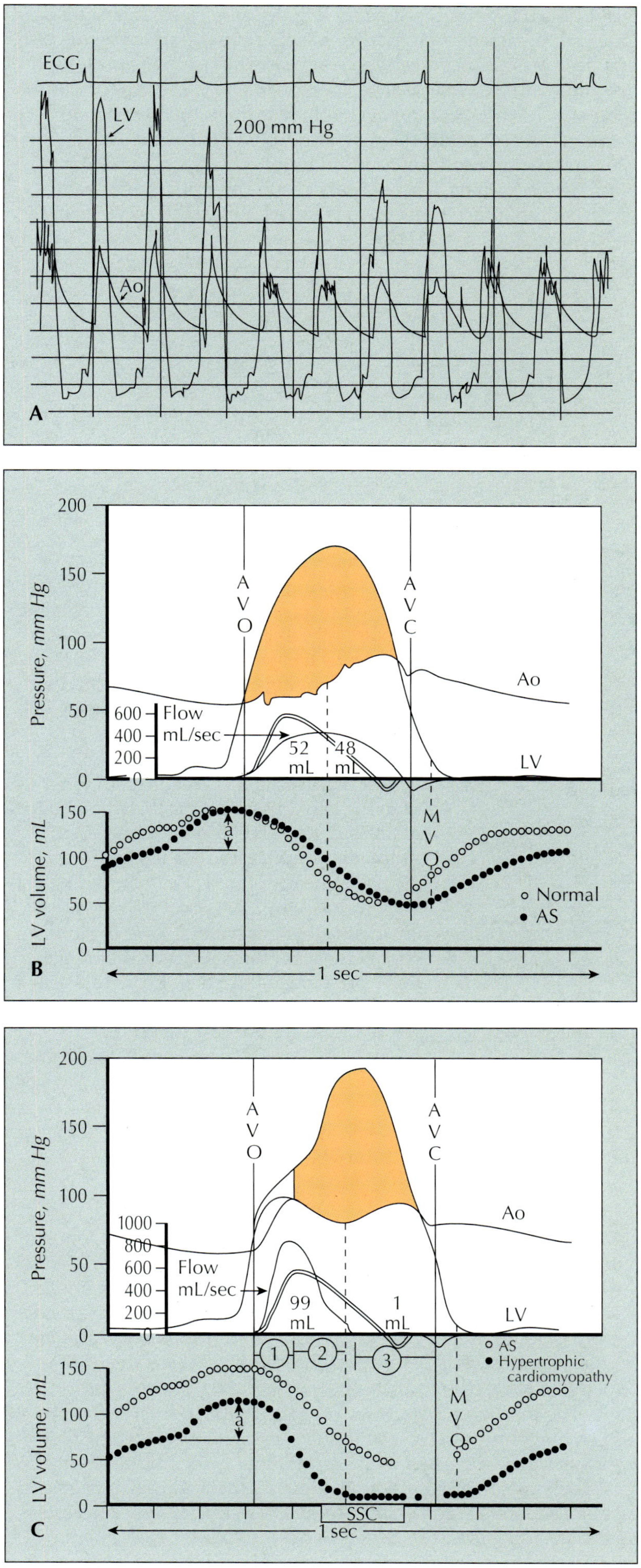

FIGURE 5-21. Left ventricular (LV) pressure gradients in hypertrophic destructive cardiomyopathy. LV–aortic (Ao)pressure gradients may not be due to aortic valve disease. Significant intraventricular gradients can occur in patients with hypertrophic cardiomyopathy and must be differentiated from those of aortic valve stenosis. In some patients, these two conditions may coexist. Maneuvers in the cardiac catheterization laboratory help to identify this finding. Echocardiography may not be able to differentiate this entity with certainty.

A, Simultaneous LV and aortic pressures recorded with a pigtail catheter and side arm of a femoral artery sheath with fluid-filled transducers. Note the large transvalvular gradient in the initial beats at the left of the illustration with LV pressure exceeding 220 mm Hg. The aortic upstroke is rapid. There is a spike and dome-like pattern to the aortic pressure. LV end-diastolic pressure is elevated at 24 mm Hg. As the LV catheter is pulled back, the LV gradient is obliterated while the catheter remains underneath the aortic valve. Note the two beats at the far right side in which aortic and LV pressures are equal, indicating a transventricular and not transvalvular gradient [10].

There are several mechanisms to augment intraventricular gradients: decreasing LV end-diastolic volume, lowering left atrial filling pressure, and prolonging the length of diastole. LV gradients can be augmented by increasing the force or duration of ventricular contraction or decreasing aortic outflow resistance. In addition, four common maneuvers have been used in the cardiac catheterization laboratory to induce intraventricular gradients: Valsalva maneuver, administration of nitroglycerin, post-extrasystolic potentiation, or isoproterenol infusion. Brockenbrough, Braunwald, and Morrow described hemodynamic characteristics of patients with hypertrophic cardiomyopathy in 1961 and identified important differences between valvular stenosis and discrete subvalvular transventricular pressure gradients. Criley and Siegel [11] provided an excellent physiologic demonstration of the differences in aortic pressure gradients for aortic valvular stenotic hypertrophic transventricular pressure gradients.

B, In patients with aortic stenosis (AS), an increase in arterial pulse pressure accompanies a rise in LV peak systolic pressure after premature ventricular contractions. An example of a patient with discrete AS demonstrates the slow aortic pressure upstroke and late ventricular emptying, divided equally over half the systolic period. Aortic flow velocity measured by flow meter (*thin line identified by arrow*) demonstrated evenly distributed ejection velocity over the two halves of the LV ejection period, with 52 and 48 mL of blood ejected over the first and second half of the ejection period.The *thick line* denotes filling velocity in AS.

C, In contrast, in patients with hypertrophic subaortic stenosis (hypertrophic obstructive cardiomyopathy), premature ventricular contractions are followed by narrowing of the arterial pulse pressure in association with increasing LV systolic pressure. This finding, known as the Brockenbrough-Braunwald sign, is characteristic of an early forceful LV ejection producing decreased filling of the postpotentiated beat.

This figure shows a dynamic pressure gradient in a patient with hypertrophic cardiomyopathy. The outflow tract gradient in this patient is associated with rapid arterial pressure upstroke and nearly complete LV ejection in the first one third of systole. Compared with AS, nearly all blood is ejected in the first half of systole, 99 mL, with only 1 mL remaining to be ejected in the last half of the LV ejection period. *Numbered circles 1, 2, and 3* represent the three phases of ejection from the LV and discrete alterations in the pressure and waveform due to intracavitary obstruction with intraventricular pressure gradient development [10]. *(continued)*

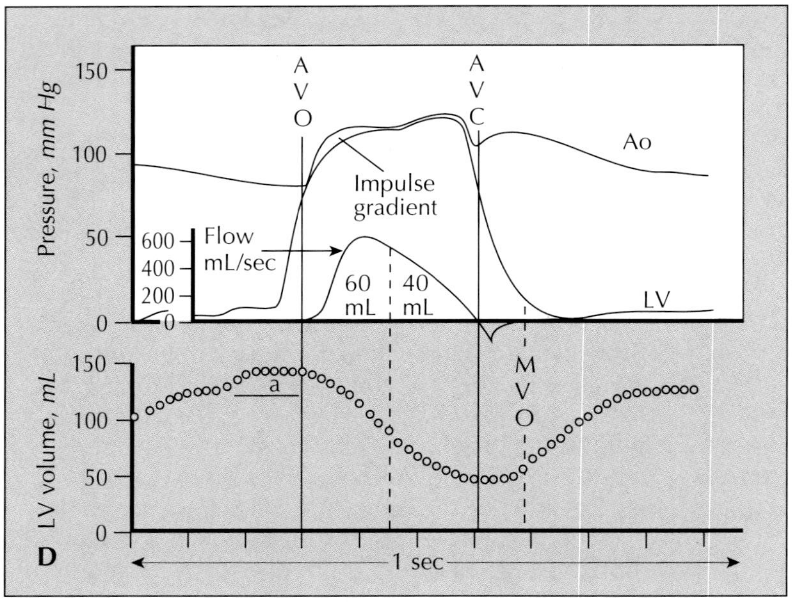

FIGURE 5-21. (*continued*) The *thin line identified by the arrow* donates LV ejection velocity in hypertrophic cardiomyopathy. The *thick line* denotes LV ejection velocity in AS. **D**, Relationship of aortic and LV pressure with LV volume and filling over a normal cardiac cycle for comparison with that of hypertrophic cardiomyopathy and AS in the previous sections. a—atrial contribution to ventricular filling; AVC—aortic valve closure; AVO—aortic valve opening; MVO—mitral valve opening; SSC—onset of septal anterior motion and septal contact. (Part A *adapted from* Kern [10]; parts B and C *adapted from* Criley and Siegel [11].)

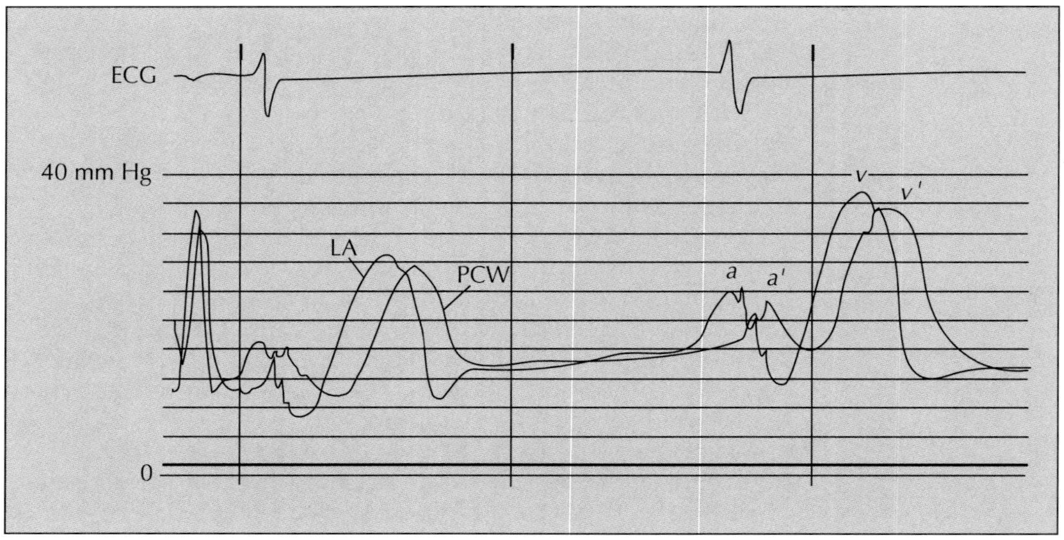

FIGURE 5-22. Pulmonary capillary wedge (PCW) pressure in the assessment of mitral valve (MV) disease. The PCW pressure has been commonly accepted as an accurate reflection of left atrial (LA) pressure in the assessment of MV disease. This figure shows the simultaneous recording of LA and PCW pressures in a patient with mild mitral regurgitation. The PCW pressures were obtained through an 8-F balloon-tipped pulmonary artery catheter, which is directed into the right heart and pulmonary artery with the balloon inflated. After appropriate flushing through the fluid-filled transducer system, the PCW pressure is obtained after the balloon is advanced into a position wedging the catheter in a small pulmonary artery branch. The LA pressure was obtained through a 7-F Brockenbrough catheter and transseptal technique using similar transducers. Both transducers were matched for zero and equiphasic pressure responses. Normal LA pressure waves precede PCW pressure by 40 to 120 ms in timing and often have a slightly higher pressure compared with the PCW pressure due to a minimal loss of pressure transmission through the pulmonary capillaries. The tracings are otherwise nearly identical in their timing and waveforms. Mean PCW and LA pressures are identical in this patient. Note the influence of the arrhythmia on both the LA and PCW pressure in this patient. The first beat is a sinus beat, whereas the next beat is an ectopic atrial contraction , which has a prolonged PR interval and produces a larger *v* wave [4]. *a—a* wave of PCW; *a′—a* wave of LA; *v—v* wave of PCW; *v′—v* wave of LA pressure. ECG—electrocardiogram. (*Adapted from* Kern [4].)

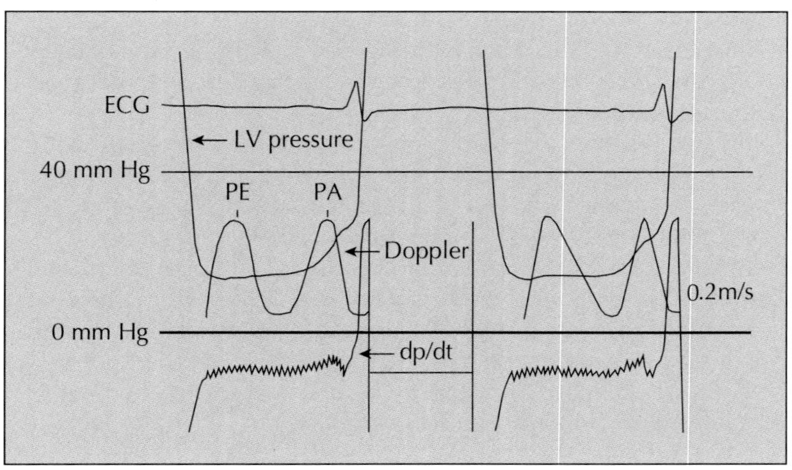

FIGURE 5-23. Simultaneous left ventricular pressure and Doppler mitral inflow velocity illustrate the early and late filling phases of flow through the mitral valve, which corresponds to the *v* and *a* waves, respectively. The peak early filling (PE) wave corresponds to the descent of the *v* wave of the atrial and pulmonary capillary wedge pressures. The peak atrial (PA) filling wave is the flow velocity increase due to atrial contraction and produces the *a* wave. The timing of these flow velocities corresponds to the pressure changes and can be seen in the simultaneous overlay of left ventricular pressure over the Doppler flow velocity (the change in pressure/time of left ventricular pressure (dP/dt) is also shown as part of a separate study). The alterations in mitral flow thus influence the *v* and *a* pressure waves in hemodynamic assessment of mitral valve disease [4]. (*Adapted from* Kern [4].)

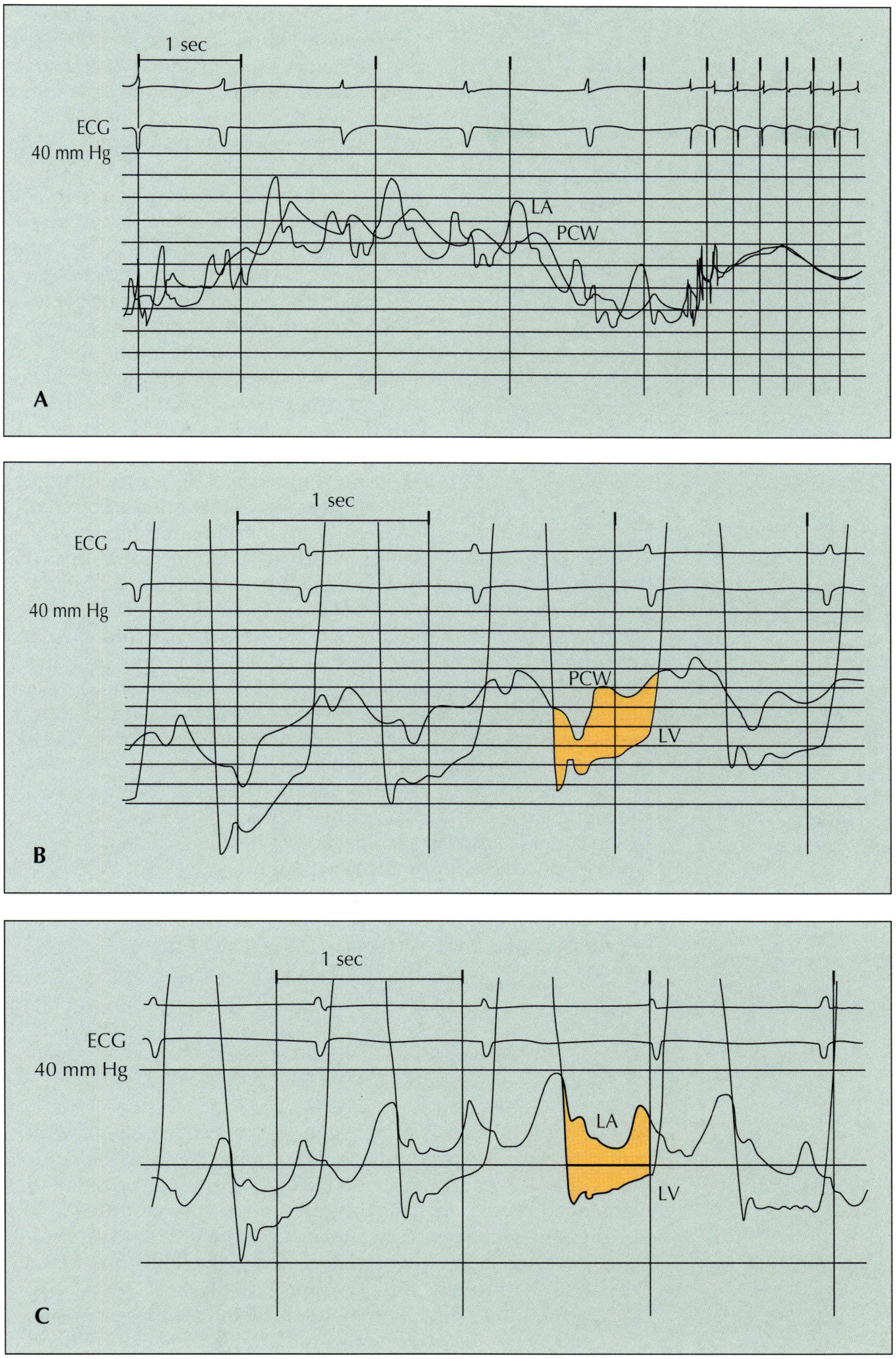

FIGURE 5-24. A, Although pulmonary capillary wedge (PCW) pressure is generally accepted for assessment of left atrial (LA) pressure in the examination of mitral valve hemodynamics, at times, PCW pressure is not satisfactory. An overly damped PCW pressure may provide an equivalent mean pressure to LA pressure; however, the phasic waveforms may obscure the precise diagnosis of mitral stenosis. In a patient in whom mitral stenosis was present, LA and PCW pressure on a 0- to 40-mm Hg pressure scale were measured. Note the identical matching of mean pressures at the far left, but disparity between the phasic waveforms. *A* large *v* wave is present on the LA pressure, which is not appreciated on the damped wedge pressure. Despite multiple catheter manipulations and flushing of the transducer system, the PCW pressure could not be improved [10].

B, Simultaneous PCW and left ventricular (LV) pressure recording demonstrates a mitral valve gradient but a poor PCW waveform. The precision with which mitral valve stenosis was assessed in this individual was not satisfactory and required transseptal assessment [10].

C, Direct LA pressure measured with transseptal catheter and LV pressure. Note the improved fidelity of the pressure gradient, the waveforms identifying both the *a* and *v* wave, and the consistent gradient over the cardiac cycles. This gradient assessment was necessary before valvuloplasty. PCW pressure could not be relied on to identify a satisfactory resolution of the pressure gradient in this procedure [10]. ECG—electrocardiogram. (*Adapted from* Kern [10].)

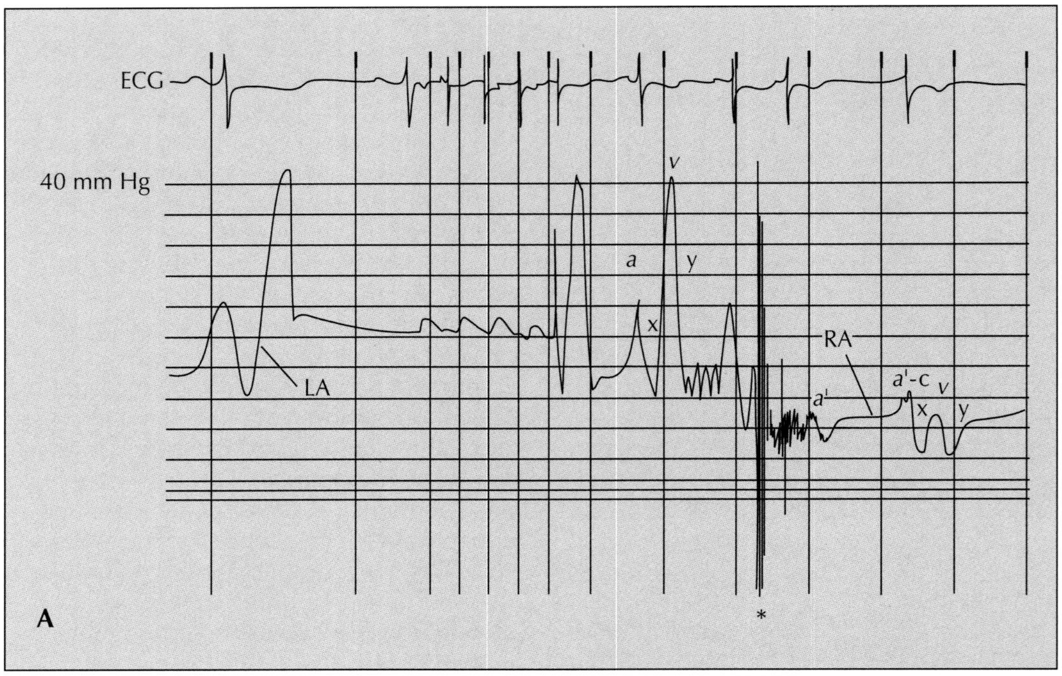

Figure 5-25. Analysis of *v* waves in the assessment of mitral regurgitation. The atrial and ventricular filling patterns demonstrated by transmitral Doppler flow translate into *a* and *v* waves on left atrial (LA) and right atrial (RA) pressures. **A,** Transseptal LA pressure during pullback from the LA to RA. Large *a* and *v* waves are demonstrated. The *v* waves represent mitral regurgitation in a patient with mild aortic stenosis. The *v* wave of 40 mm Hg is twice the mean LA pressure of 20 mm Hg. Note that the *a* and *v* waves in the RA pressure are diminutive relative to the left side. Pressure artifact from the catheter as it crosses the septum (*asterisk*) is easily seen and the continuous pressure recording accurately reflects the transatrial pressure gradient. The height of the *v* wave is sensitive but not specific for mitral regurgitation. The *v* waves are often associated with significant mitral regurgitation, ventricular septal defects, and other conditions of altered compliance and pressure-volume relationships within the atrial and ventricular chambers [4].

B, Two pressure-volume curves of the LA indicate differences in *v* waves, noted by *black circles,* depending on cardiac output. In the top curve, increasing pressure is obtained with increasing flow or volume in the LA. A large *v* wave can be associated with a small increase in pressure. Likewise, the higher compliance of the LA in the lower curve would yield a much smaller *v* wave. Pharmacotherapy with vasodilators often lowers pressure, thus reducing the *v* wave. Cardiac catheterization data acquired in this fashion provide an accurate reflection of the hemodynamic responses obtained during the procedure. *a*—*a* wave of PCW; *a'*—*a* wave of PCW; *a'*-c—*a* wave + c wave of RA pressure; c—c wave of RA pressure; ECG—electrocardiogram; x—x descent after *a* wave; y—y descent after *v* wave. (Part A *adapted from* Kern [4].)

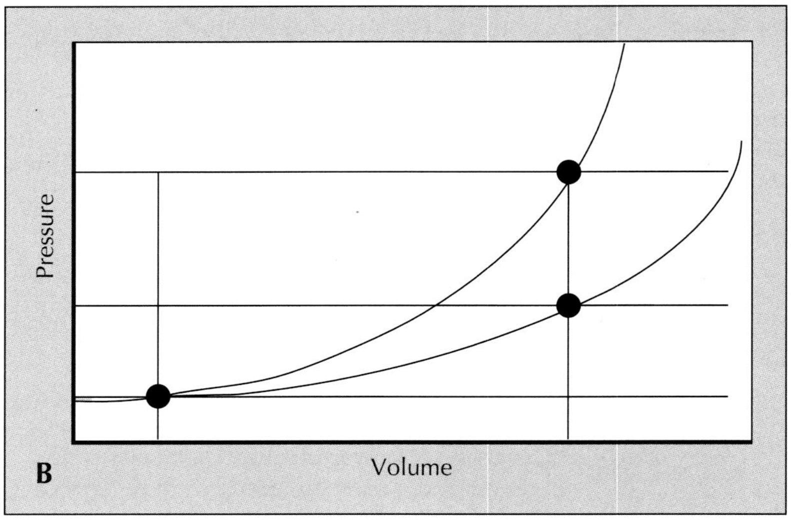

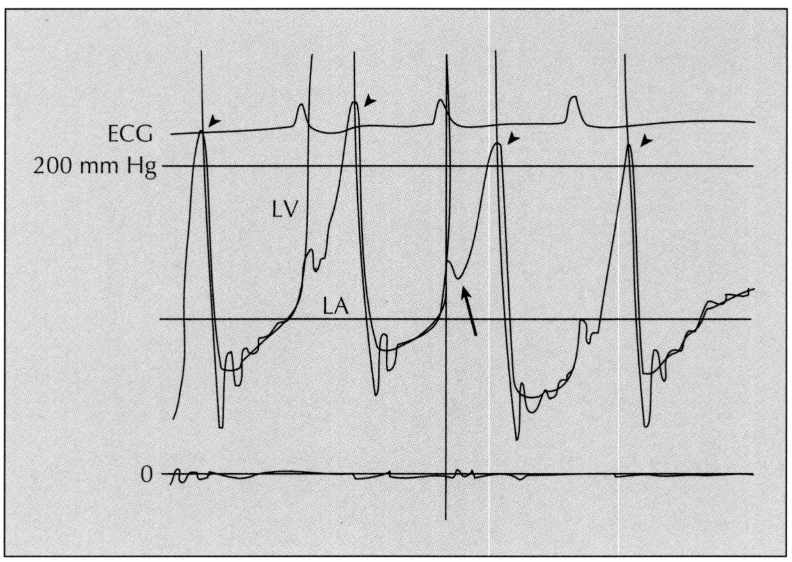

Figure 5-26. The *v* wave of mitral regurgitation. In patients with significant mitral regurgitation without mitral stenosis, the regurgitant volume is transmitted into the left atrium (LA) without obstruction of backflow. This transmission of flow produces a large pressure wave occurring at the end of ventricular systole. The LA pressure is rapidly decompressed to the left ventricular (LV) pressure during the initial part of diastole.

This figure shows directly measured LA and LV pressures via transseptal technique and demonstrates large *v* waves and identically matching LA and LV pressures in early diastole and over the diastolic period. The electrocardiogram (ECG) shows atrial fibrillation, thus no *a* wave is apparent. The LV systolic upstroke is obscured on beat three. A C notch (*arrow*) and large *v* waves (*arrowheads*) are apparent on the LA tracing [10]. ECG—electrocardiogram. (*Adapted from* Kern [10].)

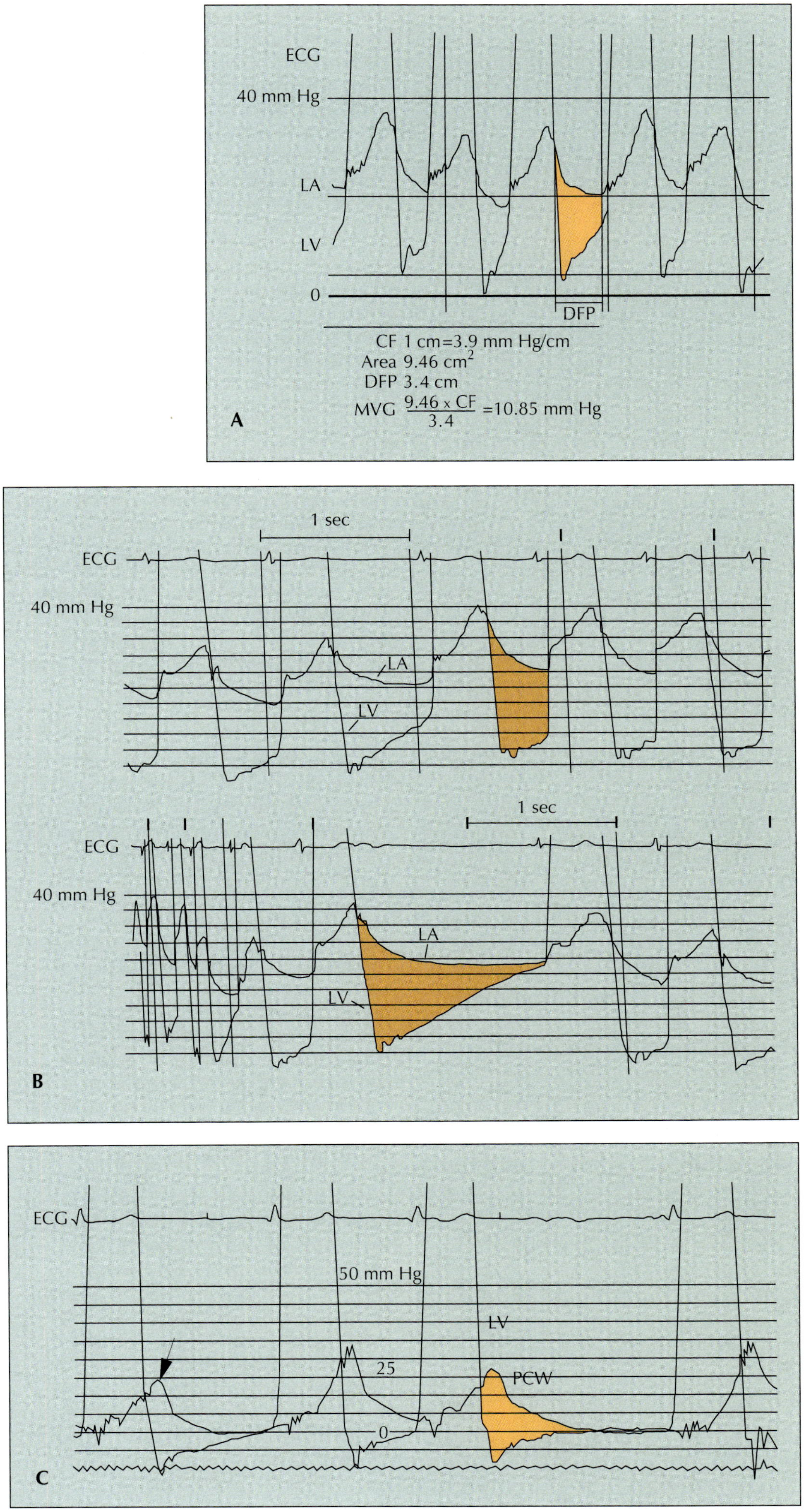

FIGURE 5-27. Hemodynamics of mitral stenosis. In the cardiac catheterization laboratory, mitral stenosis is assessed by comparison of left atrial (LA) and left ventricular (LV) pressures during diastole. The diastolic filling period (DFP) is used to compute the mitral valve gradient (*orange area* in *A, B, and* C).

A, In this patient, LA and LV pressures are simultaneously measured. LA pressure was obtained via the transseptal approach. A correction factor (CF) for the paper scale is used to compute the area of the mitral gradient. The mitral valve gradient (MVG) is computed using the standard Gorlin formula corrected for paper scale and speed. The DFP is important in the assessment of MVGs. Patients who are in atrial fibrillation require the planimetry and average of valve gradients over at least 10 cardiac cycles [4].

B, The influence of long RR intervals on the mitral gradient is well appreciated. The *top panel* shows short RR interval with the gradient (*orange area*) compared with the *lower panel* with a long RR interval. The Gorlin formula is best applied in patients in sinus rhythm without mitral regurgitation, normal LV function, and no other concomitant valve lesions. The effect of heart rate on MVG may be important as demonstrated in the *top panel*. A short RR interval has an MVG of 22 mm Hg with reduced mitral valve area. On beat two with a long RR interval, the MVG was calculated at 29 mm Hg with end-diastolic pressure equilibration. These factors are evident at cardiac catheterization and should be considered in the computation of mitral valve stenosis [10].

C, Mitral stenosis as assessed by pulmonary capillary wedge (PCW) pressure is different from that obtained with the LA pressure in a patient in atrial fibrillation. PCW and LV pressures are measured simultaneously with fluid-filled systems. Note the delay in *v* wave (arrow) relative to the LV downstroke and the rapid equilibration of pressure by mid-diastole in this patient. Phase shifting of the *v* wave to the downstroke of the LV pressure further reduces the LV/PCW pressure gradient. Transseptal assessment of pressure in this individual is probably not needed because the PCW pressure is low and satisfactory for assessing the clinical importance of mitral stenosis under resting conditions [9]. ECG—electrocardiogram; RR interval—time from R wave to R wave of following beat. (Part A *adapted from* Kern [4]; parts B and C *adapted from* Kern [10].)

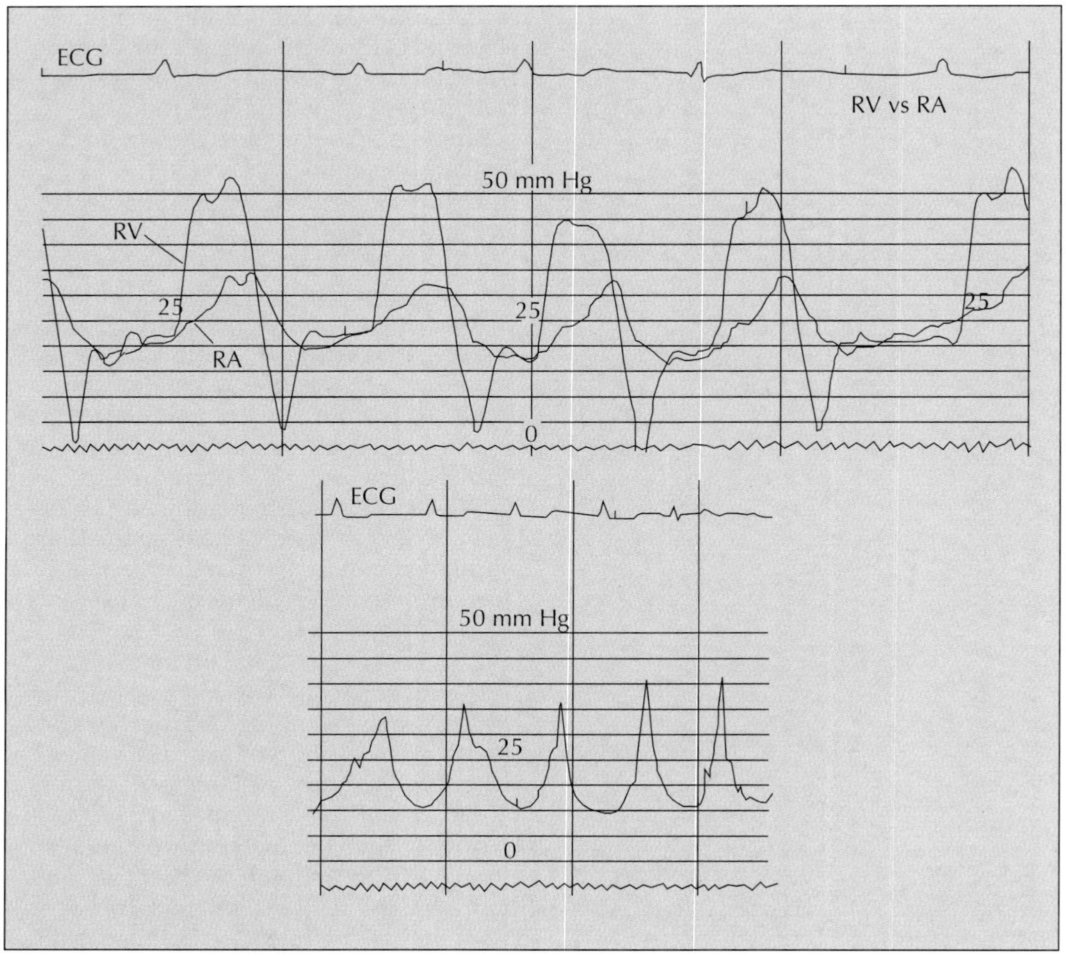

Figure 5-28. Tricuspid regurgitation. In patients with tricuspid regurgitation, characteristic waveforms are identified in the catheterization laboratory. The regurgitation of blood into the right atrium (RA) produces large systolic (*v*) waves in the atrial pressure. The summed regurgitant wave, also called the S wave, is proportional to the severity of regurgitation in most patients. As on the pulmonary wedge pressure, the depths of the *v* waves on the right side of the heart are determined by the pressure-volume characteristics of the chamber. Thus, severe angiographic regurgitation may also be present when small *v* waves are registered. In this patient, right ventricular (RV) and RA pressures are simultaneously obtained with two catheters through fluid-filled transducer systems. The pressure scale is 0 to 50 mm Hg. Large *v* waves can be seen on the RA pressure during RV systole. The tricuspid regurgitation in this patient is severe. Transmission of the venous pulse of the regurgitation can be detected in the femoral vein shown in the lower panel. The large *v* waves are also well appreciated during physical examination of the neck [10]. ECG—electrocardiogram. (*Adapted from* Kern [10].)

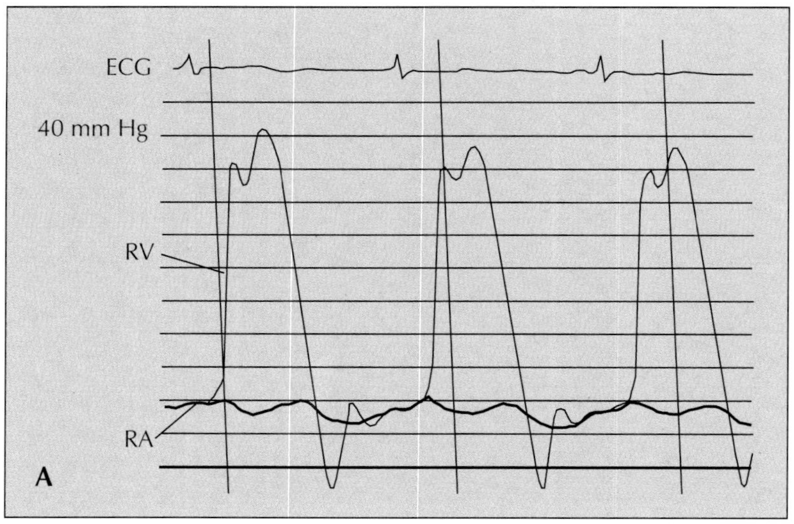

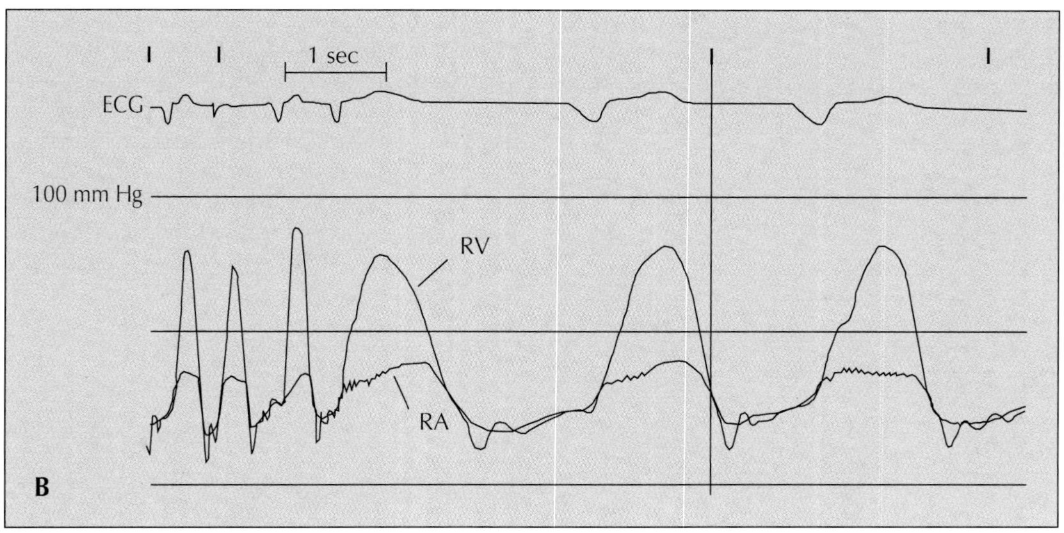

Figure 5-29. A, Mildly elevated right ventricular (RV) pressure with normal right atrial (RA) pressure. Note the correspondence of simultaneous *a* and *v* waves. The pressure scale is 0 to 40 mm Hg. This normal tracing should be used for comparison with Fig. 5-30 *B* demonstrating pulmonary hypertension and severe tricuspid regurgitation. The normal hemodynamic recordings of tricuspid valve function should be identified in the interpretation of abnormal waveforms [4].

B, Elevated RV pressure in a patient with marked pulmonary hypertension and tricuspid regurgitation. The pressure scale is 0 to 100 mm Hg. The RA pressure increases corresponded to the systolic regurgitation of blood into the RA chamber. Note that the RA pressure mean is approximately 20 mm Hg, with a systolic regurgitant wave covering all of the RV systolic ejection period and a *v* wave peaking immediately before the RV pressure downslope. This patient had severe multivalvular regurgitation and pulmonary hypertension, evidenced by physical examination and Doppler echocardiography, and confirmed by hemodynamic studies [10]. ECG—electrocardiogram. (Part A *adapted from* Kern [4]; part B *adapted from* Kern [10].)

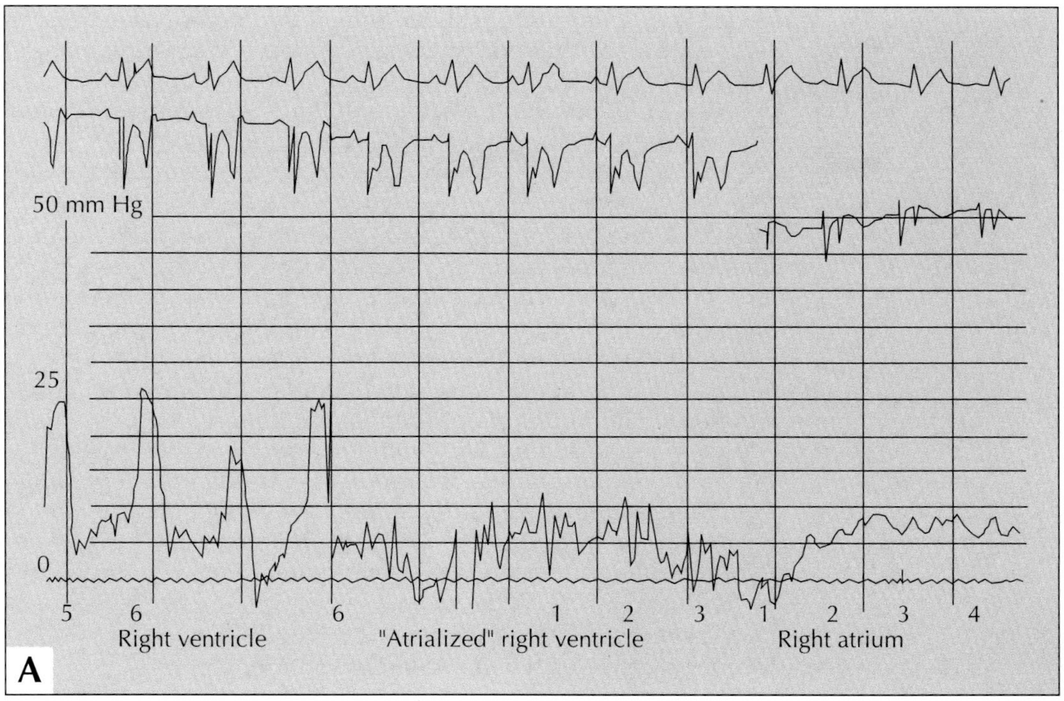

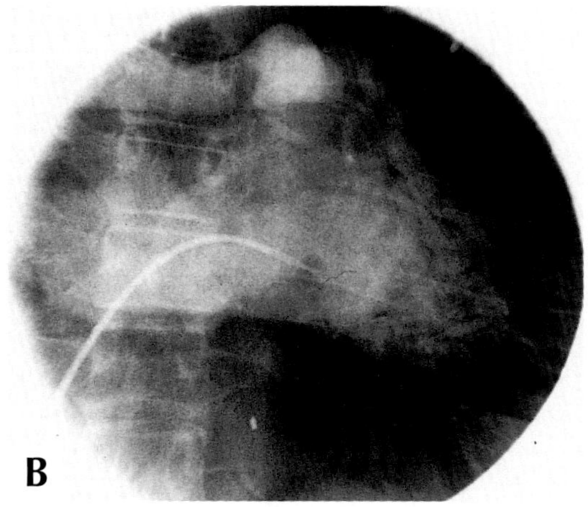

B

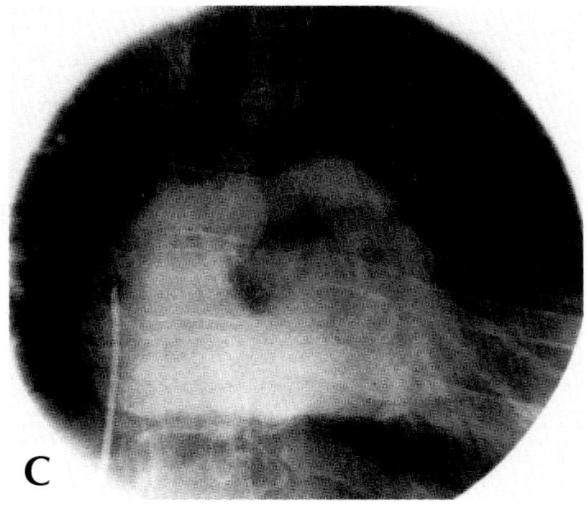

C

Figure 5-30. Congenital anomalies associated with valvular heart disease. In the assessment of valvular heart disease, various types of congenital anomalies may be coexistent in the adult patient. The cardiac catheterization laboratory is appropriately suited for sophisticated evaluation of the complex anomalies that may be associated with valvular heart disease. In particular, congenital lesions such as ventricular septal defect, atrial septal defect, tetralogy of Fallot, and other common cardiac anomalies may be associated with valvular or myopathic dysfunction. These findings are often associated with characteristic waveforms of tricuspid or mitral regurgitation. Intracardiac shunts may also be present.

During diagnostic studies for symptomatic palpitations in a young patient, two-dimensional and transesophageal echocardiography demonstrated abnormalities of the tricuspid and mitral valves and right atrium, the abnormal septal motion consistent with right ventricular volume overload, and an ostium secundum septal defect. A cardiac shunt was estimated by contrast echocardiography at 1.4:1. Right and left heart catheterization was performed with standard technique to assess both hemodynamics and intracardiac shunts. **A,** Right ventricular catheter pullback pressure tracing with a simultaneous intracardiac electrogram in this patient. The intracavity electrogram and hemodynamic recordings were obtained with a Zucker pacing end-hole Dacron catheter. On right ventricular electrocatheter pullback from the right ventricle to the right atrium, the right ventricular electrogram maintains its configuration while the right ventricular pressure changes into an atrialized pressure waveform. The further withdrawal of the catheter then changes the right ventricular electrogram to an atrial electrogram while maintaining atrial pressure. The transition to atrial pressure with simultaneous ventriculogram is a classic finding of Ebstein's anomaly as identified in the cardiac catheterization laboratory [10].

B, Right ventriculography in this patient demonstrated a small ventricular chamber with a markedly displaced tricuspid valve caudally and anteriorly into the right ventricular cavity [10].

C, The right atrial angiogram demonstrated the large atrial chamber and location of the tricuspid valve. Ebstein's anomaly is thus precisely described using catheterization techniques [10]. (*Adapted from* Kern [10]; with permission.)

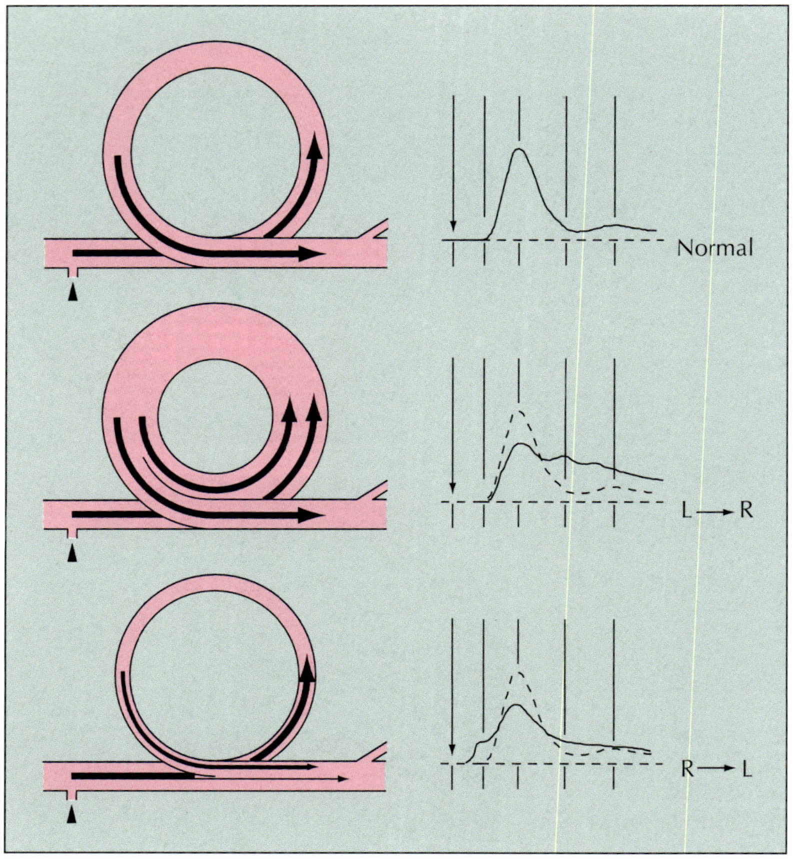

FIGURE 5-31. Intracardiac shunts. Some valvular lesions of heart disease are associated with intracardiac shunts. Intracardiac shunts are evaluated by five methods: oximetry, indocyanine green dye dilution curves, angiography, radioisotope tracers, and contrast studies with transesophageal and transthoracic Doppler echocardiography. In patients with normal cardiac circulation, the injected indicator circulates through the pulmonary circulation (*top loop*) to the systemic circulation producing a normal transit time curve of the indicator. In patients with left-to-right (L ← R) shunts (*middle panel*), the indicator is not cleared rapidly, recirculating through the pulmonary system. This increase in pulmonary flow produces a diminution in the peak of the circulatory curve and recirculation signal on the downstroke of the dilution curve. In patients with right-to-left (R →L) shunt (*bottom panel*), there is a decrease in the pulmonary blood flow relative to the systemic flow and a portion of the indicator passes directly to the arterial circulation resulting in an early appearance of the indicator on the upstroke of the indicator curve. The indicator passes directly to the arterial circulation via the defect without passing through the lungs and arrives at the arterial sampling site early before the major deflection. This technique is commonly used to accurately document right-to-left and left-to-right shunting.

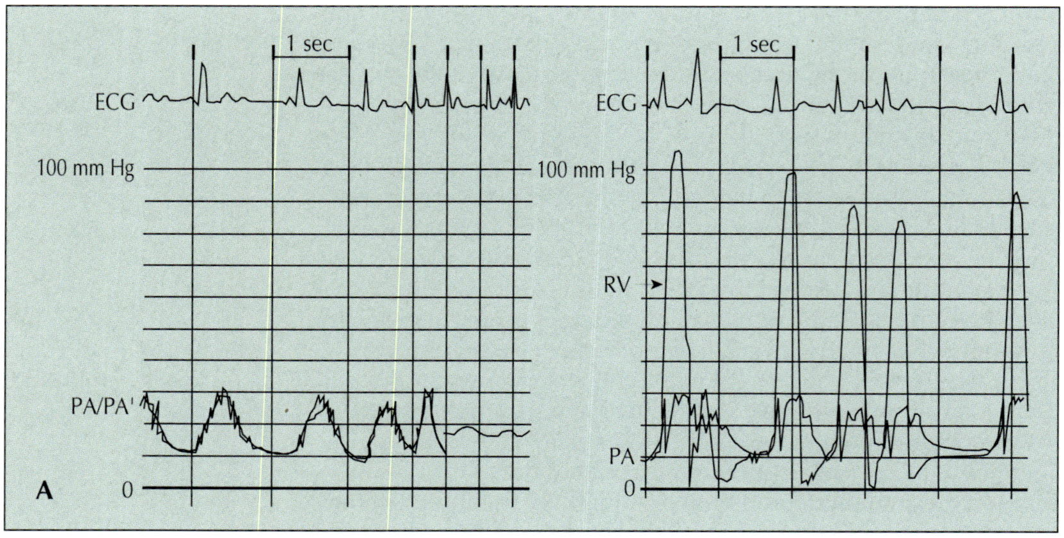

FIGURE 5-32. Pulmonary valve disease. Although pulmonary stenosis is readily detectable on physical examination and by Doppler ultrasound, confirmation of the precise location of the obstruction of right ventricular (RV) outflow may be required. At times branch pulmonary stenosis may be confused with valvular pulmonary stenosis. These entities may be differentiated by hemodynamic study with multiple catheters in the pulmonary artery (PA) and RV.

A, In the assessment of pulmonary valve (PV) stenosis, two catheters were placed in the pulmonary artery as indicated by PA and PA′. The pressures are matched in their phasic waveform and mean pressure on a 0- to 100-mm Hg pressure scale. On catheter pullback, an RV pressure is matched against the PA pressure and the findings are consistent with PV stenosis. (*continued*)

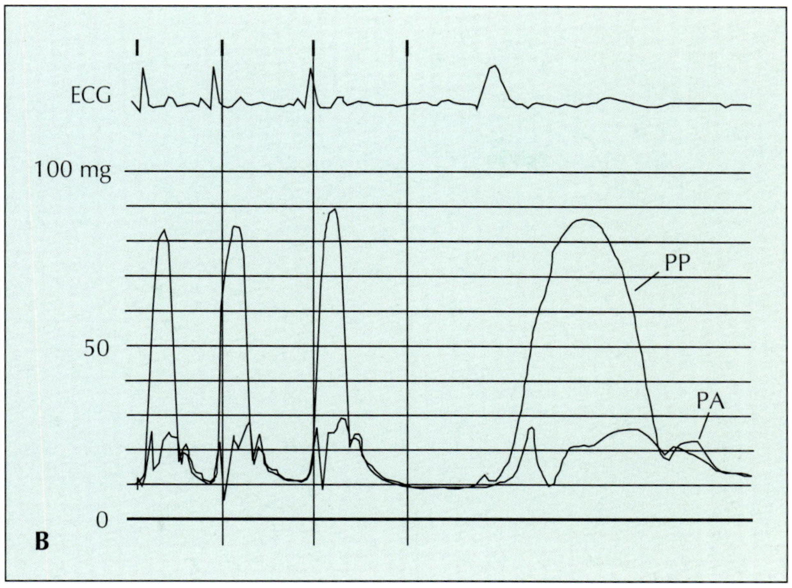

Figure 5-32. (*continued*) **B,** On slow pullback of the RV catheter, it can be appreciated that there is a subvalvular chamber complicating the assessment of the PV lesion. This patient did not have valvular but had supravalvular pulmonary stenosis in which the tracing labeled PP is a proximal PA pressure obtained above the PV but below the area of narrowing. The area of narrowing was due to a prior PA banding proximal to the bifurcation of the left and right pulmonary arteries. Pressures in the distal pulmonary arteries (PA) of 34/12 mm Hg were distinctly lower than pressure obtained proximal to the site of narrowing (PP), 85/12 mm Hg. RV pressure of 95/10 mm Hg (as shown in *panel A, right side*) was one clue to the important differentiation of this entity. Angiography was consistent with pulmonary outflow obstruction without identification of valvular stenosis [10]. ECG—electrocardiogram. (*Adapted from* Kern [10].)

References

1. Grossman W, ed: *Cardiac Catheterization and Angiography*, edn 3. Philadelphia: Lea & Febiger; 1986.
2. Pepine CJ, ed: *Diagnostic and Therapeutic Cardiac Catheterization*. Baltimore: Williams & Wilkins; 1989.
3. Yang SS, Bentivoglio LG, Maranhao V, Goldberg H, eds: *Cardiac Catheterization Data to Hemodynamic Parameters*, edn 3. Philadelphia: FA Davis; 1978.
4. Kern MJ, ed: *The Cardiac Catheterization Handbook*, edn 2. St. Louis: Mosby-Year Book; 1994.
5. Krone J, Morton MJ, eds: *Complications of Cardiac Catheterization and Angiography: Prevention and Management*. Mount Kisco, NY: Futura Publishing; 1989.
6. Friesinger GC, Adams DF, Bourassa MG, *et al.*: Optimal resources for examination of the heart and lungs: cardiac catheterization and radiographic facilities. *Circulation* 1983, 68:893A–930A.
7. Tilkian AG, Daily EK: *Cardiovascular Procedures: Diagnostic Techniques and Therapeutic Procedures*. St. Louis; Mosby-Year Book; 1986.
8. Croft CH, Lipscomb K: Modified technique of transseptal left heart catheterization. *J Am Coll Cardiol* 1985, 5:904.
9. Pujadas G: *Coronary Angiography in the Medical and Surgical Treatment of Ischemic Heart Disease*. New York: McGraw-Hill; 1980.
10. Kern MJ: *Hemodynamic Rounds: Interpretation of Cardiac Pathophysiology from Pressure Waveform Analysis*. New York: Wiley-Liss; 1993.
11. Criley JM, Siegel RJ: Has "obstruction" hindered our understanding of hypertrophic cardiomyopathy? *Circulation* 1985, 72:1148–1154.

Aortic Valve Stenosis

6

CHAPTER

Shahbudin H. Rahimtoola

Aortic stenosis (AS) is now the most common valve lesion for which patients undergo diagnostic cardiac catheterization-angiography and valve replacement. The most common causes of AS are calcific (degenerative), congenital, and rheumatic. With the decline in the incidence of rheumatic fever and rheumatic valve disease in developed countries, calcific AS accounts for over half of the patients undergoing valve replacement for AS. Recent evidence suggests that calcific AS may be the result of an immune reaction to antigens present in the valve. Calcific AS is the most common cause of AS in the older patient population.

With the increased performance of checkups in healthy people and the increasing use of Doppler ultrasound, mild and even moderate AS is being detected more often in asymptomatic persons. In patients with severe AS, the classic clinical presentation includes angina, syncope, and symptoms of heart failure.

AS is usually easy to diagnose by clinical evaluation (history, physical examination, electrocardiography, and chest radiography). Doppler ultrasound is the single most important noninvasive test and is useful in diagnosing and evaluating the severity of AS. A common clinical problem is distinguishing moderate from severe AS even after clinical evaluation and Doppler ultrasound. Cardiac catheterization-angiography remains an extremely important diagnostic procedure and should be performed in most patients before valve surgery. Associated significant obstructive coronary artery disease is present in approximately one half of patients older than 35 to 40 years of age.

The outcome with medical treatment in patients with severe AS, especially in those with symptoms, is very poor. Patients with severe AS need interventional therapy. Catheter balloon valvuloplasty is a useful technique in children and young adults in whom the main lesion is commissural fusion(s) in a congenitally abnormal valve. It has a limited role in the calcified valve of the older patient whether the etiology is congenital, rheumatic, or degenerative. Valve replacement for severe AS relieves symptoms, reduces left ventricular hypertrophy, improves left ventricular size and function in those in whom it was abnormal preoperatively, and improves survival.

Etiology

ETIOLOGY OF AS
Congenital
Acquired
Rheumatic
Calcific (degenerative)
Rare causes
Obstructive infective vegetations
Homozygous type II hyperlipoproteinemia
Paget's disease of bone
Systemic lupus erythematosus
Rheumatoid involvement
Ochronosis (alkaptonuria)
Irradiation

Figure 6-1. Etiology of aortic stenosis (AS). The three most common causes of AS are congenital, rheumatic, and calcific (degenerative) [1,2]. Calcific AS is seen in patients 35 years of age or older and may be the result of calcification of a congenital or rheumatic valve, or calcification of a normal valve that has undergone degenerative changes. Data suggest that calcific AS may represent an autoimmune reaction to antigens present in the valve [3].

The other causes of AS are rare. Obstructive infective vegetations usually result from large exuberant vegetations (*eg*, those seen in fungal endocarditis). Atherosclerotic AS occurs most frequently in patients with severe hypercholesterolemia and is observed in children with homozygous type II hyperlipoproteinemia. Other rare cause of AS include Paget's disease of the bone, systemic lupus erythematosus, rheumatoid involvement, ochronosis, and irradiation.

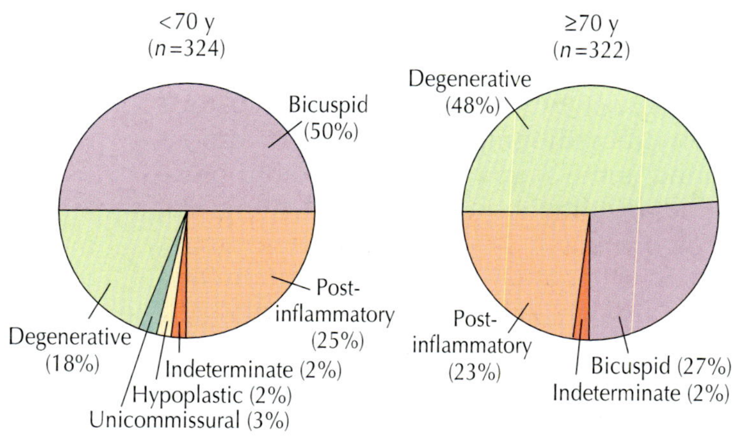

Figure 6-2. Percentages of valve lesions. At the present time, calcific AS in the older patient is the most common valve lesion requiring valve replacement [4]. According to Passik *et al.* [5], among patients under 70 years of age, congenital bicuspid valves accounted for one half of the surgical cases, and degenerative changes were the cause in 18%. Conversely, in patients 70 years of age or older, degenerative changes accounted for almost one half of the surgical cases and a congenital bicuspid valve for approximately one quarter of the cases. (*Adapted from* Passik and coworkers [5].)

CONFIGURATION OF AORTIC VALVE IN ISOLATED AS IN RELATION TO AGE

	AGE, y		
NUMBER OF VALVE CUSPS	≤15, %	15–65, %	>65, %
Unicuspid	60	10	0
Bicuspid	20	60	10
Tricuspid	15	25	90
Uncertain	5	5	0

Figure 6-3. Isolated AS related to age. Pathologic examination of the number of cusps involved in patients with isolated AS shows that under the age of 15 years, 60% were unicuspid. Between the ages of 15 and 65, 60% were bicuspid. Above the age of 65, 90% were tricuspid [6]. (*Adapted from* Roberts [6].)

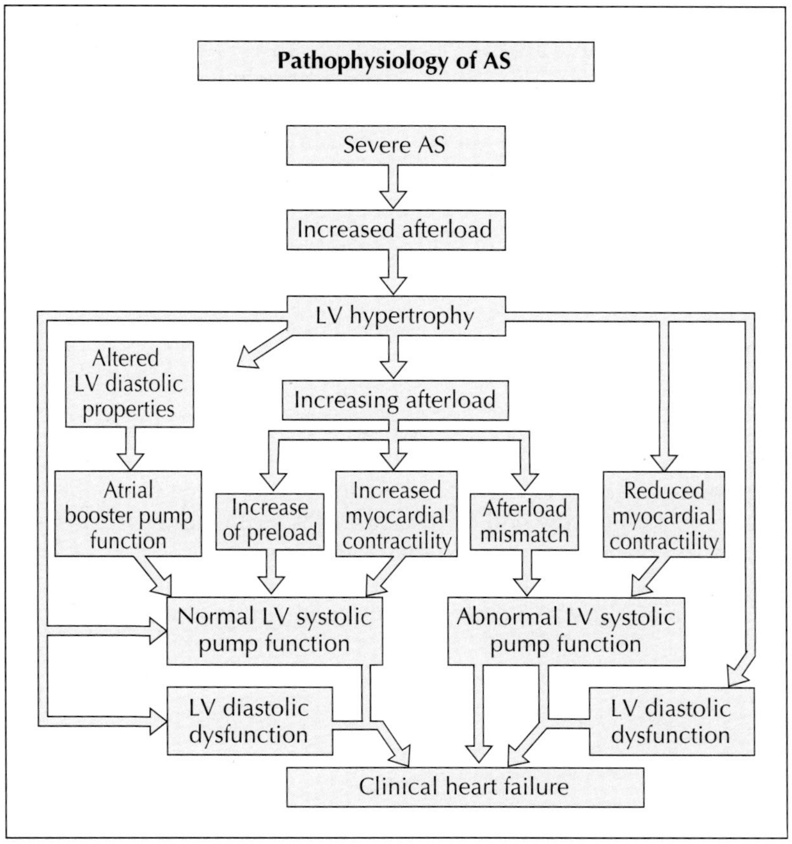

FIGURE 6-4. Pathophysiology of AS. With reduction in the aortic valve area (AVA), energy is dissipated during the transport of blood from the left ventricle (LV) to the aorta. The AVA has to be reduced by 50% of normal before a measurable gradient can be demonstrated. When a pressure gradient develops between the LV and the ascending aorta, LV pressure rises and LV wall stress (afterload) increases. This could result in an impairment of LV function. The heart responds by becoming hypertrophied and myocardial stress remains normal. LV mass in patients with severe AS undergoing valve replacement averages 229 g/m^2 (normal mass, 105 g/m^2) [7]; at autopsy, LVs weighing as much as 1000 g have been reported. LV volume remains within the normal range; therefore, there is considerable thickening of the LV wall. As a result of the LV hypertrophy, LV systolic pump function remains normal. LV hypertrophy may alter the LV diastolic properties and there is increased resistance to LV filling. As a result, LV end-diastolic pressure is elevated; but this cannot be used as a measure of LV failure. Powerful atrial contraction produces the required LV filling [8,9] and fiber length (atrial booster pump function). Because atrial systole occupies only a small part of the cardiac cycle, there is only a transient increase in left atrial pressure; therefore, mean left atrial pressure remains in the normal range [8] or is only minimally increased.

As LV afterload continues to increase, the LV uses two additional compensatory mechanisms, namely, increase of preload and increase of myocardial contractility. Both of these help maintain normal LV systolic pump function.

When the limit of the preload reserve has been reached (afterload mismatch) [10] or myocardial contractility is reduced, LV systolic pump function becomes abnormal.

Clinical heart failure is usually a result of abnormal LV systolic pump function; diastolic dysfunction may also be present in some patients (*see* Fig. 6-13). Clinical heart failure in those with normal systolic pump function is a result of LV diastolic dysfunction. (© Copyright SH Rahimtoola, MB, FRCP, MACP.)

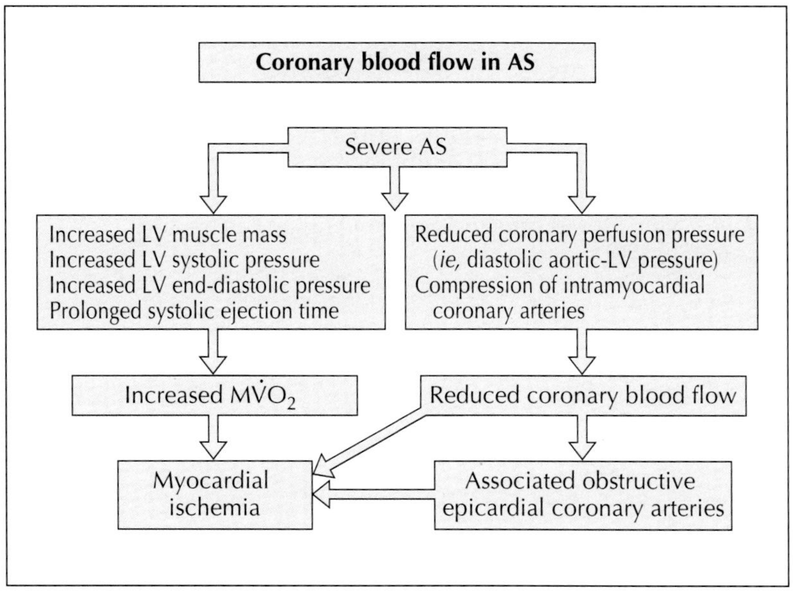

FIGURE 6-5. Coronary blood flow in AS. In severe AS, myocardial oxygen demands ($M\dot{V}O_2$) are increased because of increased muscle mass (hypertrophy), increases in left ventricular (LV) pressures, and prolongation of the systolic ejection time. Total coronary blood flow is increased; however, coronary blood flow per 100 g of LV mass is reduced [11] because of a reduction of the diastolic aortic-LV pressure gradient and compression of the coronary arteries as they traverse the myocardium from the epicardium to the endocardium to supply the subendocardial myocardial region. Thus, these patients have myocardial ischemia, particularly in the subendocardial region. Because coronary reserve, *ie*, the ability of the coronary blood flow to increase with vasodilatation, is significantly reduced [12], the myocardial ischemia can be markedly exacerbated on effort. Associated obstructive coronary artery disease (*see* Fig. 6-36) can be expected to further exacerbate the myocardial ischemia. (© Copyright SH Rahimtoola, MB, FRCP, MACP.)

Natural History and Prognosis

NATURAL HISTORY OF MILD AS

	10 Y, %	20 Y, %	25 Y, %
Mild	88	63	38
Moderate	4	15	25
Severe	8	22	38

Figure 6-6. Natural history of AS. One hundred forty-two patients with an aortic valve area (AVA) greater than 1.5 cm^2, documented by cardiac catheterization, had a comparatively benign clinical course [13]. At the end of 20 years, 63% continued to have mild AS and only 22% had severe disease. This clinical course is better than the outcome after any interventional therapy and, therefore, an AVA of greater than 1.5 cm^2 should be considered mild AS. (*Adapted from* Horstkotte and Loogen [13].)

MODERATE AS

Patients, *n*	44
AVA, *cm^2*	0.95–1.4
Died:	
1 y, %	3
10 y, %	14.5
Events at 10 y, %	65

Figure 6-7. Moderate AS. According to Turina *et al.*, mortality at the end of 1 year was 3% and at the end of 10 years was 14.5% in 44 patients with moderate AS, *ie*, an aortic valve area (AVA) of 0.95 to 1.4 cm^2 [14]. At the end of 10 years, 65% of the patients had had an event. This indicates that patients with an AVA of 1.0 to 1.4 cm^2 will not have quite as benign a course as those patients with an AVA of greater than 1.5 cm^2. (*Adapted from* Turina and coworkers [14].)

AVERAGE SURVIVAL IN SYMPTOMATIC PATIENTS WITH SEVERE AS

VARIABLE	AUTOPSY DATA, *y*	POST CARDIAC CATHETERIZATION, *mo*
Overall	3	23
Angina	5	45
Syncope	3	27
Heart failure	<2	11

Figure 6-8. Severe AS. The outcome in patients with severe AS is lethal. The classic study by Ross and Braunwald [15] (a retrospective of autopsy data) and a more recent study by Horstkotte and Loogen [13] of patients followed after cardiac catheterization reveal remarkably similar data. After the onset of symptoms, the overall average survival times in the two studies were 3 years and 23 months, respectively. The average survival times after the onset of angina were 5 years and 45 months, respectively, and for syncope, 3 years and 27 months, respectively. The onset of heart failure carries an extremely ominous prognosis with almost all patients being dead within 2 years and 1 year, respectively. (*Adapted from* Horstkotte and Loogen [13] and Ross and Braunwald [15].)

Grading Severity

SUGGESTED GRADING OF THE DEGREE OF AS

AS	AVA, cm^2	AVA INDEX, cm^2/m^2
Mild	>1.5	>0.9
Moderate	1.1–1.5	>0.6–0.9
Severe	≤1.0	≤0.6

Figure 6-9. Grading criteria for AS. Many different criteria have been used to define severe AS; aortic valve areas (AVAs) have ranged from 0.5 or less to 1 cm^2 [16]. Another common criterion is the peak systolic gradient of 50 mm Hg or greater obtained by cardiac catheterization studies [17]. The systolic gradient is determined by the stroke volume and systolic ejection time, both of which are dependent on the loading conditions of the left ventricle (LV), resistance in the arterial system, and the contractile state of the LV. Moreover, the stenotic valve area is inversely related not to the mean systolic gradient but to the square root of the mean systolic gradient. Thus it seems best to define severe AS in terms of valve area.

Based on the natural history studies cited in the previous section, patients with an AVA greater than 1.5 cm^2 should be considered to have mild AS and patients with AVAs of 1.1 to 1.5 cm^2 should be considered to have moderate AS. Based on a natural history study [18] and a hemodynamic study [19], patients with an AVA index of 0.63 cm^2/m^2 or less or an AVA of 0.75 to 1.0 cm^2 (less than 0.4 to 0.6 cm^2/m^2) are considered to have severe AS [16].

The optimum AVA in any individual is determined significantly by body size and the need for a certain cardiac output; therefore, valve area is best corrected for body size. Many institutions simply list AVA not corrected for body size. In patients with an average body size, one can use the valve areas expressed in square centimeters (listed in this figure) as appropriate guidelines for grading the severity of AS. However, it is important to index the AVA to body size. In these circumstances, patients with AVA index greater than 0.9 cm^2/m^2 are considered to have mild AS, and patients with an AVA index of 0.4 to 0.6 cm^2/m^2 or less are considered to have severe AS.

Patients with AVA values that are at borderline between moderate and severe grades (*eg*, 0.9 to 1.1 cm^2; 0.55 to 0.65 cm^2) should be considered individually. Because errors may creep into the calculations of AVA in an individual patient, it may be important to consider the clinical condition of the patient as well as other relevant findings, such as the degree of hypertrophy, when determining whether a patient has severe AS. (*Adapted from* Rahimtoola [16].)

Clinical Manifestations

CLINICAL PRESENTATION

- Asymptomatic
- Symptomatic
  - Angina pectoris
  - Syncope, presyncope
  - Heart failure symptoms
  - Aborted sudden death
  - Others
    - Arrhythmias
    - Gastrointestinal bleeding
    - Result of systemic emboli

Figure 6-10. Clinical presentation. With the increasing performance of checkups in healthy people and the increasing use of Doppler ultrasound, many asymptomatic patients are being diagnosed with AS. The classic symptoms of AS are angina pectoris, syncope or presyncope, and symptoms related to clinical heart failure [1,2]. Typical angina pectoris occurs with or without associated coronary disease and results from an imbalance between myocardial oxygen demand and supply; rarely, it results from calcium emboli to the coronary arteries. The absence of angina in a patient with severe AS does not exclude associated significant obstructive coronary artery disease. Syncope is the result of reduced cerebral perfusion. Syncope occurring on effort is caused by either systemic vasodilatation in the presence of fixed or inadequate cardiac output, an arrhythmia, or both. The systemic vasodilatation in excess of the cardiac output may be related to inappropriate baroreceptor response. Syncope at rest is usually caused by transient ventricular tachyarrhythmia from which the patient recovers spontaneously. Other possible causes of syncope include transient atrial fibrillation or transient atrioventricular block during which the ventricle is deprived of the powerful atrial booster pump function and/or the ventricular rate is slow. Dyspnea on exertion, orthopnea, paroxysmal nocturnal dyspnea, and pulmonary edema result from various grades and duration of pulmonary venous (and left atrial) hypertension. These may be a result of left ventricular systolic dysfunction, diastolic dysfunction, or both. Systemic venous congestion with enlargement of the liver and peripheral edema results from increased systemic venous pressure and salt and water retention. Patients may present with aborted sudden death. Sudden cardiac death occurs in 5% or fewer of patients with AS. It occurs only in those with severe AS, most of whom have had some cardiac symptoms before the "sudden death" episode.

There is an increased incidence of gastrointestinal bleeding in patients with AS. This may be idiopathic or due to angiodysplasia, most commonly of the right colon, or other vascular malformations. Patients may suffer a systemic embolus; their presentation depends on the vascular bed that is obstructed by the embolus.

PHYSICAL EXAMINATION FOR AS

	SEVERITY OF AS		
	MILD	MODERATE	SEVERE
Arterial pulse	Normal	Slowly rising	Parvus et tardus
Jugular venous pulse	Normal	Normal	Usually normal
Carotid thrill	±	±	±
Cardiac impulse	Normal	Heaving	Heaving, sustained
Precordial thrill	±	±	Palpable *a* wave Usually ++
Auscultation			
S_4	-	±	++
ESC	+	±	-
Peak of ESM	Early systole	Mid systole	Late systole
S_2	Normal	Normal or single	Single or paradoxic

FIGURE 6-11. Physical examination. The findings on physical examination in patients with mild AS are an ejection systolic click (ESC) and ejection systolic murmur (ESM) that peak in early systole. The ESC may be absent if the valve is calcified or is rigid. These patients may have a carotid or precordial thrill.

Patients with severe AS display characteristic physical findings. The arterial pulse, which is best felt over the carotid or the suprasternal notch, shows a slowly rising pulse that takes longer to reach peak (parvus et tardus) (*see* Fig. 6-13C). The jugular venous pulse is normal and a carotid thrill may be present. The cardiac impulse is left ventricular (LV) in type; it is heaving and sustained. Often a powerful presystolic wave (*a* wave) is felt. A precordial systolic thrill is often present. On auscultation, there is an S_4 gallop, the ESC is absent, the ESM peaks in late systole, and the S_2 is single. S_2 is at times paradoxic, but this usually occurs in the presence of associated left bundle branch block or LV failure. In addition, there is usually a faint diastolic murmur of minimal aortic regurgitation. In the presence of congestive heart failure, the jugular venous pressure is often increased, the LV is dilated, there is an S_3, and the ESM may be very soft or absent. Frequently, a holosystolic murmur of mitral regurgitation is present. The findings on physical examination resemble those of heart failure from a variety of causes, *eg*, a cardiomyopathy, rather than AS. The physical findings in moderate AS are between those seen in mild and severe AS.

CASE STUDIES

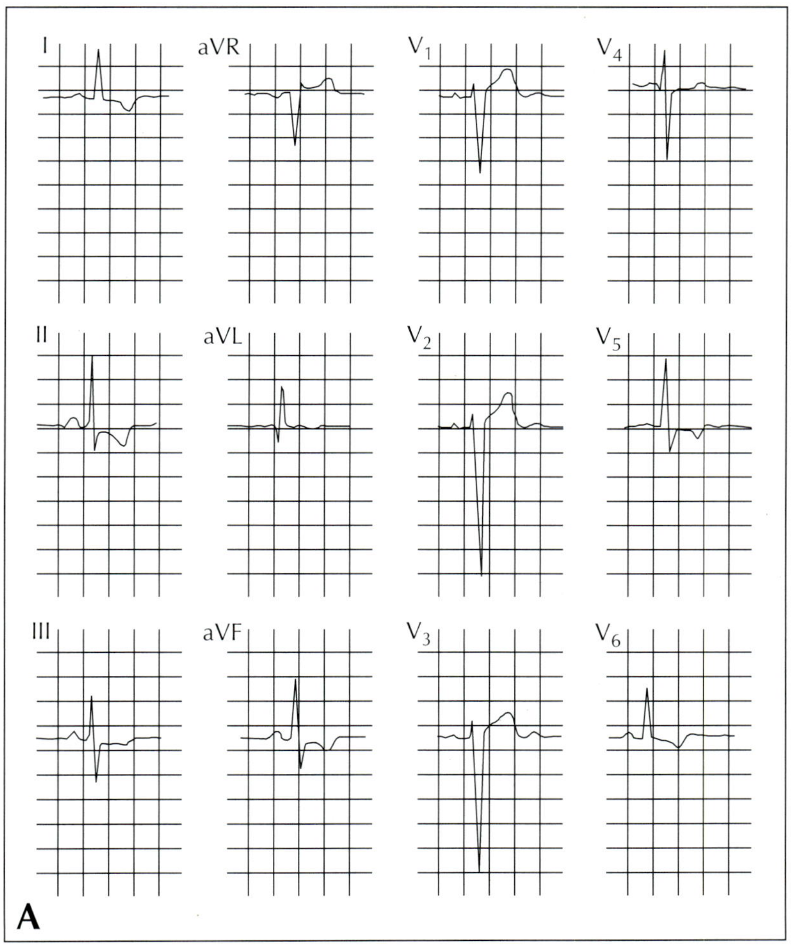

Figure 6-12. Electrocardiographic (ECG), chest radiographic, and Doppler ultrasound data diagnostic of AS. **A,** The ECG shows ST-segment depression and T-wave inversion in leads I, aVL, V_5 to V_6. A left atrial P-wave abnormality is present with P waves of 0.12 sec in lead II. The terminal segment of the P wave was negative in lead V_1. ECG standardization is mV=10 mm. The usual voltage criteria for left ventricular (LV) hypertrophy are not met in this case; this occurs in a small percentage of patients with severe AS. (*continued*)

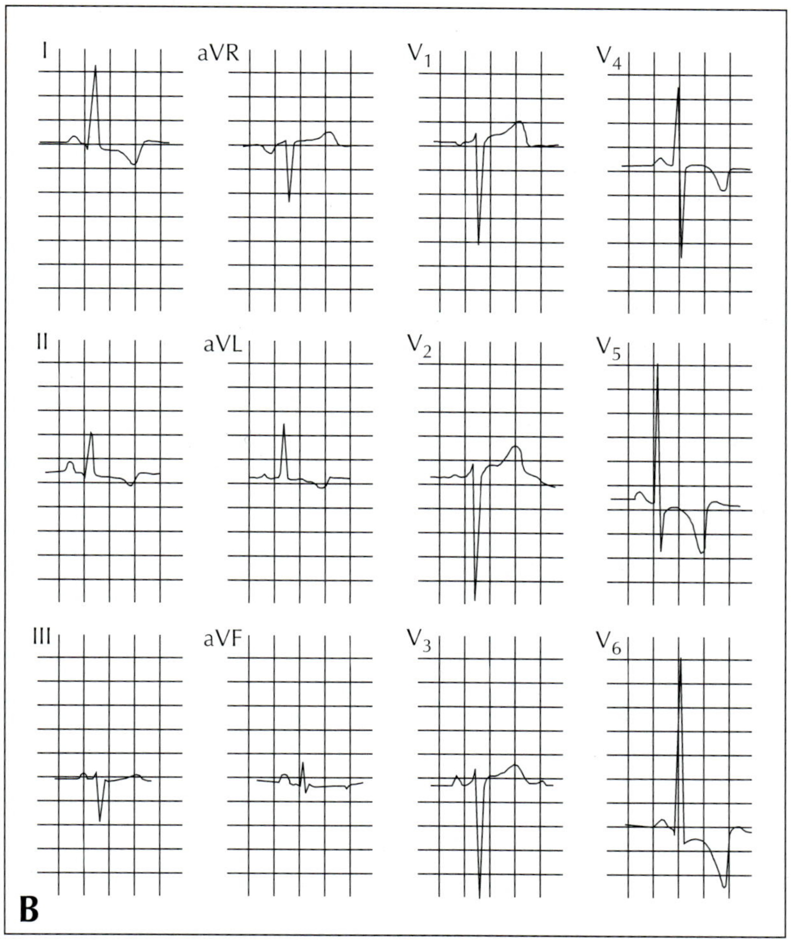

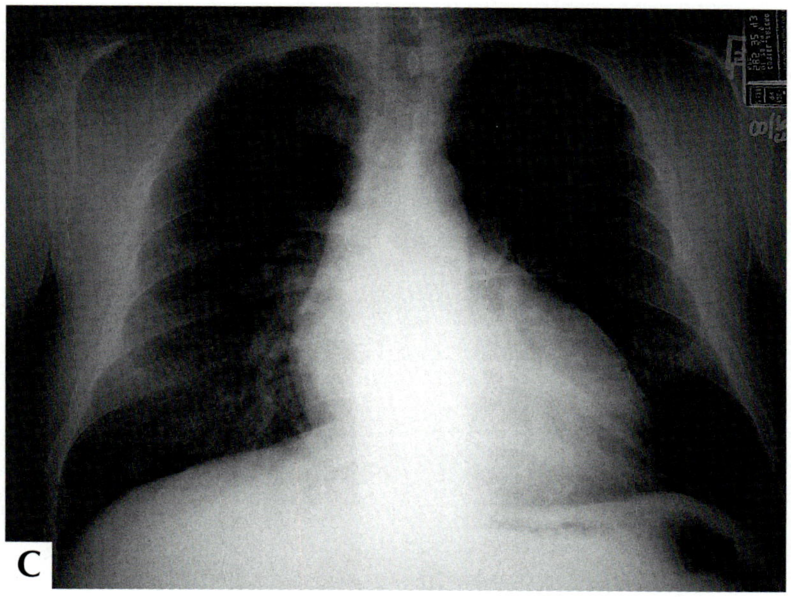

FIGURE 6-12. *(continued)* **B**, A more classic ECG example of AS is from a 63-year-old symptomatic patient with severe AS. The ECG shows marked voltage criteria for LV hypertrophy with ST-segment depression and T-wave inversion in leads I, aVL, V_5, and V_6. There is also T-wave inversion in leads II and V_4.

C, Chest radiography (posteroanterior view) shows an increased heart size (cardiothoracic ratio, 0.53) and normal pulmonary vasculature. The cardiac silhouette is typical for LV hypertrophy associated with severe AS. Calcification of the aortic valve would be best appreciated in the lateral view of the chest.

D, Two-dimensional and Doppler ultrasound data in a 36-year-old patient with symptoms of angina, presyncope, and shortness of breath, confirm normal LV size (dimension and volumes) and normal LV systolic function (ejection fraction and fractional shortening). The LV is hypertrophied (increased septal and posterior wall thickness). The aortic valve was calcified and there was a trace of aortic regurgitation. The peak and mean systolic aortic valve gradients were 103 and 46 mm Hg, respectively, and the calculated aortic valve area was 0.62 cm^2. There was no other valvular abnormality. The patient refused surgery.

This is a young patient with classic severe AS and a calcified valve. The valve lesion is likely a congenital one and the valve is likely to be bicuspid. There is considerable LV hypertrophy and the LV size and systolic pump function are normal (*see* the Pathophysiology section in this chapter). EPSS—E-point septal separation.

D. ECHOCARDIOGRAPHIC/DOPPLER DATA

LV	DATA
End-diastolic dimension, *mm*	50
End-systolic dimension, *mm*	35
Fractional shortening, *%*	30
EPSS, *mm*	7
Interventricular septal thickness, *mm*	12
Posterior wall thickness, *mm*	12
End-diastolic volume, *mL*	96
End-systolic volume, *mL*	42
Ejection fraction	0.56
AORTIC VALVE	
Aortic valve	Calcified
Aortic regurgitation	Trace
Peak systolic gradient, *mm Hg*	103
Mean systolic gradient, *mm Hg*	46
Aortic valve area, *cm^2*	0.62

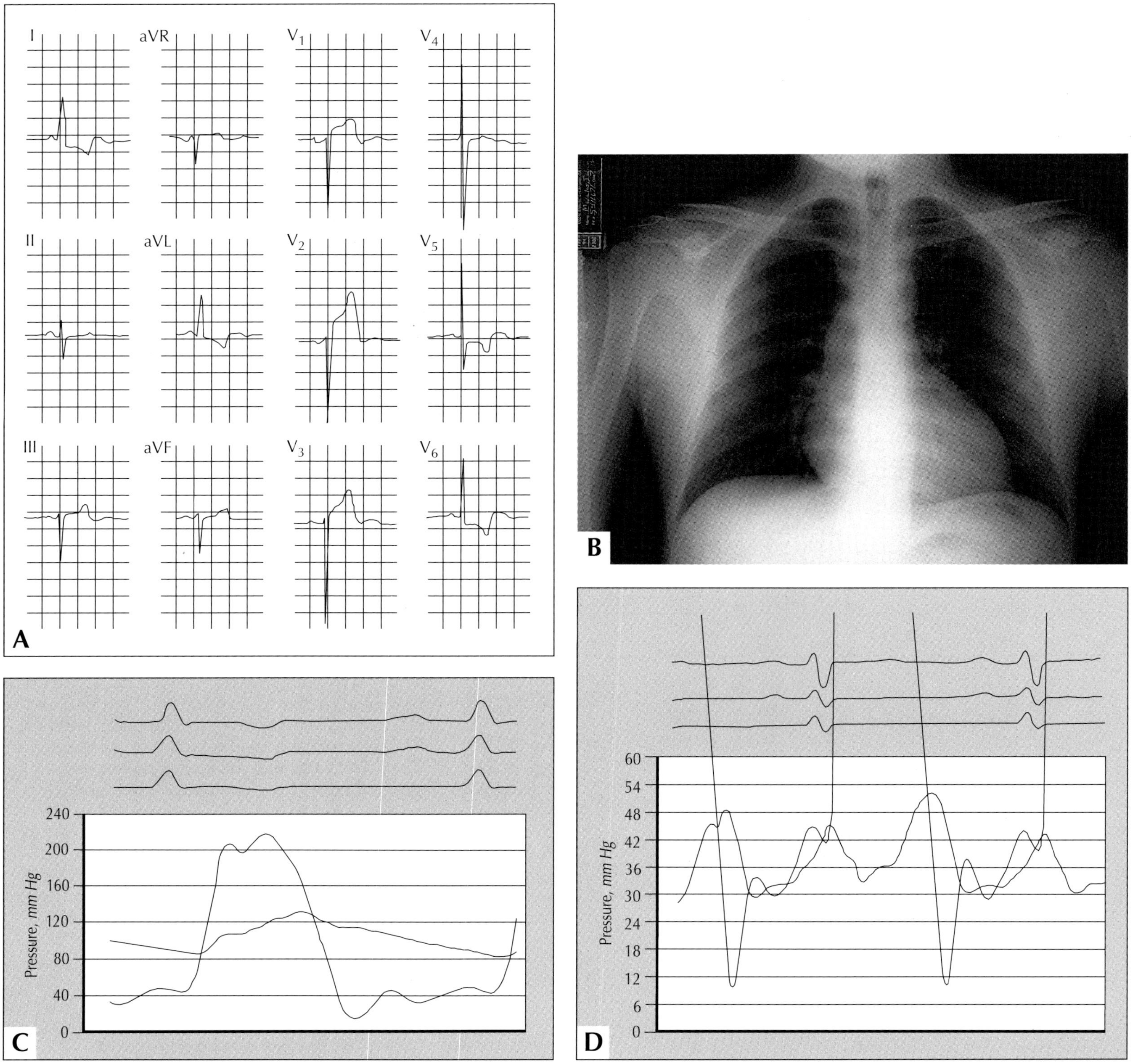

FIGURE 6-13. Electrocardiograph (ECG), chest radiographic, left ventricular (LV) and ascending aorta pressure pulses, LV diastolic pulmonary artery wedge (PAW) pressure pulses, and hemodynamic-LV function data. This 61-year-old man had recent onset of symptoms of mild shortness of breath on exertion.

A, The ECG shows voltage criteria for LV hypertrophy and ST depression with *T*-wave inversion in leads I, aVL, V_5, and V_6. The LV voltage criteria in this patient are less marked than in the patient demonstrated in Fig. 6-12. ECG standardization is 1 mV=10 mm.

B, Chest radiography (posteroanterior view) shows a considerably enlarged cardiac silhouette (cardiothoracic ratio, 0.58) and some increase in the pulmonary vasculature. The aortic knob is small.

C, The ascending aortic pressure tracing shows a characteristic parvus et tardus pulse and the anacrotic notch is low on the ascending limb of the pressure pulse. There is a large systolic pressure gradient between the LV and ascending aortic pressure tracing.

D, LV diastolic pressure shows an early dip with rapid rise of pressure (square root sign) and subsequent elevation of LV diastolic pressure by a large *a* wave due to powerful atrial contraction. The PAW pressure tracing shows huge *a* and *v* waves. *(continued)*

E. HEMODYNAMIC AND LV DATA IN 61-YEAR-OLD PATIENT

AREA ASSESSED	DATA
Pressures, *mm Hg*	
Right atrium	
a wave	12
v wave	10
Mean	8
RV (systolic/diastolic–end-diastolic)	66/6–10
Pulmonary artery	
Systolic	66
Diastolic	36
Mean	52
PAW	
a wave	46
v wave	50
Mean	38
LV (systolic/diastolic–end-diastolic)	224/8–40
Ascending aorta	
Systolic	128
Diastolic	84
Mean	104
Peak systolic gradient	96
Mean systolic gradient	58
Cardiac output (Fick), *L/min*	5.1 (2.6 L/min/m^2)
AVA, cm^2	0.4 (0.2 cm^2/m^2)
LV	
End-diastolic volume, *mL*	210 (105 mL/m^2)
End-systolic volume, *mL*	115 (57 mL/m^2)
Ejection fraction	0.45
Posterior wall thickness, *mm*	15
Aortic regurgitation	1+
Mitral regurgitation	1+
Coronary arteriography	Normal coronary arteries; left-dominant system

FIGURE 6-13. (*continued*) **E**, Hemodynamic and LV data show marked elevation of LV end-diastolic and PAW pressures. The pulmonary artery and right ventricular (RV) pressures are moderately increased. Both peak and mean systolic gradients are large, and the aortic valve area (AVA) is very small. The LV systolic pump function is mildly reduced (ejection fraction is 0.45). However, the LV is only mildly dilated (end-diastolic volume index 105 mL/m^2) and there is severe ventricular hypertrophy (wall thickness, 15 mm). There is a 1+ regurgitation at both the aortic and mitral valves. The aortic valve was calcified. Coronary arteriography showed normal arteries in a left-dominant system. The left main coronary artery is 5 mm in length.

This is an older patient with very severe AS and minimal symptoms. There is severe LV hypertrophy and some LV enlargement. The LV has exceeded the limit of preload reserve [10], and now there is LV systolic pump dysfunction.

However, the LV diastolic pressure pulse exhibits changes compatible with severe resistance to LV filling (probably due to the severe LV hypertrophy), and there are marked elevations of LV end-diastolic and PAW pressures and moderate elevations of pulmonary artery and RV pressures. These findings suggest strongly that there is significant LV diastolic dysfunction in addition to the mild LV systolic dysfunction (*see* the Pathophysiology section in this chapter).

There is a left-dominant coronary artery system, which is seen in 25% of patients with isolated AS as compared with a 9% incidence in control patients [20]. The left main coronary artery is short (5 mm). The left main coronary artery in AS is shorter in those with a left-dominant system (6.2±1.3 mm) than in those with right dominance (9.9±0.7 mm) [20]. This anatomic information is important if myocardial protection during open heart surgery involves cannulating the left coronary artery [20].

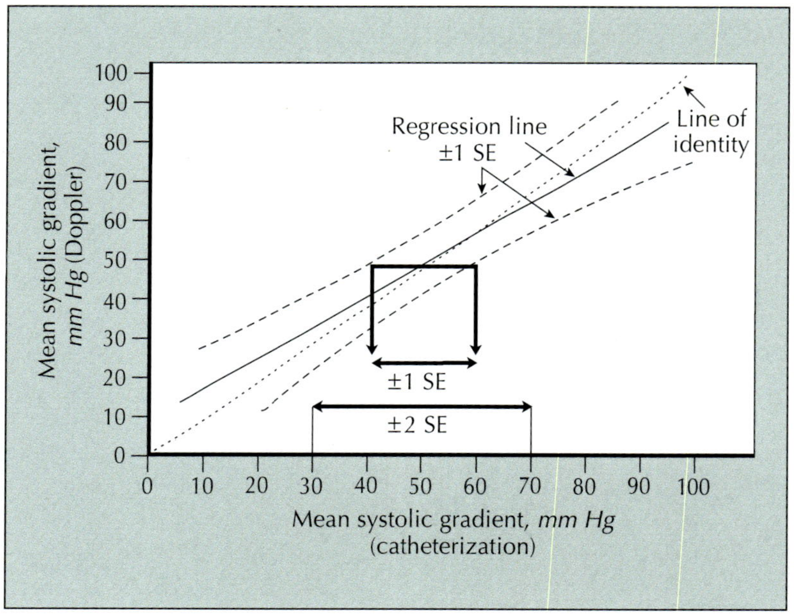

FIGURE 6-14. Relationship between aortic valve gradient and area. Doppler ultrasound is the single most useful noninvasive test available for AS. Estimates of aortic valve gradient from these tests are used frequently in evaluating the severity of AS; therefore, a perspective on the relationship of the valve gradients and valve areas obtained by echocardiography to those obtained by cardiac catheterization studies is appropriate.

A hypothetical relationship of Doppler-derived mean systolic valve gradient to that obtained by cardiac catheterization is depicted. The regression equation of this relationship and its standard error is shown. Even though the gradients by Doppler and cardiac catheterization are identical at 50 mm Hg, the 2 SE value is ± 20 mm Hg. Thus, when the Doppler gradient is 50 mm Hg, the 95% confidence limit predicts the gradient by cardiac catheterization is likely to be between 30 and 70 mm Hg. This figure does not necessarily state whether one or the other technique is more accurate but simply shows the relationship between the two. Thus it becomes important to consider the data that are available showing the 2 SE of the regression equation estimate. (*Adapted from* Rahimtoola [16].)

RELATIONSHIP BETWEEN DOPPLER AND CARDIAC CATHETERIZATION GRADIENT AND VALVE AREAS IN AS

		2 SE OF REGRESSION EQUATION ESTIMATE	
STUDY	PATIENTS, *n*	MEAN AORTIC VALVE GRADIENT, *mm Hg*	AORTIC VALVE AREA, *cm²*
Currie *et al.**	100	20	—
Skjaerpe *et al.*	30	18	—
	16–30	—	0.20 to 0.42
Krafchek *et al.*	39	18	—
Currie *et al.**	62	16	—
Smith *et al.*	40	12	—
Yeager *et al.*	58	22	—
Zoghbi *et al.*	39	—	0.22 to 0.30
Otto *et al.*	48	24	0.80
Teirstein *et al.*	30	16	0.34
Come *et al.*†	31	—	0.32
Oh *et al.**	100	20	0.38
Nishimura *et al.**	55	—	0.20 to 0.34
Come *et al.*†	30	—	0.36
Davidson *et al.*	20	22	—
Range		±12 to ±24	±0.20 to ±0.80

*Same medical center.
†Same medical center.

FIGURE 6-15. Doppler and catheterization studies. The studies cited [16] show that the 2 SE of the regression equation estimate for the mean aortic valve gradient ranges from ±12 to ±24 mm Hg. Two studies from the Mayo Clinic, one by Currie *et al.* [21] and one by Oh *et al.* [22], examined 100 consecutive patients in the cardiac catheterization laboratory in a blinded manner simultaneously with Doppler ultrasound and cardiac catheterization. The 2 SE of the regression equation in both studies was 20 mm Hg. Data are much less definitive with regard to the regression equation of the aortic valve area relationship. These range from ±0.20 to ±0.80 cm^2. An average may be taken to be about 0.3 to 0.4 cm^2. (*Adapted from* Rahmitoola [16].)

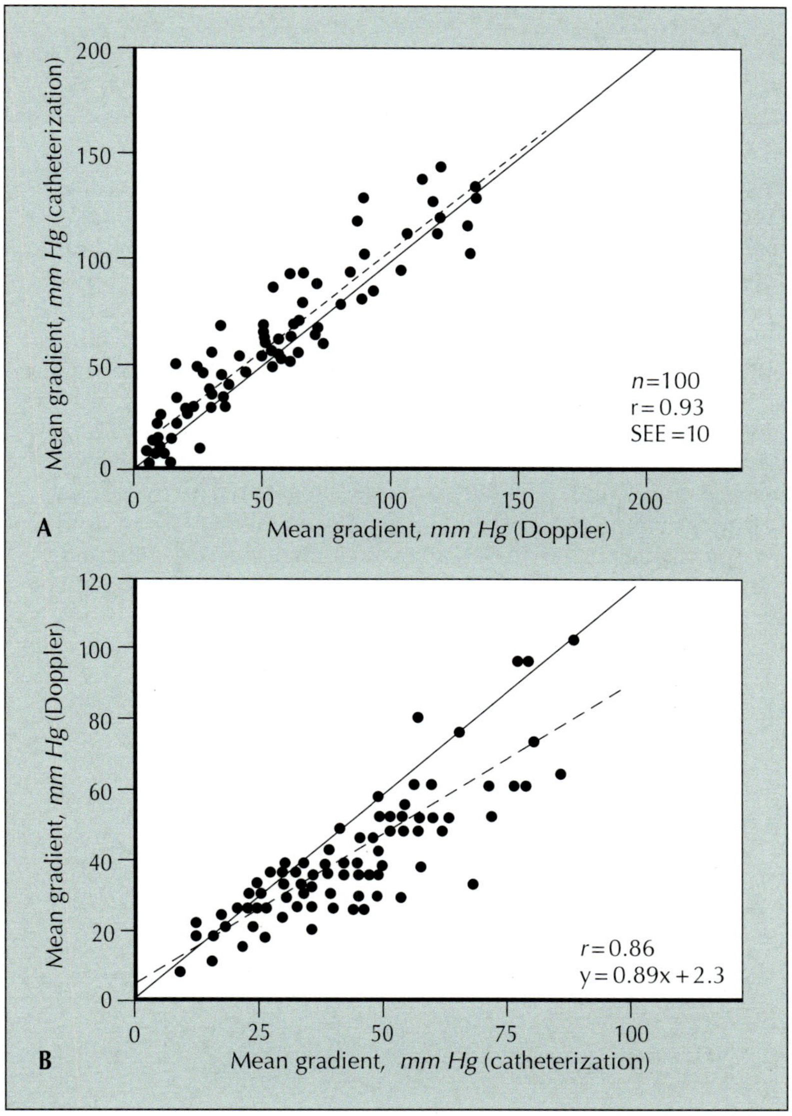

FIGURE 6-16. Relationship between mean systolic gradient by Doppler and cardiac catheterization in the studies of Currie *et al.* [21](*top panel*) and Oh *et al.* [22](*bottom panel*). The following can be observed: 1) The relationship varies in the same excellent medical center from one time to another and 2) even though the regression equation may at one time be almost identical to the line of identity, there is a considerable spread of actual values along that regression equation. SEE—standard error of the estimate.(*adapted from* Currie and coworkers [21]; and Oh and coworkers [22].)

SUGGESTED CONSERVATIVE GUIDELINES FOR RELATING DOPPLER GRADIENT TO SEVERITY OF AS IN ADULTS WITH NORMAL CARDIAC OUTPUT

PEAK GRADIENT, *mm Hg*	MEAN GRADIENT, *mm Hg*	SEVERE AS
≥80	≥70	Highly likely
60–79	50–69	Probable
<60	<50	Uncertain

FIGURE 6-17. Guidelines for assessing AS severity. Given the frequency with which the Doppler gradient is used to assess the severity of AS, one needs to consider guidelines for gradients [16]. Furthermore, because at times gradients and valve areas from cardiac catheterization findings are not or cannot be obtained, one must be very conservative with Doppler guidelines because they may result in very serious procedures (aortic valve replacement) being performed. Because the 2 SE of the regression equation relating mean Doppler gradient to cardiac catheterization is 20 mm Hg, one can assume in the presence of peak gradient of 80 mm Hg or greater, or a mean gradient of 70 mm Hg or more, that AS is highly likely to be severe, particularly in the presence of a normal cardiac output. When the peak gradient is 60 to 79 mm Hg and the mean gradient is 50 to 60 mm Hg, AS is most probably severe. On the other hand, when the peak gradient is less than 60 mm Hg or the mean gradient is less than 50 mm Hg, AS may be mild, moderate, or severe depending on the stroke volume and the systolic ejection time. (*Adapted from* Rahimtoola [16].)

STEPS IN CLINICAL DECISION MAKING IN PATIENTS WITH VALVULAR HEART DISEASE

1. Complete clinical evaluation
   - History
   - Physical examination
   - Electrocardiogram
   - Chest radiograph
2. Diagnose and assess severity of disease
   - All valves
   - Ventricular function
   - Hemodynamic effects
   - Coronary artery disease
   - Other cardiovascular disease
   - Effects of other body organs
   - Other organ diseases
3. List questions that need answering
4. Be reasonably certain these questions need to be answered
5. Perform test(s) most likely to provide these answers in one's own institution with the following criteria:
   - Reliably
   - Accurately
   - Lowest risk to patient
   - Reasonable (or lowest) cost
6. Review results of test(s)
7. Make an overall assessment of patient
8. Make recommendations regarding management

FIGURE 6-18. Steps in clinical decision making in patients with AS [16]. The first step is a complete clinical evaluation that includes history, physical examination, electrocardiography, and chest radiography. At the end of the clinical evaluation, the severity of disease of all cardiac valves, ventricular function, hemodynamic effects, coronary artery disease, other cardiovascular disease, and disease of other organs must be diagnosed and assessed. Before proceeding to additional testing, it is important to list the question(s) that must be answered. Test(s) are then performed that are most likely to provide these answers in *one's own institution* with the following criteria being kept in mind: reliability, accuracy, lowest risk to the patient, and reasonable (lowest) cost. Test results are then reviewed as they become available and an overall evaluation and assessment of the patient is made. Finally, recommendations regarding management are made. (*Adapted from* Rahimtoola [16].)

CLINICAL DECISION MAKING FOR AS

VARIABLE STUDIED	AFTER CLINICAL EVALUATION, %	AFTER DOPPLER ULTRASOUND EVALUATION, %
Diagnosis of AS		
Sensitivity	78	100
Specificity	92	92
Accuracy of diagnosis		
Including severity	48	65
Moderate or severe AS	100	100

FIGURE 6-19. Sensitivity and specificity of diagnosing AS. In a prospective blinded study of consecutive patients with valvular heart disease [23], the sensitivity and specificity of diagnosing of AS after clinical evaluation were 78% and 92%, respectively. After Doppler echocardiography, the sensitivity and specificity of diagnosing AS were 100% and 92% respectively. In addition to merely diagnosing AS, if the accuracy of assessing the severity of AS is included, then the accuracy of clinical evaluation fell to 48%, and that of Doppler echocardiography to 65%. On the other hand, if AS is merely diagnosed and determined to be moderate or severe, then both clinical evaluation and Doppler echocardiography were 100% accurate. Several conclusions can be drawn from this study: 1) Clinical evaluation is very sensitive, highly specific, and reasonably accurate in diagnosing AS and assessing its severity as moderate or severe; 2) Doppler ultrasound improves this only to a slight extent; 3) The reason clinical evaluation and Doppler echocardiography do not have a 100% specificity is the occasional inability to distinguish mild AS from turbulence across a normal or slightly diseased aortic valve; and 4) The other difficulty in diagnosis by clinical evaluation and by Doppler ultrasound is being able to separate accurately all patients with moderate AS from those with severe AS. (*Adapted from* Kotlewski [23].)

AVA BEFORE AND AFTER CBV

		AORTIC VALVE AREA, *cm²*	
STUDY	PATIENTS, *n*	PRE-CBV	POST-CBV
MSAV registry	492	0.5±0.18	0.82±0.30
NHLBI registry	636	0.5±0.2	0.8±0.3

Figure 6-20. Registry studies. Catheter balloon valvuloplasty (CBV) for severe AS in children and young adults gives generally good to excellent results when the stenosis is largely a result of commissural fusion. This is because in these patients CBV produces an increase in aortic valve area (AVA) by commissural splitting and stretching of the valve tissue. As a result, CBV is the procedure of first choice in selected children and in young adults with severe AS [24].

In the United States, this procedure in adults has been largely evaluated in older patients with calcified valves [25]. CBV in calcific AS, particularly in the older patient population, usually does not yield good results. This is because CBV increases AVA by fracture of the calcified leaflet and by displacement and stretching of rigid valve cusps [26]; commissural separation may also occur.

Two large registry studies in the United States, the Mansfield Scientific Aortic Valve (MSAV) registry [27] and the National Heart, Lung, and Blood Institute (NHLBI) registry [28] have demonstrated that on an average, AVA increases from 0.5 to 0.8 cm^2. About 70% of patients or more continue to have AVA of less than 1 cm^2. Most patients with an AVA larger than 1 cm^2 after CBV have a larger AVA before valvuloplasty. (*Adapted from* Holmes and coworkers [27] and Otto and coworkers [28].)

CBV FOR CALCIFIC SEVERE AS IN NHLBI REGISTRY

AREA ASSESSED	DATA
Patients, *n*	674
Age, *y*	78±9
LV ejection fraction: normal or mildly reduced, %	64
Mortality after CBV, %	
1 y	45
2 y	65
3 y	77
LV systolic function, % (3-y mortality)	
Normal	69
Severely reduced	91
Cardiac cause of death, %	70

Figure 6-21. Three-year results from the NHLBI registry [28]. The average age of these patients was 78±9 years. The left ventricular (LV) ejection fraction was normal or mildly reduced in two thirds of the patients. The actuarial mortality rates at 1, 2, and 3 years were 45%, 65%, and 77%, respectively. At the end of 3 years, the mortality rate in those with normal LV systolic function was 69% and in those in whom it was severely reduced the rate was 91%. The major cause of death after catheter balloon valvuloplasty (CBV) was cardiac related. (*Adapted from* Otto and coworkers [28].)

MAJOR REASONS FOR HIGH MORTALITY AFTER CBV FOR CALCIFIC SEVERE AS

Most patients (≥70%) have residual aortic valve stenosis (AVA ≤1.0 cm^2)

Myocardium supplied by obstructive CAD is usually not revascularized

Associated comorbid factors

Figure 6-22. Reasons for high mortality rate. The result of catheter balloon valvuloplasty (CBV) for calcific AS in the older patient population is very poor beyond the first few months. The first of three major reasons for the high mortality [24] in these patients is that most patients have residual severe AS, *ie*, they have an aortic valve area (AVA) of 1 cm^2 or less. Second, approximately 50% of such patients can be expected to have obstructive coronary artery disease (CAD) (*see* Fig. 6-36) and usually this is not relieved by percutaneous transluminal coronary angiography or coronary bypass surgery. Thus, many patients at the end of the procedure still have severe AS and associated obstructive CAD; they can be expected to have a high mortality that will be similar to that of a natural history of this condition. Finally, most patients have associated comorbid factors that would have a negative impact on late survival. (*Adapted from* Rahimtoola [24].)

SUGGESTED INDICATIONS FOR CATHETER BALLOON VALVULOPLASTY IN PATIENTS WITH CALCIFIC SEVERE AS*

Bridge procedure to eventual AVR
- Cardiogenic shock
- Moderate to severe heart failure
- Emergent/urgent need for noncardiac therapeutic procedures (*eg*, operation)

Patient with limited life span
- Noncardiac reasons (*eg*, carcinoma)
- Cardiac reason(s) other than AS

Others
- Patient at extremely high risk for AVR
- AVR not desirable for noncardiac reasons or cardiac causes other than aortic stenosis
- Patient refuses surgery

Therapeutic test in rare instances: Patients with small stroke volume and small valve gradient with valve stenosis suspected to be severe but severity is in doubt even after provocative diagnostic tests

*Caution should be exercised in recommending this procedure in asymptomatic patients.

FIGURE 6-23. Indications for catheter balloon valvuloplasty (CBV). In older patients with severe calcific AS, CBV is largely a palliative procedure [24]. The major indication is as a "bridge" procedure to subsequent early aortic valve replacement (AVR). It is of benefit in patients in cardiogenic shock, those in moderate to severe heart failure, and those who are in emergent or urgent need for a noncardiac therapeutic procedure, *eg*, an abdominal operation. The modest improvement in aortic valve area usually improves the hemodynamics and the clinical state of the patients in cardiogenic shock and heart failure so that they become better candidates for subsequent early AVR. However, it must be emphasized that CBV is considered to be a palliative procedure and AVR should not be unduly delayed. CBV also makes the patients better candidates for emergent noncardiac surgery. The second main group of indications is for patients with a limited life span, either due to noncardiac disease (*eg*, carcinoma with a short life expectancy) or cardiac disease other than AS. The third major group includes those whom the surgeon and cardiologist consider to be at "extremely" high risk for AVR or in whom AVR is considered not desirable because of noncardiac or cardiac reasons other than AS. Finally, it can be considered in the occasional patient who refuses cardiac surgery.

On rare occasions, CBV can be considered as a "therapeutic" test. A small group of patients with left ventricular dysfunction have a small stroke volume and a small gradient with valve stenosis suspected to be severe on clinical grounds. If the severity of AS is in doubt after provocative diagnostic tests, then CBV can be considered as a procedure that will determine whether improving the aortic valve area modestly results in a significant improvement of stroke volume and a major increase of valve gradient. If it does, then the patient should undergo AVR; if it does not, then the patient most likely has left ventricular dysfunction due to causes other than AS. (*Adapted from* Rahimtoola [24].)

RESULTS OF AORTIC VALVE REPLACEMENT

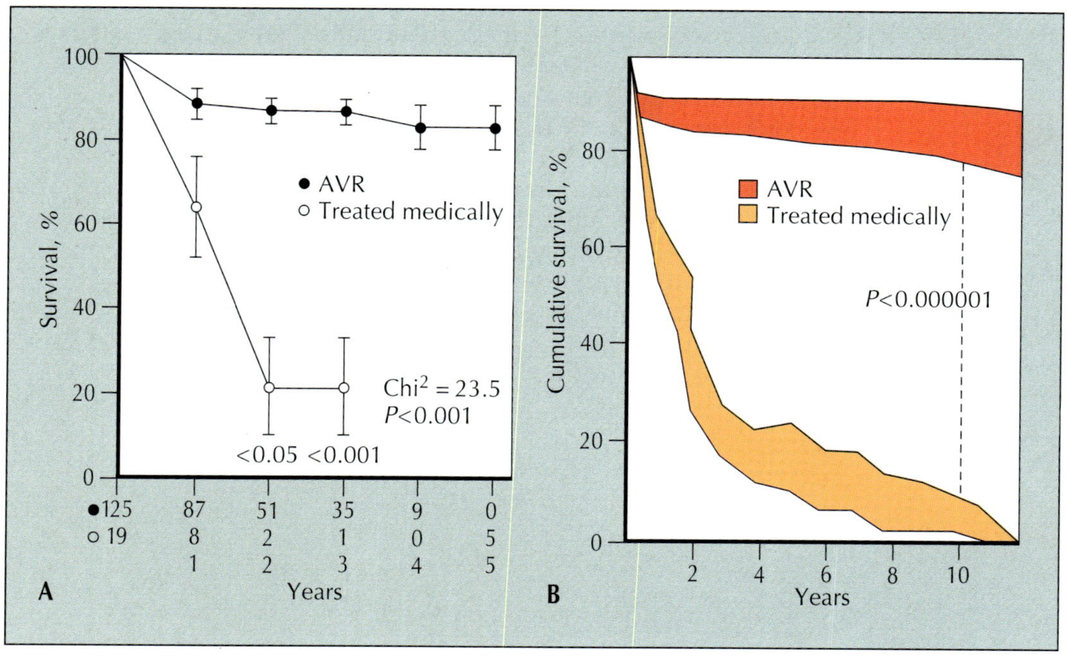

FIGURE 6-24. Comparative results of aortic valve replacement (AVR) and medical treatment. There are no prospective randomized trials of AVR in severe AS, and there are unlikely to be any in the near future. Two studies have compared the results of AVR with those of medical treatment during the same time period in symptomatic patients with normal left ventricular systolic pump function. **A** and **B,** In the two studies shown[13,29], patients who had AVR had a much better survival than those treated medically. These differences in survival between those treated medically and surgically are so large that there is a great deal of confidence that AVR significantly improves the survival of those with severe AS. (Part A *adapted from* Schwarz and coworkers [29]; part B *adapted from* Horstkotte and Loogen [13].)

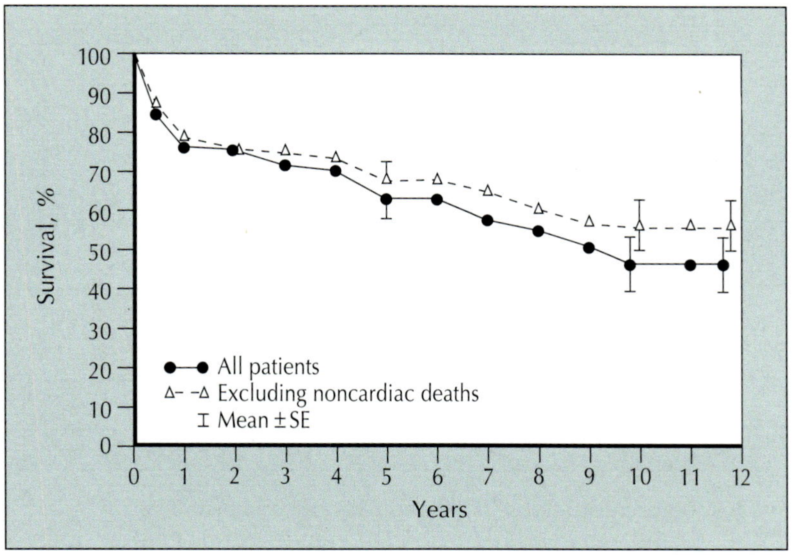

FIGURE 6-25. Survival in older patients. Among patients 60 years of age and older who had aortic valve replacement in the 1960s and 1970s, the 12-year survival rate was approximately 50%. Excluding noncardiac deaths it was 60% [30]. There is a high initial operative mortality because these patients had surgery a couple of decades ago. Nevertheless, 12-year survival is still encouraging. If one keeps in mind that the average age of these patients at the time of surgery was 68 years, at 12 years of follow-up, one is evaluating survival in patients whose average age is 80 years. These data are consistent with the hypothesis that valve replacement in patients aged 60 years of age and older appears to eliminate the expected long-term mortality of patients not undergoing valve replacement for severe AS. (*Adapted from* Murphy and coworkers [30].)

LONG-TERM SURVIVAL FOLLOWING AVR

Severe AS + LV dysfunction + clinical CHF	
Average follow-up, *y*	6
Median follow-up, *y*	5
Actuarial 7-y survival	
All patients, %	67±11
Operative survivors, %	84±10

FIGURE 6-26. Long-term survival. Patients with severe AS, left ventricular (LV) systolic dysfunction, and clinical heart failure have been followed in the study by Smith *et al.* [31] for an average of 6 years (median follow-up of 5 years) after aortic valve replacement (AVR). By actuarial analysis, the 7-year survival rate of all patients was 67% and that of AVR survivors 84% [32]. Most of these patients were operated on in the late 1960s and 1970s; the operative mortality at that time was higher than at the present time. Natural history data elucidated earlier indicate that most patients who are in clinical heart failure would be dead within a period of 1 to 2 years. The extremely encouraging long-term survival indicates that AVR almost certainly prolongs the life of patients with severe AS and LV systolic dysfunction who are in clinical heart failure. (*Adapted from* Rahimtoola and coworkers [32].)

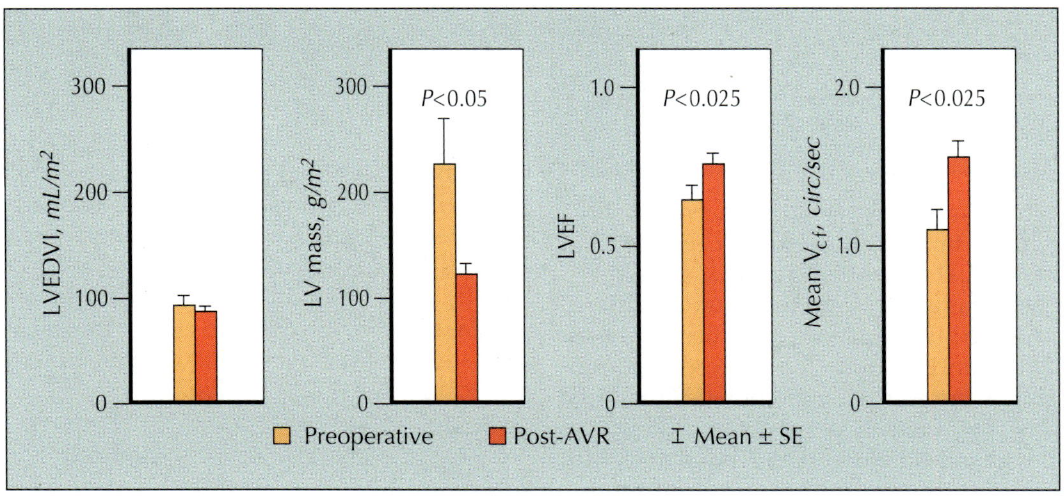

FIGURE 6-27. Effects of successful, uncomplicated aortic valve replacement (AVR) in severe AS. Data in patients with normal left ventricular (LV) systolic function who have undergone successful, uncomplicated AVR and were restudied approximately 18 months after surgery indicate that there is marked reduction in LV hypertrophy (mass) and an improvement in LV systolic pump function, as demonstrated by increases in LV ejection fraction (LVEF) and mean velocity of circumferential fiber shortening (mean V_{cf}) [7]. LVEF improves, even though it was within the normal range preoperatively and probably represents a response to a reduction of afterload, and hence, to a reduction of LV systolic stress. In such patients, there is a further reduction of LV mass at up to 10 years of follow-up [33]. circ—circumferences; LVEDVI—left ventricular end-diastolic volume index. (*Adapted from* Pantely and coworkers [7].)

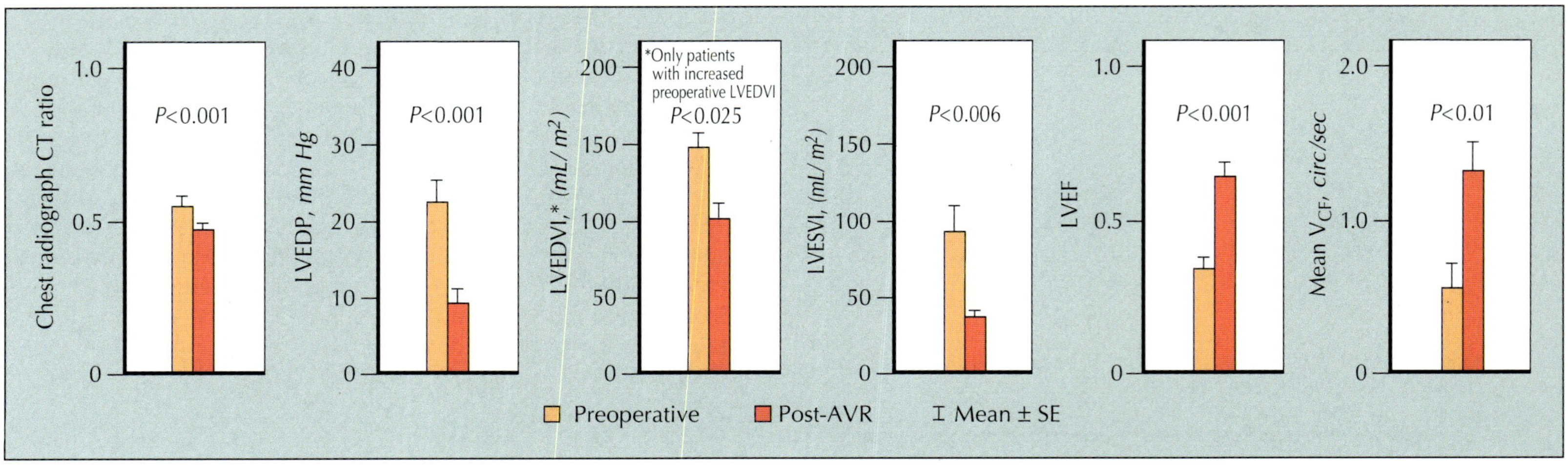

FIGURE 6-28. Results of aortic valve replacement (AVR) in patients with severe AS, left ventricular (LV) systolic dysfunction, and clinical heart failure. AVR has a marked beneficial effect [32]. There is a reduction in the cardiothoracic (CT) ratio on the chest radiograph and a large reduction in LV end-diastolic pressure (LVEDP). Patients in whom the LV end-diastolic volumes were increased preoperatively showed reductions in LV end-diastolic volume index (LVEDVI) and a marked reduction in LV end-systolic volume index (LVESVI). There is improvement in LV systolic pump function as demonstrated by increases in LV ejection fraction (LVEF) and mean velocity of circumferential fiber shortening (V_{cf}). circ—circumferences. (*Adapted from* Smith and coworkers [31].)

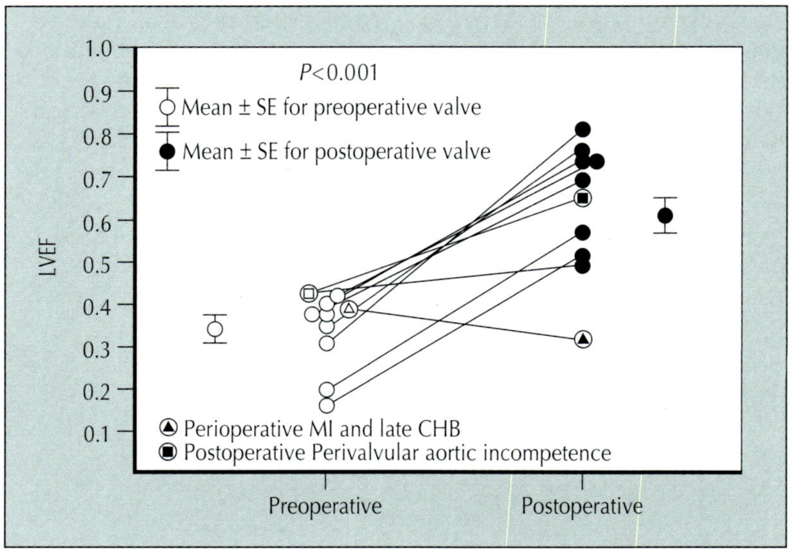

FIGURE 6-29. Ejection fraction after aortic valve replacement (AVR). Examination of changes in left ventricular (LV) ejection fraction (LVEF) in each individual patient who had LV systolic dysfunction and clinical heart failure showed that after AVR the LVEF improved from 0.34 to 0.63 [31]. All but one patient showed an improvement in LVEF. The only patient who showed a deterioration suffered a perioperative myocardial infarction (MI) and had complete heart block (CHB), and the only patient who showed only a small increase had had an MI before AVR. Note that LVEF normalized in two thirds of the patients, and in the two patients with the lowest LVEFs (0.18 and 0.19), LVEF normalized in both.

These data indicate that there is no lower limit of LVEF at which time these patients become inoperable. Data also indicate that the lower the LVEF, the more urgent the need for AVR. (*Adapted from* Smith and coworkers [31].)

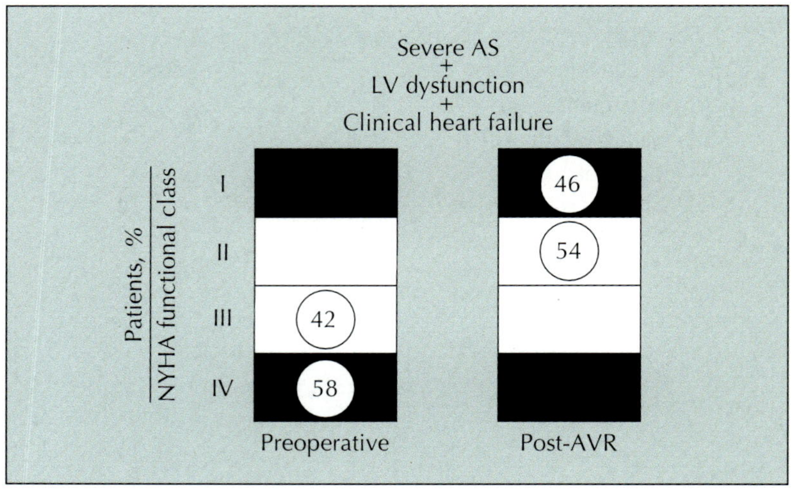

FIGURE 6-30. Changes in the New York Heart Association (NYHA) functional class in patients who had severe AS, left ventricular (LV) systolic dysfunction, and clinical heart failure [31]. Preoperatively, 42% and 58% of the patients were in functional classes III and IV, respectively. After aortic valve replacement (AVR), none of the survivors were in classes III and IV, 54% were in class II, and 46% were in class I, that is, they were totally asymptomatic. (*Adapted from* Smith and coworkers [31].)

OLDER PATIENTS

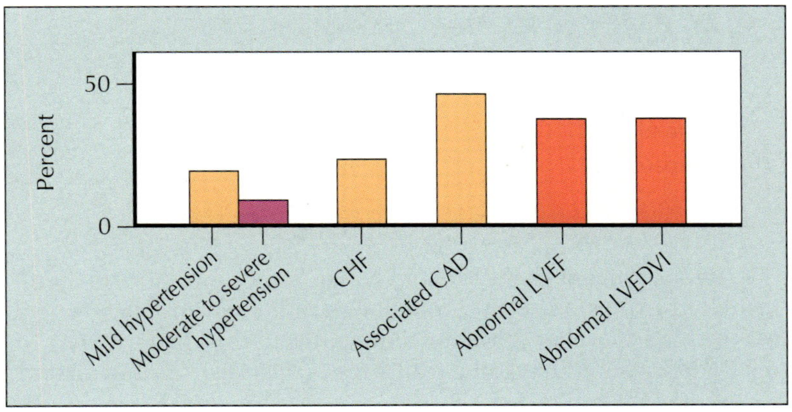

FIGURE 6-31. Clinical aspects in older patients. Patients 60 years of age or older with severe AS have a clinical presentation [30] that is somewhat different from that seen in younger patients. Twenty percent of older patients have associated mild systemic hypertension, and 10% have moderate to severe systemic hypertension. Approximately 20% to 25% of these patients present in clinical heart failure (CHF). Forty-five percent have associated significant obstructive coronary artery disease (CAD). About one third of patients have a reduced left ventricular (LV) ejection fraction (LVEF) at rest and an abnormally increased LV end-diastolic volume index (LVEDVI). The vast majority of patients with severe AS 60 years of age and older will not be in CHF and will have normal LV systolic pump function; only one half will have significant obstructive CAD.

The following are physical findings in the older patients with critical AS that are frequently different from those seen in the younger patients: 1) Because many of them have changes in their arterial walls that make the arteries less elastic and more rigid, the peripheral pulse often does not exhibit the parvus et tardus character that is present in the younger patient population; and in fact the pulse may be normal or may rise fairly rapidly; 2) systolic thrills in the carotid artery and the precordium are present less frequently; 3) the incidence of an S_4 is also lower; 4) the systolic ejection click is almost never present; 5) the murmur is often atypical inasmuch as it is a "cooing" type of murmur that is frequently heard best, and at times only heard, at the cardiac apex; 6) usually, they do not have marked electrocardiographic changes of LV hypertrophy. (*Adapted from* Murphy and coworkers [30].)

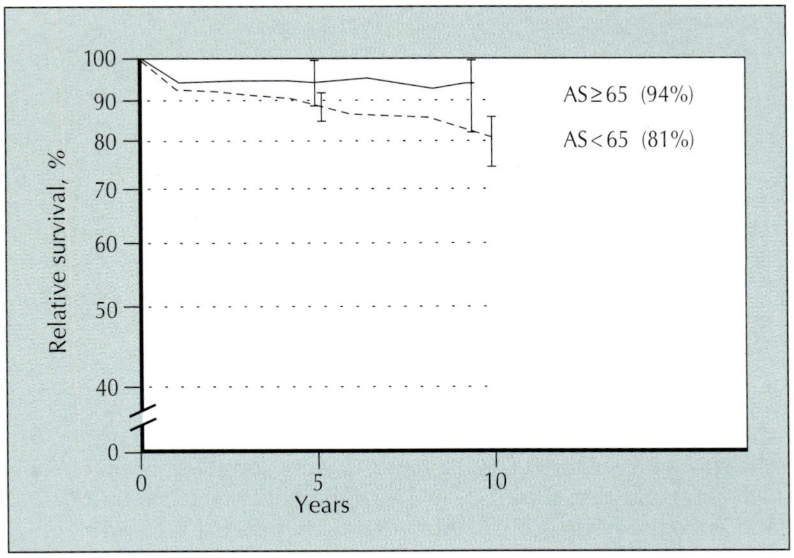

FIGURE 6-32. Long-term survival. Data from the Karolinska Institute in Sweden [34] have provided an interesting perspective on the long-term survival after aortic valve replacement (AVR) in patients aged 65 years or older. Investigators have examined the relative survival, *ie*, they compared the survival of the patient who had undergone AVR with another age- and gender–matched person in the same population. Patients under the age of 65 had a relative survival of 81%, which is significantly lower than 100%. Patients who underwent AVR at 65 years or older had a relative survival of 94% at the end of 10 years; this was not significantly different from 100%. These data indicate that survival after AVR for AS in patients aged 65 and over is identical to an age- and gender-matched individual in the population who does not have AS and that the late relative survival of patients 65 years of age or older is much better than that of patients under the age of 65. (*Adapted from* Lindblom and coworkers [34].)

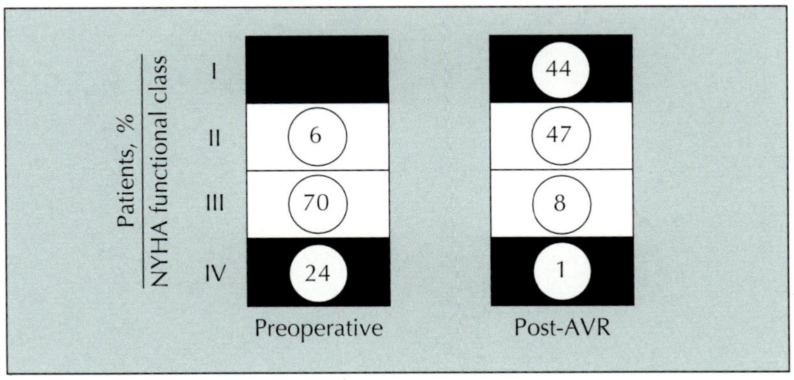

FIGURE 6-33. Pre- and postoperative New York Heart Association (NYHA) functional class in patients 60 years of age and older [30]. Before surgery, 94% of the patients were in functional classes III and IV. Postoperatively only 1% of the survivors were in class IV and 8% were in class III. Ninety-one percent of the patients were in either classes I or II.

Patients aged 60 to 65 years with severe AS have more marked abnormalities of left ventricular function on exercise [35]. Their AS progresses at a much faster rate than in the younger patient population. After aortic valve replacement (AVR), they have an excellent long-term survival that is not different from an age- and gender-matched general population without AS. They also get an excellent long-term functional result, with 91% of the patients being either in class I or II. These data indicate that one should be aggressive about performing AVR in this age group. (*Adapted from* Murphy and coworkers [30].)

SEVERE AS IN PATIENTS ≥60 Y: GENDER DISTRIBUTION AND CHAMBER PROPERTIES			
	LV SYSTOLIC FUNCTION		
	SUBNORMAL, %	NORMAL, %	SUPERNORMAL, %
Gender			
Men (n=29)	64	22	14
Women (n=34)	18	41	41
LV chamber size	Increased	Normal	Normal to decreased
Chamber geometry (R/Th ratio)	Increased	Normal to decreased	Decreased
Afterload (end-systolic stress)	Increased	Normal	Decreased
Diastolic pressures	Markedly increased	Increased	Increased

FIGURE 6-34. Differences based on gender. It appears that women 60 years of age and older with severe AS have significantly different left ventricular (LV) chamber characteristics compared with men [36]. Overall, despite a similar degree of AS and symptomatic status, women had better LV systolic pump function, achieved a smaller end-systolic chamber size, and generated more LV pressure.

Forty-one percent of the women had a "supernormal" function (increased LV systolic pump function parameters) and had a small, thick-walled chamber (end-diastolic radius to thickness [R/Th] ratio) and lower end-systolic wall stress. (*Adapted from* Carroll and coworkers [36].)

ASSOCIATED OBSTRUCTIVE CORONARY ARTERY DISEASE

ISOLATED AVR: INCIDENCE OF ASSOCIATED CAD			
	VA COOPERATIVE STUDY [38]	MAYO CLINIC [39]	MGH [40]
Patients, n	643	618	64
Patients with CD, n (%)	312 (49)	321 (52)	37 (58)
1VD, %	17	22	27
2VD, %	17	14	19
3VD, %	15	17	13
Additional LMCAD, %	—	5	3

FIGURE 6-35. Incidence of associated coronary artery disease (CAD) with aortic valve replacement (AVR). Two large studies, the Veterans Administration (VA) cooperative study [37] and the Mayo Clinic study [38], showed that the incidence of associated CAD was approximately 50%. About one third of the patients with obstructive CAD had single-vessel disease (1VD), another third had two-vessel disease (2VD), and another third had three-vessel disease (3VD). Data from the Massachusetts General Hospital (MGH) [39] indicate that in patients 80 to 89 years of age the incidence of associated CAD was 58%. Additional left main CAD (LMCAD) was present in 3% to 5% of the patients. (*Adapted from* Sethi and coworkers [37], Mullany and coworkers [38], and Levinson and coworkers [39].)

EFFECT OF CABG AND AVR ON OPERATIVE MORTALITY AND LATE SURVIVAL

	1982–1983	1967–1976					
PROCEDURE	OPERATIVE MORTALITY, %	OPERATIVE MORTALITY, %	ALL PATIENTS, %*	1VD†	2VD†	3VD†	LMCAD†
AVR + No CAD	1.4	4.5	63	—	—	—	—
AVR + CAD + CABG	4.0	6.3	49	38	28	34	11
AVR + CAD + No CABG	9.4	10.3	36	65	22	13	1

*10-y survival.
† Incidence of associated CAD.

FIGURE 6-36. Effect of coronary bypass grafting (CABG) on survival. Data from Mullany *et al.* [38] indicate that the operative mortality in patients without coronary artery disease (CAD) undergoing aortic valve replacement (AVR) was 1.4%; this was increased to 4% if the patients had CAD and underwent CABG. If they had associated CAD and no CABG performed at the time of AVR, operative mortality increased markedly to 9.4%. Examination of the 10-year survival in patients who had undergone AVR from 1967 to 1976 indicates that the best survival was in patients who had no associated CAD. However, those who had associated CAD and underwent CABG had a better 10-year survival than those who did not undergo CABG for CAD. It should be noted that patients who underwent CABG in addition to AVR had a 45% incidence of either three-vessel (3VD) CAD, or left main CAD (LMCAD); whereas in patients who did not undergo CABG, 65% had one-vessel disease (1VD). Thus if the patients who had undergone CABG had in fact not undergone CABG, then their 10-year survival would have been expected to be much lower than in those who did not undergo CABG in this study. In view of this, it becomes imperative that the patients who have significant obstructive CAD undergo CABG at the same time as AVR. Therefore, an issue that has to be considered is who should undergo coronary arteriography prior to AVR. 2VD—two-vessel disease. (*Adapted from* Mullany and coworkers [38].)

INDICATIONS FOR CORONARY ARTERIOGRAPHY

- Patients ≥35 y
- Patients <35 y
  - LV dysfunction
  - Symptoms or signs suggesting CAD
  - One or more risk factors for premature CAD (excluding gender)

FIGURE 6-37. Suggested indications for coronary arteriography before valve surgery [16]. All patients 35 years of age and older should undergo coronary arteriography before aortic valve surgery. In patients under the age of 35 years, coronary arteriography should be performed if they have left ventricular (LV) dysfunction, have signs or symptoms that suggest the presence of associated coronary artery disease (CAD), or if they have one or more risk factors for premature CAD (excluding gender). (*Adapted from* Rahimtoola [16] with permission.)

MEDICAL TREATMENT OF AS

- Antibiotic prophylaxis
  - Infective endocarditis
  - Recurrent rheumatic carditis
- Restrict activities
  - Severe exercise
  - Competitive sports
- Arrhythmias
  - Prevent and/or control
  - Restore sinus rhythm, if possible
- Cardiac medications (use only if essential)
  - Avoid negative inotropic and pro-arrhythmic agents if possible
  - Diuretics—use cautiously
  - Arteriolar and venodilators—use cautiously
- Follow-up
  - Mild AS: Every 2–5 y
  - Moderate AS: Every 6–12 mo
  - Develop symptoms: Immediate

FIGURE 6-38. Medical treatment of AS. All patients need antibiotic prophylaxis for prevention of infective endocarditis; those with rheumatic valve disease should also receive it for prevention of recurrences of rheumatic carditis. Patients with severe AS should undergo valve surgery (*see* Fig. 6-39). Others should have their activities restricted, *ie*, they should not undertake severe or vigorous exercise and competitive sports. Arrhythmias should be prevented if possible, particularly ventricular tachyarrhythmias and atrial arrhythmias, because of loss of atrial contraction that can produce a fall of cardiac output. Restoration of sinus rhythm should be a priority. In general, cardiac medications should only be used if there are specific indications for their use. Negative inotropic and proarrhythmic agents, by depressing left ventricular (LV) function and reducing cardiac output and arterial pressure, may be deleterious. Diuretics and vasodilators, if they lower cardiac output and arterial pressure, may be deleterious. Follow-up should include clinical evaluation (history, physical examination, electrocardiography, chest radiography) and Doppler echocardiography with quantitative assessment of LV size and function. Patients with mild AS should have follow-up every 2 to 5 years depending on the calculated aortic valve area. Patients with moderate AS should have follow-up every 6 to 12 months depending on the calculated aortic valve area. Patients who develop symptoms related to AS should have an "immediate" follow-up visit. (© Copyright SH Rahimtoola, MB, FRCP, MACP.)

INDICATIONS FOR SURGERY FOR SEVERE AS
All symptomatic patients
LV function normal: As soon as possible
LV dysfunction: Urgent
Heart failure: Emergent
Asymptomatic patients
All patients
Alternative strategy
All patients with AVA ≤0.75 cm^2
Patients with AVA 0.76–1.0 cm^2
LV dysfunction
Associated significantly obstructive CAD
Patients ≥60–65 y
Severe LV hypertrophy
Painless ischemia
Significant arrhythmias
LV dysfunction on exercise

FIGURE 6-39. Indications for surgery for severe AS. Symptomatic patients with severe AS should have aortic valve surgery (usually valve replacement) unless there is a specific contraindication to its performance. The urgency of surgery depends on the state of left ventricular (LV) function and the severity of the symptoms. For example, if there is LV dysfunction, the procedure is urgent; in the presence of heart failure or cardiogenic shock, it is usually an emergency.

Probably all asymptomatic patients with severe AS should have valve surgery. An alternative strategy is to perform surgery on all patients with aortic valve areas (AVAs) of 0.75 cm^2 or less. In patients with small or large body size an equivalent value after correcting for body size may need to be determined (*see* Fig. 6-9). For patients with valve areas of 0.76 to 1.0 cm^2 surgery is performed in those at "higher risk." These include patients with LV dysfunction, associated significantly obstructive coronary artery disease (CAD), age 60 to 65 years or older, severe LV hypertrophy, painless ischemia, significant arrhythmias, and significant LV dysfunction on exercise. (© Copyright SH Rahimtoola, MB, FRCP, MACP.)

REFERENCES

1. Braunwald E: Valvular heart disease. In *Heart Disease*, edn 5. Edited by Braunwald E. Philadelphia: WB Saunders; 1997:1007–1077.
2. Rahimtoola SH: Valvular heart disease. In *Internal Medicine*, 4th ed. Edited by Stein J (Cardiology Section edited by O'Rourke RA). St. Louis: Mosby-Year Book; 1994:202–234.
3. Olsson N, dalsgaaro C-J, Haegerstrand A, *et al.*: Accumulation of T lymphocytes and expression of interleukin-2 receptors in nonrheumatic stenotic aortic valves. *J Am Coll Cardiol* 1994, 23:1162–1170.
4. Selzer A: Changing aspects of the natural history of valvular aortic stenosis. *N Engl J Med* 1987, 31:91–98.
5. Passik CS, Ackerman DM, Pluth JR, Edwards WD: Temporal changes in the causes of aortic stenosis: a surgical pathological study of 646 cases. *Mayo Clin Proc* 1987, 62:119–123.
6. Roberts WC: The structural basis of abnormal cardiac function: a look at coronary, hypertensive, valvular, idiopathic myocardial, and pericardial heart disease. In *Cardiovascular Physiology*. Edited by Levine JJ. New York: Grune & Stratton; 1976.
7. Plantely G, Morton MJ, Rahimtoola SH: Effects of successful, uncomplicated valve replacement on ventricular hypertrophy, volume, and performance in aortic stenosis and aortic incompetence. *J Thorac Cardiovasc Surg* 1978, 75:383–391.
8. Braunwald E, Frahm CJ: Studies on the Starling's law of the heart. IV. Observations on the hemodynamic functions of the left atrium in man. *Circulation* 1961, 24:633–642.
9. Stott DK, Marpole DGF, Bristow JD, *et al.*: The role of left atrial transport in aortic and mitral stenosis. *Circulation* 1970, 41:1031–1041.
10. Ross J Jr: Afterload mismatch and preload reserve: a conceptual framework for the analysis of ventricular function. *Prog Cardiovasc Dis* 1976, 18:255–264.
11. Johnson LL, Sciacca RR, Ellis K, *et al.*: Reduced left ventricular myocardial blood flow per unit mass in aortic stenosis. *Circulation* 1978, 57:582–590.
12. Marcus ML, Doty DB, Horatzka LF, *et al.*: Decreased coronary reserve: a mechanism for angina pectoris in patients with aortic stenosis and normal coronary arteries. *N Engl J Med* 1982, 307:1362–1366.
13. Horstkotte D, Loogen F: The natural history of aortic valve stenosis. *Eur Heart J* 1988, 9(suppl E):57–64.
14. Turina J, Hess O, Sepulcri F, Krayenbuehl HP: Spontaneous course of aortic valve disease. *Eur Heart J* 1987, 8:471–483.
15. Ross J Jr, Braunwald E: Aortic stenosis. *Circulation* 1968, 36 (suppl IV):61–67.
16. Rahimtoola SH: Perspective on valvular heart disease: update II. In *Era in Cardiovascular Medicine*. Edited by Knoebel S. New York: Elsevier; 1991:45–70.
17. Braunwald E, Morrow AG: Obstruction to left ventricular outflow: current criteria for the selection of patients for operation. *Am J Cardiol* 1963, 12:53–59.
18. Frank S, Johnson A, Ross J Jr: Natural history of valvular aortic stenosis. *Br Heart J* 1973, 35:41–46.
19. Tobin JR Jr, Rahimtoola SH, Blundell PE, Swan HJC: Percentage of left ventricular stroke workloss: a simple hemodynamic concept for estimation of severity in valvular aortic stenosis. *Circulation* 1967, 35:868–879.
20. Murphy ES, Röosch J, Rahimtoola SH: Frequency and significance of coronary arterial dominance in isolated aortic stenosis. *Am J Cardiol* 1977, 39:505–509.
21. Currie PJ, Seward JB, Reeder GS, *et al.*: Continuous-wave Doppler echocardiographic assessment of severity of calcific aortic stenosis: a simultaneous Doppler-catheter correlative study in 100 adult patients. *Circulation* 1985, 71:1162–1169.
22. Oh JK, Taliercio CP, Holmes DR Jr, *et al.*: Prediction of the severity of aortic stenosis by Doppler aortic valve area determination: prospective Doppler-catheterization correlation in 100 patients. *J Am Coll Cardiol* 1988, 11:1227–1234.

23. Kotlewski A, Kawanishi DT, McKay CR, *et al.*: The relative value of clinical examination, echocardiography with Doppler and cardiac catheterization with angiography in the evaluation of aortic valve disease. In *Surgery for Heart Valve Disease*. Edited by Bodnar E. London: ICR Publishers; 1990:66–72.
24. Rahimtoola SH: Catheter balloon valvuloplasty for severe calcific aortic stenosis: a limited role. *J Am Coll Cardiol* 1994, 23:1076–1078.
25. Kulick DL, Kawanishi DT, Reid CL, Rahimtoola SH: Catheter balloon valvuloplasty in adults. Part I. Aortic stenosis. *Curr Probl Cardiol* 1990, 15:359–395.
26. McKay RG, Safian RD, Lock JE, *et al.*: Balloon dilation of calcific aortic stenosis in elderly patients: post mortem, intraoperative, and percutaneous valvuloplasty studies. *Circulation* 1986, 74:119–125.
27. Holmes DR Jr, Nishimura RA, Reeder GS: In-hospital mortality after balloon valvuloplasty: frequency and associated factors. *J Am Coll Cardiol* 1991, 17:189–192.
28. Otto CM, Mickel MC, Kennedy JW, *et al.*: Three-year outcome after balloon aortic valvuloplasty: insights into prognosis of valvular aortic stenosis. *Circulation* 1994, 89:642–650.
29. Schwarz F, Banmann P, Manthey J, *et al.*: The effect of aortic valve replacement on survival. *Circulation* 1982, 66:1105–1110.
30. Murphy ES, Lawson RM, Starr A, Rahimtoola SH: Severe aortic stenosis in the elderly: state of left ventricular function and result of valve replacement on ten-year survival. *Circulation* 1981, 64(suppl II):184–188.
31. Smith N, McAnulty JH, Rahimtoola SH: Severe aortic stenosis with impaired left ventricular function and clinical heart failure: results of valve replacement. *Circulation* 1978, 58:255–264.
32. Rahimtoola SH, Starr A: Valvular surgery. In *Congestive Heart Failure: Current Research and Clinical Applications*. Edited by Braunwald E, Mock M, Watson J. New York: Grune & Stratton; 1982:303–316.
33. Monrad ES, Hess OM, Murakami T, *et al.*: Time course of regression of left ventricular hypertrophy after aortic valve replacement. *Circulation* 1988, 77:1345–1355.
34. Lindblom D, Lindblom U, Qvist J, Lundström H: Long-term relative survival rates after heart valve replacement. *J Am Coll Cardiol* 1990, 15:566–573.
35. Bache RJ, Wang Y, Jorgensen CR: Hemodynamic effects of exercise in isolated valvular aortic stenosis. *Circulation* 1971, 44:1003–1013.
36. Carroll JD, Carroll EP, Feldman T, *et al.*: Sex-associated differences in left ventricular function in aortic stenosis of the elderly. *Circulation* 1992, 86:1099–1107.
37. Sethi GK, Miller DC, Sonchek J, *et al.*: Clinical, hemodynamic and angiographic predictors of operative mortality in patients undergoing single valve replacement. *J Thorac Cardiovasc Surg* 1987, 93:884–887.
38. Mullany CJ, Elveback ER, Frye RL, *et al.*: Coronary artery disease and its management: influence on survival in patients undergoing aortic valve replacement. *J Am Coll Cardiol* 1987, 10:66–72.
39. Levinson JR, Akins CW, Buckley MJ, *et al.*: Octogenarians with aortic stenosis: outcome after aortic valve replacement. *Circulation* 1989, 80 (suppl I):49–56.

Aortic Valve Regurgitation

7

CHAPTER

Shahbudin H. Rahimtoola

Aortic regurgitation (AR) may be acute or chronic. The most common causes of acute AR are infective endocarditis and prosthetic valve dysfunction. Mild acute AR needs no specific therapy except for the underlying disorder that caused the AR. Severe acute AR is usually a medical emergency; it can be diagnosed by clinical evaluation (history, physical examination, electrocardiography, and chest radiography). Doppler ultrasound (transthoracic and, in particular, transesophageal), is the single most useful test to diagnose acute AR, assess its severity and its effects on the left ventricle, and diagnose its etiology. Bedside hemodynamic monitoring is recommended in most, if not all, patients with moderate or severe acute AR. In such patients, vasodilators, especially intravenous nitroprusside, are an important addition to the therapeutic armamentarium. Surgery is the cornerstone of the most definitive therapy currently available for severe acute AR, especially if the patient is in clinical heart failure.

The most common causes of chronic AR are aortic root/annular dilatation (often called idiopathic) and congenital bicuspid valve. The incidence of rheumatic AR has declined greatly. Chronic AR is usually easy to diagnose by clinical evaluation. Doppler ultrasound is the single most important noninvasive test and is useful to diagnose and evaluate the severity of AR. A common clinical problem is distinguishing moderate from severe AR after clinical evaluation and Doppler ultrasound. Cardiac catheterization or angiography remains an extremely important diagnostic procedure and should be performed in most patients before valve surgery. Associated significant obstructive coronary artery disease is present in up to one half of patients over the age of 35 to 40 years.

Vasodilators have proven to be of great value in patients with chronic severe AR. It is palliative therapy in the symptomatic patient. Nifedipine reduces or delays the need for valve surgery in the asymptomatic patient with normal left ventricular systolic pump function. Valve replacement for severe AR relieves symptoms, reduces left ventricular volume and hypertrophy, and improves left ventricular systolic function in selected patients.

Acute Aortic Regurgitation

ETIOLOGY OF ACUTE AR

Infective endocarditis
Prosthetic valve dysfunction
Dissection of the aorta
Systemic hypertension
Trauma

Figure 7-1. Etiology of acute aortic regurgitation (AR). The two most common causes of acute AR are infective endocarditis and prosthetic valve dysfunction [1]. Other causes include dissection of the aorta, systemic hypertension, and trauma [2,3]. AR associated with dissection of the aorta indicates that the dissection involves the ascending aorta down to the aortic root/annulus. AR associated with systemic hypertension is usually mild and transient; it is associated with severe elevation of aortic pressure and when the systemic hypertension is controlled, the AR disappears.

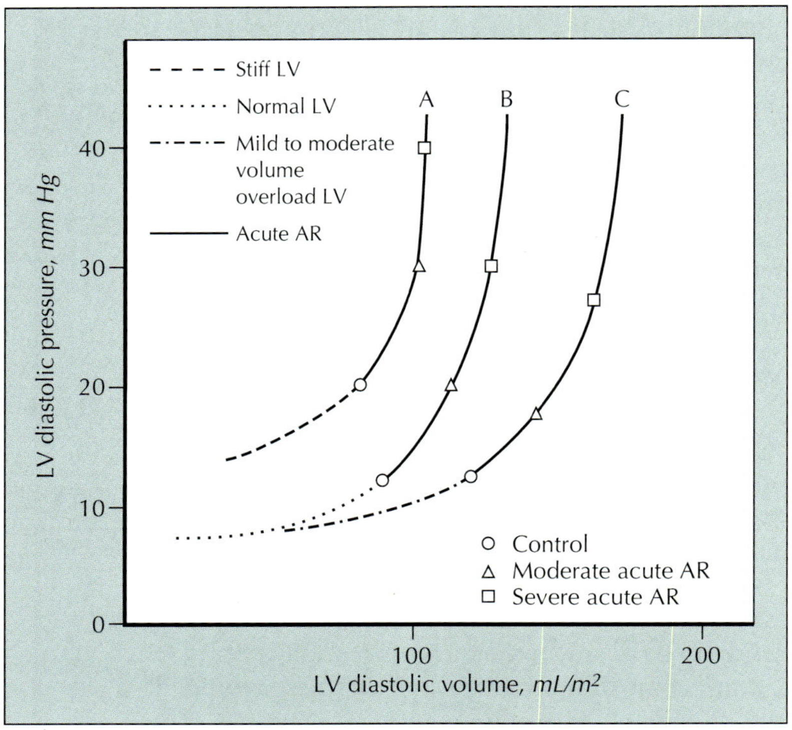

Figure 7-2. Pathophysiology of acute AR. The left ventricular (LV) diastolic pressure-volume (P-V) relationship plays an important role in the pathophysiology of acute AR [4]. Two issues must be considered. First is the limited ability of the LV to dilate acutely. As a result, the volume overload of acute AR produces a rapid increase of LV diastolic pressure (*curve B*). Second is the LV diastolic P-V relationship before the onset of acute AR. If the LV is already stiff or less compliant than normal from an associated lesion (*eg*, aortic stenosis or systemic hypertension), then the LV diastolic pressure rises more precipitously as a result of the volume overload of acute AR (*curve A*) than if the LV is normal (*curve B*). On the other hand, if the LV is somewhat dilated from a previous lesion (*eg*, mild AR [*curve C*]), then, with acute AR, the LV pressure rises more gradually initially but may subsequently rise to the same high levels as those with a normal or stiff LV. (*Adapted from* Rahimtoola [4].)

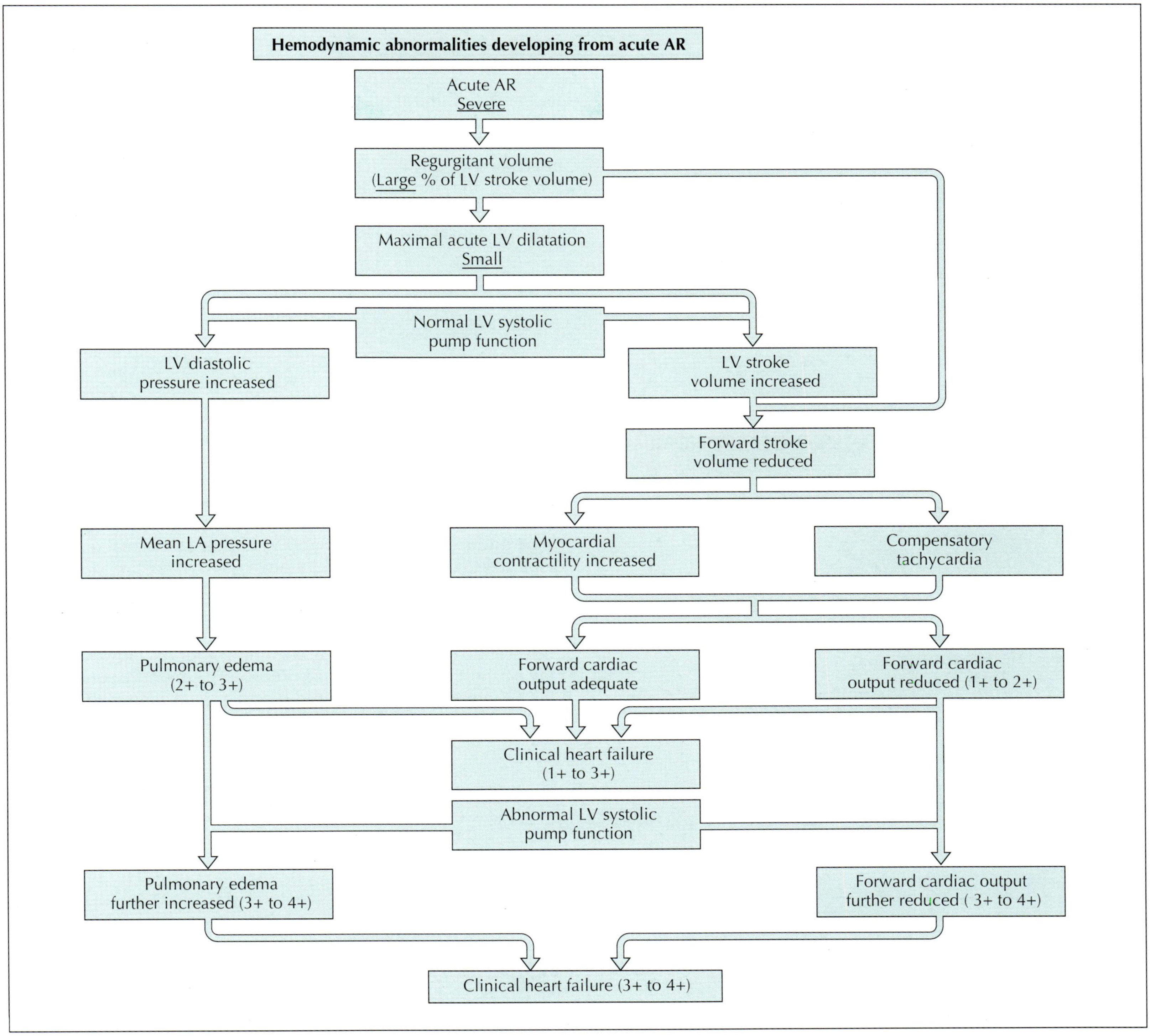

FIGURE 7-3. Hemodynamic abnormalities. Mild acute AR (*eg*, when associated with systemic hypertension) produces little or no hemodynamic abnormality. Increasing severity of regurgitation produces greater degrees of hemodynamic abnormalities, and severe AR often produces the clinical picture of heart failure.

Severe acute AR results in a large volume of regurgitant blood in the left ventricle (LV) in diastole. In an acute situation, the LV end-diastolic volume can only increase mildly (no more than 20% to 30%) and the LV diastolic pressure-volume relationships are particularly important (*see* Fig. 7-2). The LV systolic pump function is initially normal (*see* Fig. 7-6). The increased LV diastolic pressure results in increases in mean left atrial (LA) and pulmonary venous pressures and produces varying degrees of pulmonary edema [5]. The normal LV systolic pump function in the presence of LV dilatation results in an increase in LV stroke volume. However, a large percentage of the LV stroke volume is returned to the LV in diastole; as a result, the forward stroke volume is reduced. The LV uses two mechanisms, an increase of myocardial contractility and, importantly, a compensatory tachycardia to maintain an adequate forward cardiac output. As a result, initially the forward cardiac output may be appropriate. However, if the compensatory mechanisms are inadequate, forward cardiac output is reduced. The pulmonary edema with or without an adequate cardiac output produces the picture of clinical heart failure. Subsequently, LV systolic pump function may become abnormal; when that occurs, the pulmonary edema is further increased and the forward cardiac output is further reduced, leading to more severe manifestations of clinical heart failure. (© Copyright SH Rahimtoola, MB, FRCP, MACP)

ACUTE AR CLINICAL PRESENTATION

Relating to preexisting disorders
  eg: infective endocarditis
Relating to AR
  Asymptomatic
  Symptomatic: Clinical heart failure symptoms

FIGURE 7-4. Clinical presentation of acute AR. Patients with acute AR have signs relating to preexisting disorders that have caused the acute AR. For example, patients may have peripheral signs of infective endocarditis. The other clinical presentations are those related to the AR itself. If the AR is mild, the patient is usually asymptomatic. In the symptomatic patient, the symptoms are those of clinical heart failure.

PHYSICAL EXAMINATION IN ACUTE SEVERE AR

Tachycardia
Arterial pulse
  Increased rate of rise
  Systolic pressure normal
  Diastolic pressure normal to decreased
Clinical signs of heart failure
LV hyperdynamic
S_1 soft
S_2 soft, often single
S_3 often loud
Early or immediate diastolic murmur
Aortic systolic murmur
Austin Flint murmur

FIGURE 7-5. Physical examination. The symptomatic patient with acute severe AR usually has tachycardia. The arterial pulse shows an increased rate of pressure rise. However, systolic pressure is usually normal unless there is very severe heart failure, and diastolic pressure is normal or may be decreased. The usual clinical signs of heart failure may be present. On examination of the precordium, the left ventricular (LV) impulse is normal or slightly displaced to the left; it is usually not hyperdynamic. S_1 is soft, S_2 is often single and is soft unless pulmonary hypertension is present, and there is a loud S_3 gallop. S_4 gallop is absent. There is the usual murmur of AR; this is an early or immediate blowing decrescendo diastolic murmur beginning after A_2. However, it may be short and soft if the ascending aortic pressure equalizes with LV pressure in early or mid-diastole. An Austin Flint murmur, if present, occurs only in mid-diastole.

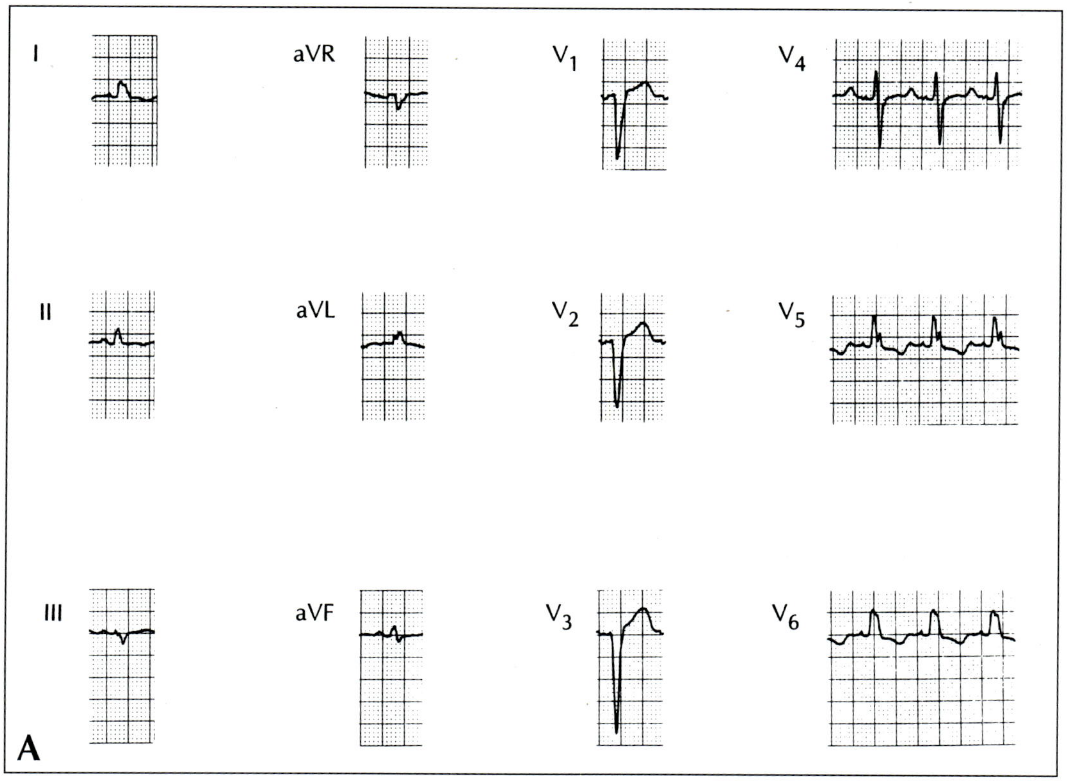

FIGURE 7-6. Diagnostic work-up in a patient with an unusual presentation for AR. This patient is a 49-year-old man who had no known cardiac disease. He had a colonoscopy for diarrhea *without* prophylactic antibiotics; a polyp was seen and was biopsied; the biopsy material grew *Enterococcus faecalis*. Approximately 3 weeks later, he presented in heart failure and blood cultures grew *E. faecalis*.

The patient's electrocardiogram demonstrated two rhythms at different times: **A,** Left bundle branch block and sinus rhythm. (*continued*)

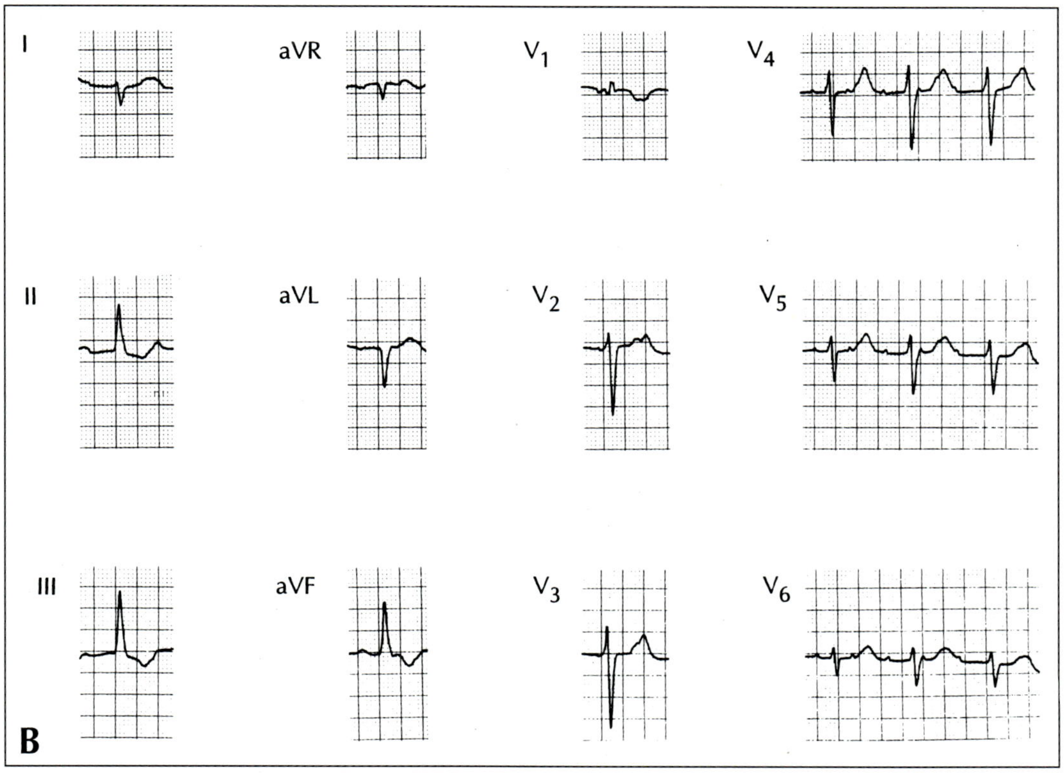

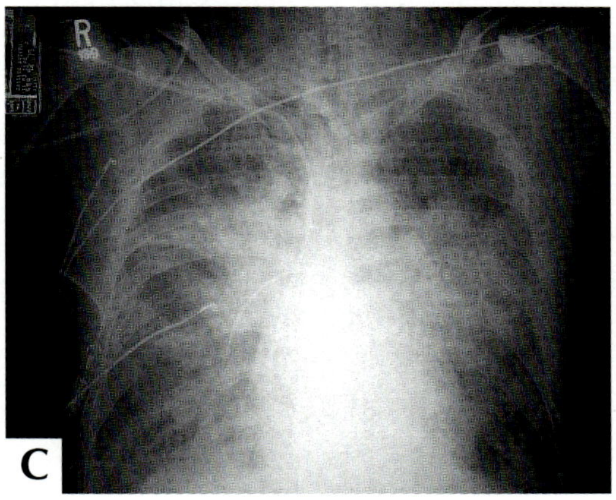

Figure 7-6. (*continued*) **B,** Right bundle branch block with right axis deviation and complete heart block. **C,** Portable chest radiograph (anteroposterior view) showed acute pulmonary edema and normal heart size. **D,** Hemodynamic studies demonstrated that blood pressure was normal; the mean pulmonary artery (PA) wedge pressure (PAWP) was elevated at 47 mm Hg, as was the PA diastolic pressure; and the cardiac output and index were normal. On 45%, fraction inspired oxygen, the systemic and PA oxygen saturations were 91% and 57%, respectively. The patient was agitated. With sedation (fentanyl and Versed), intravenous nitroprusside, dopamine, and Lasix, the mean PAWP was 23 mm Hg, the PA diastolic pressure was 27 mm Hg, and there was much clinical improvement. **E,** Coronary arteriography demonstrated normal coronary arteries. Aortography showed severe (4+) AR vegetations and a large abscess. Left ventricular (LV) volumes and ejection fraction calculated from the left ventricle (LV) opacified from the aortogram showed volumes in the upper range of normal and a normal ejection fraction. The LV was not entered with the cardiac catheter.

This patient subsequently underwent urgent valve surgery, which confirmed the preoperative diagnoses. The underlying cardiac lesion was a congenital bicuspid, partly calcified, aortic valve that was initially likely stenotic (or possibly regurgitant), a diagnosis that had not been made before the colon biopsy and the endocarditis.

D. BEDSIDE HEMODYNAMIC MANIFESTATIONS OF SEVERE, ACUTE AR IN A 49-YEAR-OLD PATIENT

ARTERY/OUTPUT	BEFORE THERAPY	AFTER THERAPY
Systemic artery pressure, *mm Hg*		
Systolic	117	95
Diastolic	75	52
Mean	90	71
PAWP, *mm Hg*		
Mean	47	23
PA pressure, *mm Hg*		
Systolic	70	40
Diastolic	47	27
Mean	59	33
Cardiac output, *L/min*	5.3	—
Cardiac index, *L/min/m³*	2.8	—

E. CORONARY ARTERIOGRAPHY IN A 49-YEAR-OLD MAN WITH SEVERE, ACUTE AR

Coronary arteriography:
- Normal coronary arteries

Ascending aortography:
- Severe (4+) aortic regurgitation with dense complete opacification of a normal-sized LV with normal wall motion and mild (1+) mitral regurgitation

Left ventricle:

End-diastolic volume index *mL/m²*	91
End-systolic volume index *mL/m²*	41
Ejection fraction	0.54

MANAGEMENT OF ACUTE AR

- Mild AR
  - Diagnosis of AR
  - Treatment of underlying disorder
  - Diagnosis of etiology of AR
- Moderate or severe AR
  - Diagnosis of AR
  - Diagnosis of etiology of AR
  - Bedside hemodynamic monitoring
  - Treatment
    - Medical
    - Surgical

FIGURE 7-7. Disease management. In mild AR, management consists of the diagnosis of AR and its etiology, and treatment is directed at the underlying disorder. Management of severe AR, and in most instances that of moderate AR, is a four-part process consisting of diagnosing the AR, determining its etiology, providing bedside hemodynamic monitoring, and instituting treatment that is a combination of pharmacologic and surgical measures.

DIAGNOSIS OF ACUTE AR

- Clinical evaluation
  - History
  - Physical examination
  - Electrocardiography
  - Chest radiography
- Echocardiography/Doppler ultrasound
- Cardiac catheterization and angiography

FIGURE 7-8. Diagnosis of acute AR. In most instances, the diagnosis can be made by clinical evaluation, which includes the history and physical examination, electrocardiography, and chest radiography. The diagnosis by physical examination in an acutely ill patient who is in extremis may be difficult.

Transthoracic Doppler ultrasound is an important and valuable noninvasive procedure that should be used in every instance. It demonstrates the AR and its severity and provides useful information about the size and function of the left ventricle and other valvular and cardiac abnormalities. If the transthoracic method is not adequate, *eg*, and in the very ill patient, then the transesophageal method should be used.

Cardiac catheterization and angiography, including coronary angiography, may be needed to make the diagnosis and are usually performed before surgical intervention.

ETIOLOGIC DIAGNOSIS OF ACUTE AR

- Usual clinical findings of underlying lesion
- Additional laboratory tests, *eg*, blood cultures
- Doppler ultrasound/echocardiography
- Occasionally: Magnetic resonance imaging, cine CT

FIGURE 7-9. Etiologic diagnosis. Diagnosis of the etiology of AR may be made during the clinical evaluation by finding the usual clinical characteristics of the underlying lesions, *eg*, those of infective endocarditis. Additional laboratory tests are needed to confirm the diagnosis, such as blood cultures in those suspected of having infective endocarditis.

Doppler ultrasound (transthoracic and transesophageal) is also extremely valuable in diagnosing the underlying lesion, *eg*, infective endocarditis or dissection of the aorta. Its widespread availability and comparative ease of use make it the noninvasive procedure of choice, especially in the very acutely ill patient. The availability of biplane and omniplane transesophageal probes enhances its value as a diagnostic tool.

Recent data show that magnetic resonance imaging has a higher specificity than Doppler ultrasound for the diagnosis of dissection of the aorta [6] and if available should be used in all hemodynamically stable patients if the diagnosis has not been made [7]. However, biplane or omniplane transesophageal echocardiography markedly improves the specificity and diagnostic accuracy of transesophageal echocardiography. Angiography is also an effective and time-honored method of diagnosing dissection of the aorta. Cine computed tomographic (CT) scanning (including fast cine CT) may be used in selected cases.

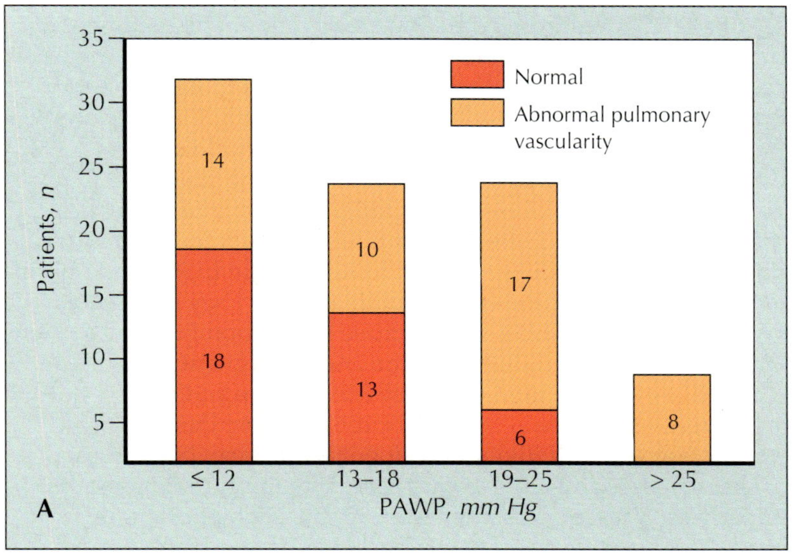

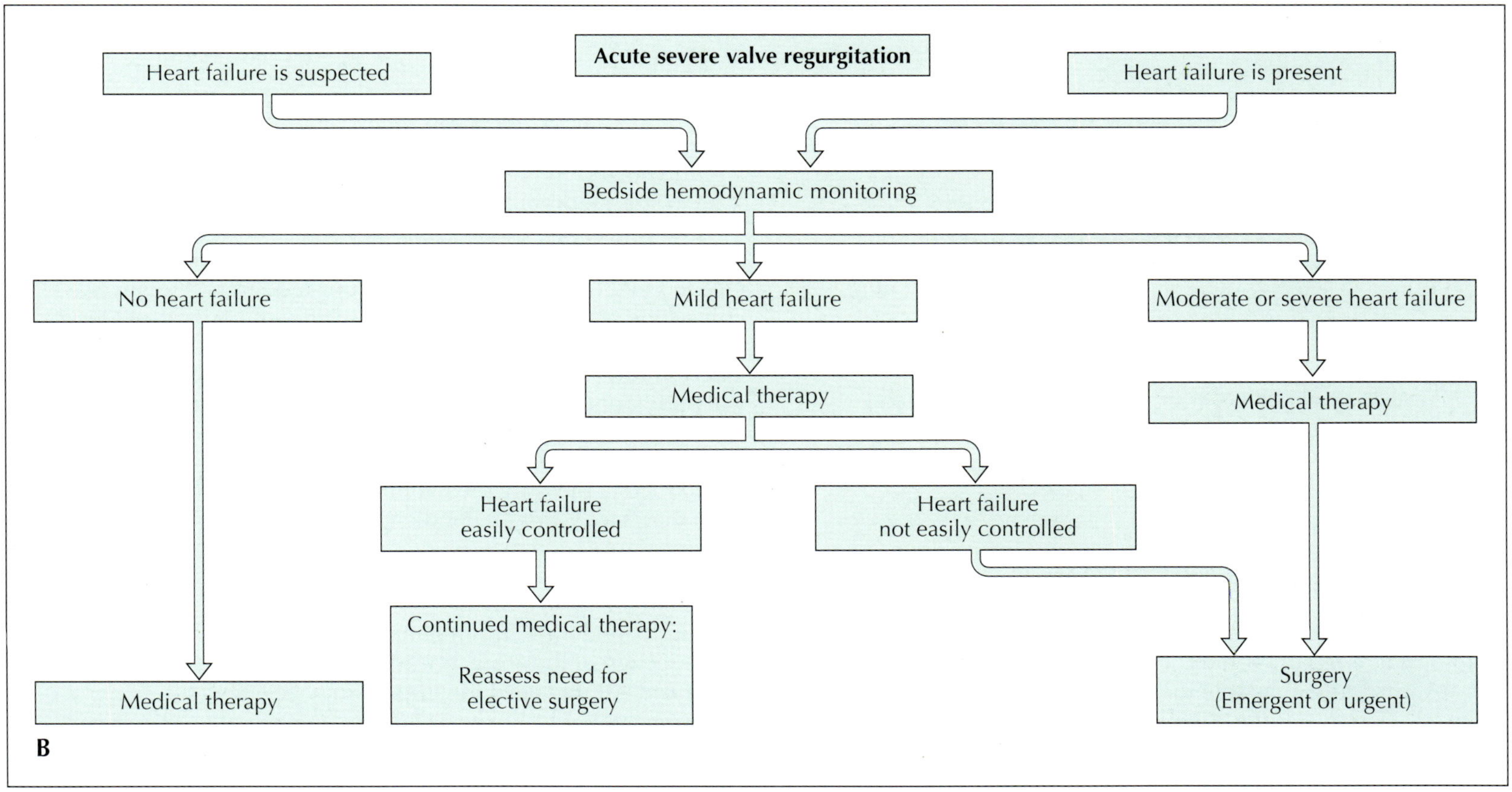

FIGURE 7-10. Hemodynamic parameters. In acute disorders affecting the left ventricle, including AR, there may be a phase lag of up to 72 hours between the rise in left atrial and pulmonary venous pressures and the appearance of pulmonary edema on the chest radiograph, thus making the chest radiograph unreliable in this situation. **A,** Data from patients with acute myocardial infarction [8]. Of 32 patients who had pulmonary artery wedge pressures (PAWP) of 12 mm Hg or less, 14 had radiographic changes that were interpreted as pulmonary edema. Treatment with diuretics in such patients could result in a fall in cardiac output [9]. Of 31 patients with PAWP of 19 mm Hg or greater, six had normal chest radiographs. In such patients, volume loading for a reduced cardiac output or hypotension may result in a further increase in left atrial pressure and pulmonary edema.

Furthermore, the optimization of filling pressures and cardiac output may not be made accurately in acute heart failure without measuring their actual value. Thus, use of balloon flotation catheters for hemodynamic monitoring is recommended in almost all patients. **B,** This procedure can be used to determine which therapies should be instituted.

If the AR is mild and there are no significant hemodynamic abnormalities, the balloon flotation catheter can be withdrawn. If the AR is moderate to severe and significant hemodynamic abnormalities are present, the balloon flotation catheter is left in place to guide therapy in the management of these acutely ill patients [4]. If the hemodynamic abnormalities are mild, the patient is treated medically. If these abnormalities are easily controlled, medical therapy is continued and periodic reassessments are made to determine the need for elective surgery. If the hemodynamic abnormalities are not easily corrected or the hemodynamic abnormalities initially are moderate or severe, surgery is undertaken either emergently or urgently. (Part A *adapted from* Kostuk and coworkers [8]; part B *adapted from* Rahimtoola [4].)

TREATMENT OF HEART FAILURE IN ACUTE AR

- Correct or control altered pathophysiologic state
  - Reduce pulmonary venous pressure
    - Diuresis
    - Vasodilation
    - Control heart rate and maintain sinus rhythm (digitalis, cardioversion, antiarrhythmics)
  - Increase cardiac output
    - Reduction of AR (vasodilators)
    - Inotropic stimulation (digitalis, dobutamine)
- Correct or control underlying disease or disorder
  - Antibiotics for infective endocarditis
  - Pharmacologic therapy for systemic hypertension
  - Surgery for valve regurgitation in infective endocarditis, prosthetic valve dysfunction, dissection of the aorta, trauma

FIGURE 7-11. Two-pronged treatment direction. The treatment of heart failure in acute severe AR is directed toward correcting or controlling the altered pathophysiologic state [1]. Based on the pathophysiology (*see* Figs. 7-2 and 7-3), the goals are to reduce pulmonary venous pressure toward normal and to increase cardiac output. Measures successful in reducing pulmonary venous pressure are diuresis, vasodilation, and controlling heart rate and maintaining sinus rhythm. Vasodilators (intravenous nitroprusside for an acute, severe condition) are useful and important in the management of these patients [10]. They reduce left ventricular (LV) volumes and increase LV ejection fraction and left atrial pressure. Regurgitant fraction and regurgitant volumes are reduced; as a result, the forward stroke volume and cardiac output are increased. If there is LV systolic dysfunction, then inotropic stimulation, *eg*, with digitalis or dobutamine, may be necessary.

Therapy is also directed toward correcting or controlling the underlying disease or disorder. Appropriate antibiotic therapy is needed for infective endocarditis and pharmacologic therapy for systemic hypertension. (*Adapted from* Rahimtoola [1].)

TIMING OF SURGERY IN HEART FAILURE DUE TO ACUTE AR

LESION	TIMING OF SURGERY
Dissection of aorta	Emergent
Infective endocarditis	Emergent, urgent, elective
Prosthetic valve dysfunction	Emergent, urgent, elective
Trauma	Emergent, urgent, elective

FIGURE 7-12. Timing of surgery. Surgical therapy (valve replacement or valve repair) is the cornerstone of the most definitive therapy currently available for heart failure in patients with acute AR [4,11,12]. If the AR is due to the dissection of the aorta, cardiac surgery is an emergency even if the AR is mild or moderate, because the AR indicates involvement of the dissection down to the region of the aortic valve root/annulus. The indications for surgery in infective endocarditis usually depend on whether there is clinical heart failure, the type of infecting organism, and the response to therapy. Infective endocarditis due to special organisms (*eg*, fungi) can only rarely be controlled by pharmacologic therapy, and surgery is almost always needed. For these and some other conditions, valve surgery may be needed even if the AR is only mild or moderate. However, it must be recognized that in 90% to 95% of patients needing surgery for endocarditis, the indication for valve surgery is heart failure. When the heart failure is a result of prosthetic valve dysfunction or trauma, the need for surgery can be an emergency, an urgent situation, or elective.

Prosthetic valves are inherently stenotic. When AR is added, it produces a pressure plus volume overload on the left ventricle (LV) that the LV cannot handle very well acutely. Furthermore, valve regurgitation may be a sign of degeneration of biologic prosthetic valves or of prosthetic endocarditis; in both conditions, valve surgery is usually needed even if the valve regurgitation is mild to moderate. Trauma may result in AR from valve damage or dissection of the aorta. If trauma produces dissection of the aorta and AR, the need for surgery may be emergent.

In some patients, the heart failure can be easily controlled completely with pharmacologic therapy. The LV and left atrium are able to dilate and adapt to the volume overload; there are no hemodynamic abnormalities and LV function is normal. In such instances, surgical therapy may be delayed, perhaps for a considerable period of time.

Chronic Aortic Regurgitation

ETIOLOGY

ETIOLOGY OF CHRONIC AR

Aortic root/annular dilatation
Congenital bicuspid valve
Previous infective endocarditis
Rheumatic disease

Figure 7-13. Etiology of chronic AR. Aortic root/annular dilatation presumably due to medial disease is the single most common cause of chronic AR leading to aortic valve replacement in the United States [3]. In various series, it has accounted for 41% to 56% of the cases; it is referred to as idiopathic in some reports. In such patients, approximately 40% to 62% of the valves from various series showed myxomatous changes. Other common causes include congenital bicuspid valve, previous infective endocarditis, and rheumatic disease.

CHRONIC AR IN ASSOCIATION WITH OTHER DISEASE

Congenital lesions
Connective tissue disease
Autoimmune diseases
Various forms of aortitis and arteritis
Syphilis

Figure 7-14. Chronic AR in association with other diseases [2,3].

PATHOPHYSIOLOGY

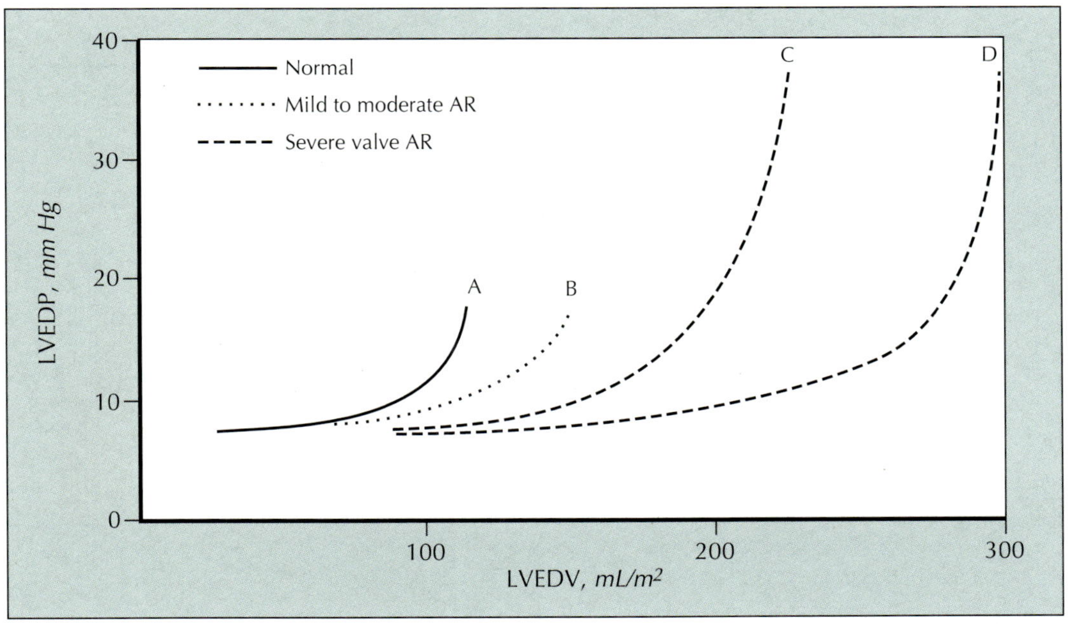

Figure 7-15. Left ventricular (LV) diastolic pressure-volume (P-V) relationships: effects of chronic valve regurgitation. In chronic AR, as opposed to acute AR, the AR becomes severe over a period of time; and therefore, the LV diastolic P-V relationships are different from those seen in acute AR (*see* Fig. 7-2). If the AR is mild to moderate, the LV end-diastolic volume (LVEDV) is increased moderately, the LV diastolic P-V curve is moved to the right (*curve B*) of normal (*curve A*), and the LV end-diastolic pressure (LVEDP) is usually normal. In severe AR, the LV diastolic P-V curves are moved to the right (*curves C* and *D*). If the LV systolic pump function is normal, the LVEDV can be quite large without significant elevation of LVEDP (*curve C*). However, if the LVEDV increases further, the LVEDP will be increased. If LV systolic pump dysfunction supervenes, the LV diastolic P-V curve relationships are moved even further to the right (*curve D*) with quite marked LV dilatation and increases in LVEDP. (*Adapted from* Rahimtoola [4].)

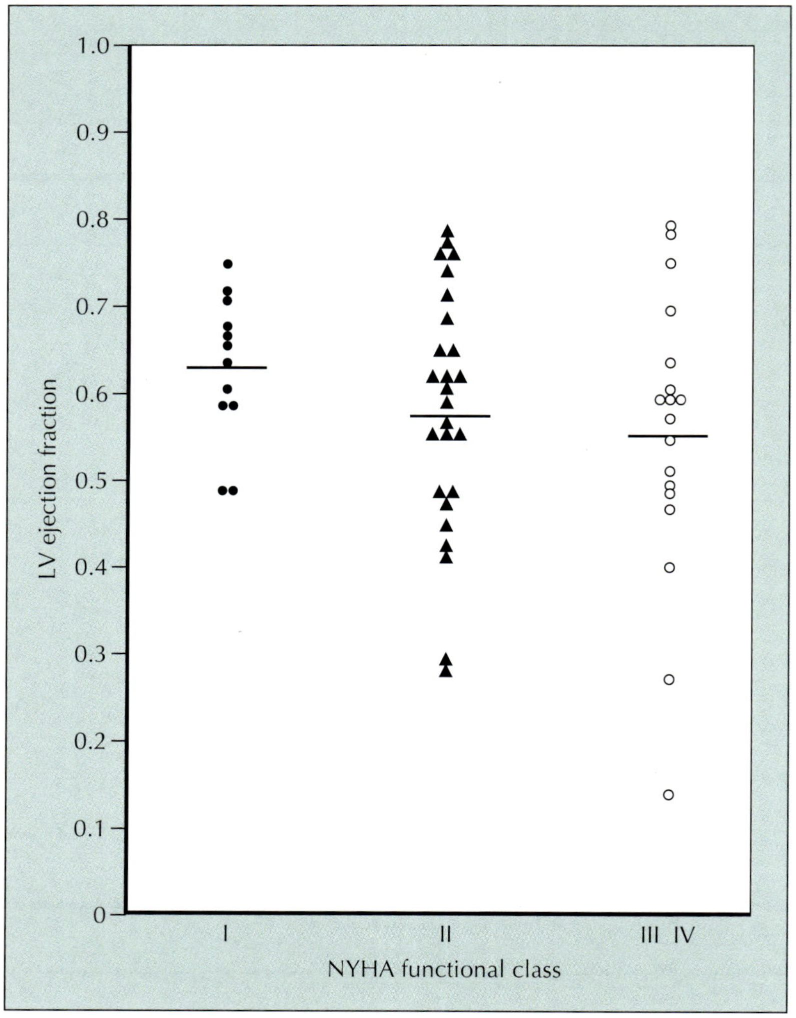

FIGURE 7-16. Left ventricular (LV) ejection fraction in patients with chronic AR [13]. Most asymptomatic patients (New York Heart Association [NYHA] functional class I) have normal LV systolic pump function as do most patients who are mildly symptomatic (class II). However, some patients with only mild symptoms may have LV systolic pump dysfunction at rest. Patients who are moderately to severely symptomatic (classes III and IV) may have either normal or abnormal LV systolic pump function. In those with normal LV systolic pump function, the symptoms are probably due to LV diastolic dysfunction (*see* Fig. 7-17). These patients will have a much better survival rate after valve surgery, even if they are severely symptomatic, than those who are severely symptomatic and have abnormal LV systolic pump function (*see* Fig. 7-35). (*Adapted from* Karaian and coworkers [13].)

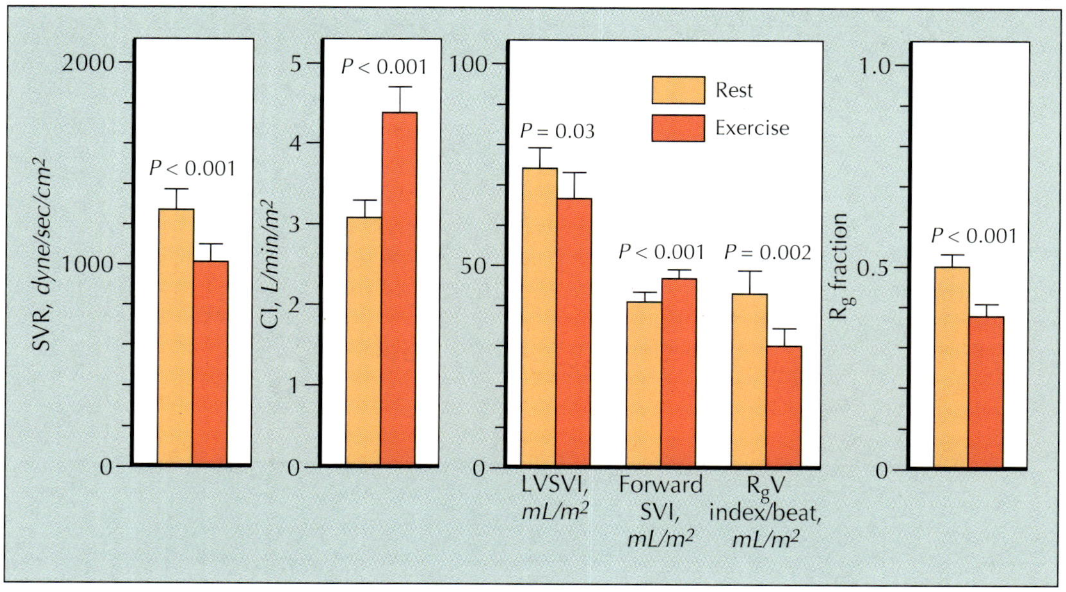

FIGURE 7-17. Effect of dynamic exercise on chronic AR. Dynamic exercise produces interesting changes in cardiac hemodynamics in patients with chronic AR [14]. On exercise, there is a fall of systemic vascular resistance (SVR). The total left ventricular (LV) stroke volume index (LVSVI) may decrease slightly but not significantly so. Because of the fall in SVR, the body is able to redistribute the LV stroke volume; the regurgitant volume (R_gV) and regurgitant (R_g) fraction (R_gV as a fraction of LV stroke volume) are significantly reduced. As a result, forward stroke volume index (SVI) is increased and the tachycardia associated with the exercise results in a marked increase in forward cardiac output and the body's need of an increased cardiac output of exercise is met. In chronic AR there is a reserve mechanism; the body is able to increase the forward cardiac output at the expense of the R_gV without a change, or even a fall, in total LV stroke volume. CI—cardiac index. (*Adapted from* Kawanishi and coworkers [14].)

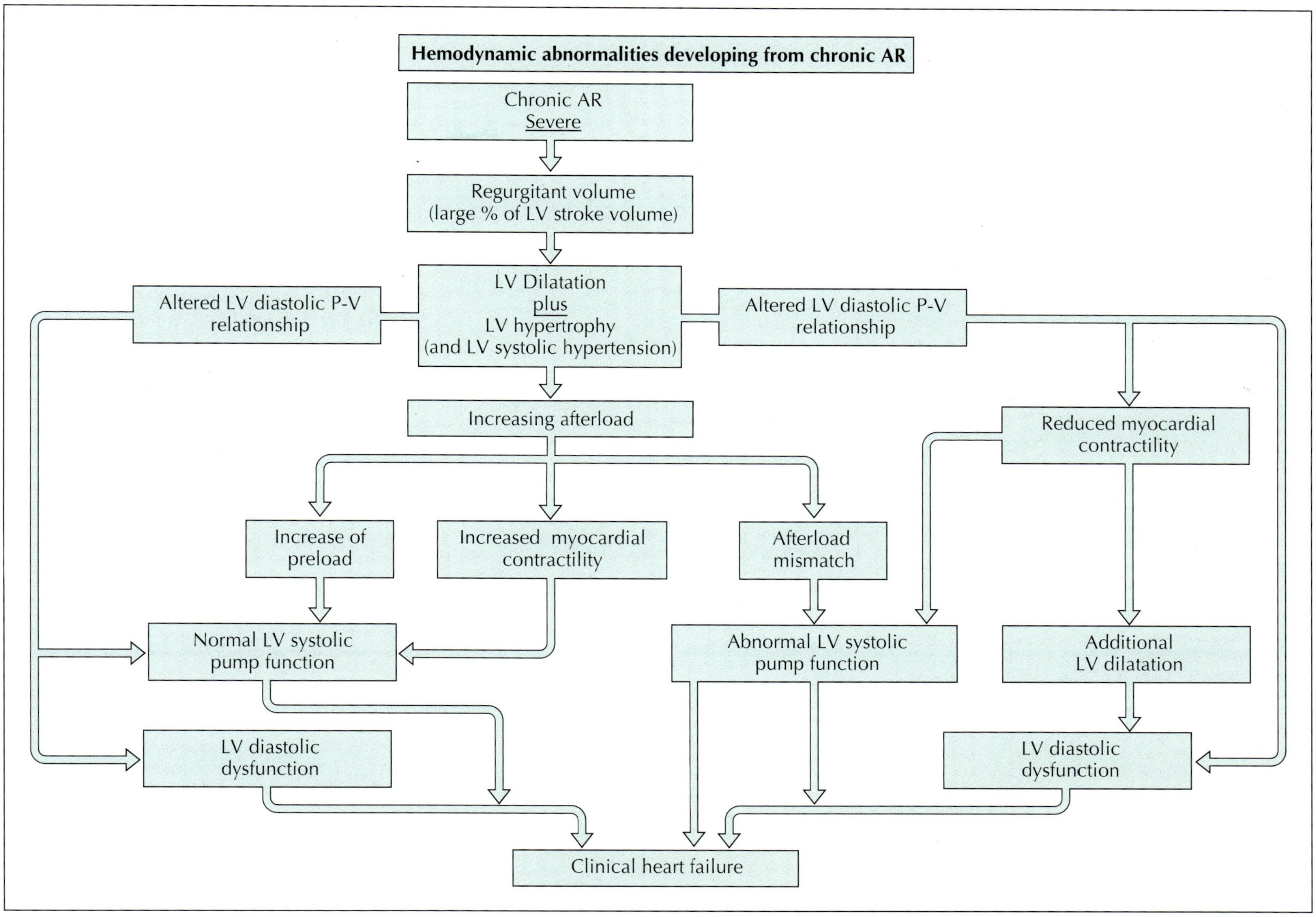

FIGURE 7-18. Hemodynamic abnormalities. Severe chronic AR results in a large regurgitant volume (a large percentage of left ventricular [LV] stroke volume). The LV responds by dilating (average LV end-diastolic volume in patients undergoing surgery, 205 mL/m^2) [15]; the dilatation is proportional to the regurgitant volume. The subsequent large LV stroke volume results in the production of LV systolic hypertension. Both of these increase LV wall stress (afterload), which could result in an impairment of LV function. The heart responds by becoming hypertrophied (average LV mass in patients undergoing valve surgery 222 g/m^2) [15]; myocardial stress remains normal and LV systolic pump function remains normal. There is an alteration of the LV diastolic pressure-volume (P-V) relationship (*see* Fig. 7-15). However, some patients with normal LV systolic pump function become symptomatic because of the abnormal LV diastolic function.

As LV afterload (a result of LV dilatation, hypertrophy, and systolic hypertension) continues to increase, the LV uses two additional compensatory mechanisms, namely, increase of preload and increase of myocardial contractility. Both of these help maintain normal LV systolic pump function.

When the limit of preload reserve has been reached (afterload mismatch) [16] or myocardial contractility is reduced, LV systolic pump function becomes abnormal. The additional LV dilatation also results in further alteration of the LV diastolic P-V relationship (*see* Fig. 7-15).

Clinical heart failure is usually a result of the abnormal LV systolic pump function; diastolic dysfunction may also be present in some patients. Clinical heart failure in those with normal LV systolic pump function is a result of LV diastolic dysfunction. (© Copyright SH Rahimtoola, MB, FRCP, MACP.)

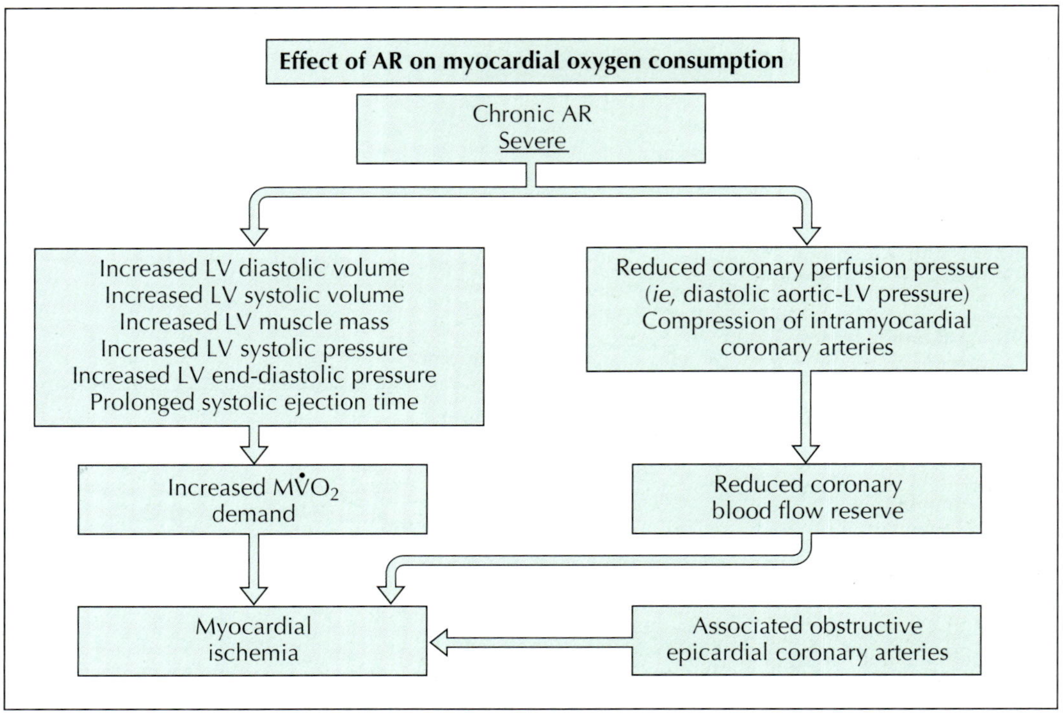

FIGURE 7-19. Effect of AR on myocardial oxygen ($M\dot{V}O_2$) consumption. In severe AR, $M\dot{V}O_2$ is increased because of increases in left ventricular (LV) diastolic and systolic volumes, LV muscle mass (hypertrophy), and LV pressures; as well as prolongation of systolic ejection time. Total coronary blood flow is increased. However, coronary reserve, *ie*, the ability of the coronary blood flow to increase with vasodilatation, is significantly reduced [17], probably because of a reduced diastolic aortic-LV pressure gradient and compression of intramyocardial coronary arteries. Therefore, myocardial ischemia is often present on stress in these patients. Associated obstructive coronary artery disease (*see* Fig. 7-40) can be expected to further exacerbate the myocardial ischemia. (© Copyright SH Rahimtoola, MB, FRCP, MACP.)

NATURAL HISTORY AND PROGNOSIS

PROGNOSIS IN CHRONIC AR

COURSE OF DISEASE	MORTALITY, %
Mild AR	Normal
Moderate AR: 10 y	15
Severe, symptomatic AR	
5 y	25
10 y	50
Angina, 4 y	≤100
Heart failure, 2–3 y	50–70

FIGURE 7-20. Prognosis in AR. If mild AR does not progress, patients can be expected to have a life expectancy that is not significantly different from normal. Their major risk is development of infective endocarditis and its complications. Patients with moderate AR, if it does not progress, also can be expected to have an excellent prognosis; however, it does progress and the mortality rate at 10 years is approximately 15%. Patients with severe AR who are symptomatic have 5- and 10-year mortality rates of 25% and 50%, respectively [18]. Almost all patients who develop angina are dead within a period of 4 years. In those in heart failure, the mortality rates at the end of 2 to 3 years are approximately 50% to 70%, respectively [19].

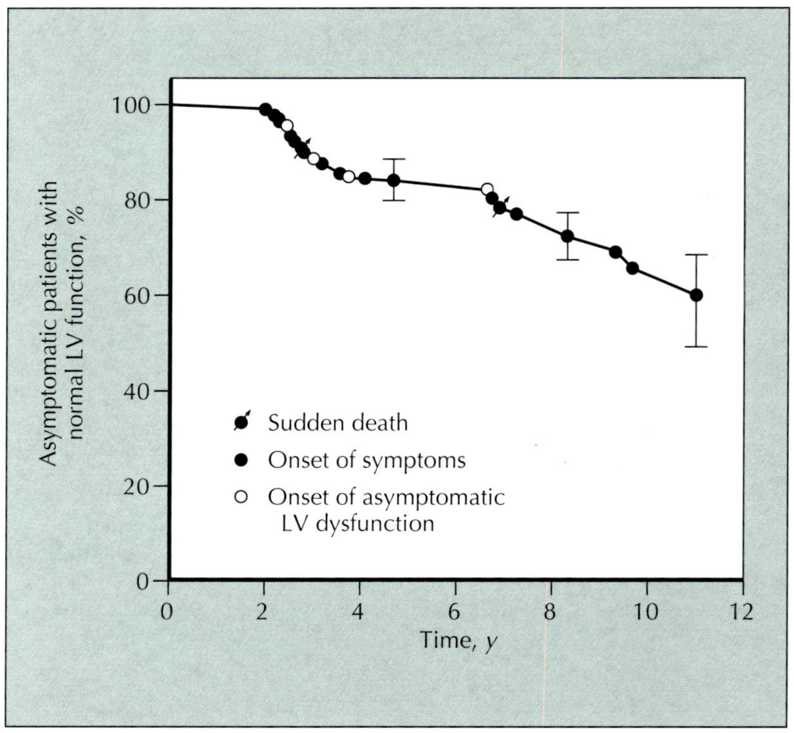

FIGURE 7-21. Natural history. The classic natural history study of Bonow *et al.* [20] from the National Institutes of Health prospectively evaluated 104 patients with severe AR who were initially asymptomatic and had normal left ventricular (LV) systolic pump function at rest. At the end of 11 years, 42% of them had become either symptomatic (19 patients), or had developed LV dysfunction (four patients) or had died suddenly (two patients); 11 of the 19 patients who had become symptomatic also developed LV dysfunction. In other words, the development of the adverse cardiac events occurs at a rate of just under 4% per year. (*Adapted from* Bonow and coworkers [20].)

PREDICTORS OF ADVERSE CARDIAC EVENTS IN CHRONIC SEVERE AR

PREDICTORS OF ADVERSE CARDIAC EVENTS	LIKELIHOOD OF SYMPTOMS OF LV DYSFUNCTION OR DEATH, %/Y
LV end-diastolic dimension, *mm*	
≥70	10
<70	2
LV end-systolic dimension, *mm*	
≥50	19
40–49	6
<40	0

FIGURE 7-22. Predictors of adverse cardiac events. Patients who are asymptomatic develop adverse events at a relatively low rate (*see* Fig. 7-21). However, in such patients it is appropriate to look for markers that are predictors of the development of adverse cardiac events. Of patients with a left ventricular (LV) end-diastolic dimension of 70 mm or greater on M-mode echocardiography, the linearized rate of an adverse event is 10% per year. In those with an end-systolic dimension of 50 mm or greater, the linearized rate of an adverse event is 19% per year [20]. Other predictors include an LV end-diastolic volume index of 150 mL/m^2 or greater [21]). In the study of Bonow *et al.* [20] two patients suffered sudden death and both of them had an LV end-diastolic dimension of 80 mm or greater. (*Adapted from* Bonow and coworkers [20].)

CLINICAL MANIFESTATIONS

CLINICAL PRESENTATION OF AR

- Asymptomatic
- Symptomatic
  - Pounding of the head
  - Tachycardia
  - Angina pectoris
  - Heart failure symptoms

FIGURE 7-23. Clinical presentation. Many patients with severe AR are asymptomatic. They may complain of pounding of the head or palpitations. Palpitations are a result of the awareness of the beating of a dilated LV that undergoes a large volume change in systole, during either sinus beats or postectopic beats. Angina pectoris occurs in about 20% of patients and may be present even when the coronary arteries are normal. Angina associated with syphilitic AR may be due to associated osteal stenosis of the coronary arteries. In such patients, angina often occurs at rest and is difficult to control.

The main symptoms of severe AR are those of heart failure. These result from elevated pulmonary venous pressure and include dyspnea on exertion, orthopnea, and paroxysmal nocturnal dyspnea. When congestive heart failure occurs, patients may also complain of fatigue, weakness, and swelling of the feet.

MURMUR OF AR

An early or immediate, blowing, decrescendo, diastolic murmur beginning after A_2 (S_2)

FIGURE 7-24. AR murmur. The sine qua non diagnostic clinical sign of AR is the murmur of AR. It is an early or immediate blowing decrescendo diastolic murmur beginning after A_2 (S_2).

USEFUL SIGNS OF CHRONIC, SEVERE AR

- de Musset's sign
- Traube's sign
- Duroziez's sign
- Quincke's sign

FIGURE 7-25. Useful signs in chronic, severe AR [2,3]. These include de Musset's sign, Traube's sign, Duroziez's sign, and Quincke's sign.

PHYSICAL EXAMINATION IN AR

AREA ASSESSED	SEVERITY OF AR: MILD	MODERATE	SEVERE
Arterial pulse	Normal	Corrigan's 1+ to 2+	Corrigan's 3+
Arterial pressure			
Systolic	Normal	Increased 1+ to 2+	Increased 3+
Diastolic	Normal	Decreased 1+ to 2+	Decreased 3+ to 4+
Pulse pressure	Often normal	Increased 1+ to 2+	Increased 3+ to 4+
Cardiac impulse	Often normal	Hyperdynamic	Very hyperdynamic, visible; chest may rock
Precordial thrill			
Systolic	—	±	±
Diastolic	—	—	±
Auscultation			
S_4	—	—	—
S_1	Normal	Often soft	Soft
S_2	Normal	Normal or single	Often single
S_3	—	+	2+ to 3+
ESM	±	+	1+ to 2+
AoDM	+	++	3+ to 4+
Austin Flint murmur	—	—	±

FIGURE 7-26. Physical examination in AR. The main finding on physical examination in patients with mild chronic AR is the aortic regurgitant murmur.

Patients with chronic severe AR display characteristic physical findings. The arterial pulse shows an abrupt distention with a rapid rise and a quick collapse (Corrigan's pulse). The systolic arterial pressure is increased, the diastolic pressure is reduced, and Korotkoff's sounds persist down to 0 mm Hg. Even in such instances, however, the recorded intra-arterial pressure rarely falls below 30 mm Hg. As a result of the changes in systolic and diastolic pressures, the pulse pressure is increased. The jugular venous pressure is normal unless heart failure is present.

On inspection, the chest may rock and the cardiac impulse may be visible. The cardiac impulse is hyperdynamic. There may be a systolic thrill at the base of the heart, over the carotids, and in the suprasternal notch. This results from a very large LV stroke volume across a diseased aortic valve. A diastolic thrill usually signifies severe AR. S_1 is usually soft because the mitral valve leaflets are close to each other at the end of systole or the valve is prematurely closed. This is exaggerated if the PR interval is prolonged. S_2 is usually single because the aortic valve does not close properly or the LV ejection time is prolonged; P_2 may not be heard. There is usually an S_3 gallop but no S_4.

The sine qua non of AR is an early or immediate decrescendo blowing aortic diastolic murmur (AoDM) beginning after A_2 (S_2). It is best heard with the diaphragm of the stethoscope at the left sternal border, or, in difficult instances, by having the patient sit up and lean forward and by auscultating in held respiration at the end of a deep inspiration.

In severe AR, the murmur may be holodiastolic. When it is soft, its intensity can be increased by doing isometric exercise such as a hand grip that increases aortic diastolic pressure. At times, this murmur is best heard along the right sternal border, which should draw attention to the possibility that the cause of AR is aortic root disease. There is usually an ejection systolic murmur due to an increased LV stroke volume across the diseased aortic valve.

In many patients with severe AR, an Austin Flint murmur is present [22]. This is a presystolic or mid-diastolic murmur heard at the cardiac apex, originating at the mitral valve when blood enters the LV simultaneously from the aorta and left atrium. When an Austin Flint murmur is heard, two inferences can be drawn: 1) it signifies that the AR is severe, and 2) it requires that associated mitral stenosis be excluded. ESM—ejection systolic murmur.

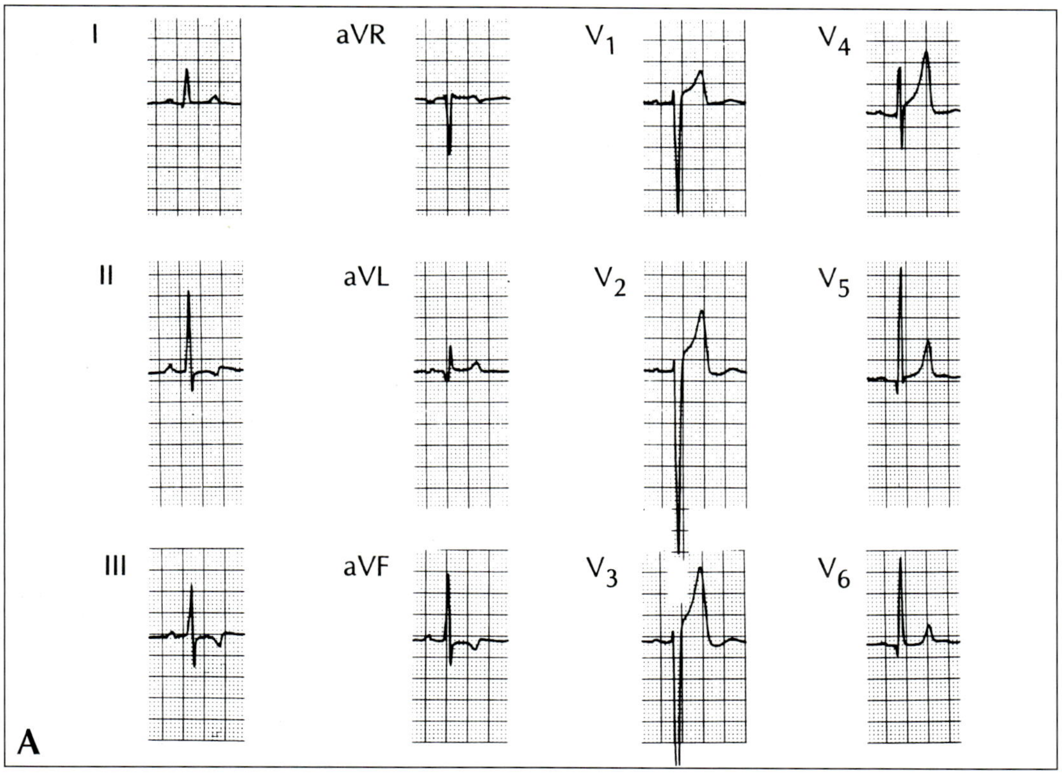

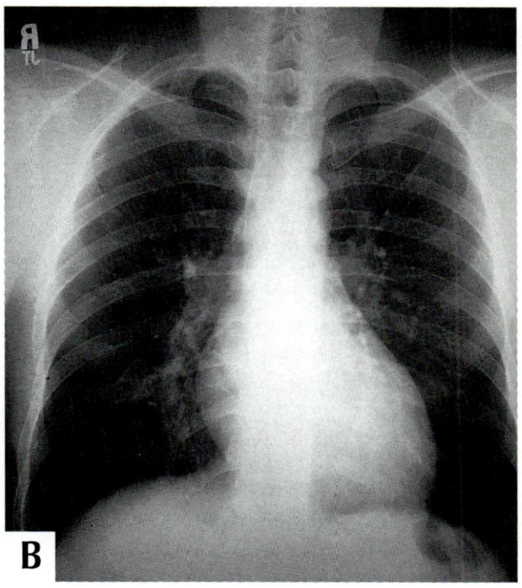

C. DOPPLER ULTRASOUND DATA IN A 25-YEAR-OLD PATIENT

AREA ASSESSED	DATA
LV	
End-diastolic dimension, *mm*	70
End-systolic dimension, *mm*	50
Fractional shortening, *%*	29
E-point septal separation, *mm*	11
Interventricular septal thickness, *mm*	9
Posterior wall thickness,*mm*	9
Aortic valve	
Aortic regurgitation (two jets seen)	4+

FIGURE 7-27. Electrocardiographic (ECG), chest radiographic, Doppler ultrasound, and hemodynamic and angiographic data from a 25-year-old man. The patient was asymptomatic and on examination for another minor noncardiavascular symptom a cardiac murmur was heard. On clinical examination, he had the classic signs of isolated, chronic severe AR.

A, Left ventricular (LV) hypertrophy on ECG with T-wave inversions present only in the inferior leads. With a more "vertical" heart in the thorax, it is not uncommon to see ECG changes associated with LV hypertrophy in the inferior leads. **B,** Chest radiography (posteroanterior view) reveals an enlarged cardiac silhouette (cardiothoracic ratio 0.50) and normal pulmonary vasculature. **C,** Doppler ultrasound data confirm a dilated LV with normal fractional shortening and severe AR. **D,** Hemodynamic and angiographic data show wide pulse pressure, an elevated LV end-diastolic pressure, and normal cardiac output. The LV is dilated and LV systolic pump function is normal. There is 4+ AR.

His ventricular size and volume were at the level that is associated with a higher rate of clinical deterioration (see Fig. 7-22). It would have been better to do additional testing that included an exercise test to document his symptomatic status and a right heart catheterization to determine LV filling pressure on exercise. When these are abnormal, the patient should be considered for surgery.

D. HEMODYNAMIC AND ANGIOGRAPHIC DATA IN A 25-YEAR-OLD PATIENT

AREA ASSESSED	DATA
Pressures, *mm Hg*:	
Right atrium	
a wave	6
v wave	9
Mean	6
Right ventricle	
(Systolic/diastolic—end-diastolic)	24/2–10
LV	
(Systolic/diastolic—end-diastolic)	140/2–16
Ascending aorta	
Systolic	140
Diastolic	50
Mean	90

AREA ASSESSED	DATA
Pulmonary artery	
Systolic	24
Diastolic	12
Mean	16
Pulmonary artery wedge	
a wave	16
v wave	12
Mean	10
Cardiac output	6.2 L/min
	3.7 L/min/m^2
LV	
End-diastolic volume	285 mL; 169 mL/m^2
End-systolic volume	116 mL; 69 mL/m^2
Ejection fraction	0.59
AR	4+

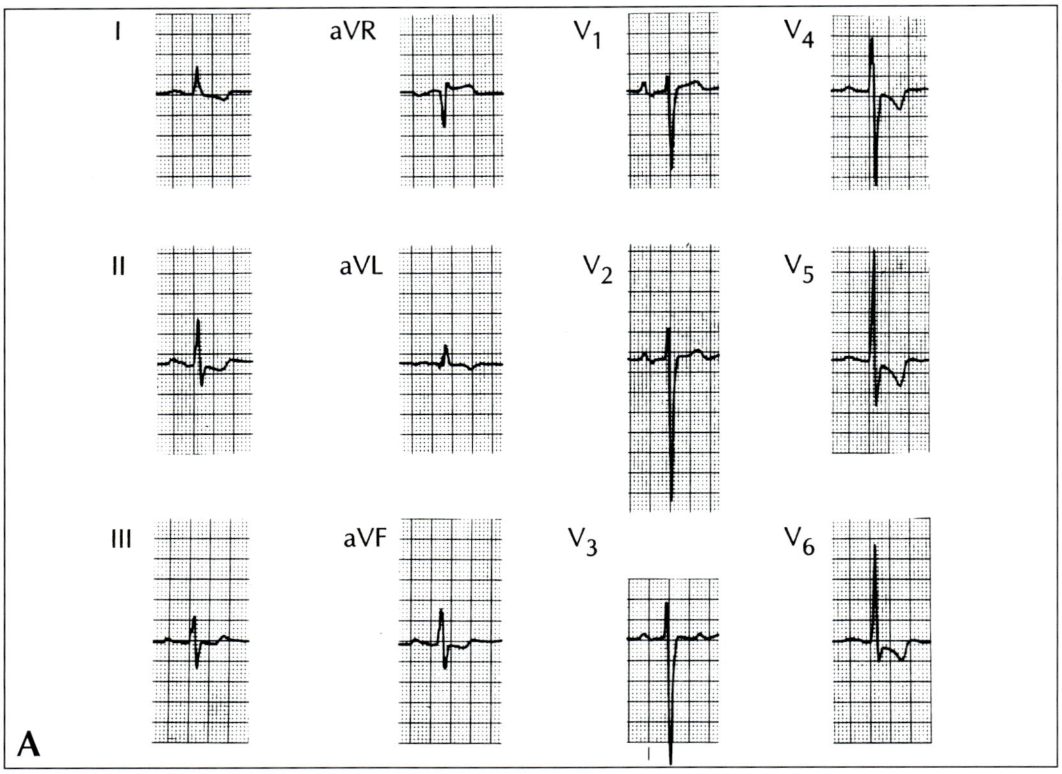

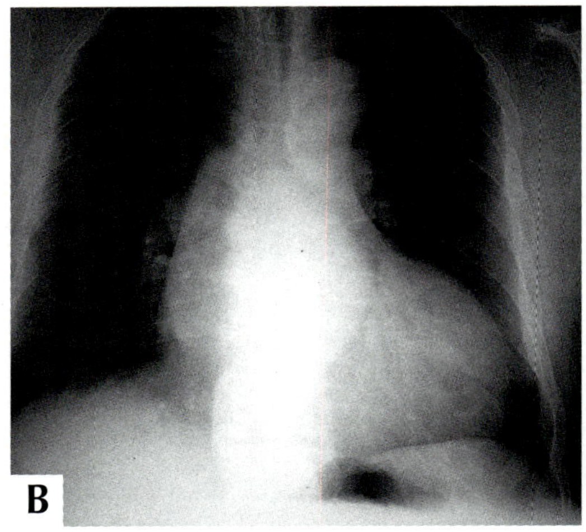

C. DOPPLER ULTRASOUND DATA IN A 61-YEAR-OLD PATIENT

AREA ASSESSED	DATA
LV	
End-diastolic dimension, *mm*	61
End-systolic dimension, *mm*	53
Fractional shortening, *%*	19
E-point septal separation, *mm*	16
Interventricular septal thickness, *mm*	13
Posterior wall thickness, *mm*	13
LV Wall motion	abnormal
Aortic valve	Thickened valve, partly calcified with preserved cusp motion; AR 3+
Left atrium, *mm*	50
Ascending aorta, *mm*	50

FIGURE 7-28. Electrocardiographic (ECG), chest radiographic, Doppler ultrasound, and hemodynamic and left ventricular (LV) function data from a 61-year-old man who was asymptomatic and not known to have cardiac disease. Two months before hospital admission, he started to notice shortness of breath on exertion. A few days before admission he was admitted to another hospital in acute pulmonary edema with sinus rhythm and was treated with digitalis, diuretics, and vasodilators. He improved considerably and was transferred to our hospital. He was New York Heart Association functional class III.

A, The ECG shows LV hypertrophy with ST depression and T-wave inversion. The P wave was wide (0.16 s), and there was first-degree atrioventricular block (PR is 0.24 s). **B,** Considerable cardiomegaly is demonstrated on the chest radiograph (cardiothoracic ratio 0.67), and there was left atrial enlargement, a dilated ascending aorta, and a prominent aortic knob. The pulmonary vasculature shows pulmonary congestion, interstitial edema at the bases, and some fluid in the minor fissure. **C,** Doppler ultrasound findings included dilated LV with reduced motion function and thickened walls. The aortic valve was thickened and calcified, and there was 4+ AR. The left atrium and aorta were dilated. (*continued*)

D. HEMODYNAMIC DATA IN A 61-YEAR-OLD PATIENT

AREA ASSESSED	DATA
Pressures, *mm Hg*	
Right atrium	
a wave	6
v wave	5
Mean	4
Right ventricle	
(Systolic/diastolic—end-diastolic)	40/2–6
Pulmonary artery	
Systolic	40
Diastolic	20
Mean	26
Pulmonary artery wedge	
a wave	24
v wave	36
Mean	22
LV	
(Systolic/diastolic—end-diastolic)	150/0–20
Ascending aorta	
Systolic	150
Diastolic	64
Mean	96
Cardiac output (Fick)	3.4 L/min 1.8 L/min/m^2
LV	
End-diastolic volume	333 mL; 178 mL/m^2
End-systolic volume	187 mL; 100 mL/m^2
Ejection fraction	0.43
Aortic regurgitation	4+
Mitral regurgitation	1+
Coronary arteriography	Normal coronary arteries Left dominant system L main: Normal LAD: Proximal luminal irregularities Cx: Obtuse marginal 1, a large vessel with 70% proximal stenosis Distal Cx totally occluded RCA: Normal

FIGURE 7-28. (*continued*) **D,** Hemodynamic data: the LV end-diastolic pressure and pulmonary artery wedge pressure were elevated. The ascending aortic pressures indicated systolic hypertension and wide pulse pressure. The cardiac index was reduced. The LV was considerably dilated and there was abnormal LV systolic pump function. The severity of AR was 4+, and mitral regurgitation measured 1+. There was also single-vessel coronary artery disease involving the left circumflex (Cx) coronary artery system.

This is a patient with isolated, severe chronic AR, the etiology likely being a congenitally abnormal valve. The LV is large and there is mild systolic pump dysfunction (ejection fraction 0.43). Although the patient is out of frank pulmonary edema, the LV filling pressures are elevated and the chest radiograph indicates milder forms of pulmonary edema, and there is LV systolic pump dysfunction. The patient needs aortic valve replacement on an urgent basis and single-vessel coronary bypass surgery. LAD—left anterior descending; RCA—right coronary artery.

SENSITIVITY AND SPECIFICITY OF AR DIAGNOSIS

Perform complete clinical evaluation
- History
- Physical examination
- Electrocardiogram
- Chest radiograph

Diagnose and assess severity of disease
- All valves
- Ventricular function
- Hemodynamic effects
- Coronary artery disease
- Other cardiovascular disease

Effects on other body organs
- Other organ diseases

List questions that need answering

Be reasonably certain these questions need to be answered

Perform test(s) most likely to provide these answers in one's own institution with the following criteria:
- Reliably
- Accurately
- Lowest risk to patient
- Reasonable (or lowest) cost

Review results of test(s)

Make an overall assessment of patient

Make recommendations regarding management

FIGURE 7-29. Steps involved in clinical decision making in patients with AR [23]. The first step is a complete clinical evaluation that includes history, physical examination, electrocardiogram, and chest radiograph. At the end of the clinical evaluation, the severity of disease of all cardiac valves, ventricular function, hemodynamic effects, coronary artery disease, other cardiovascular disease, as well as disease of other organs must be diagnosed and assessed. Before proceeding to additional testing, it is important to list the question(s) that must be answered and to be reasonably certain that these questions need to be answered. Tests that are most likely to provide these answers in *one's own institution* are then performed, with the following criteria being kept in mind: reliability, accuracy, lowest risk to the patient, and reasonable (lowest) cost. The test results are then reviewed as they become available and an overall evaluation and assessment of the patient is made. Finally, recommendations regarding management are made. (*Adapted from* Rahimtoola [23].)

CLINICAL DECISION MAKING IN AR

VARIABLE STUDIED	AFTER CLINICAL EVALUATION, %	AFTER DOPPLER ULTRASOUND EVALUATION, %
Diagnosis of AR		
Sensitivity	66	79
Specificity	76	74
Accuracy of diagnosis		
Including severity	43	57
Moderate or severe AR	91	100

FIGURE 7-30. Sensitivity and specificity of AR diagnosis. In a prospective blinded study of patients with valvular heart disease, the sensitivity and specificity of diagnosing AR after clinical evaluation were 66% and 76%, respectively [24]. After Doppler ultrasound, the sensitivity and specificity of diagnosing AR were 79% and 74%, respectively. In addition to merely diagnosing AR, if one includes the accuracy of assessing the severity of AR, then the accuracy of clinical evaluation is 43% and that of Doppler ultrasound is 57%. If one demanded only that one diagnose AR and determine whether it is moderate or severe, then both clinical evaluation and Doppler ultrasound improve markedly; the accuracy was 91% and 100%, respectively. Several conclusions can be drawn from this study: 1) The sensitivity and specificity of clinical evaluation and Doppler ultrasound in diagnosing AR are not as high as for aortic stenosis (*see* Chapter 6). 2) The reason for this is that auscultation for the murmur of AR in mild AR may be difficult. On the other hand, Doppler ultrasound findings are frequently diagnostic of mild AR in normal patients. 3) The other difficulty in diagnosis by clinical evaluation and by Doppler ultrasound is being able to separate accurately all patients with moderate AR from those with severe AR. (*Adapted from* Kotlewski and coworkers [24].)

LONG-TERM RESPONSE TO HYDRALAZINE IN 19 SYMPTOMATIC PATIENTS WITH CHRONIC SEVERE AR

	HYDRALAZINE		
	INITIAL	LATE	*P* VALUE
Follow up, *mo*		11±3	
Treadmill time			
(Bruce protocol), *min*	6.3±2.6	7.8±2.8	0.04
Ultrasound			
LV end-diastolic dimension, *mm*	64±12	61±11	
LV end-systolic dimension, *mm*	44±9	42±9	
Fractional shortening, %	31±6	30±7	
Radionuclide ventriculography			
Rest LVEF	0.54±0.12	0.52±0.13	
Exercise LVEF	0.52±0.10	0.49±0.14	
Ascending aortic pressure, *mm Hg*	95±10	86±10	0.006
Cardiac output, *L/min*	4.8±1.1	5.9±1.2	0.0006
Systemic resistance, $dynes \cdot sec \cdot cm^{-5}$	1511±334	1125±218	0.00007
LV function at angiography			
EDVI, mL/m^2	161±64	174±60	
ESVI, mLm^2	76±45	78±48	
Ejection fraction	0.55±0.13	0.59±0.17	

FIGURE 7-31. Response to hydralazine. In moderate and severely *symptomatic* patients with chronic severe AR, an arterial dilator, hydralazine, reduced pulmonary artery wedge pressure at rest, increased stroke volume index and cardiac index, and reduced systemic vascular resistance [25]. On exercise, there was a reduction of mean arterial pulmonary artery wedge pressures, an increase of cardiac index, and a reduction of systemic vascular resistance [25]. These beneficial effects were the result of reduction of regurgitant volume, regurgitant fraction, and left ventricular (LV) end-diastolic and end-systolic volumes; there was a small increase in LV ejection fraction (LVEF) [25]. As a consequence of these findings, it became important to evaluate the role of long-term arterial dilator therapy in patients with chronic severe AR [25].

Shown here are the results in symptomatic patients with chronic severe AR of long-term (11 months) maximum-dose hydralazine therapy in addition to digitalis plus diuretic therapy [23]. An improvement in exercise capacity was associated with increased cardiac output and reduced arterial pressure and systemic vascular resistance. There were no significant changes in echocardiographic LV dimensions or fractional shortening, radionucleotide LVEF at rest and during exercise, and LV volumes and LVEF calculated from contrast ventriculography. However, analysis of individual patient data showed that major benefits in exercise capacity and cardiac output were present in 37% of patients and that major reductions in LV volume and LVEF were present in only 21% of patients. Furthermore, these beneficial effects could not be predicted from the baseline clinical, hemodynamic, exercise, or LV function data. These findings, combined with the known beneficial effects of valve replacement (*see* Figs. 7-35 through 7-39) suggest that long-term hydralazine therapy is of limited value in most patients with symptomatic severe AR who are candidates for valve surgery. Valves are mean ± standard deviation. EDVI—end-diastolic volume index; ESVI—end-systolic volume index. (*Adapted from* Rahimtoola [23].)

LONG-TERM VASODILATOR THERAPY IN CHRONIC AR

	HYDRALAZINE (2-Y STUDY), %	NIFEDIPINE (1-Y STUDY), %
Decrease of SBP	NS	13
Decrease of LVEDVI		
1 y	NS	19
2 y	14	—
Increase of LVEF		
1 y	0.028	0.12
2 y	0.028	—
Decrease of LV mass	—	19
Discontinued therapy	33	3
Completed trial	46	97

FIGURE 7-32. Long-term vasodilator therapy. Two prospective, randomized, double-blind, controlled studies in asymptomatic patients have compared hydralazine with placebo and nifedipine with placebo in 80 and 72 patients, respectively. The hydralazine study was of 2 years' duration and included patients with normal left ventricular (LV) systolic function, patients with moderate and severe AR, as well as asymptomatic and minimally symptomatic patients [26]. The nifedipine study was a 1-year study and included only asymptomatic patients with normal LV systolic function [27]. Interestingly, the hydralazine study did not show a significant decrease of systolic blood pressure (SBP), whereas the nifedipine study showed an SBP reduction of 13%. There was a 14% reduction in LV end-diastolic volume index (LVEDVI) with hydralazine at the end of 2 years, but the change at 1 year was not statistically significant. The nifedipine study showed a 19% reduction in LVEDVI at the end of 1 year. The hydralazine study showed an increase of LV ejection fraction (LVEF) at the end of 1 year by 0.028, whereas the nifedipine study showed an increase of LVEF by 0.12. The nifedipine study showed a 19% decrease in LV mass. A possible reason for the greater beneficial effects of nifedipine was that 33% of the hydralazine-treated patients discontinued therapy and only 46% completed the trial. On the other hand, only 3% of the patients on nifedipine discontinued therapy and 97% completed the trial. NS—not statistically significant. (*Adapted from* Greenberg and coworkers [26] and Scognamiglio and coworkers [27].)

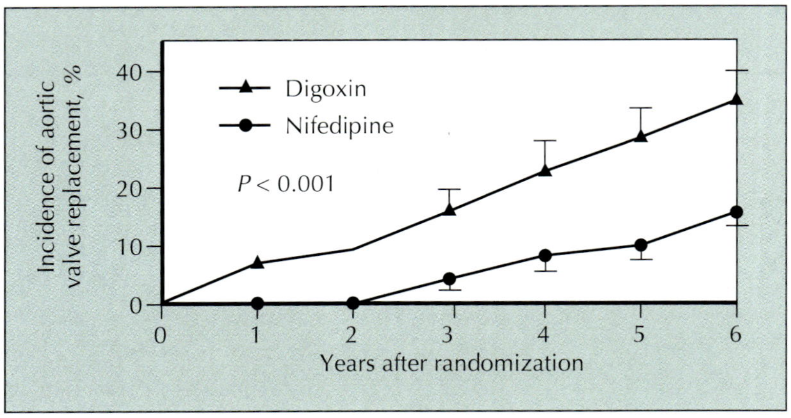

FIGURE 7-33. Long-term nifedipine therapy. The role of *long-term* slow-release nifedipine therapy in *asymptomatic* patients with severe AR and normal left ventricular (LV) systolic pump function was evaluated in 143 asymptomatic patients in a prospective randomized trial. The patients were followed at 6-month intervals. By actuarial analysis, at 6 years, 34±6% of patients in the digoxin group underwent valve replacement versus 15±3% of those in the nifedipine group [28]. In the digoxin group, aortic valve replacement (AVR) was performed in 20 patients because of LV systolic dysfunction (ejection fraction less than 0.50) in 75%, LV systolic dysfunction plus symptoms in 10%, and symptoms in 15%. In the nifedipine group, all six patients underwent AVR because of development of LV dysfunction. In addition, all 26 patients who underwent AVR also had an increase in LV end-diastolic volume index of at least 15%.

This randomized trial demonstrates that long-term vasodilator therapy with nifedipine reduces or delays the need for AVR in asymptomatic patients with severe AR and normal LV systolic pump function. Slow-release nifedipine therapy should be used in all such patients unless there is a specific contraindication to such therapy. (*Adapted from* Scognamiglio and coworkers [28].)

RESULTS OF AORTIC VALVE REPLACEMENT

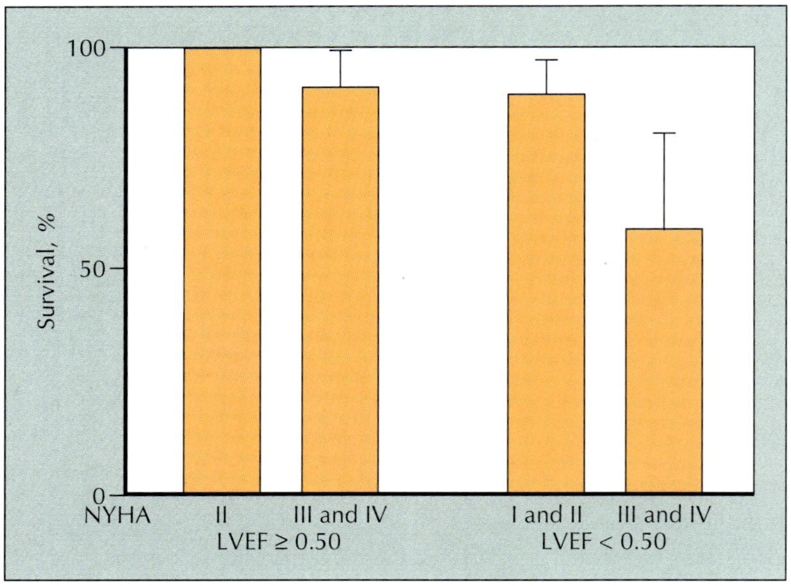

FIGURE 7-34. Five-year survival rates after aortic valve replacement (AVR). The 5-year survival after AVR for chronic severe AR is determined by the state of left ventricular (LV) systolic pump function and the New York Heart Association (NYHA) functional class of the patient [29]. The 5-year survival rates in patients with normal LV systolic pump function (LV ejection fraction [LVEF] 0.50 or greater), who were in NYHA functional class II or III/IV, were 100% and 90%, respectively. In those with abnormal LV systolic pump function (LVEF less than 0.50) who are either asymptomatic or minimally symptomatic (NYHA classes I and II), the 5-year survival rate was 88%. The 5-year survival rates in these three subgroups were not statistically significantly different. Only patients who had reduced LVEF and were moderately or severely symptomatic (NYHA classes III and IV) had a lower 5-year survival of 63%. (*Adapted from* Greves and coworkers [29].)

EFFECT OF AVR ON LV FUNCTION IN PATIENTS WITH AR

	NORMAL VALVE	BEFORE AVR	AFTER AVR, *Y*	
			1.6±0.5	8.1±2.9
LVEDVI, *mL/m²*	93±14	225±49	123±36	111±53
LVESVI, *mL/m²*	31±9	99±35	51±30	46±47
LVEF, %*	67±7	57±11	61±9	64±14
LV muscle mass index, *g/m²*	85±9	191±36	128±29	113±35

*Changes not statistically significant.

FIGURE 7-35. Effect of aortic valve replacement (AVR) in patients with normal left ventricular (LV) systolic function who had undergone successful AVR and were restudied at an average of 1.6 and 8.1 years after surgery [30]. There is a marked reduction in LV end-diastolic and end-systolic volume indices (LVEDVI and LVESVI) and a marked reduction in LV hypertrophy (mass) at an average of 1.6 years after AVR. Interestingly, LV end-diastolic volume and LV mass undergo further slow reductions on late follow-up (up to an average of 8.1 years) after AVR, provided that LV systolic pump function was normal preoperatively [31]. Because LV ejection fraction (LVEF) was normal preoperatively and the postoperative change was small, the increases in LVEF were not statistically significant. (*Adapted from* Monrad and coworkers [30].)

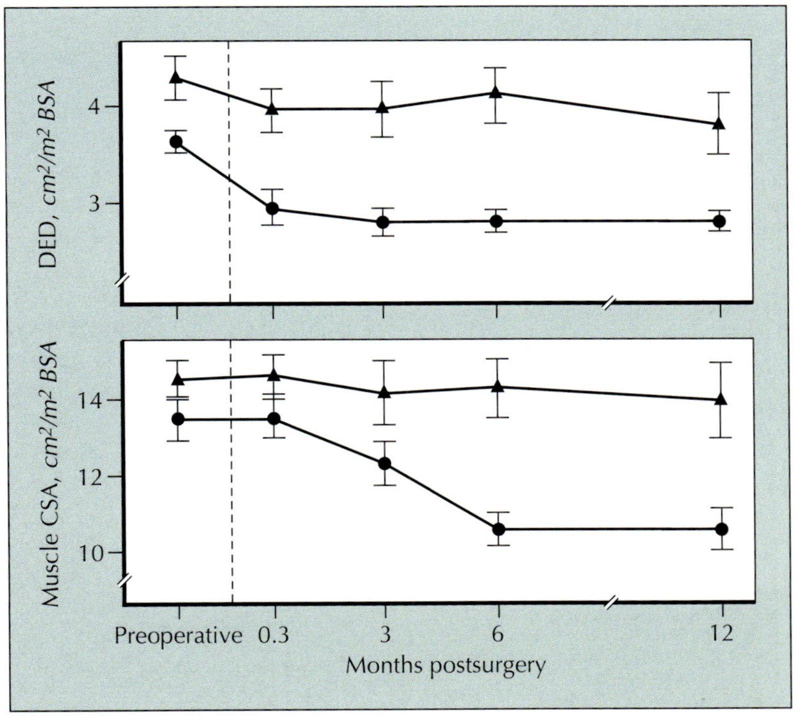

FIGURE 7-36. Aortic valve replacement (AVR) and systolic pump function. This study demonstrates that patients who underwent AVR and had normal left ventricular (LV) systolic pump function (fractional shortening on M-mode echocardiography of 34±6%; *circles*) had less LV dilatation and hypertrophy [32]. Furthermore, after AVR, they had a rapid reduction in LV dimension and hypertrophy regressed progressively over a 6-month period. In contrast, patients who had abnormal LV systolic pump function (fractional shortening of 27±6%; *triangles*) had larger LV dimensions and greater degree of LV hypertrophy preoperatively. Furthermore, after AVR, over a 12-month period there were no significant reductions in either LV dimension or LV hypertrophy (mass). BSA—body surface area; CSA—cross sectional area; DED—end-diastolic dimension.(*Adapted from* Gaasch and coworkers [32].)

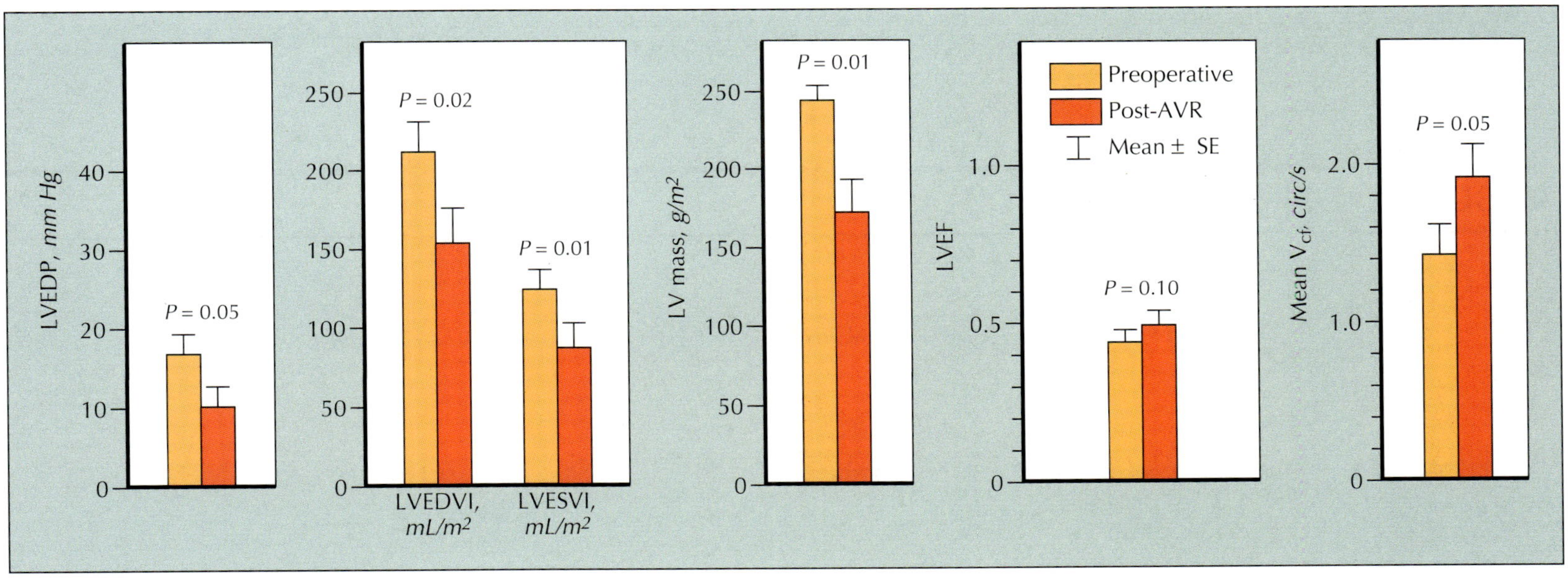

FIGURE 7-37. Effects of aortic valve replacement (AVR) on severe AR and left ventricular (LV) dysfunction. Patients who have abnormal LV systolic pump function undergo important changes in LV size and function over a 2-year period [33]. These patients had significant reductions in LV end-diastolic pressure (LVEDP), LV end-diastolic and end-systolic volume indices (LVEDVI and LVESVI) and LV hypertrophy (mass). LV systolic pump function was improved as demonstrated by increases in mean velocity of circumferential fiber (V_{cf}) shortening; however, LV ejection fraction (LVEF) in this study increased mildly and this change was not statistically significant.

However, it appears that these patients have no further changes in LV size, hypertrophy [31], or LVEF, which is different from those who have normal LV systolic function preoperatively (*see* Figs. 7-36 and 7-39). circ—circumferences. (*Adapted from* Clark and coworkers [33].)

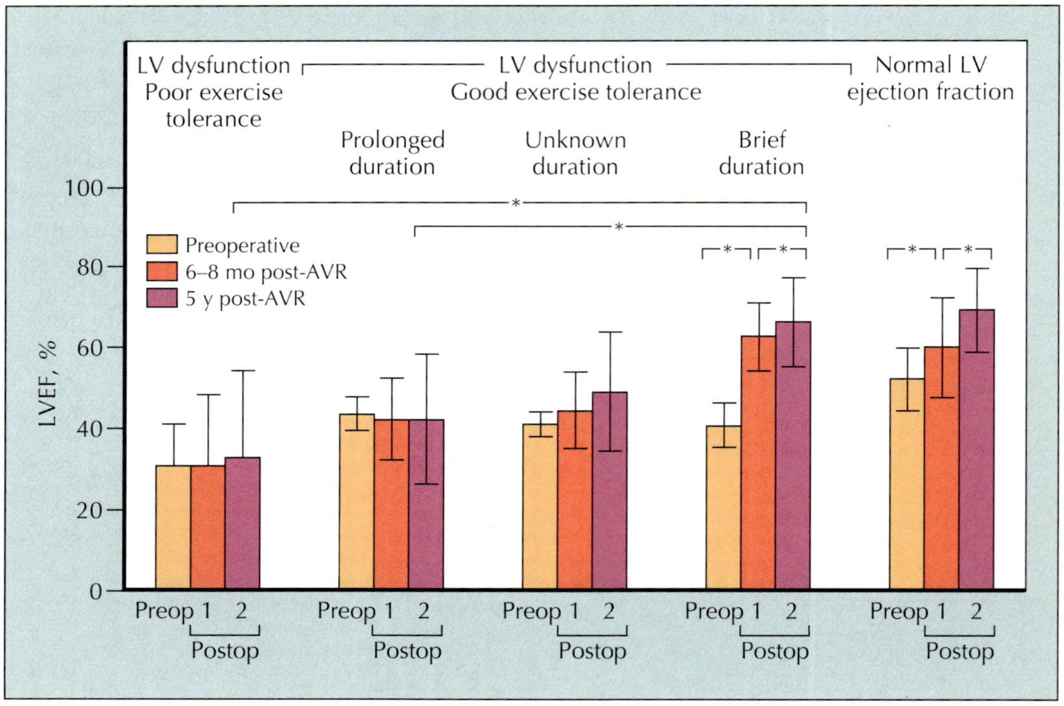

FIGURE 7-38. Left ventricular (LV) function, exercise tolerance, and aortic valve replacement (AVR). This important study by Bonow *et al.* [31] from the National Institutes of Health showed that patients who have normal LV ejection fractions (LVEF) preoperatively show an improvement in LVEF at the end of 6 to 8 months after AVR and have further improvement in LVEF at an average of 5 years after AVR. At the other extreme, patients with LV dysfunction who have poor exercise tolerance have no improvement of LVEF either early or late after AVR. Patients with LV dysfunction and good exercise tolerance are shown in the center of the figure. As long as the LV dysfunction was of brief duration (less than 12 to 14 months) before AVR, LVEF normalized and improved to the same levels as in those patients who had normal LVEF preoperatively. Patients who had LV dysfunction of prolonged duration (more than 12 to 14 months) had no significant change in LVEF either early or late after AVR.

The implication of this study is that patients who are asymptomatic with normal LV function should have a follow-up assessment of symptoms and of LV systolic pump function at a minimum of every 12 months. The actual frequency of follow-up should be partly dependent on the time lag after LV dysfunction or symptoms are discovered. *Asterisks* denote significant differences. *T-bars* indicate ± SEM. (*Adapted from* Bonow and coworkers [31]; with permission.)

ASSOCIATED CORONARY ARTERY DISEASE

ISOLATED AORTIC VALVE REPLACEMENT: INCIDENCE OF ASSOCIATED CAD

	VA COOPERATIVE STUDY [34]	MAYO CLINIC	MGH
Total patients, *n*	643	618	64
CAD patients, *n*	312	321	37
Patients with CAD, %	49	52	58
1VD	17	22	27
2VD	17	14	19
3VD	15	17	13
Additional LMCAD, %	—	5	3

FIGURE 7-39. Incidence of coronary artery disease (CAD). Two large studies, the Veterans Administration (VA) Cooperative Study [34] and the Mayo Clinic data [35], showed that the incidence of associated CAD was approximately 50%. About one third of the patients with obstructive CAD had single-vessel disease (1VD), another third had two-vessel disease (2VD), and a third had three-vessel disease (3VD). Data from Massachusetts General Hospital (MGH) [36] indicate that in patients 80 to 89 years of age the incidence of associated CAD was 58%. Additional left main CAD (LMCAD) was present in 3% to 5% of the patients. (*Adapted from* Sethi and coworkers [34]; Mullany and coworkers [35]; and Levinson and coworkers [36].)

EFFECT OF CBS AND AVR ON OPERATIVE MORTALITY AND LATE SURVIVAL

	1982–1983	1967–1976					
				INCIDENCE OF ASSOCIATED CAD, %			
	OPERATIVE MORTALITY, %	OPERATIVE MORTALITY, %	ALL PATIENTS,%*	1VD	2VD	3VD	LMCAD
AVR + no CAD	1.4	4.5	63	—	—	—	—
AVR + CAD + CBS	4.0	6.3	49	38	28	34	11
AVR + CAD + no CBS	9.4	10.3	36	65	22	13	1

* 10-y survival, %

FIGURE 7-40. Operative mortality and late survival. Data of Mullany *et al.* [35] indicate that the operative mortality in patients undergoing aortic valve replacement (AVR) if they had no coronary artery disease (CAD), was 1.4%; this was increased to 4% if the patients had CAD and underwent coronary bypass surgery (CBS). On the other hand if they had associated CAD and had no CBS performed at the time of AVR, operative mortality increased markedly to 9.4%.

Examination of the 10-year survival in patients who had undergone AVR from 1967 to 1976 indicates that the best survival was in patients who had no associated CAD. However, those who had associated CAD and underwent CBS had a better 10-year survival than those who did not undergo CBS for CAD. It should be noted that patients who had CBS in addition to AVR had 45% incidence of either three-vessel coronary artery disease (3VD) or left main coronary artery disease (LMCAD), whereas in patients who did not undergo CBS, 65% had one-vessel disease (1VD). Thus, if the patients who had undergone CBS had in fact not undergone CBS, their 10-year survival without CBS would have been expected to be much lower than those who in fact did not undergo CBS in this study.

In view of this, it becomes imperative that the patients who have significantly obstructive CAD must undergo CBS at the same time as AVR. Therefore, an issue that has to be considered is who should undergo coronary arteriography before AVR. 2VD—two-vessel disease. (*Adapted from* Rahimtoola [23] and Mullany and coworkers [35].)

INDICATIONS FOR CORONARY ARTERIOGRAPHY BEFORE VALVE SURGERY

Patients ≥ 35 y
Patients < 35 y
- Left ventricular dysfunction
- Symptoms or signs suggesting CAD
- One or more risk factors for premature CAD (excluding gender)

FIGURE 7-41. Suggested indications for coronary arteriography before valve surgery [23]. All patients 35 years of age and over should undergo coronary arteriography before aortic valve surgery. In patients under the age of 35 years, coronary arteriography should be performed if they have left ventricular dysfunction or signs or symptoms that suggest the presence of associated coronary artery disease (CAD), or if they have one or more risk factors for premature CAD (excluding gender). (*Adapted from* Rahimtoola [23].)

MEDICAL TREATMENT OF AR

- Antibiotic prophylaxis
  - Infective endocarditis
  - Recurrent rheumatic carditis
- Restrict activities (moderate/severe AR)
  - Severe exercise
  - Competitive sports
- Arrhythmias
  - Prevent or control
  - Restore sinus rhythm, if possible
- Cardiac medications
  - Asymptomatic
    - Mild AR: None
    - Moderate AR: ? Nifedipine
    - Severe AR: Nifedipine
  - Severe AR symptomatic (while waiting for surgery)
    - Normal LV function: Nifedipine
    - LV dysfunction:
    - Digitalis
    - Hydralazine ± nitrates
    - Diuretics, if needed
  - Severe AR plus heart failure
    - Digitalis, diuretics
    - Hydralazine + nitrates
    - IV nitroprusside, if IV therapy needed
- Follow-up
  - Mild AR: Every 2–5 y
  - Moderate AR: Every 1–2 y
  - Severe AR: Every 6–12 mo
  - Develop symptoms: Early or "immediate"

FIGURE 7-42. Medical treatment of AR. All patients need antibiotic prophylaxis for the prevention of infective endocarditis; those with rheumatic valve disease should also receive it for prevention of recurrences of rheumatic carditis. Patients with mild AR do not need to have their activities restricted. Those with moderate and severe AR should ideally have their activities restricted, *ie*, they should not undertake severe or vigorous exercise and competitive sports. Arrhythmias should be prevented if possible, particularly tachy- and bradyarrhythmias. Atrial fibrillation is usually a result of associated mitral valve disease or left ventricular dysfunction. Restoration of sinus rhythm should be a priority.

In general, cardiac medications should only be used if there are specific indications for their use. The asymptomatic patient with mild AR requires no specific therapy. Patients with severe AR and normal left ventricular (LV) ejection fraction should receive slow-release nifedipine therapy (*see* Figs. 7-32 and 7-33). Although not studied specifically at this time, in view of the very favorable results with slow-release nifedipine therapy in severe AR, consideration should be given to using nifedipine therapy in patients with moderate AR and a moderately dilated LV.

Patients with severe AR who are symptomatic should undergo aortic valve replacement. While waiting for surgery, it would be reasonable to treat patients who have normal LV function with nifedipine; those who have LV dysfunction should receive digitalis [37], diuretics if needed, and vasodilators. In those who have abnormal LV systolic function, hydralazine could be used (*see* Fig. 7-31). Large doses of hydralazine (more than 100 mg twice daily) are needed in AR [38]. If the patient also has elevations of left atrial pressure, sublingual nitrates could be combined with the hydralazine therapy.

Patients with severe AR who are also in heart failure need digitalis, a diuretic, and vasodilators. For oral vasodilator therapy, a combination of hydralazine and nitrates is recommended in those who have abnormal LV systolic function. However, if the hemodynamic abnormalities are moderate or severe, intravenous (IV) vasodilator therapy may be needed; and in that instance, nitroprusside is the drug of choice.

In patients with AR, follow-up should include clinical evaluation (history, physical examination, electrocardiogram, chest radiograph) and Doppler ultrasound with quantitative assessment of LV size and function. Patients with mild AR should have follow-up every 2 to 5 years. Patients with moderate AR should have follow-up every 1 to 2 years. Those with severe AR should have follow-up every 6 to 12 months (*see* Figs. 7-33 and 7-38). Patients who develop symptoms that are related to AR should have an early or "immediate" follow-up visit.

INDICATIONS FOR VALVE REPLACEMENT/VALVE REPAIR IN CHRONIC SEVERE AR

SYMPTOMATIC PATIENTS

LV function normal: as soon as possible
LV dysfunction: urgent
Heart failure: emergent
Individualize if:
  Very severe LV dysfunction (LVEF ≤0.20)
  Severe LV dilatation (LVEDD ≥80 mm; LVEDVI ≥ 300 mL/m^2)
  Small R_gV (R_gV/EDV ≤0.14)

ASYMPTOMATIC PATIENTS

LV dysfunction (LVEF ≤0.50)
Normal LV function
  Associated severe obstructive CAD
  Other valve disease needing cardiac surgery
  Any of the following (Additional testing needed):
    LVEDD ≥70 mm
    LVESD ≥50 mm
    LVEDVI ≥150 mL/m^2 *plus* PAWP on exercise ≥20 mm Hg

FIGURE 7-43. Indications for valve repair or replacement. Symptomatic patients with chronic severe AR are candidates for valve replacement. At the present time, various forms of valve repair appear to have encouraging early results. Symptomatic patients with severe AR should have valve surgery unless there is a specific contraindication to its performance. The urgency of surgery depends on the state of left ventricular (LV) function and severity of symptoms. For example, if there is LV dysfunction the procedure is urgent; and in selected patients with heart failure, surgery is a relatively emergent procedure. In aortic stenosis there is no lower level of LV ejection fraction (LVEF) at which the patient becomes inoperable; indeed the lower the LVEF the more urgent the need for valve surgery (*see* Chapter 6). However, in AR there comes a time when valve surgery is associated with a much higher operative mortality and the postoperative results are not very satisfactory. The precise level at which this occurs has not been well defined. General guidelines are that one should individualize the performance of surgery in the presence of very severe LV dysfunction (LVEF 0.20 or less), in the presence of severe LV dilatation (probably LV end-diastolic dimension [LVEDD] 80 mm or more, or LV end-diastolic volume index [LVEDVI] 300 mL/m^2 or more) [39], and in patients who have a large LV with a small regurgitant volume (R_gV) (the ratio of R_gV to end-diastolic volume [EDV] probably 0.14 or less) [40].

Asymptomatic patients with severe chronic AR should undergo valve surgery in the presence of LV dysfunction (LVEF less than 0.50). In those with normal LV function, surgery is recommended in the presence of associated severe obstructive coronary artery disease that needs to be bypassed or if the patient is undergoing cardiac surgery for any other valve disease. In others, it is prudent to follow patients with changes in LV size and function. LVEDD on M-mode echocardiography of 70 mm or more, LV end-systolic dimension (LVESD) of 50 mm or greater, or LVEDVI of at least 150 mL/m^2 are markers of subsequent higher incidence of an adverse event, *ie*, these patients are at significant risk of developing symptoms or developing LV systolic dysfunction over the next 5-year period. Therefore, it is recommended that such patients should have an exercise study with a right heart balloon flotation catheter; if the pulmonary artery wedge pressure (PAWP) on exercise is 20 mm Hg or more, serious consideration should be given to undertaking valve surgery provided there is experience and skill in performing valve surgery at an acceptable and low risk at the institution where the procedure is to be performed.

REFERENCES

1. Rahimtoola SH: Recognition and management of acute aortic regurgitation. *Heart Disease and Stroke* 1993, 2:217–221.
2. Braunwald E: Valvular heart disease. In *Heart Disease*, edn 5. Edited by Braunwald E. Philadelphia: WB Saunders; 1997:1007–1076.
3. Rahimtoola SH: Valvular heart disease. In *Internal Medicine*, edn 4. Edited by Stein J (Cardiology Section edited by O'Rourke RA). St. Louis: Mosby-Year Book; 1994:202–234.
4. Rahimtoola SH: Management of heart failure in valve regurgitation. *Clin Cardiol* 1992, 15(suppl I):22–27.
5. DeMots H, Rahimtoola SH, McAnulty JH, Murphy ES: Pulmonary edema. In *Cardiac Emergencies*. Edited by Mason DT. Baltimore: Williams & Wilkins; 1978:173–223.
6. Nienaber CA, von Kodolitsch Y, Nicholas V, *et al.*: The diagnosis of thoracic aortic dissection by noninvasive imaging procedures. *N Engl J Med* 1993, 328:1–9.
7. Cigarroa JE, Isselbacher EM, De Sanctis RW, Eagle KA: Diagnostic imaging in the evaluation of suspected aortic dissection: old standards and new directions. *N Engl J Med* 1993, 328:35–43.
8. Kostuk W, Barr JW, Simon AL, Ross J Jr: Correlations between the chest film and hemodynamics in acute myocardial infarction. *Circulation* 1973, 48:624–632.
9. Kiely J, Kelly DT, Taylor DR, Pitt B: The role of furosemide in the treatment of left ventricular dysfunction associated with acute myocardial infarction. *Circulation* 1973, 48:581–587.
10. Chatterjee K, Parmley WW, Swan HJC, *et al.*: Beneficial effects of vasodilator agents in severe mitral regurgitation due to dysfunction of subvalvular apparatus. *Circulation* 1973, 48:684–690.
11. Richardson JV, Karp RB, Kirklin JW, Dismukes WE: Treatment of infective endocarditis: a 10-year comparative analysis. *Circulation* 1978, 58:589–597.
12. Rahimtoola SH: Valvular heart disease: a prospective. *J Am Coll Cardiol* 1983, 1:199–215.
13. Karaian CH, Greenberg BH, Rahimtoola SH: The relationship between functional class and cardiac performance in patients with chronic aortic insufficiency. *Chest* 1985, 88:553–557.
14. Kawanishi DT, McKay CR, Chandraratna PAN: Cardiovascular response to dynamic exercise in patients with chronic symptomatic mild-to-moderate and severe aortic regurgitation. *Circulation* 1986, 73:62–72.

15. Pantely G, Morton MJ, Rahimtoola SH: Effects of successful, uncomplicated valve replacement on ventricular hypertrophy, volume, and performance in aortic stenosis and aortic incompetence. *J Thorac Cardiovasc Surg* 1978, 75:383–391.
16 Ross J Jr: Afterload mismatch and preload reserve: a conceptual framework for the analysis of ventricular function. *Prog Cardiovasc Dis* 1976, 18:255–264.
17. Nittenburg A, Foult JM, Antony I, *et al.*: Coronary flow and resistance reserve in patients with chronic aortic regurgitation, angina pectoris, and normal coronary arteries. *J Am Coll Cardiol* 1988, 11:478–486.
18. Rapaport E: Natural history of aortic and mitral valve disease. *Am J Cardiol* 1975, 35:221–227.
19. McKay CR, Rahimtoola SH: Natural history of aortic regurgitation. In *Chronic Aortic Regurgitation*. Edited by Gaasch WH, Levine HJ, Kluwer Academic Publications; 1980:1–17.
20. Bonow RO, Lakatos E, Maron BJ, Epstein SE: Serial long-term assessment of the natural history of asymptomatic patients with chronic aortic regurgitation and normal left ventricular systolic function. *Circulation* 1991, 84:1625–1635.
21. Siemienczuk D, Greenberg B, Morris C, *et al.*: Chronic aortic insufficiency: factors associated with progression to aortic valve replacement. *Ann Intern Med* 1989, 110:587–592.
22. Schaefer RA, McAnulty JH, Starr A, Rahimtoola SH: Diastolic murmurs in the presence of Starr-Edwards mitral prosthesis: with emphasis on the genesis of the Austin Flint murmur. *Circulation* 1975, 51:402–409.
23. Rahimtoola SH: Perspective on valvular heart disease: update II. In *Era in Cardiovascular Medicine*. Edited by Knoebel S, Dack S. New York: Elsevier Publishing; 1991:45–70.
24. Kotlewski A, Kawanishi DT, McKay CR, *et al.*: The relative value of clinical examination, echocardiography with Doppler and cardiac catheterization with angiography in the evaluation of aortic valve disease. In *Surgery for Heart Valve Disease*. Edited by Bodnar E. London: ICR Publishers; 1990:66–72.
25. Rahimtoola SH: Vasodilator therapy in chronic severe aortic regurgitation. *J Am Coll Cardiol* 1990, 16:430–432.
26. Greenberg B, Massie B, Bristow JD, *et al.*: Long-term vasodilator therapy of chronic aortic insufficiency: a randomized double-blinded, placebo-controlled clinical trial. *Circulation* 1988, 78:92–103.
27. Scognamiglio R, Rasoli G, Ponchia A, Dalla-Volta S: Long-term nifedipine unloading therapy in asymptomatic patients with chronic severe aortic regurgitation. *J Am Coll Cardiol* 1990, 16:424–429.
28. Scognamiglio R, Rahimtoola SH, Fasoli G, *et al.*: Nifedipine in asymptomatic patients with severe aortic regurgitation and normal left ventricular function. *N Engl J Med* 1994, 331:689–694.
29. Greves J, Rahimtoola SH, McAnulty JH, *et al.*: Preoperative criteria predictive of late survival following valve replacement for severe aortic regurgitation. *Am Heart J* 1981, 101:300–308.
30. Monrad ES, Hess OM, Murakami T, *et al.*: Time course of regression of left ventricular hypertrophy after aortic valve replacement. *Circulation* 1988, 77:1345–1355.
31. Bonow RO, Dodd JT, Maron BJ, *et al.*: Long-term serial changes in left ventricular function and reversal of ventricular dilatation after valve replacement for chronic aortic regurgitation. *Circulation* 1988, 78:1108–1120.
32. Gaasch WH, Carroll JD, Levine HJ, Criscitiello MG: Chronic aortic regurgitation: prognostic value of left ventricular end-systolic dimension and end-diastolic radius/thickness ratio. *J Am Coll Cardiol* 1983, 1:775–782.
33. Clark DG, McAnulty JH, Rahimtoola SH: Valve replacement in aortic insufficiency with left ventricular dysfunction. *Circulation* 1980, 61:411–421.
34. Sethi GK, Miller DC, Sonchek J, *et al.*: Clinical, hemodynamic and angiographic predictors of operative mortality in patients undergoing single valve replacement. *J Thorac Cardiovasc Surg* 1987, 93:884–887.
35. Mullany CJ, Elveback ER, Frye RL, *et al.*: Coronary artery disease and its management: influence on survival in patients undergoing aortic valve replacement. *J Am Coll Cardiol* 1987, 10:66–72.
36. Levinson JR, Akins CW, Buckley MJ, *et al.*: Octogenarians with aortic stenosis: outcome after aortic valve replacement. *Circulation* 1989, 80(suppl I):49–56.
37. Crawford MH, Wilson RS, O'Rourke RA, Vittitoe JA: Effect of digoxin and vasodilators on left ventricular function in aortic regurgitation. *Int J Cardiol* 1989, 23:385–393.
38. McKay CR, Nanna M, Kawanishi DT, *et al.*: Importance of internal controls, statistical methods, and side-effects in acute vasodilator trials: a study of hydralazine kinetics in patients with aortic regurgitation. *Circulation* 1985, 72:865–872.
39. Taniguchi K, Nakano S, Hirose H, *et al.*: Preoperative left ventricular function: minimal requirement for successful late results of valve replacement for aortic regurgitation. *J Am Coll Cardiol* 1987, 10:510–518.
40. Levine HJ, Gaasch WH: Ratio of regurgitant volume to end-diastolic volume: a major determinant of ventricular response to surgical correction of chronic volume overload. *Am J Cardiol* 1983, 52:406–410.

MITRAL STENOSIS

8

CHAPTER

David T. Kawanishi and Shahbudin H. Rahimtoola

Mitral stenosis (MS) in adults is almost invariably the late result of rheumatic carditis. Particularly in Western countries, a prior episode of acute rheumatic carditis may have been clinically inapparent or misdiagnosed. Nonetheless, the cause of virtually all MS in young and middle-aged adults is the pathologic process initiated by a bout of rheumatic carditis. The reduction of the effective mitral valve orifice results from a combination of fusion of the commissures and chordae tendineae, retraction of the chordae, and thickening of the leaflets. The leaflets, subvalvular apparatus, and annulus may be calcified. Only certain strains of *Streptococcus* organisms can cause rheumatic fever, which initiates this process. The mitral valve is the most frequently involved valve although the aortic and tricuspid valves may also be affected; each of these valves may become stenotic or regurgitant.

In Western countries, the patient presents with MS after a long period of latency following the episode(s) of rheumatic carditis. This may be due to the slow indolent nature of the pathologic process as well as the hemodynamics of blood flow through stenotic orifices in which significant narrowing must occur before flow rates change appreciably and a pressure gradient develops. However, the clinical presentation may be precipitated earlier by physiologic or pathologic conditions associated with increased flow rates or reduced diastolic filling times. For example, pregnancy, exercise, atrial fibrillation with rapid ventricular rate, fever, and hyperthyroidism are common settings for the initial presentation of MS. In less developed areas of the world, MS develops more rapidly after the initial episode of rheumatic carditis.

The symptoms and signs of MS result from an elevated pulmonary venous pressure, which is a consequence of the increased left atrial pressure upstream from the stenotic mitral valve. A reduced cardiac output may also contribute to the initial clinical presentation. When pulmonary arterial hypertension is sustained and severe or when tricuspid regurgitation develops, the signs of right heart failure may be present. The diagnosis of MS is usually easily made by clinical evaluation of the patient (history, physical examination, electrocardiography, and chest radiography); Doppler ultrasound is the most useful noninvasive test.

The patient with severe MS usually obtains marked symptom relief by maneuvers aimed at reducing left atrial–pulmonary venous pressures. Patients with severe MS need interventional therapy, either catheter balloon commissurotomy, surgical valve repair, or valve replacement. If the valve is mobile and nonthickened, then catheter balloon commissurotomy is the procedure of choice in centers with skill and experience; otherwise, open surgical commissurotomy or valve repair is the procedure of choice. If the valve is not suitable for repair, valve replacement is performed.

Etiology and Pathophysiology

CAUSES OF MS

CAUSE	INVOLVED STRUCTURE(S): LEAFLET	CHORDAE	COMMISSURES	OTHER
Rheumatic fever	+	+	+	
Congenital	+	+		Single papillary muscle
Active infective endocarditis	+			Vegetation
Neoplasm				Mass, pulmonary vein obstruction
Massive annular calcification	+	0	0	Rigid annulus
Systemic lupus erythematosus	+	+	+	Verrucous vegetations may extend into papillary muscles
Carcinoid tumor				Atrial septal defect or lung tumor to affect left heart
Methysergide therapy	+	+		Serotonin agonist/antagonist
Hunter-Hurler syndromes				Mucopolysaccharide deposits
Fabry's disease				Aramide trihexoxide deposits
Whipple's disease				PAS-positive macrophage deposits
Rheumatoid arthritis	+	+	+	PAS-positive plasma cell infiltrate

Figure 8-1. Causes of mitral stenosis (MS). The most frequent etiology of MS is chronic rheumatic valve disease. In a series of 1414 patients with mitral valves excised at the time of valve replacement between December 1962 and January 1984, 404 had isolated MS [1]. Pathologic examination of 705 stenotic mitral valves in this series, which included multivalve disease, showed the cause to be rheumatic in all [1].

Congenital MS is usually caused by the single papillary muscle syndrome or related conditions in which the entire mitral apparatus is malformed. The mitral leaflets are fibrotic; the chordae tendineae are short and thick, are frequently fewer than normal in number, and are abnormally inserted into the leaflets as well as into the (often single) papillary muscle. Other congenital anomalies may be present; these include bicuspid aortic valve, ventricular septal defect, coarctation of the aorta, and subaortic stenosis [2]. Presentation of hypoplastic and atretic MS is limited to the neonatal period.

Active infective endocarditis produces MS when a large vegetation obstructs the mitral orifice [3]. Obstruction of the mitral orifice or the pulmonary veins may also produce an "MS-like" pathophysiology. The most common tumor is a left atrial myxoma [2,4]. Calcification of the mitral annulus usually results in mitral regurgitation. However, when the calcification is very extensive, it may be associated with stenosis; this has been attributed at least in part to rigidity of the annular ring with minimal leaflet or subvalvular involvement. A mean mitral valve gradient of 18 mm Hg has been reported in association with only 1+ mitral regurgitation [5]. Systemic lupus erythematosus may result in verrucous vegetations on any endocardial surface, but they are most commonly located in the angles of the valve and may extend into the chordae or papillary muscle. The lesions usually do not result in impairment of valve function, but marked scarring during healing may lead to deformity sufficient to require valve replacement [6,7]. MS has also been described in the setting of carcinoid tumor and methysergide therapy, which share in common a higher than normal level of serotonin or serotonin-like substances and a laying down of avascular fibrous tissue on the valve cusps and chordae. Mucopolysaccharidoses of the Hunter-Hurler phenotype, aramide trihexoxide deposition, Fabry's disease, Whipple's disease, and other conditions associated with periodic acid-Schiff (PAS)–positive amyloid-type deposition such as that which occurs rheumatoid arthritis [2] rarely cause MS.

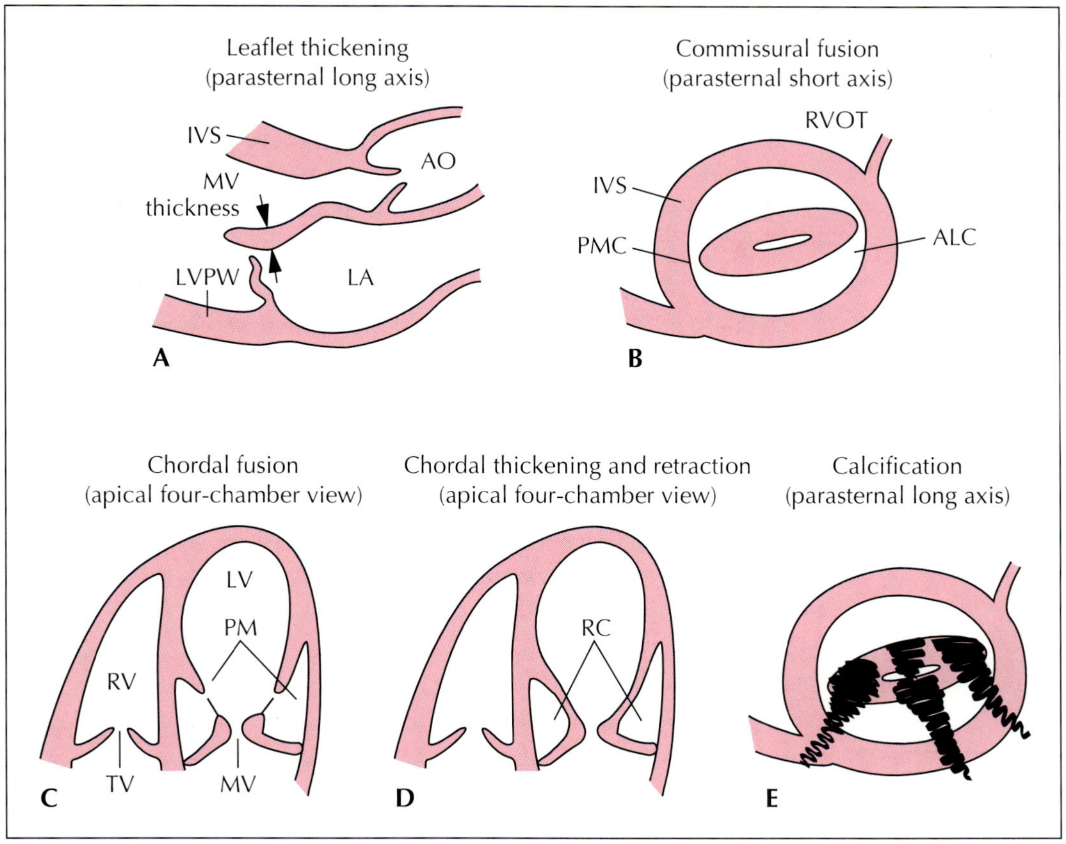

FIGURE 8-2. Morphologic changes in rheumatic MS that are seen on two-dimensional echocardiography [1,8] (*see* Chapter 3). **A,** Increased thickness of the mitral valve (MV), particularly at the tips. In more severe disease the entire valve leaflet is involved. As the thickening and fibrosis involves progressively more of the leaflet, it becomes less pliable and the "doming" of the midportion of the leaflet diminishes progressively. When the valve is rigid, the leaflets may appear to move only a little if at all and the entire leaflet remains straight throughout diastole. **B,** Fusion of the posteromedial commissure (PMC) and the anterolateral commissure (ALC). When the process is more extensive, it may involve the surface of the cusps themselves. **C** and **D,** Subvalvular changes, including fusion of the chordae tendineae and retraction of the chordae (RC); a "thickening" and a "matting together" of all the subvalvular apparatus may occur as the scarring process becomes progressively more extensive. Fusion of otherwise normally mobile structures contributes to a narrowing of the orifice resulting in the commonly described "fish-mouth" or "buttonhole" appearance typically associated with this disorder. **E,** Chronic scarring, calcification of the leaflets, and commissures may occur.

It has been suggested that the fusion process be subdivided into four categories characterized by involvement of 1) commissures, 2) cusps, 3) chordae, and 4) a combination of 1, 2, and 3. The state of pathologic change at the time of disease detection may have implications for the rate of clinical deterioration during subsequent follow-up [9]. AO—aortic outflow tract; IVS—interventricular posterior wall; PM—papillary muscles; RV—right ventricle; RVOT—RV outflow tract; TV—tricuspid valve.

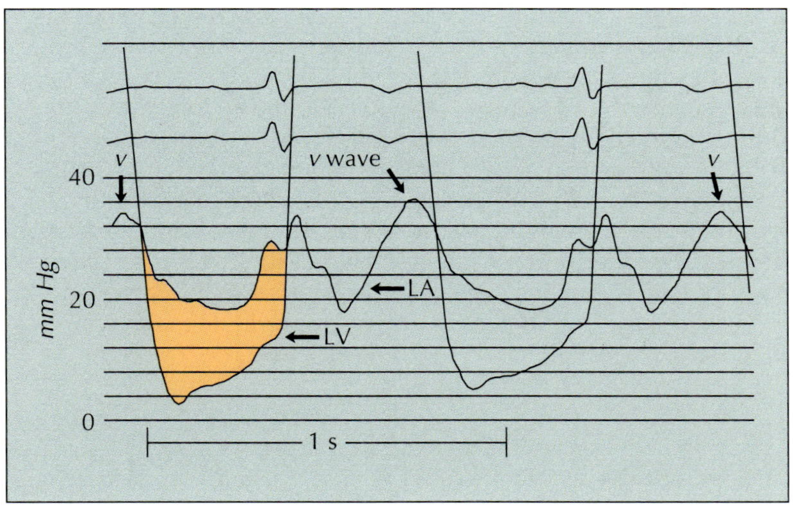

FIGURE 8-3. Simultaneous left atrial (LA) and left ventricular (LV) pressures in a patient with MS illustrate the hemodynamic hallmark of MS, *ie*, a pressure gradient in diastole between the LA and LV (*orange area*). There is a gradient between the LA and LV throughout diastole. The presystolic rise in LA pressure due to atrial systole results in an increase of the pressure gradient between the two chambers. In patients with atrial fibrillation, a similar pressure gradient exists throughout diastole; however, the presystolic rise in the LA pressure recording is not present. Note also that the height of the *v* wave is increased. Overall, the LV diastolic pressure is normal and the mean LA pressure is elevated. With an increase in flow such as that which occurs with exercise, the stenotic mitral valve (MV) is not able to accommodate the increase in volume of flow without an increase of the pressure gradient (*see* Fig. 8-4), which results in an increase of LA pressure with exercise. Typically with severe MS, this elevation of LA pressure may result in severe elevations of systolic pulmonary arterial pressure, often above 70 mm Hg, and occasionally into the systemic range. This is often associated with the decline in exercise tolerance and functional capacity of patients with MS. As the degree of stenosis increases, at any given level of flow across the MV the gradient progressively increases and severe pressure elevations may be present even at rest. In the most severe conditions, the cardiac output may be reduced because this may be the only mechanism left to keep the LA and pulmonary vascular pressures in the tolerable range [10].

Note that because the higher LA pressure crosses the LV pressure tracing at a higher point than normal, a delay in closure of the MV results. This is the reason for the loud S_1. A similar but opposite relationship exists at the beginning of diastole. The higher the LA pressure, the earlier it will exceed LV pressure and the earlier the opening of the MV. This is the reason for the narrowing of the interval between the S_2 and the opening snap (mitral opening sound) with more severe MS.

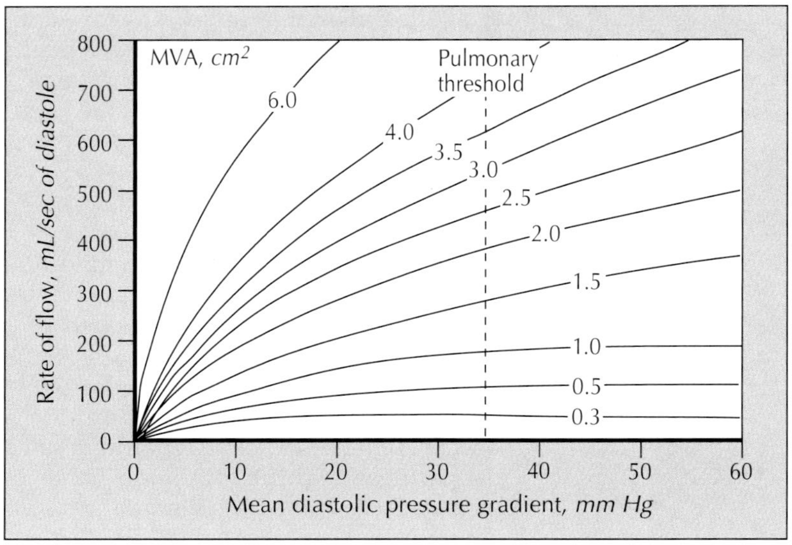

FIGURE 8-4. The relationship of the mean diastolic pressure gradient across the mitral valve as a function of the rate of mitral blood flow for various mitral valve areas (MVAs) determined by the Gorlin formula. Each line represents the relationship between flow and the gradient for a given size of mitral valve orifice. As the MVA decreases from 6.0 to 0.3 cm^2, the pressure gradient rises more rapidly with any increase in trans-mitral flow. The increase of the pressure gradient is a function of the square of valve area but is linear with the *rate of diastolic flow* [11]. The *dashed line* shows the mean diastolic pressure gradient of 34 mm Hg; it indicates the pressure gradient at which most patients would be expected to manifest (frank) pulmonary edema.

When the MVA is 2 cm^2, as flow is increased to 400 mL per diastolic second, the pressure gradient rises rapidly. In the most severe stenosis, with an MVA of 1.0 cm^2 or less, the absolute volume of flow the valve can accommodate is markedly reduced and, thus, may result in a "fixed" cardiac output.

As the MVA is reduced to 2.5 cm^2, high rates of flow can be achieved with mild increases in the pressure gradient. Between valve areas of 2.5 and 1.5 cm^2, progressive increases in flow are associated with mild to moderate increases in gradient, and thus most patients are asymptomatic or minimally symptomatic. With valve areas below 1.5 cm^2, the ability to increase flow is progressively reduced and the pressure gradient across the valve also rises progressively, which will lead to progressive increases in symptoms; these become more marked at valve areas of 1.0 cm^2 or less. (*Adapted from* Wallace [12].)

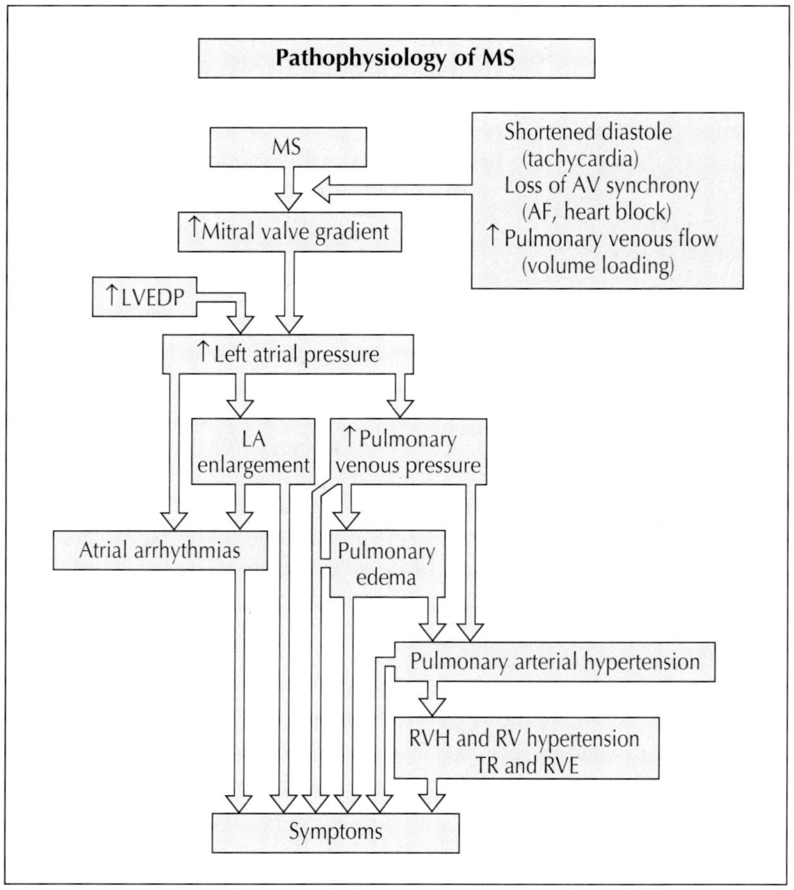

FIGURE 8-5. Pathophysiology of MS. MS results in a diastolic pressure gradient between the left atrium (LA) and the left ventricle (LV). The actual gradient depends on the mitral valve area (MVA) and the mitral valve *flow per diastolic second* (*see* Fig. 8-4). As a result, there is an elevation of LA pressure and, therefore, also of pulmonary venous pressure. Physiologic and pathologic changes—such as tachycardia and atrial fibrillation (AF) (which shorten diastole and may also result in loss of effective atrial contraction) or pregnancy, volume loading, and left-to-right shunts (at ventricular and aortopulmonary levels), which increase pulmonary venous flow—increase the mitral valve gradient and LA and pulmonary venous pressures. An increased LV end-diastolic pressure (LVEDP) also results in further increase of LA pressure.

An elevated LA pressure has several important effects, including enlargement of the LA, atrial arrhythmias, and an increase of pulmonary venous pressure. Pulmonary venous hypertension may result in pulmonary edema and pulmonary arterial hypertension. Pulmonary arterial hypertension and right ventricular (RV) hypertension result in RV hypertrophy (RVH) and may result in tricuspid regurgitation (TR) and RV enlargement (RVE). All of these changes contribute to producing symptoms. In addition, a fixed or even reduced cardiac output (*see* Fig. 8-4) also contribute to the symptomatic state of the patient. AV—atrioventricular. (© Copyright SH Rahimtoola, MB, FRCP, MACP.)

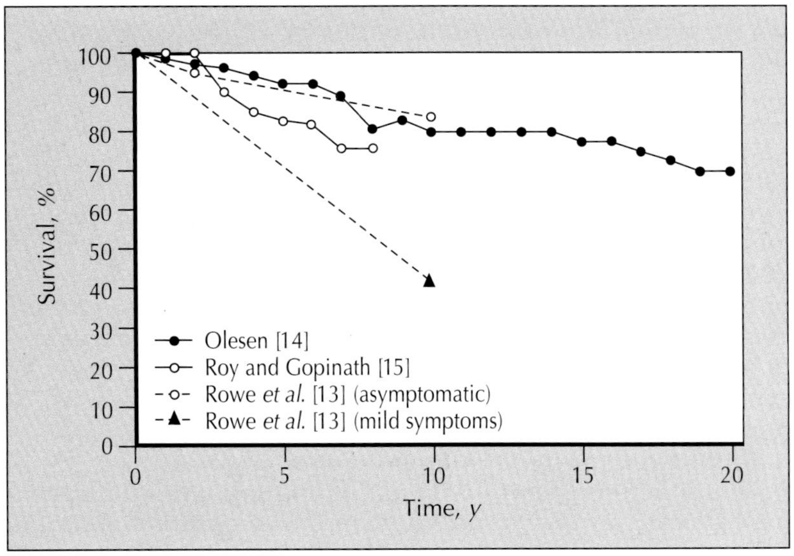

FIGURE 8-6. Survival of patients with MS who initially were asymptomatic or had mild symptoms and were treated medically. In the study by Rowe *et al.* [13], 130 (52%) of 250 patients with "auscultatory MS" who presented between 1925 and 1947 were asymptomatic; their 10-year survival rate was 84%. In the 42% of patients who had mild symptoms on clinical presentation, 10-year survival was 42% [13]. The data of Olesen [14] show the survival in 57 (21%) of 271 symptomatic MS patients who had New York Heart Association functional class II symptoms. Their 10- and 20-year survival rates were 34% and 14%, respectively. Survival data of Roy and Gopinath [15] also show similar survival in patients with class II symptoms.

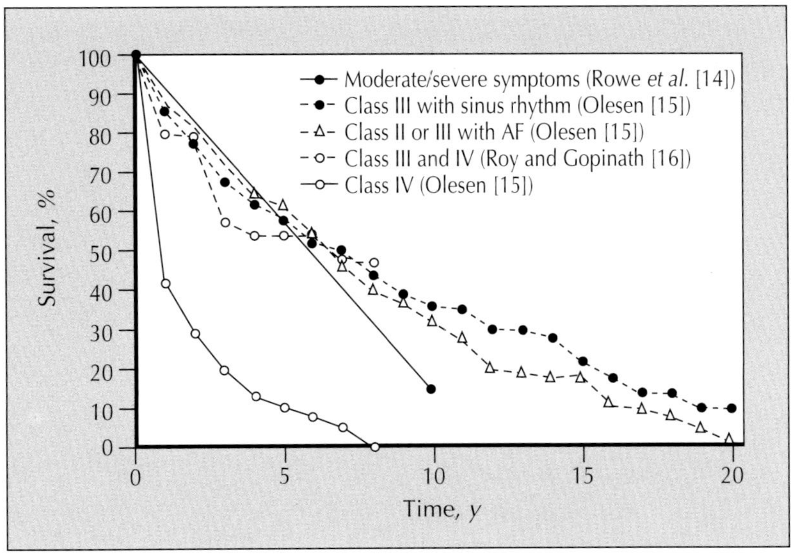

FIGURE 8-7. Survival of patients with MS and moderate or severe symptoms. Patients who were in New York Heart Association functional class IV [14] had a 42% 1-year survival, and all patients died within 8 years. The other four survival curves show patients who were in functional classes II through IV; their survival curves are similar with 5-, 10-, and 15-year approximate survival rates of 60%, 40%, and 20%, respectively. At 20 years, less than 10% of the patients were still alive [13–15]. Thus, survival in this group of patients with more advanced symptoms is much worse than that of patients who were initially asymptomatic or minimally symptomatic (*see* Fig. 8-6).

Clinical Manifestations

CLINICAL MANIFESTATIONS OF MS

- Asymptomatic
- Symptomatic
  - On exertion
    - Diminished activity tolerance or pace of activity
    - Fatigue
    - Dyspnea on exertion
    - Wheezing
    - Cough
    - Palpitations
    - Feeling faint
    - Presyncope/syncope
    - Chest pain/angina
  - At rest
    - Paroxysmal nocturnal dyspnea
    - Cough
    - Orthopnea
    - Palpitations
    - Sequelae of embolism: cerebral, coronary, gastrointestinal, extremities
    - Chest pain/angina
    - Hemoptysis
    - Peripheral edema
    - Ascites
    - Hoarseness (Ortner's syndrome)
    - Symptoms of endocarditis

FIGURE 8-8. Clinical manifestation of MS. Patients with MS usually have a long asymptomatic period; some patients with severe MS may even be asymptomatic.

The early symptoms of MS usually occur on exertion and are a result of tachycardia and either an increased flow across the mitral valve or an inability to increase flow (*see* Figs. 8-4 and 8-5). Patients complain of a diminished activity tolerance. This may be an actual reduction in activity levels or a more subtle diminution of the pace of activity or early onset of fatigue despite maintenance of near normal activities. A detailed history may be required [2,16]. Symptoms associated with elevation of pulmonary venous pressure and pulmonary congestion are dyspnea on exertion, wheezing, or cough. Symptoms related to an inadequate cardiac output and lower levels of perfusion in response to exercise, such as dizziness and muscle aches, may be present. Dizziness associated with palpitations may be due to an arrhythmia. Chest pain indistinguishable from angina may also occur [17]. This may be due to the pressure load on the right ventricle as a result of pulmonary arterial hypertension [18], concomitant coronary artery disease, or embolism of thrombotic material into a coronary artery. In some individuals, the etiology is obscure. At times, the first symptom may occur at rest, *eg*, when a systemic embolus is the first clinical manifestation of MS.

Symptoms at rest may also be the result of an elevated pulmonary venous pressure. When the patient assumes the supine position, the increased venous return may lead to marked elevation of left atrial (LA) pressures due to difficulty in increasing the flow of blood through the severely stenotic mitral valve. Palpitations may be the result of sinus tachycardia or more often an arrhythmia, especially atrial fibrillation. Systemic embolism is not uncommon and occurs particularly in patients with either paroxysmal or established atrial fibrillation. Hemoptysis appearing as an abrupt, often profuse hemorrhage may be an early manifestation of MS. In this situation, it results from an acute elevation of LA and, consequently, of pulmonary venous pressures at a time when the pulmonary veins are thin walled and dilated and have yet to undergo wall thickening in response to chronic, sustained, or recurrent pressure elevations that result after MS has been present for several years; this was described by Paul Wood in his classic treatise on MS [17]. Hemoptysis may also be observed as blood-tinged sputum secondary to edematous bronchial mucosa or associated with attacks of paroxysmal nocturnal dyspnea; pink sputum may be seen with the frothy effluence of acute pulmonary edema. Frank hemoptysis may also occur with pulmonary infarctions in patients with MS who have persistent heart failure.

Patients may complain of peripheral edema, increased abdominal girth, and nausea when right heart failure or tricuspid regurgitation develops. Hoarseness resulting from compression of the left (recurrent) laryngeal nerve by an enlarged LA, enlarged tracheobronchial lymph nodes, or dilated pulmonary artery is recognized as Ortner's syndrome [16]. Symptoms associated with any of the complications of MS, *eg*, infective endocarditis, may also be the cause for the clinical presentation of patients with MS (*see* Fig. 8-14).

PHYSICAL SIGNS OF MS

EXAMINATION	SIGN
General	Low cardiac output: pink-purple facies, peripheral cyanosis, cool extremities
Arterial	Small-volume pulse
	Absent or reduced pulse in any vascular territory
Venous	Jugular venous distension
	Hepatojugular reflux
	Prominent *a* wave
	Prominent *v* wave
Cardiac palpation	Inconspicuous apical impulse
	Palpable mitral valve closure (S_1)
	Palpable diastolic thrill at apex
	Palpable pulmonic valve closure (P_2)
	RV lift
Auscultation	Accentuated S_1
Cardiac	Opening snap
	Diastolic rumbling murmur
	Presystolic murmur
	Accentuated P_2
	Pulmonic ejection click
	Pulmonic regurgitation (Graham-Steell) murmur
	RV S_4/S_3
Pulmonary	Egophony at tip of left scapula
	Rales

FIGURE 8-9. Physical signs of MS. In severe MS with a low cardiac output at rest, hypoperfusion may be suggested on general inspection of the patient; a characteristic pink-purple complexion was described by Wood [17]. The extremities may be cool and cyanotic. In such severe cases, the small stroke volume results in a perceptibly diminished pulse volume. An elevated right atrial (RA) pressure is apparent from distention of the jugular veins, or such distention may be elicited by compression of the abdomen. The elevated RA pressure is a result of fluid retention associated with heart failure, right ventricular (RV) hypertension, or tricuspid regurgitation. The *a* wave is prominent in the presence of RV hypertension and the *v* wave is prominent with tricuspid regurgitation.

Palpation of the precordium may reveal an inconspicuous apical impulse, and mitral valve closure may be felt (a palpable S_1). A loud diastolic rumbling murmur may be felt as a thrill at the apex; this can be better appreciated if the apex is brought more into proximity of the chest wall by placing the patient in the left lateral decubitus position. With pulmonary arterial hypertension or RV dilatation, a parasternal RV lift may be present. When the RV is markedly dilated, the left ventricular (LV) apical impulse may be displaced posteriorly and the RV impulse may be mistaken for the LV apex. Also in the presence of severe pulmonary arterial hypertension, pulmonic valve closure (P_2) may be palpable in the second left parasternal intercostal space.

On auscultation, a loud S_1, an opening snap, and a mid-diastolic rumbling murmur with presystolic accentuation are considered the cardinal signs of MS [2,16] (*see* Fig. 8-10). With pulmonary arterial hypertension, the intensity of P_2 is increased; in severe pulmonary arterial hypertension, a pulmonary ejection click and a diastolic murmur of pulmonary valve regurgitation may be present (Graham Steell murmur). Auscultation of the posterior chest rarely reveals an area of egophony at the lower tip of the left scapula; a result of marked left atrial enlargement [18]. Rales may be present when there is pulmonary congestion or pulmonary edema.

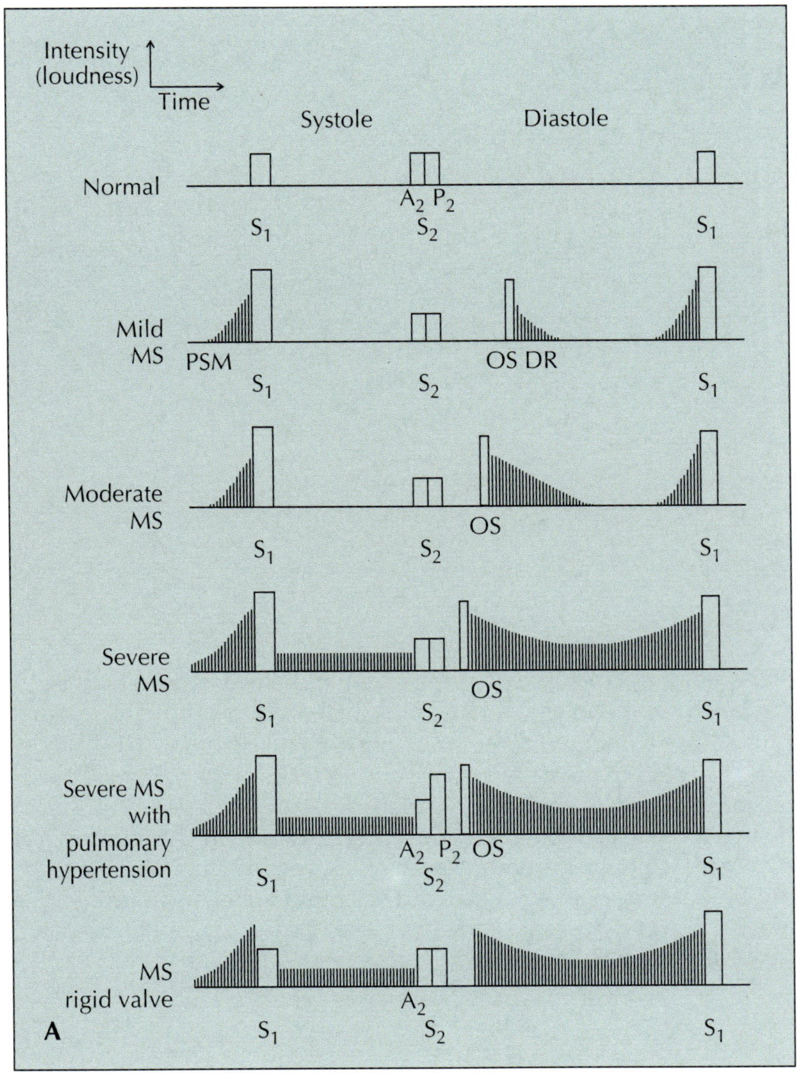

FIGURE 8-10. A, The classic auscultatory signs of MS in patients in sinus rhythm. These include a presystolic murmur, a loud S_1, an opening snap (OS), and a mid-diastolic murmur (DR, low-pitched, decrescendo diastolic rumble). These signs may be accentuated or at times may only be heard by placing the patient in the left lateral decubitus position.

Importantly, these signs are helpful in assessing the severity of the MS; as the MS becomes more severe, the S_2-OS interval is shortened and the length of the mid-diastolic rumble is increased. In mild MS, the S_2–OS interval is long and the diastolic murmur is short. In moderate MS, the S_2–OS interval is shorter and although the diastolic murmur is longer at rest, there is usually a gap between the end of the murmur and the onset of the presystolic murmur. When the MS is severe, the S_2–OS interval is short (usually 0.04 second) and the diastolic murmur is a full-length murmur. With pulmonary arterial hypertension, P_2 is increased in intensity. In the presence of a rigid mitral valve (with or without calcification), S_1 is soft and the OS is usually not heard. With severe MS and also with a rigid valve, a holosystolic murmur of mitral regurgitation is often present. (*continued*)

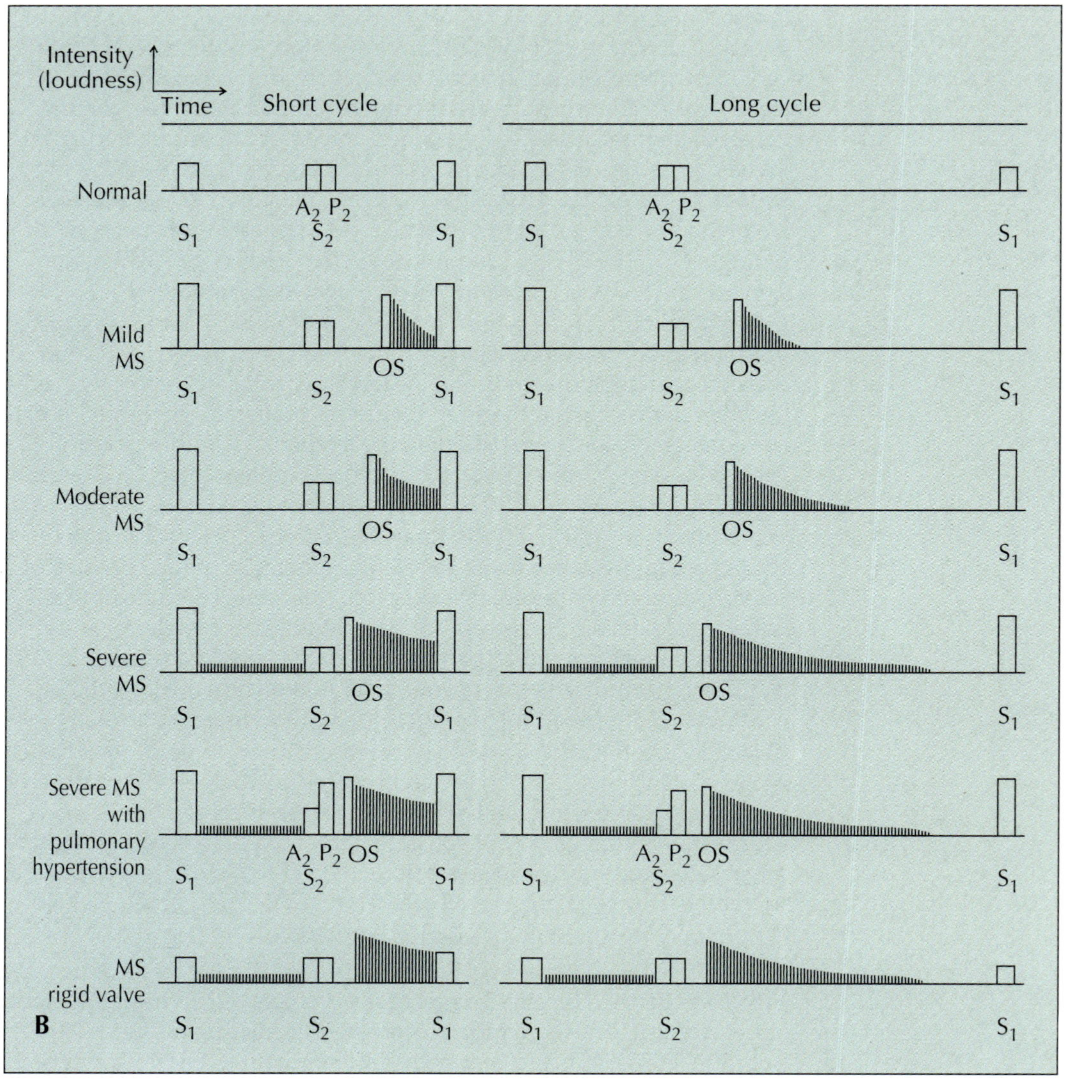

FIGURE 8-10. (*continued*) **B,** The classic auscultatory signs of MS in atrial fibrillation (AF). The auscultatory findings are much more variable on a beat-to-beat basis in AF. The presystolic murmur is usually absent. The loud S_1 and the OS are still heard. In the short cycles, the duration of diastole is short and the mid-diastolic rumble occupies the whole of diastole (*left panel*). In the long cycles (*right panel*) the duration of the mid-diastolic murmur is related to the severity of MS (*panel A*). As the MS becomes more severe, the length of this murmur is increased (*see* pressure tracings in MS with AF, Fig. 8-24). In AF, with a slow ventricular response and very long R-R intervals, the diastolic rumble may not occupy the whole diastolic period and the presystolic murmur is absent. Thus, one may get the impression that the MS is moderate rather than severe. Increasing the heart rate, *eg*, with brief physical exertion, may produce more characteristic auscultatory findings. Alternatively, when the ventricular rate in AF is rapid or in short cycles, the auscultatory findings may suggest a more severe degree of MS than is really the case (*left panel*).

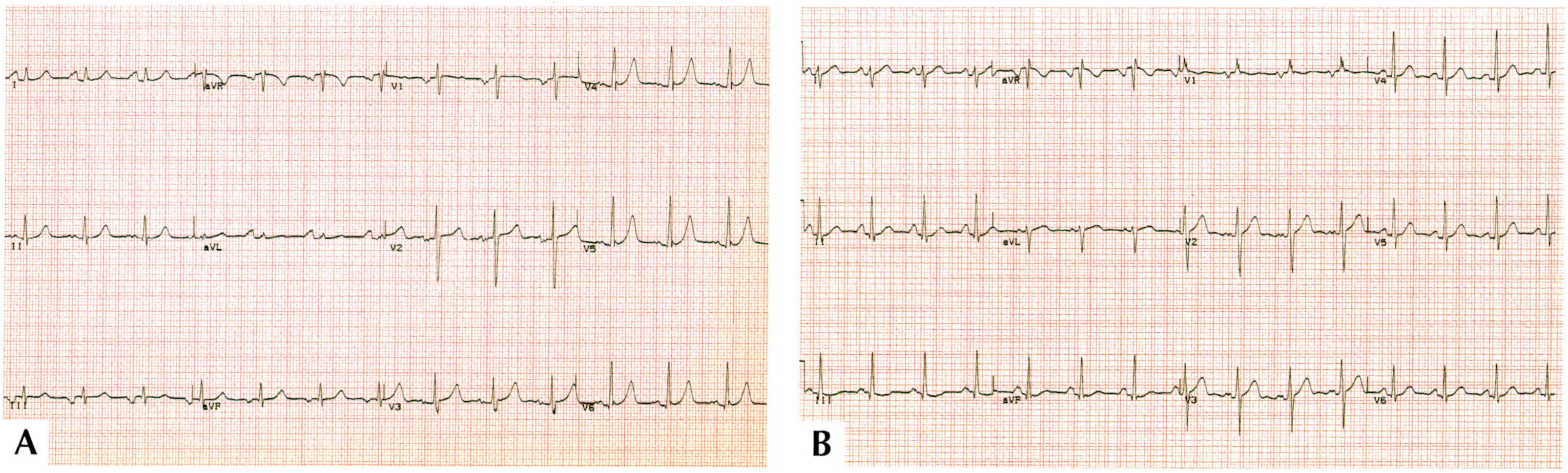

FIGURE 8-11. Electrocardiographic (ECG) signs in MS. **A,** The ECG findings from a patient with MS and regular sinus rhythm is normal except for signs of left atrial (LA) enlargement, that is, a P wave widened to 0.12 second or more. In lead II, the P wave has a double peak often characterized by an M-shaped configuration. In lead V_1, the late negative portion of the P wave is characteristically increased in both width and depth. The P-wave changes are also called "P mitrale."

B, ECG from a patient with MS, sinus rhythm, and signs of right ventricular (RV) hypertrophy. In addition to the findings of LA enlargement, which are described in *A* and are also present here, the height of the P wave in lead II is increased to 3 mm; the P wave thus shows combined right atrial and LA enlargement. The QRS axis is shifted to the right (+105°) and in lead V_1 the QRS width is normal but shows an RS pattern indicating RV hypertrophy. This degree of RV hypertrophy on the ECG is seen with chronic and severe elevations of pulmonary arterial pressure. In this patient pulmonary artery pressure was 68/32 mm Hg, mean 46 mm Hg; mean LA and right atrial pressures were 28 and 7 mm Hg, respectively. (*continued*)

Clinical Decision Making

STEPS IN CLINICAL DECISION MAKING IN PATIENTS WITH VALVULAR HEART DISEASE

Complete clinical evaluation
History
Physical examination
Echocardiography
Electrocardiogram
Chest radiograph
Diagnose and assess severity of disease
  All valves
  Ventricular function
  Hemodynamics effects
  Coronary artery disease
  Other cardiovascular disease
  Effects on other body organs
  Other organ diseases
List questions that need answering
Be reasonably certain these questions need to be answered
Perform test(s) most likely to provide these answers in one's own institution with the following criteria:
  Reliably
  Accurately
  Lowest risk to patient
  Reasonable (or lowest) cost
Review results of test(s)
Make an overall assessment of patient
Make recommendation regarding management

Figure 8-16. Steps in clinical decision making in patients with MS [21]. The first step is a complete clinical evaluation that includes history, physical examination, electrocardiography, and chest radiograph. At the end of the clinical evaluation, the severity of disease of all cardiac valves, ventricular function, hemodynamic effects, coronary artery disease, other cardiovascular disease, and diseases of other organs must be diagnosed and assessed. Before proceeding to additional testing, it is important to list the questions that must be answered and to be reasonably certain that these questions need to be answered. Tests are then performed that are most likely to provide these answers in *one's own institution* with the following criteria being kept in mind: reliability, accuracy, lowest risk to the patient, and reasonable (lowest) cost. Results are then reviewed as they become available and an overall evaluation and assessment of the patient is made. Finally, recommendations regarding management are made. (*Adapted from* Rahimtoola [21].)

CLINICAL DECISION MAKING FOR MS

	CLINICAL EVALUATION, %	ECHOCARDIOGRAPHIC/ DOPPLER EVALUATION, %
Diagnosis of MS		
Sensitivity	86	94
Specificity	87	89
Accuracy of diagnosis		
Including severity	44	52
For moderate to severe stenosis	92	97

Figure 8-17. Diagnostic sensitivity and specificity of clinical evaluation methods. In a prospective blinded study of consecutive patients with valvular heart disease, the sensitivity and specificity of the clinical evaluation (history, physical examination, electrocardiogram, chest radiograph) for making the diagnosis of MS were 86% and 87%, respectively [22]. After Doppler ultrasound, the sensitivity and specificity for diagnosing MS were 95% and 89%, respectively. If determining the severity of MS were required in addition to determining merely whether it is present or absent, the accuracy of the clinical evaluation was 44% and that of Doppler ultrasound was 52%. If one demanded only that MS be diagnosed and determined to be moderate or severe, then both the clinical evaluation and Doppler ultrasound improved markedly; the accuracies were 92% and 97%, respectively.

Several conclusions can be drawn from this study: 1) the clinical evaluation is highly sensitive and specific in making the diagnosis of MS; 2) the sensitivity is increased moderately by Doppler ultrasound, whereas specificity is not increased markedly and; 3) the clinical evaluation and Doppler ultrasound are highly accurate for diagnosing moderate or severe MS. The major difficulty is in separating mild from moderate MS and moderate from severe MS. (*Adapted from* Kawanishi [23].)

INDICATIONS FOR CORONARY ARTERIOGRAPHY

Patients ≥35 y

Patients <35 y

- LV dysfunction
- Symptoms or signs suggesting CAD
- ≥ risk factors for premature CAD (excluding gender)

FIGURE 8-18. Suggested indications for coronary arteriography before valve surgery [21]. All patients 35 years of age and older should undergo coronary arteriography before valve surgery. In patients under the age of 35 years, coronary arteriography should be performed if they have left ventricular (LV) dysfunction, have signs or symptoms that suggest the presence of associated coronary artery disease (CAD), or if they have one or more risk factors for premature CAD (excluding male gender). (*Adapted from* Rahimtoola [21].)

TREATMENT

CATHETER BALLOON COMMISSUROTOMY

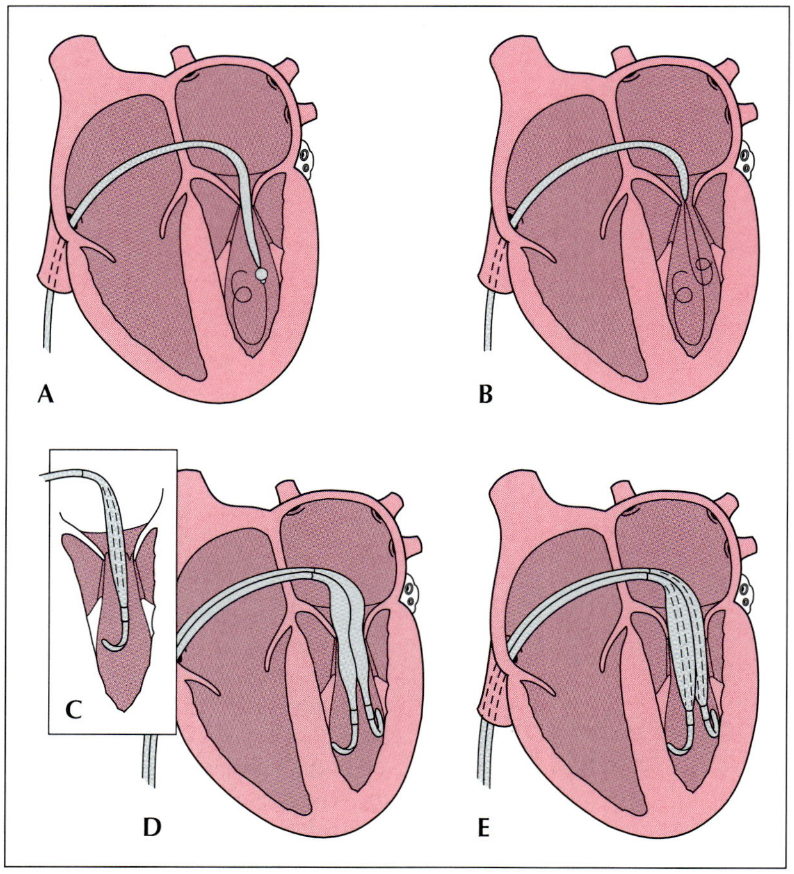

FIGURE 8-19. Catheter balloon commissurotomy (CBC) by the double-balloon technique [23,24]. **A,** The placement of the catheter and the guidewire in the left ventricle (LV) by the transseptal technique. The second guidewire is then placed in the LV (**B**). There is the stepwise insertion of each balloon over its own guidewire (**C**) with positioning across the mitral valve and subsequent inflation, which produces a "waist" in the balloons (**D**). Splitting of the fused commissures results in the expansion of the "waist" (**E**). (*Adapted from* Kawanishi and coworkers [23].)

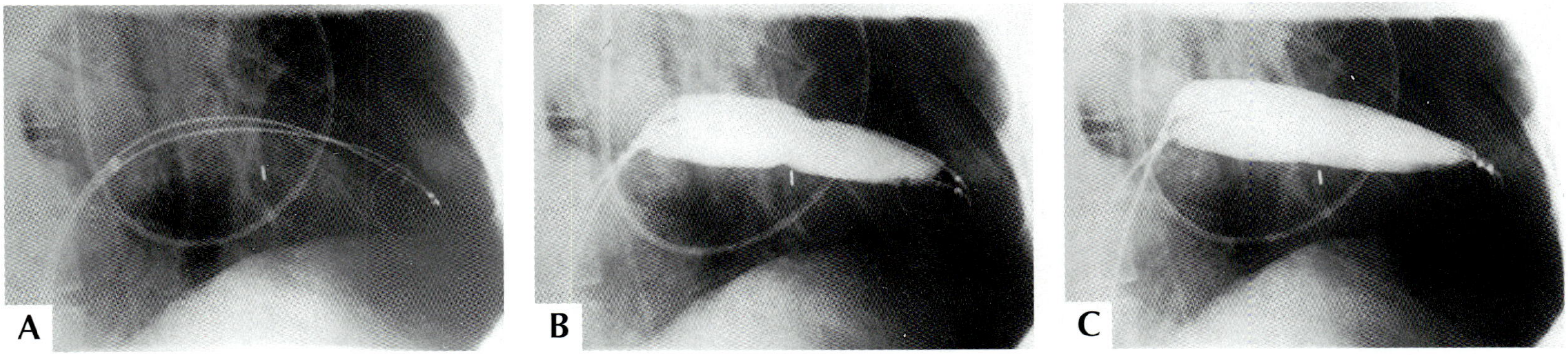

FIGURE 8-20. Cineradiographs of a double-balloon catheter balloon commissurotomy. **A,** The guidewires have been advanced across the interatrial septum from the right to left atrium, then across the mitral valve with the ends curled at the apex of the left ventricle (LV). Alternatively, the ends of the wires could have been advanced across the aortic valve into the ascending and then into the descending aorta. A balloon has been advanced over each guidewire. Note that the standard 5.5-cm long balloons must be positioned carefully, the distal marker at the sharp tip of the catheters is very near the LV apex, whereas the proximal marker just clears the interatrial septal puncture site. Further, unless calcification of the mitral valve or of the annulus is present, it may be difficult to know when the balloons are positioned properly with their center at the valve. **B,** Partial inflation of the balloons reveals that they are positioned properly with the "waist," or indentation of their outer margins, being very nearly at the center of each balloon. This point is located just to the left of the linear metal marker in the center of the image.

C, With full inflation of the balloons, the "waist" is no longer visible, suggesting that the valve commissures have been separated and the orifice has increased in size. Note also the proximity of the tips of the catheters to the LV apex during full balloon inflation and the straightening and rigidity of the balloons at this time. Perforation of the LV is one of the complications with use of this technique.

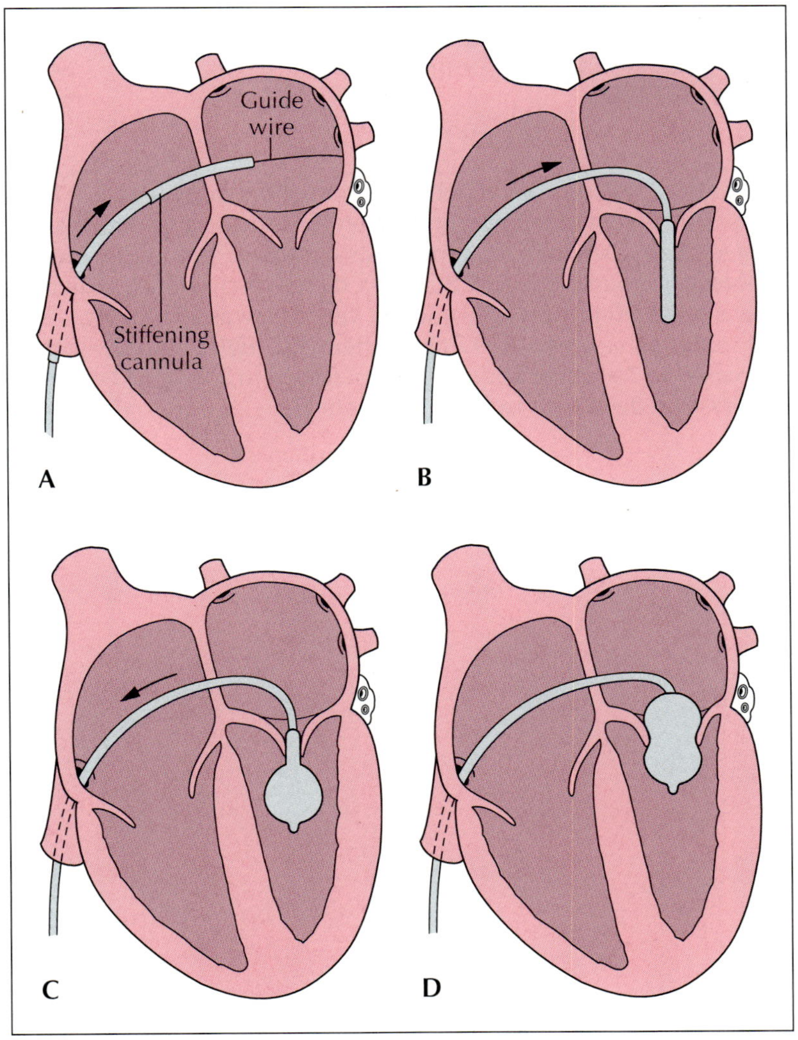

FIGURE 8-21. Inoue balloon technique for catheter balloon commissurotomy [25]. A transseptal puncture is performed (**A**) and the deflated Inoue balloon catheter is placed across the mitral valve into the left ventricle (LV) (**B**). Stepwise inflation of first the front then the rear of the Inoue balloon is performed (**C**). Inflation of the middle of the Inoue balloon and final expansion at the "waist" (**D**) suggests that enlargement of the valve orifice has occurred. The staged inflation of the various parts of this balloon are depicted. (*Adapted from* Inoue and coworkers [25].)

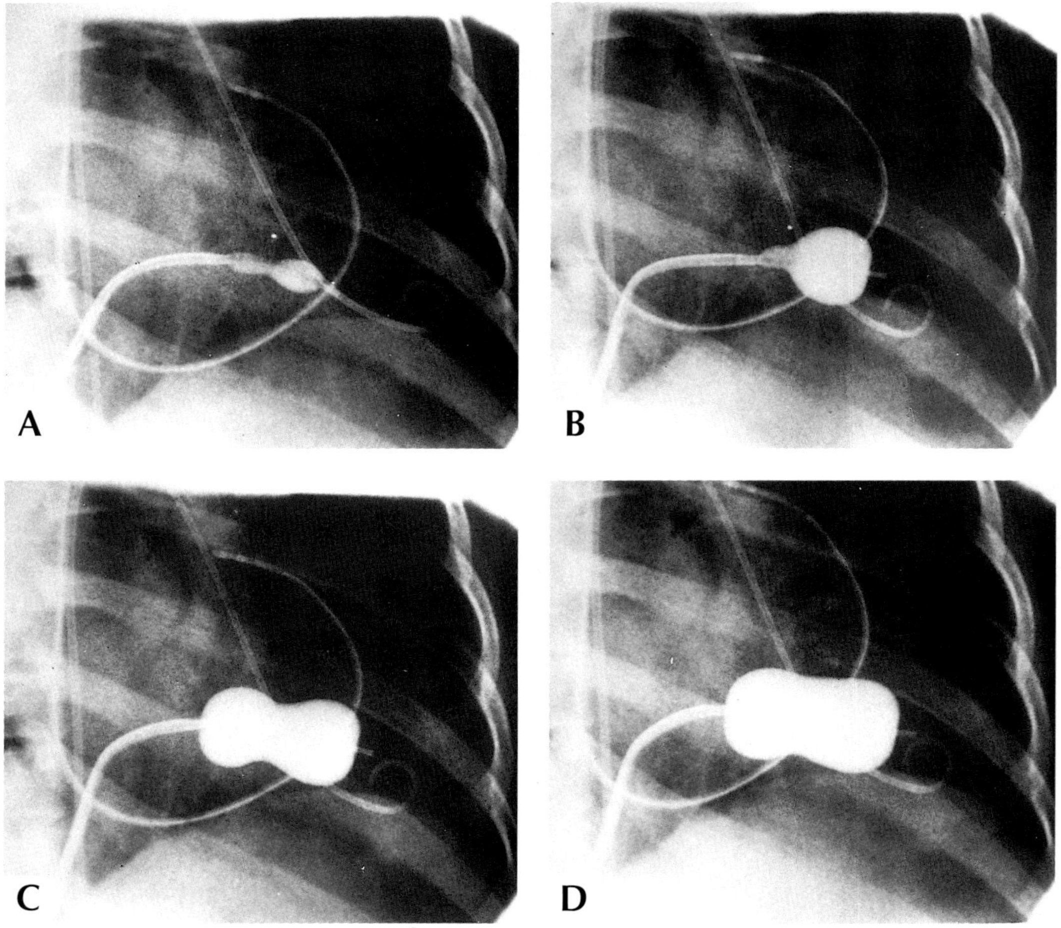

FIGURE 8-22. Cineradiographs of the Inoue technique for catheter balloon commissurotomy. **A,** The first portion of the balloon to inflate is the bulbous front. This may be inflated partially even before the balloon is advanced across the mitral orifice because the tendency of the balloon to float with the bloodstream may facilitate passage across the mitral valve. The rounded tip of the balloon catheter reduces markedly, or even eliminates, inadvertent puncture of the left ventricle.

B, As inflation continues, the front end inflates fully and the balloon is pulled back so that it sits snugly against the valve. The valve plane against which the front end of the balloon is being pulled is even with the small radiopaque center dot in this picture.

C, The rear or proximal end of the balloon inflates, creating a dumbbell shape with the center positioned precisely in the valve. As inflation is continued, the "waist" of the dumbbell begins to enlarge. Before insertion, each balloon is calibrated such that a known inflation volume results in a known waist diameter.

D, When fully inflated, the waist expands to the desired dilating diameter, resulting in commissural splitting and enlargement of the mitral valve orifice.

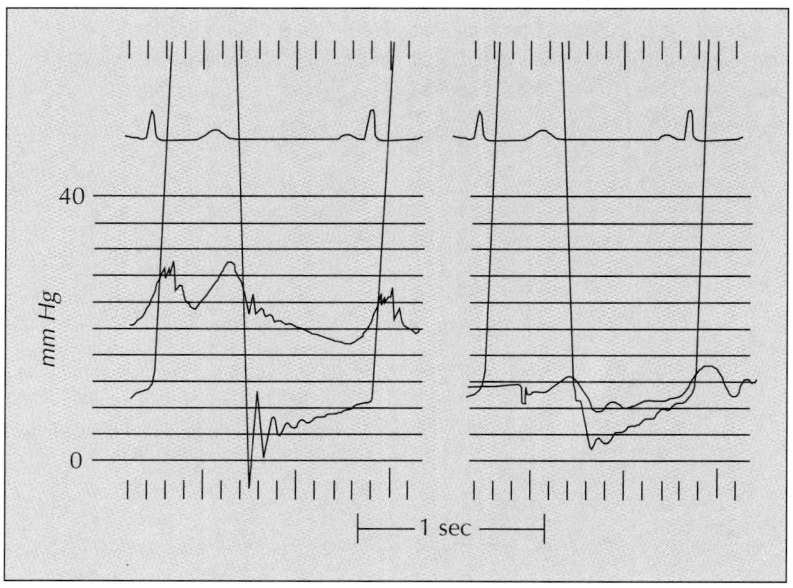

FIGURE 8-23. Results of balloon dilatation of the mitral valve. After successful balloon dilatation of the stenotic mitral valve, there is an immediate reduction in the mitral valve gradient. Before catheter balloon commissurotomy (CBC) (*left*), the mean diastolic gradient between the left atrium (LA) and left ventricle was 15 mm Hg and mitral valve area was 0.7 cm^2. After CBC (*right*), the gradient decreased to 3 mm Hg and the area increased to 2.0 cm^2. The mean LA pressure decreased from 24 to 12 mm Hg.

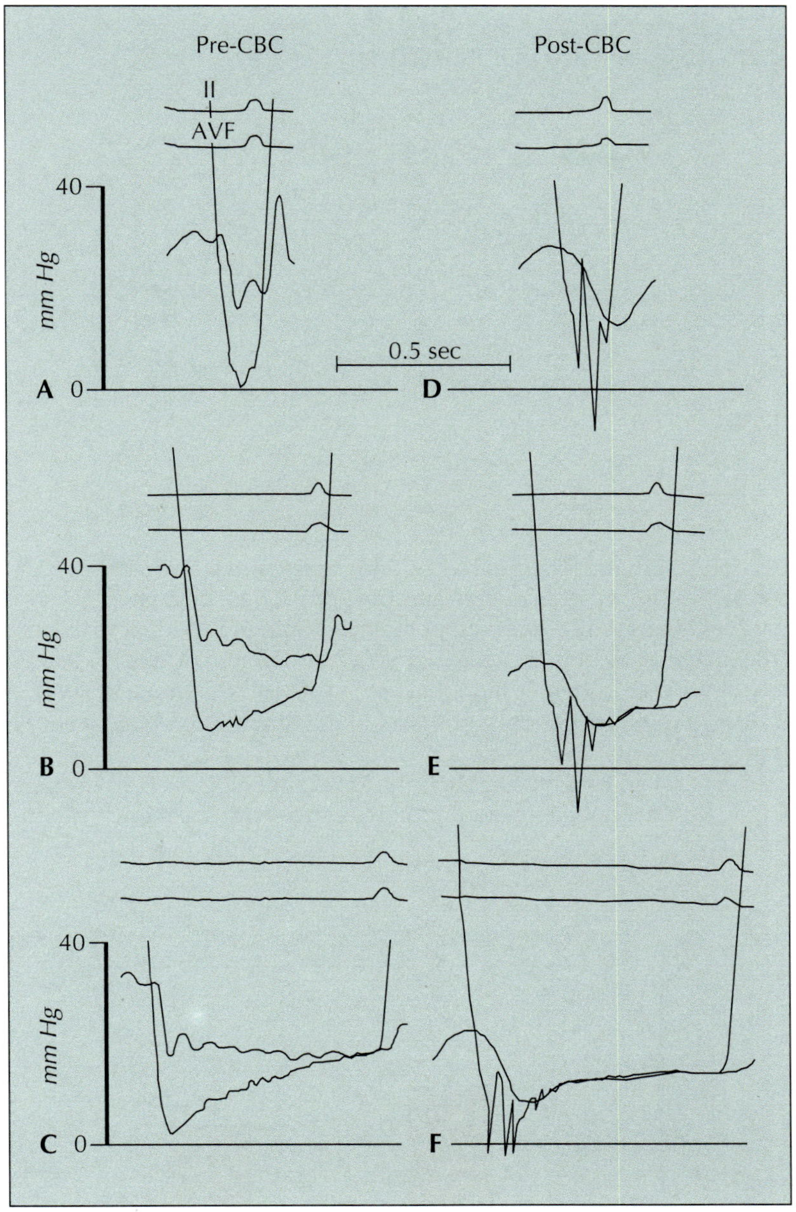

FIGURE 8-24. Left atrial (LA) and left ventricular (LV) pressures before (**A–C**) and after (**D–F**) catheter balloon commissurotomy (pre-CBC and post-CBC). Because of atrial fibrillation in this patient, there is the large variation of the gradient pre-CBC, which is dependent on the length of diastole (*panels A–C*). The mean gradient averaged over 10 or more beats was 26 mm Hg and the calculated mitral valve area (MVA) was 0.6 cm^2, 0.4 cm^2/m^2. The gradient is exaggerated during the short cycles (*panel A*) but during long cycles (*panel C*), the additional time afforded for flow results in a diminution of the gradient.

After successful CBC (*panels D–F*), the mean gradient was reduced to 18 mm Hg, and MVA had increased to 2.6 cm^2 (1.5 cm^2/m^2). During the short cycles (*panel D*), there is a gradient, but it is not large because the LA pressure has fallen, and in the long cycles a gradient is only present in the very early part of diastole (*panel F*).

IMMEDIATE RESULTS OF CBC FOR MS DOUBLE-BALLOON TECHNIQUE

STUDY	PATIENTS, *n*	MVA, cm^2 PRE-CBC	MVA, cm^2 POST-CBC	INCREASE IN MVA, cm^2
Al Zaibag *et al.* [24]	9	0.7	2.0	1.3
Babic *et al.* [28]	72	1.2	2.3	1.1
McKay, *et al.* [31]	12	1.0	2.4	1.4
Chen *et al.*[32]	23	0.8	1.9	1.1
McKay *et al.* [42]	24	1.0	2.2	1.2
Block *et al.* [30]	22	0.8	1.7	0.9
Palacios *et al.*[40]	78	0.9	1.9	1.0
Vahanian *et al.* [44]	200	1.1	2.2	1.1
NHLBI Valvuloplasty Participants [27]	557	1.0	2.0	1.0

FIGURE 8-25. Results of catheter balloon commissurotomy (CBC). The double-balloon technique has been reported to produce an increase in mitral valve area (MVA) from an average of 1.0 to 2.0 cm^2 [26,27]. Initially described by Al Zaibag *et al.* in 1986 [24], most investigators have followed a similar technique in which the two balloons are advanced antegrade through a transseptal puncture and then antegrade across the mitral valve (*see* Figs. 8-19 and 8-20). An exception is the series by Babic *et al.* [28], in which the balloons were introduced into the femoral arteries and advanced in a retrograde manner over guidewires across the aortic valve into the left ventricle and back across the mitral valve into the left atrium. The technique of Babic *et al.* [28] also requires the puncture of the atrial septum for insertion of guidewires. An alternative technique that avoids the transseptal puncture entirely has also been described by Stefanadis *et al.* [29]. There is the suggestion that a smaller MVA may result when the technique is used in very diseased and rigid valves as in the report by Block *et al.* [30]. (*Adapted from* Kulick and coworkers [26] and NHLBI Valvuloplasty Participants [27].)

RESULTS OF SINGLE-CENTER STUDIES COMPARING DOUBLE-BALLOON AND INOUE CBC

	DOUBLE BALLOON			INOUE BALLOON		
STUDY	PATIENTS, *n*	PRE-CBC MVA, *cm*²	POST-CBC MVA, *cm*²	PATIENTS, *n*	PRE-CBC MVA, *cm*²	POST-CBC MVA, *cm*²
Bassand *et al.* [33]	161	1.00±0.30	2.00±0.50	71	1.10±0.20	2.00±0.50
Abdullah *et al.* [37]	60	0.90±0.20	2.10±0.50	60	0.80±0.20	1.90±0.40
Kasper *et al.* [38]	23	1.10±0.30	2.20±0.80	22	1.20±0.40	1.70±0.70
Ruiz *et al.* [39]	322	0.88±0.24	2.41±0.63	85	0.89±0.21	1.84±0.38
Sharma *et al.* [34]	230	0.83±0.18	2.10±0.45	120	0.83±0.17	2.16±0.39
Rihal *et al.* [35]	33	1.17±0.32	2.24±0.74	28	1.05±0.35	1.73±0.57
Park *et al.* [36]	61	0.90±0.20	2.00±0.50	59	0.90±0.30	1.90±0.50

FIGURE 8-26. Results of seven series comparing the immediate results of the double-balloon technique and the Inoue balloon catheter for performance of catheter balloon commissurotomy (CBC) [33–39]. Each series was from a single medical center. *Only* in the Park *et al.* series [36] was the selection of technique randomly assigned.

In all series, the initial mitral valve area (MVA) was similar for the two groups receiving the different techniques of CBC. In two large series, the final MVA was similar. However, in the other four series, including one large study and the randomized trial, the final MVA with the Inoue balloon was smaller than with use of the double-balloon technique. The final MVA after successful CBC may be related to the size of the valve and the body. Thus, in smaller patients, successful CBC even in the morphologically ideal valve for CBC may not be able to achieve final MVA with the double-balloon technique that is greater than that achieved with the Inoue balloon. Indeed, in smaller patients, one should not attempt to obtain a very large MVA with CBC.

In general, in the United States, the MVA after CBC is on an average larger with the double-balloon technique than with the Inoue balloon technique.

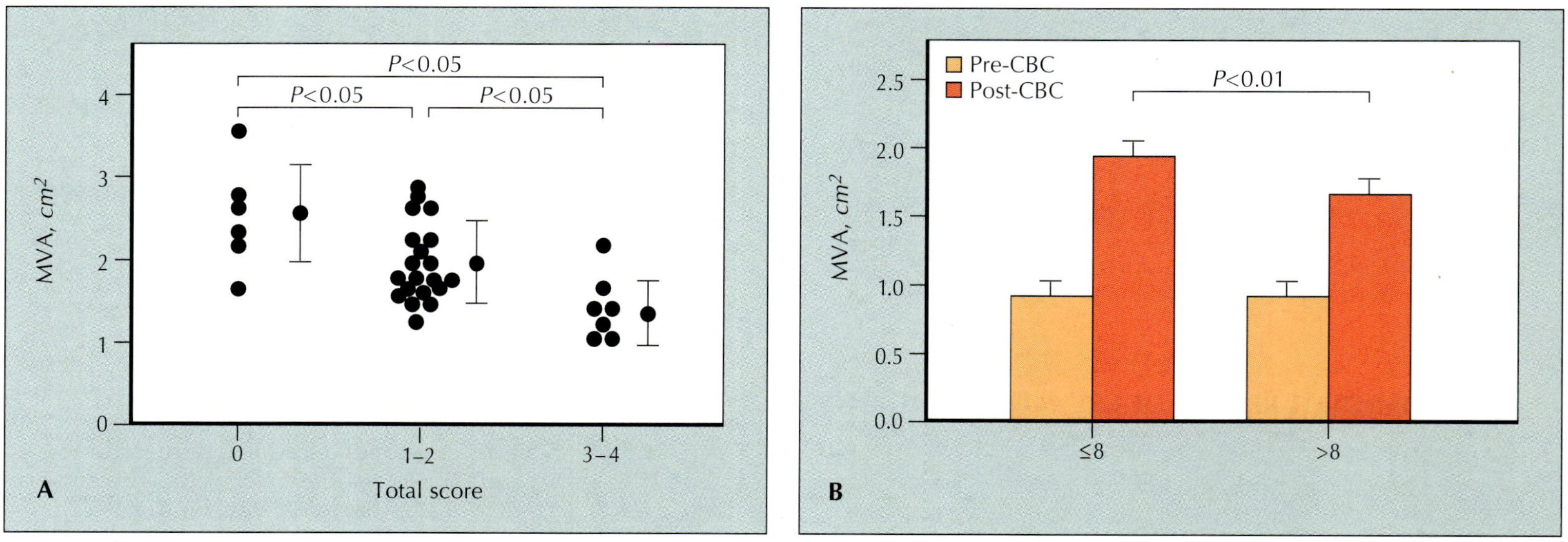

FIGURE 8-27. Quantitative and nonquantitative scoring for catheter balloon commissurotomy (CBC). Two series of patients using two different echocardiographic scoring systems show a smaller postprocedure mitral valve area (MVA) as the echocardiographic score increases.

A, In this series of 33 patients the morphologic features of leaflet mobility and thickness were scored using a quantitative system to measure the extent of leaflet motion and thickness of the valve [8]. The maximum score was 4. With a score of 2 or less, 83% of patients had an MVA post-CBC of 2.0 cm² or greater, whereas 83% of patients with a score of 3 or more had an MVA post-CBC of 2.0 cm² or less.

B, Similar results were obtained using a nonquantitative scoring system and assigning a score on a scale of 1 to 4 for leaflet mobility, thickness, subvalvular disease, and calcification. The maximum score was 16. The pre-and post-CBC MVA for patients with a score of 8 or less and greater than 8 are shown [40]. The MVA after CBC was significantly less (P<0.01) in those with a pre-CBC score of more than 8 when compared with those with a pre-CBC score of 8 or less. (Part A *adapted from* Reid and coworkers [8]; part B *adapted from* Palacios and coworkers [40].)

COMPLICATIONS OF CBC FOR MS

STUDY*	PATIENTS, *n*	TECHNIQUE	SUCCESS, %	MORTALITY, %	COMPLICATIONS, %			
					TAMPONADE	MR	ASD	TE
Nobuyoshi	106	Inoue	98	0	2	5	5	0
Hung	219	Inoue	99	0.5	0	6	15	1.4
Nar	200	Inoue	90	0.5	1	2	11	2
Fawzy	60	Inoue	95	0	2	0	0	0
Feldman	162	Inoue	95	0	1	11	6	0.6
Fer	527	Inoue	98	0	1.5	2	12	0.6
Herman	74	Double	89	2.7	5.4	8	18	2.7
NHLBI	591	Double	97	3.0	4.0	14	10	4.0
Tuzcu	161	Double	77	0	0.6	6	11	—
Cohen	146	Double	93	0.6	4.0	1	—	2.0

FIGURE 8-28. Reported procedural complications of the Inoue balloon and the double-balloon techniques [41]. Mortality with the double-balloon technique is usually due to tamponade or left ventricular perforation. The latter has not been reported with the Inoue balloon technique. Mitral regurgitation (MR) was greater than 3+. Significant atrial septal defect (ASD) was defined by many authors as a left-to-right shunt with a Qp/Qs ratio of 1.5 or greater. With skill and experience, including better selection of patients, the success rate is higher and complication rates are lower. TE—thromboembolism. (*Adapted from* Lau and coworkers [41].)

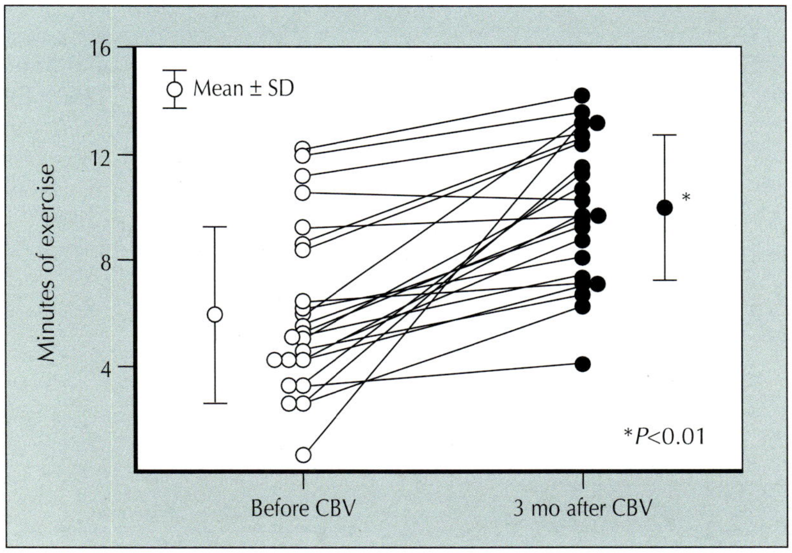

FIGURE 8-29. Exercise treadmill time before and 3 months after catheter balloon valvuloplasty (CBV) for MS with the double-balloon technique in 23 patients [42]. The mean exercise time on the Bruce protocol increased from 5.9±3.2 min to 9.8±2.9 min. A large increase was observed in 19 of 23 (83%) of patients. (*Adapted from* McKay and coworkers [42].)

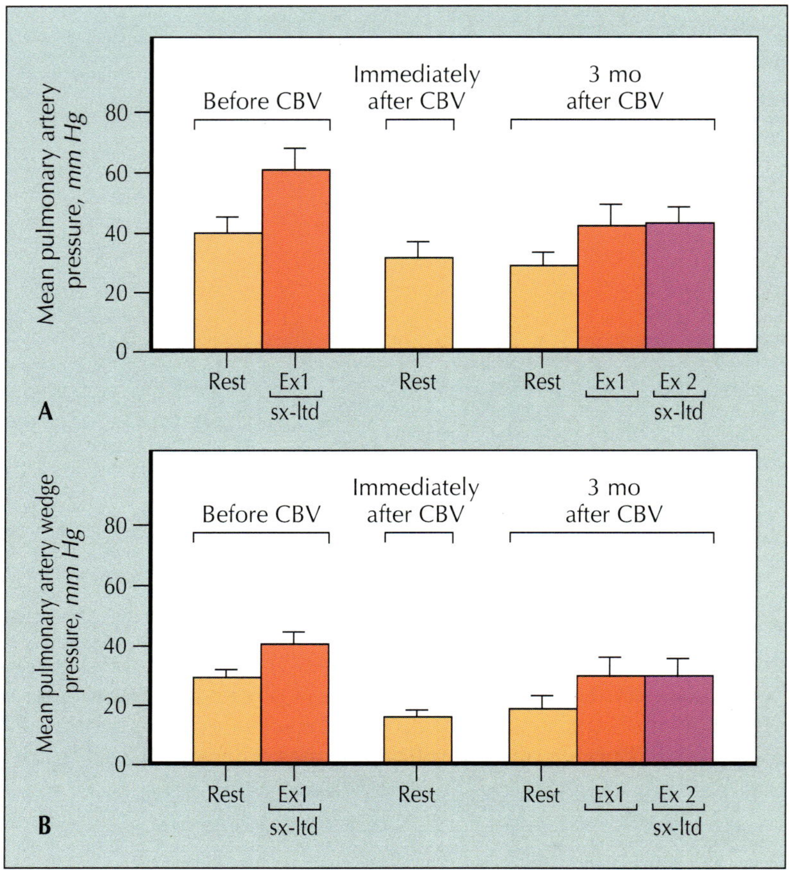

FIGURE 8-30. Pulmonary artery pressures. **A,** Mean pulmonary artery pressure at rest and during exercise before catheter balloon valvuloplasty (CBV), resting pressure immediately after CBV, and rest and exercise pressure 3 months after CBV. Exercise 1 (EX1) is the mean pulmonary artery pressure at the peak of symptom-limited (sx-ltd) supine bicycle exercise before CBV and at the same duration of exercise after commissurotomy. Exercise 2 (EX2) is the mean pulmonary artery pressure at peak of symptom-limited exercise after CBV [42]. Resting pressure fell immediately and remained lower 3 months later. The pressures at an equivalent level of exercise and even at peak exercise were lower after CBV.

B, Mean pulmonary artery wedge pressures at similar times and physiologic states as shown in *panel A*. The changes in mean pulmonary artery wedge pressure are similar to those seen with mean pulmonary artery pressures. (*Adapted from* McKay and coworkers [42].)

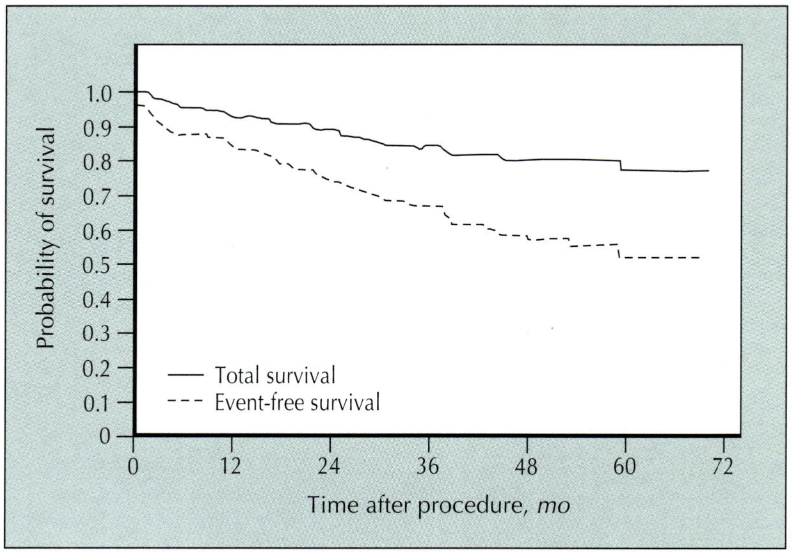

FIGURE 8-31. Actuarial estimate of survival after catheter balloon commissurotomy (CBC) [42]. Events were defined as cardiac death, mitral valve replacement, or repeat CBC. Between 1985 and 1991, 146 patients underwent the procedure, 102 (70%) with a single non-Inoue balloon. The 5-year survival rate was 76% (95% confidence interval 66% to 86%). Event-free survival at 5 years was 51% (95% confidence interval 40% to 63%). (*Adapted from* Cohen and coworkers [43].)

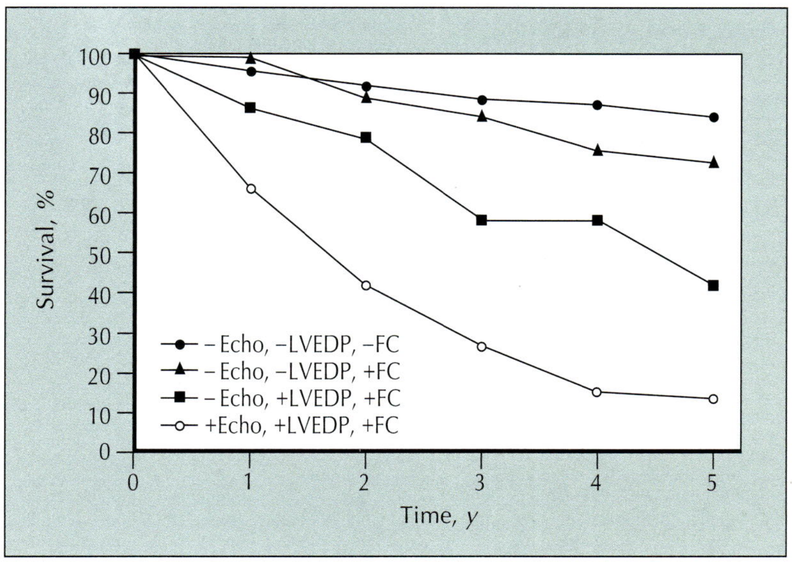

FIGURE 8-32. Survival after catheter balloon commissurotomy (CBC) according to preprocedure variables. The diminishing event-free (death, mitral valve surgery, repeat CBC) survival after CBC with the presence of ar increasing number of preprocedural high-risk variables is shown [43]. Presence (+) or absence (-) of risk factors are defined as: - echo = score of 8 c less; + echo = score above 8 (on a scale of 0 to 16); - LVEDP = left ventricula end-diastolic pressure of 10 mm Hg or less; + LVEDP = pressure above 10; - FC = New York Heart Association (NYHA) functional class II or III; + FC = NYHA class IV. In the series overall, 91% of patients had at least one grade improvement of functional class after the procedure. These data suggest that despite a "successful" procedure, the subsequent course of the patient is still strongly affected by the patient-related factors that were present before the procedure. Among postprocedure variables, survival wa significantly improved if the resultant mitral valve area (MVA) was 2.0 cm^2 or greater. However, the presence of an echocardiographic score above 8 an an LVEDP of greater than 10 mm Hg was still associated with high morbidit 5-year event-free survival with an MVA of 2.0 cm^2 or greater was 30% in th presence of both of these features. (*Adapted from* Cohen and coworkers [43].

FUNCTIONAL CLASS BEFORE AND AFTER CBC FOR MS

STUDY (TECHNIQUE)	PATIENTS, *n*	PRE-CBC AND MEAN FOLLOW-UP INTERVAL (RANGE), *mo*	NYHA FUNCTIONAL CLASS, % I	II	III	IV
McKay *et al.* [42] (DB)	24	Pre-CBC	0	12	63	25
		3	63	29	8	0
Vahanian *et al.* [44] (DB)	91	Pre-CBC	0	20	76	4
		9±3 (6–20)	64	30	6	0
Nobuyoshi *et al.* [45] (IB)	106	Pre-CBC	0	60	27	4
		9±4 (3–17)	72	26	2	0
Al Zaibag *et al.* [46]	41	Pre-CBC	0	29	71	0
		12	88	12	0	0
Block *et al.* [30]	41	Pre-CBC	0	32	68	0
		24±3	41	49	10	0
Ribeiro *et al.* [47] (IB)	66	Pre-CBC	0	5	80	15
		12	85	14	2	0
Pan *et al.* [48]	298	Pre-CBC	0	36	58	6
(268 Bifoil, 82 IB)		38±15 (6–12)	84		16	

FIGURE 8-33. A compilation of improvement in New York Heart Association (NYHA) functional class from before to after catheter balloon commissurotomy (CBC) from several series with varying lengths of follow-up [30,42,44–48]. Early results up to 12 months after CBC show that 63% to 88% of patients were asymptomatic and 90% to 98% of patients were asymptomatic or in functional class II. At a mean follow-up of 2 years or more, although most patients (90%) continue to have no more than mild functional limitation (class II or asymptomatic), the number of patients who remain asymptomatic may be declining [30]. DB—double balloon; IB—Inoue balloon.

RESULTS OF SURGERY

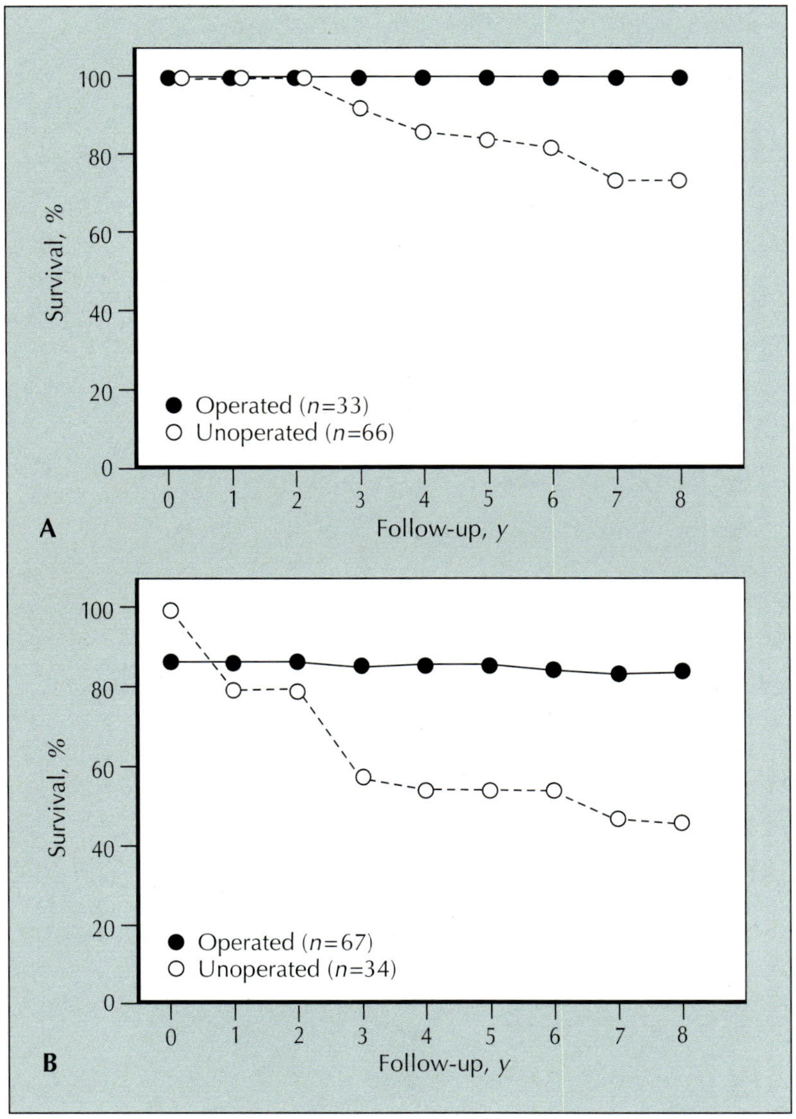

FIGURE 8-34. Survival of patients with New York Heart Association functional class II symptoms (**A**) compared with those with class III and IV symptoms (**B**) due to MS treated both medically (unoperated) and with closed surgical mitral commissurotomy (operated) [16]. There were no operative or late deaths in those with mild symptoms and no late deaths in those with class III and class IV symptoms. There is a clear improvement in survival in operated patients. The 5-year mortality with medical treatment alone in those with class III and IV symptoms approaches 50% (*see* Fig. 8-7); with surgery, there is no appreciable mortality after recovery from the procedure. (*Adapted from* Roy and Gopinath [15].)

MVA AT FOLLOW-UP AFTER SURGICAL COMMISSUROTOMY FOR MS

STUDY	TECHNIQUE	PATIENTS, *n*	MEAN FOLLOW-UP INTERVAL, *mo*	MVA, *cm²* PRETREATMENT	MVA, *cm²* FOLLOW-UP
Higgs	Closed	5	6–13	1.1	2.7
Feigenbaum	Closed	35	6–36	1.3	2.6
Mullin	Closed	21	6	1.1	2.4
Nakano	Open	30	13	0.72	2.52
			Type I, mobile	0.82	2.21
			Type II, thick with subvalvular disease	0.65	1.85
			Type III, rigid		

FIGURE 8-35. Compilation of reports of mitral valve area (MVA) at follow-up after surgical mitral valve commissurotomy [26]. A significant increase in MVA is clearly present at 13 months after either closed or open surgical commissurotomy; improvement in MVA was present as late as 36 months. As with commissurotomy using balloon catheters, the data suggest that a larger MVA is observed when the valve is more mobile and is free of subvalvular disease. (*Adapted from* Kulick and coworkers [26] and Hickey and coworkers [50].)

LATE SURVIVAL AFTER SURGICAL MITRAL COMMISSUROTOMY

STUDY	PATIENTS, *n*	TECHNIQUE	ACTUARIAL ANALYSES, *y*	LENGTH OF FOLLOW-UP MEAN (RANGE), *y*	SURVIVAL, %
Nathaniels	100	Closed	5	—	78
			10	—	62
			15	—	54
Granthan	273	Closed	—	4.4 (1–8)	87
Housman	100	Open	—	3.8 (0.8–11.3)	97
Rutledge	303	Closed	5	—	95
			10	—	82
			15	—	70
John	3724	Closed	5	—	94
			10	—	89
			20	—	78
Cohn	120	Open	—	4.4 (0.5–11.9)	95
Nakano	347	Open	—	7.5 (1–14)	95
Hickey	103	Closed	1	—	99
	236	Open	5	—	95
			10	—	87
			20	—	59
Scalia *et al.*	64	Closed	21	—	61
	103	Open	22	—	61

FIGURE 8-36. Late survival after surgical commissurotomy for MS for both closed and open techniques from several series [26,49–51]. There is a suggestion of an improvement in late survival after closed commissurotomy in the more recent series compared with the older series, *ie*, published before 1970. The data of Hickey *et al.* [50] and Scalia *et al.* [51] show that the late results after open and closed commissurotomy are comparable. In the report by Hickey *et al.* [50], all instances of "important" mitral regurgitation as judged by the surgeon in the operating room occurred only with the closed technique (closed vs the open technique 14% vs 0%, respectively). Importantly, with no or mild mitral regurgitation immediately after commissurotomy the 5-, 10-, 15-, and 20-year survival was better at 99%, 97%, 92%, and 84%, respectively, compared with survival with moderate mitral regurgitation after commissurotomy, which was 96%, 88%, 73%, and 49%, respectively [50]. Event-free survival begins to diminish between 6 and 10 years and is increased after 10 years largely due to an accelerating rate of need for reoperation [49,50]. (Adapted from Hickey and coworkers [50] and Kulick and coworkers [26].)

FUNCTIONAL CLASS BEFORE AND AFTER SURGICAL MITRAL VALVE COMMISSUROTOMY

STUDY	PATIENTS, *n*	TIME OF EVALUATION	NYHA FUNCTIONAL CLASS, %			
			I	II	III	IV
John *et al.* [49]	3724	Preop	0	1	58	41
	2587	at 5 y*	96	2	1	1
	1422	at 10 y*	66	27	5	2
	175	at 20 y*	27	54	13	6
	119†	>20 y	27	53	53	17
Hickey *et al.* [50]	274	Preop	2	28	6	0
		≥3.4 y ‡	47	37	68	12
Scalia *et al.* [51]	167 (64 closed 103 open)	Preop	1	19	8	0
		21–22 y	44	48		

*Actuarial analyses for follow-up data.
†20% were in class III or IV.
‡Functional status was "unknown" in 10%.

FIGURE 8-37. Improvement in New York Heart Association (NYHA) functional class at late follow-up in three series of patients after surgical mitral valve commissurotomy [49–51]. The data of John *et al.* [49] are the result of closed commissurotomy, in most patients using the Tubbs transventricular dilator, although 219 of the earlier procedures were done using finger fracture. At the end of 20 years, 81% of the patients were asymptomatic or mildly symptomatic. The series by Hickey *et al.* [50] is the late result after closed commissurotomy in 103 patients and open commissurotomy in 236 patients. The functional status at last follow-up of the 10% of patients not accounted for in the table was "unknown." The data of Scalia *et al.* [51] from 64 closed and 103 open commissurotomy patients indicates that after 21 to 22 years, 92% of the patients were asymptomatic or mildly symptomatic. Results of all three series show that symptoms are markedly improved in the majority of patients; 47% to 66% of patients were asymptomatic and an additional 27% to 37% were mildly symptomatic (NYHA functional class II). Note the very long follow-up (20 years or more) in the two series.

RANDOMIZED TRIALS OF CATHETER BALLOON COMMISSUROTOMY VS. SURGICAL COMMISSUROTOMY

STUDY	TIME OF FOLLOW-UP	PATIENTS, *n*	TECHNIQUE	ECHO SCORE	MVA (*cm²*)		MODERATE TO SEVERE MR, %	TE, %
					PRE	POST		
Turi *et al.* [52]								
BMC	8 mo	20	Mansfield*	7.2	0.8	1.6	5	0
SMC	8 mo	20	Tubbs dilator	8.4	0.9	1.8	5	0
Patel *et al.* [53]								
BMC	24–48 h	23	Bifoil	6	0.8	2.1	4	0
SMC	10 d	22	Logan dilator	6	0.7	1.3	4	0
Arora *et al.* [54]								
BMC	7 d	100	Mansfield*		0.8	2.4	14	0
SMC	7 d	100	Tubbs dilator		0.8	2.2	12	0
Reyes *et al.* [55]	3 y	30	Mansfield*	6.7	0.9	2.4	7	3
	3 y	30	Open commissurotomy	7.0	0.9	1.8	30	

*Double balloon.

FIGURE 8-38. Results of four randomized trials comparing balloon mitral commissurotomy (BMC) and surgical mitral commissurotomy (SMC) [52–55]. The first three compared with double-balloon technique using either balloons on two separate catheters or two balloons mounted on a single catheter (bifoil) with the closed SMC using either the Tubbs or Logan dilator. The fourth compared the double-balloon technique with open SMC via a left atrial approach.

In the study by Patel *et al.* [53], BMC resulted in a significantly larger mitral valve area (MVA) than surgery (postprocedure MVA 2.1 cm² vs 1.3 cm²). In the study of Reyes *et al.* [54], BMC also resulted in a larger MVA than open SMC at the 3-year follow-up. In the other studies, comparable results were obtained with both techniques. The risk of severe mitral regurgitation (MR) at follow-up was greater with BMC than open SMC in the Reyes study (P=0.03). The risk of thromboembolism (TE) was not significantly different between the balloon and surgical techniques in any of these studies.

RESULTS OF HEMODYNAMIC AND LV STUDIES OF MVR FOR MS

	MS	
VARIABLE	PRE-MVR	POST-MVR
Patients, *n*	33	
LV end-diastolic pressure, *mm Hg*	11±5	12±6
Mean PA wedge pressure, *mm Hg*	36±15	28±14*
Mean systolic PA pressure, *mm Hg*	54±24	42±22†
Cardiac index, *L/min/min*^{2}	2.1±1.5	2.3±0.6
LVEDVI, *mL/m*^{2}	79±18	72±24
LVESVI, *mL/m*^{2}	41±13	39±21
LVEF	0.48±0.10	0.47±0.14
Mitral regurgitant volume, *mL*	—	—
Regurgitant volume/end-diastolic volume	—	—
Mitral valve gradient *mm Hg*	15±7	8±3*
Mitral valve area, *cm*^{2}	1.2±0.4	1.8±0.6*

*P <0.001.
*P <0.01 comparing before and after MVR artery.

FIGURE 8-39. Postoperative hemodynamic and left ventricular (LV) functional studies in the Veterans Administration Cooperative Trial after mitral valve replacement (MVR) for MS. The mean pulmonary artery (PA) wedge pressure and mean PA pressure fell slightly [56]. The mean mitral valve gradient fell from an average of 15 mm Hg to 8 mm Hg and the mitral valve area (MVA) increased from 1.2 cm^2 to 1.8 cm^2. One possible reason for these modest benefits may be the inability to insert an adequate sized prosthesis in patients with severe MS [57]. The LV size and function were unchanged after MVR. LVEDVI—left ventricular end-diastolic volume index; LVEF—left ventricular ejection fraction; LVESVI—left ventricular end-systolic volume index. (*Adapted from* Crawford and coworkers [56].)

OTHER TREATMENTS

MEDICAL TREATMENT OF MS

- Prevention
  - Primary: Treatment of streptococcal group A infection
  - Secondary (antibiotic prophylaxis):
    - Recurrent rheumatic fever
    - Infective endocarditis
- Restrict activities (moderate/severe MS)
  - Severe exercise
  - Competitive sports
- Arrhythmias
  - Prevent or control
  - Restore sinus rhythm, if possible
- Cardiac medications
  - Use only if essential
  - Diuretics, vasodilators: use cautiously
  - Anticoagulants for systemic/pulmonary emboli
  - Elevated pulmonary venous pressure: diuretics
  - Heart failure: digitalis, diuretics, vasodilators
- Follow-up
  - Mild MS: every 2–5 y
  - Moderate MS: every 1–2 y
  - Develop symptoms: early or "immediate"

FIGURE 8-40. Medical treatment for MS. Early and adequate antibiotic treatment for streptococcal group A infection should prevent the occurrence of rheumatic carditis. All patients need antibiotic prophylaxis for prevention of recurrence of rheumatic fever as well as for prevention of infective endocarditis (*see* Chapter 14).

Restriction of physical activity to moderate levels helps to avoid precipitating symptoms in patients with moderate or severe MS. Both the tachycardia and increased pulmonary venous flow associated with exercise may, in the presence of moderate or large mitral valve gradients, result in elevation of left atrial pressure to levels that produce pulmonary edema.

Arrhythmias should be prevented, if possible, or controlled. Ventricular rate should be controlled in atrial fibrillation and appropriate anticoagulant therapy instituted. Sinus rhythm should be restored; in patients undergoing interventional therapy, this is usually done after completion of the intervention.

As a rule, cardiac medications should only be used if essential. Excessive diuresis with too rapid and great reduction in left atrial pressure may result in a significant reduction of flow across the mitral valve and a critical fall in a possibly already reduced cardiac output. Venodilators may have a similar deleterious effect. In the presence of a mechanical restriction to flow across the mitral valve, the patient may not be able to compensate for a fall in arterial pressures with an increase of cardiac output; therefore, arterial vasodilators should be used with great care. Patients with emboli or those at higher risk for emboli need appropriate anticoagulant therapy. Patients in congestive heart failure need digitalis and diuretics, and in selected patients, vasodilators are of benefit. In patients with atrial fibrillation, the ventricular rate is controlled with digitalis and other drugs that produce atrioventricular blockade.

The frequency of follow-up should be individualized but in general a more frequent check-up is indicated when either the MS is more severe or when symptoms develop or worsen. (© Copyright SH Rahimtoola, MB, FRCP, MACP.)

INDICATIONS FOR INTERVENTIONAL THERAPY FOR SEVERE MS*

All symptomatic patients
Asymptomatic patients†
  Pulmonary arterial hypertension
  Episodic pulmonary edema
  Atrial fibrillation
  Thromboembolism

*Catheter ballon commissurotomy/surgery.
†Individualize depending on:
  Patient characteristics
  Patient suitable for commissurotomy versus valve replacement
  Skill and experience of interventional team

FIGURE 8-41. Interventions for severe MS. All patients with symptoms due to severe MS should be treated with interventional therapy to produce an increase in mitral valve area. This may be in the form of either catheter balloon commissurotomy, surgical valve repair, or valve replacement, depending on the morphology of the valve and the skill and expertise of the interventional team.

Some asymptomatic patients may be treated appropriately with interventional therapy if *severe* MS has resulted in moderate-to-severe pulmonary arterial hypertension (either at rest or with exercise), episodic pulmonary edema, or thromboembolism, or if atrial fibrillation has supervened. When such a patient is asymptomatic, the need to intervene with a mechanical approach to enlarge the mitral valve opening should consider several factors. These include the patient's physical and psychological needs and other physical and medical limitations and whether the valve is suitable for a plastic procedure, which has the benefit of leaving the patient with his or her own tissue as opposed to requiring a valve replacement. The increased mortality and morbidity of the replacement procedure would tend to require a stronger indication to intervene than if the commissurotomy could be done. The timing of intervention when the patient is asymptomatic must also consider the skill and experience of the interventional team, whether it be the interventional cardiologist or the cardiothoracic surgeon. (© Copyright SH Rahimtoola, MB, FRCP, MACP.)

FACTORS TO BE CONSIDERED IN CHOOSING TYPE OF INTERVENTIONAL THERAPY FOR MS

Mitral valve morphology
  Low echo score
    CBC
    Surgical valve repair
  High echo score
    Surgery
    CBC in special circumstances
Mitral regurgitation
  ≥3+: Surgery
  ≤1+: CBC
  2+: Individualize (CBC vs surgery)
LA thrombus
  Surgery
  CBC in special circumstances
Need for other cardiac surgery
  Surgery
  CBC in special circumstances

FIGURE 8-42. Factors influencing choice of intervention. In determining the type of interventional therapy that should be selected, several factors should be considered in addition to the skill and experience of the interventional team. These include the mitral valve morphology, degree of mitral regurgitation, presence of left atrial (LA) thrombus, and need for other cardiac surgery.

A low echocardiographic (echo) score, irrespective of whether a quantitative or a qualitative scoring system is used, suggests that a favorable outcome may be expected from catheter balloon commissurotomy (CBC), surgical commissurotomy, or valve repair. When the echocardiographic score is high, surgery with the possible need for valve replacement is more appropriate. Even in such patients, CBC may be preferred under special circumstances, *eg*, when a surgical approach needs to be deferred or delayed, or the patient's expected life is short because of another medical disorder.

When 3+ or greater mitral regurgitation is present, surgical repair or valve replacement is more appropriate. When there is 1+ or less mitral regurgitation and the valve has a low echocardiographic score, CBC would ordinarily be the preferred treatment. With 2+ mitral regurgitation, an individualized approach is indicated, the choice of technique being weighed heavily according to the morphology of the mitral valve as well as by the skill and experience of the cardiac interventionalist and the surgical teams.

When LA thrombus is present, open surgical commissurotomy or valve replacement accompanied by thrombus removal is probably the procedure of choice. However, if treatment with anticoagulation results in resolution of the thrombus, CBC might be considered. When the patient must undergo cardiac surgery for another associated problem, the MS may be addressed at the same time. However, CBC may still be a reasonable option in certain instances, *eg*, if a patient has single-vessel coronary artery disease that is amenable to percutaneous transluminal coronary angioplasty. (© Copyright SH Rahimtoola, MB, FRCP, MACP.)

REFERENCES

1. Waller BF: Rheumatic and nonrheumatic conditions producing valvular heart disease. In *Valvular Heart Disease: Comprehensive Evaluation and Management*. Edited by Frankl WS and Brest AN. *Cardiovasc Clin* 1986, 16:3–104.
2. Braunwald E: Valvular heart disease. In *Heart Disease*, 4th ed. Edited by Braunwald E. Philadelphia: WB Saunders; 1992:1007–1018.
3. Davies JJ: *Pathology of Cardiac Valves*. London: Butterworths; 1980.
4. Fowler NO: Mitral stenosis and left atrial myxoma. In *Diagnosis of Heart Disease*. New York: Springer-Verlag; 1991:146–159.
5. Osterberger LE, Goldstein S, Khaja F, Lakier JB: Functional mitral stenosis in patients with massive mitral annular calcification. *Circulation* 1981, 64:472–476.
6. Libman E, Sacks B: A hitherto undescribed form of valvular and mitral endocarditis. *Arch Intern Med* 1924, 33:701–737.
7. Galve E, Candell-Riera J, Pigrau C, *et al.*: Prevalence, morphologic types, and evolution of cardiac valvular disease in systemic lupus erythematosus. *N Engl J Med* 1988, 817–823.
8. Reid CL, Chandraratna PAN, Kawanishi DT, *et al.*: Influence of mitral valve morphology on double-balloon catheter balloon valvuloplasty in patients with mitral stenosis: an analysis of factors predicting immediate and 3-month results. *Circulation* 1989, 80:515–524.
9. Gordon PF, Douglas PS, Come PC, Manning WJ: Two-dimensional and Doppler echocardiographic determinants of the natural history of mitral valve narrowing in patients with rheumatic mitral stenosis: implications for follow-up. *J Am Coll Cardiol* 1992, 19:968–973.
10. Braunwald E, Turi ZG: Pathophysiology of mitral valve disease. In *Mitral Valve Disease*. Edited by Ionescu MI, Cohn LH. London: Butterworths; 1985:3–10.

11. Smith DR: Clinical diagnosis and evaluation of mitral valve disease. In *Mitral Valve Disease: Diagnosis and Treatment*. Edited by Ionescu MI, Cohn LH. Boston: Butterworths; 1985:44–45.

12. Wallace AG: Pathophysiology of cardiovascular disease. In *Pathophysiology: The Biological Principles of Disease. The International Textbook of Medicine*. Edited by Smith Jr LH, Thier SO. Philadelphia: WB Saunders; 1981:1192.

13. Rowe JC, Bland EF, Sprague HB, White P: The course of mitral stenosis without surgery: ten- and twenty-year perspectives. *Ann Intern Med* 1960, 52:741–749.

14. Olesen KH: The natural history of 271 patients with mitral stenosis under medical treatment. *Br Heart J* 1962, 24:349–357.

15. Roy SB, Gopinath N: Mitral stenosis. *Circulation* 1968, 38(suppl V):68–76.

16. Rahimtoola SH: Valvular heart disease. In *Internal Medicine*, 4th ed. Edited by Stein JH. St. Louis: Mosby-Year Book; 1994:214–215.

17. Wood P: An appreciation of mitral stenosis: Part 1. Clinical features. *BMJ* 1954, 1:1051–1063; Part 2. Investigations and results. *BMJ* 1954, 1:1113–1124.

18. Ross RS: Right ventricular hypertension as a cause of precordial pain. *Am Heart J* 1961, 61:134–135.

19. Crawford MH: Iatrogenic Lutembacher's syndrome revisits [editorial]. *Circulation* 1990, 81:1422–1424.

20. Cequier A, Bonan R, Serra A, *et al*.: Left-to-right atrial shunting after percutaneous mitral valvuloplasty: incidence and long-term hemodynamic follow-up. *Circulation* 1990, 81:1190–1197.

21. Rahimtoola SH: Perspective on valvular heart disease: an update. *J Am Coll Cardiol* 1989, 14:1–23.

22. Kawanishi DT, Kotlewski A, McKay CR, *et al*.: The relative value of clinical examination, echocardiography with Doppler and cardiac catheterization with angiography in the evaluation of mitral valve disease. In *Surgery for Heart Valve Disease*. Edited by Bodnar E. London: ICR Publishers; 1990:73–78.

23. Kawanishi DT, Kulick DL, Rahimtoola SH: Catheter balloon commissurotomy for mitral stenosis. In *Techniques and Application of Interventional Cardiology*. Edited by Kulick DL, Rahimtoola SH. Chicago: Year Book Medical Publishers, 1991:325–357.

24. Al Zaibag MA, Ribeiro PA, Al Kasab S, Al Fagih MR: Percutaneous double-balloon mitral valvotomy for rheumatic mitral valve stenosis. *Lancet* 1986, 1:757–761.

25. Inoue K, Owaki T, Nakamura T, *et al*.: Clinical application of transvenous mitral commissurotomy by a new balloon catheter. *J Thorac Cardiovasc Surg* 1984, 87:394–402.

26. Kulick DL, Reid CL, Kawanishi DT, Rahimtoola SH: Catheter balloon commissurotomy in adults. Part II: Mitral and other stenoses. *Curr Probl Cardiol* 1990, 15:403–470.

27. NHLBI Valvuloplasty Participants: Multicenter experience with balloon mitral commissurotomy—NHLVI Balloon Valvuloplasty Registry report on immediate and 30-day follow-up results. *Circulation* 1992, 85:448–461.

28. Babic UU, Dorros G, Pejcic P, *et al*.: Percutaneous mitral valvuloplasty: retrograde trans-arterial double-balloon technique utilizing the transseptal approach. *Cathet Cardiovasc Diagn* 1988, 14:229–237.

29. Stefanadis C, Stratos C, Pitsavos C, *et al*.: Retrograde nontransseptal balloon mitral valvuloplasty: immediate results and long-term follow-up. *Circulation* 1992, 85:1760–1767.

30. Block PC, Palacios IF, Block EH, *et al*.: Late (two-year) follow-up after percutaneous balloon mitral valvotomy. *Am J Cardiol* 1992, 69:537–541.

31. McKay CR, Kawanishi DT, Rahimtoola SH: Catheter balloon valvuplasty (CBV)of the mitral valve in adults using a double balloon technique: early hemodynamic results. *JAMA* 1987, 257:1753–1761.

32. Chen C, Wang Y, Qing D: Percutaneous mitral balloon dilation by a new sequential single and balloon technique. *Am Heart J* 1988;116:1161–1167.

33. Bassand J-P, Schiele F, Bernard Y, *et al*.: The double-balloon and Inoue techniques in percutaneous mitral valvuloplasty: comparative results in a series of 232 cases. *J Am Coll Cardiol* 1991, 18:982–989.

34. Sharma S, Loya YS, Desai DM, Pinto RJ: Percutaneous mitral valvotomy using Inoue and double balloon techniques: comparison of clinical and hemodynamic short term results in 350 cases.*Cathet Cardiovasc Diagn* 1993, 29:18–23.

35. Rihal CS, Nishimura RA, Reeder GS, Holmes DR: Percutaneous balloon mitral valvuloplasty: comparison of double and single (Inoue) balloon techniques. *Cathet Cardiovasc Diagn* 1993, 29:183–190.

36. Park S-J, Kim J-J, Song J-K, *et al*.: Immediate and one-year results of percutaneous mitral balloon valvuloplasty using Inoue and double-balloon technique. *Am J Cardiol* 1993, 71:938–943.

37. Abdullah M, Halim M, Rajendran V, *et al*.: Comparison between single (Inoue) and double balloon mitral valvuloplasty: immediate and short-term results. *Am Heart J* 1992, 123:1581–1588.

38. Kasper W, Wollschlager H, Geibel A, *et al*.: Percutaneous mitral balloon valvuloplasty—a comparative evaluation of two transatrial techniques. *Am Heart J* 1992, 124:1562–1566.

39. Ruiz CE, Zhang HP, Macaya C, *et al*.: Comparison of Inoue single-balloon versus double-balloon technique for percutaneous mitral valvotomy. *Am Heart J* 1992, 123:942–947.

40. Palacios IF, Block PC, Wilkins GT, Weyman AE: Follow-up of patients undergoing percutaneous mitral balloon valvotomy. Analysis of factors determining restenosis. *Circulation* 1989, 79:573–579.

41. Lau K-W, Diong Z-P, Hong J-S: Percutaneous balloon mitral commissurotomy: an update. *J Inv Cardiol* 1994, 6:145–153.

42. McKay CR, Kawanishi DT, Kotlewski A, *et al*.: Improvement in exercise capacity and exercise hemodynamics 3 months after double-balloon catheter balloon valvuloplasty in the treatment of patients with symptomatic mitral stenosis. *Circulation* 1988, 77:1013–1021.

43. Cohen DJ, Kuntz RE, Gordon SPF, *et al*.: Predictors of long-term outcome after percutaneous balloon mitral valvuloplasty. *N Engl J Med* 1992, 19:1329–1335.

44. Vahanian A, Michel PC, Cormier B, *et al*.: Results of percutaneous mitral commissurotomy in 200 patients. *Am J Cardiol* 1989, 63:847–852.

45. Nobuyoshi M, Hamasaki N, Kimura T, *et al*.: Indications, complications, and short-term clinical outcome of percutaneous transvenous mitral commissurotomy. *Circulation* 1989, 809:782–792.

46. Al Zaibag MA, Ribeiro PA, Kasab SA, *et al*.: One-year follow-up after percutaneous double balloon mitral valvotomy. *Am J Cardiol* 1989, 63:126–127.

47. Ribeiro PA, Fawzy ME, Mimish L, *et al*.: Mitral restenosis and mitral regurgitation 1 year after Inoue mitral balloon restenosis and mitral regurgitation 1 year after Inoue mitral balloon valvotomy in a population of patients with pliable mitral valve stenosis. *Am Heart J* 1993, 126:136–140.

48. Pan M, Medina A, de Lezo JS, *et al*.: Factors determining late success after mitral balloon valvulotomy. *Am J Cardiol* 1993, 71:1181–1185.

49. John S, Bashi VV, Jairaj PS, *et al*.: Closed mitral valvotomy: early results and long-term follow-up of 3724 consecutive patients. *Circulation* 1983, 68:891–896.

50. Hickey MSJ, Blackstone EH, Kirklin JW, Dean LW: Outcome probabilities and life history after surgical mitral commissurotomy: implications for balloon commissurotomy. *J Am Coll Cardiol* 1991, 17:29–42.

51. Scalia D, Rizzoli G, Campanile F, *et al*.: Long-term results of mitral commissurotomy. *J Thorac Cardiovasc Surg* 1993, 105:633–642.

52. Turi ZG, Reyes VP, Raju S, *et al*.: Percutaneous balloon versus surgical closed commissurotomy for mitral stenosis: a prospective, randomized trial. *Circulation* 1991, 83:1179–1185.

53. Patel JJ, Shama D, Mitha AS, *et al*.: Balloon valvuloplasty versus closed commissurotomy for pliable mitral stenosis: a prospective hemodynamic study. *J Am Coll Cardiol* 1991, 18:1318–1322.

54. Arora R, Nair M, Kalra GS, *et al*.: Immediate and long-term results of balloon and surgical closed mitral valvotomy: a randomized comparative study. *Am Heart J* 1993, 125:1091–1094.

55. Reyes VP, Raju BS, Wynne J, *et al*.: Percutaneous balloon valvuloplasty compared with open surgical commissurotomy for mitral stenosis. *N Engl J Med* 1994, 331:961–967.

56. Crawford MH, Souchek J, Oprian CA, *et al*.: Determinants of survival and left ventricular performance after mitral valve replacement. *Circulation* 1990, 81:1173–1181.

57. Rahimtoola SH: The problem of valve prosthesis—patient mismatch. *Circulation* 1978, 58:20–24.

MITRAL REGURGITATION

9

CHAPTER

Blase A. Carabello

Clinical and basic investigations of mitral regurgitation (MR) over the past 15 years have resulted in a new understanding of the pathophysiology of the condition, new diagnostic tools to assess the disease, good clinical indexes on which to base the timing of corrective surgery, and a new understanding of the importance of the mitral valve apparatus. These advancements have led to important changes in mitral valve surgery and in improved operative results.

It is now recognized that the nature of the volume overload in MR is different from that of other left ventricular volume-overload lesions. In most volume overloads (for example, aortic regurgitation, anemia) the excess volume is pumped into the aorta, thus increasing systolic pressure. In MR the excess volume is delivered into the left atrium under normal pressure. Thus, although most left ventricular volume overloads actually constitute a combined volume and pressure overload, the volume overload of MR constitutes normal pressure or pure volume overload [1]. These differences affect the way in which the left ventricle hypertrophies in response to MR and the way in which left ventricular dysfunction develops if the regurgitation is untreated.

Diagnosis of MR has improved substantially with the advent of color-flow Doppler ultrasound. Although the physical examination can approximate lesion severity by the amount of left ventricular enlargement detected or by the presence of a third heart sound, actual quantification of the amount of MR previously rested on a left ventriculogram performed at cardiac catheterization. Now, however, color-flow Doppler ultrasound allows noninvasive visualization of the mitral regurgitant jet. Although quantification of the magnitude of the regurgitation by this technique has limitations, rough estimation of severity is possible, is a clear improvement over the physical examination alone, and can be repeated at intervals without the need for an invasive procedure [2].

There have also been advances in the proper timing of valve surgery to correct the disease. Although MR may be tolerated for years, eventually left ventricular dysfunction develops. The goal of management is to correct the MR before the occurrence of irreversible left ventricular dysfunction. Several easily obtained markers of left ventricular performance have been developed that guide the clinician in making a decision regarding the timing of surgery. The development of these markers has in part been responsible for earlier corrective surgery leading to a reduction in operative mortality and a reduction in persistent postoperative congestive heart failure.

The operation for restoring mitral competence has also been improved. Until recently, when surgery was performed, it entailed a mitral valve replacement during which the native mitral valve and its chordal attachments were removed. Although the importance of the mitral valve apparatus in maintaining ventricular performance had been alluded to four decades ago [3], only recently have we appreciated the need to preserve the mitral valve apparatus whenever possible. The advent of successful mitral valve repair instead of replacement and techniques that allow chordal preservation during replacement have led to a substantial reduction in operative mortality, improved postoperative left ventricular function, and reduced the risk of thromboembolism and the need for anticoagulants.

Thus, a new understanding of the pathophysiology of this disease, new diagnostic techniques for assessing its severity, improved indicators for the timing of surgery, and an improved operation have all led to a better outlook for patients with MR.

ETIOLOGY

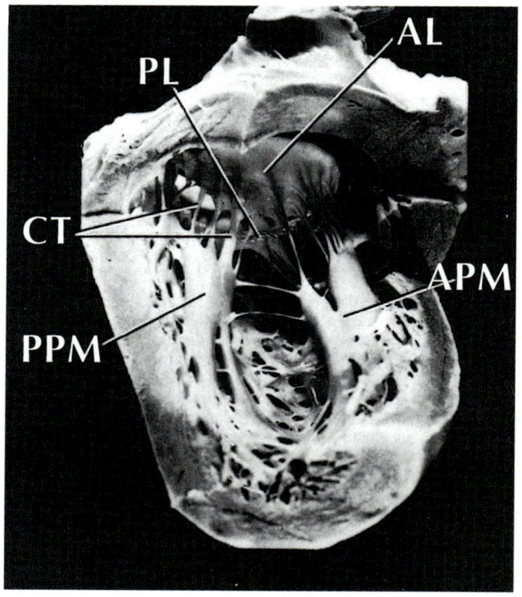

FIGURE 9-1. Structure. The mitral valve apparatus is composed of the mitral annulus, the mitral leaflets, the chordae tendineae, and the papillary muscles. Abnormalities of any of these structures can cause mitral regurgitation (MR). In this figure, the mitral valve leaflets are seen in relationship to their chordal attachments, and the chordae tendineae are seen with their attachments to the papillary muscles. AL—anterior leaflet; APM—anterior papillary muscle; CT—chordae tendineae; PL—posterior leaflet; PPM—posterior papillary muscle.(*Adapted from* Wieting and Stripling [4]; with permission.)

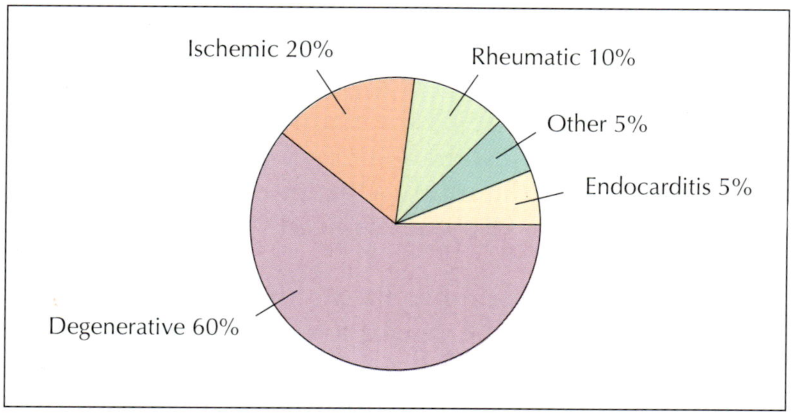

FIGURE 9-2. Relative incidence of the causes of severe primary MR evaluated at the time of autopsy or mitral valve surgery [5,6]. Whereas rheumatic heart disease was the leading cause of MR 30 years ago, degenerative mitral valve disease (mitral valve prolapse and ruptured chordae tendineae) is the leading cause of severe MR today in the developed countries of the world. This figure does not include secondary MR, in which the abnormality producing MR is a change in left ventricular geometry rather than an abnormality of the valve or valvular apparatus. Dilated cardiomyopathy is the leading cause of secondary MR.

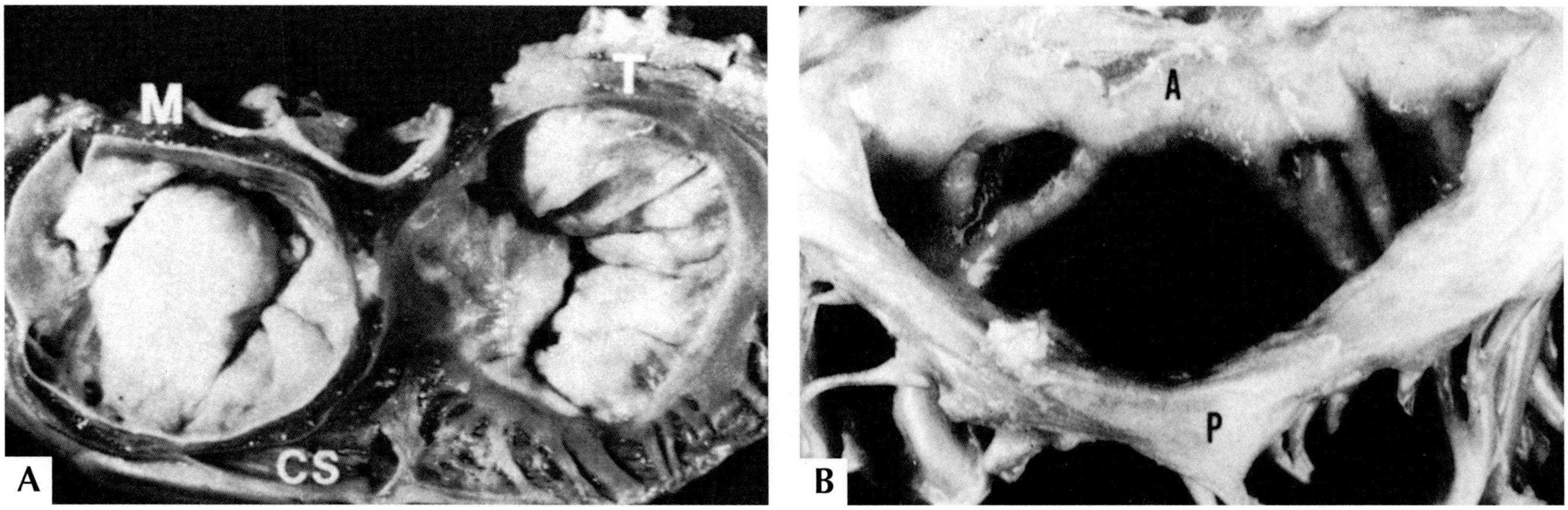

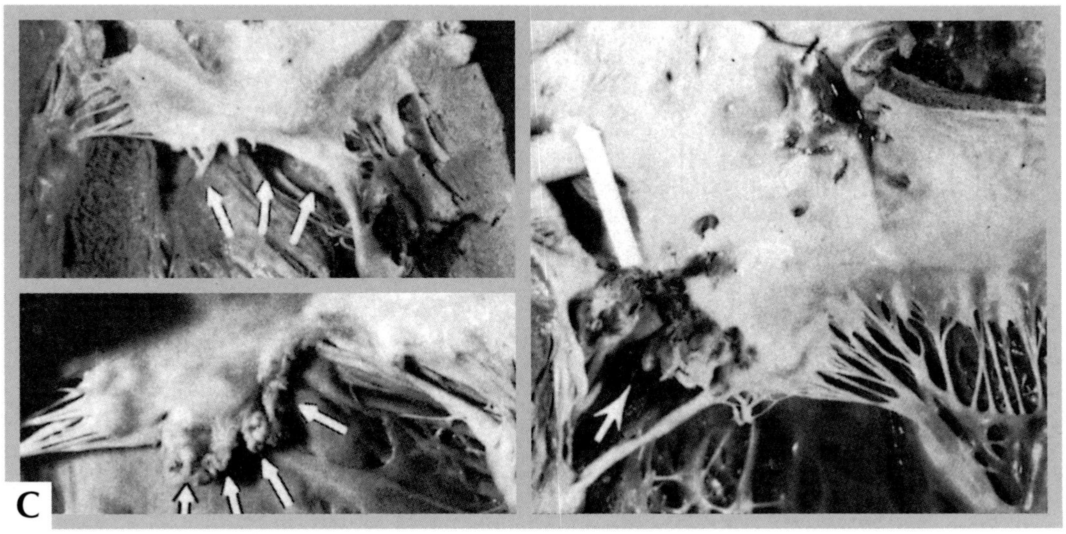

FIGURE 9-3. Mitral valve pathology. **A,** The mitral (M) and tricuspid (T) valves of a patient with severe MR due to myxomatous degeneration and mitral valve prolapse are demonstrated. A large scallop of the mitral valve is clearly seen and the patient had one ruptured chorda documented at autopsy. This type of mitral valve disease is the most common cause of MR today. **B,** Rheumatic mitral valvopathy demonstrated here is an inflammatory disease characterized by scarring and retraction of the chordae tendineae and of the leaflets. **C,** Ruptured chordae tendineae (*arrows in each panel*) due to endocarditis was the cause of severe MR in three different patients in the three panels shown. Endocarditis may also cause severe MR by infection, causing damage of the valve leaflets themselves. A—anterior; CS—coronary sinus; P—posterior. (Parts A and C *adapted from* Roberts [5]; part B *adapted from* Olson and coworkers [6]; with permission.)

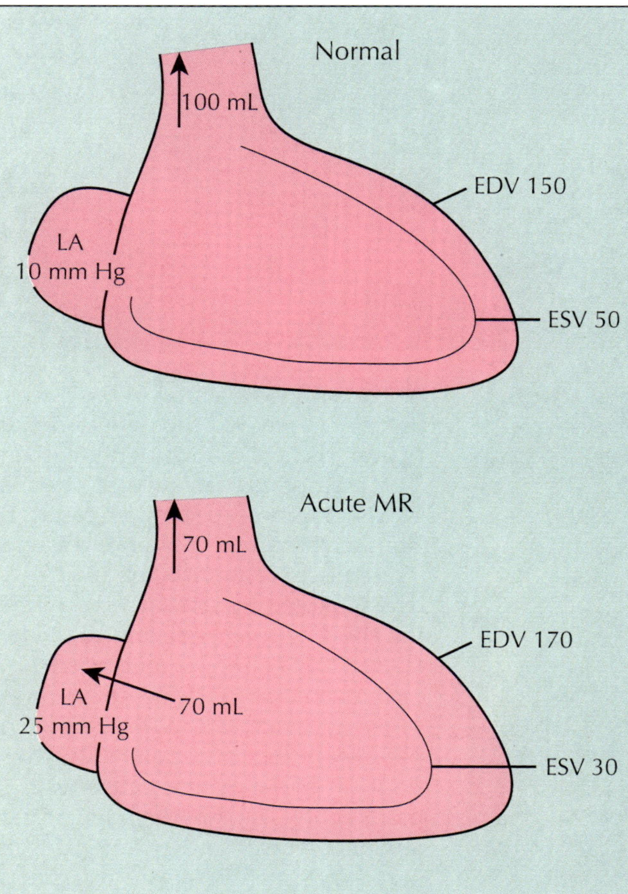

	Preload SL, μ	Afterload ESS, *Kdyne/cm²*	CF	EF	RF	FSV, *mL*
N	2.07	90	N	0.67	0.0	100
AMR	2.25	60	N	0.82	0.50	70

A

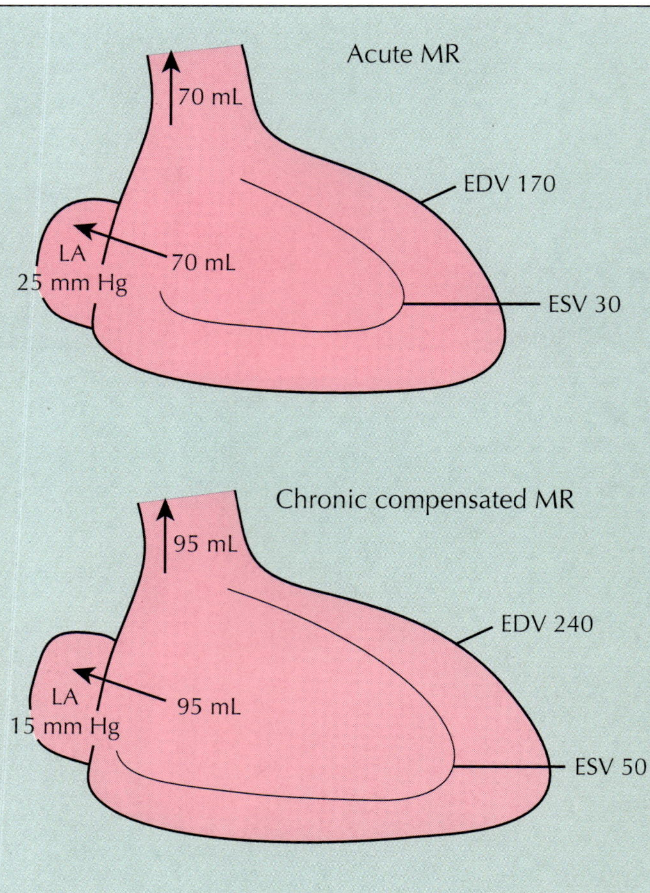

	Preload SL, μ	Afterload ESS, *Kdyne/cm²*	CF	EF	RF	FSV, *mL*
AMR	2.25	60	N	0.82	0.5	70
CCMR	2.19	90	N	0.79	0.5	95

B

FIGURE 9-4. Three pathophysiologic stages of MR. [7]. **A,** The physiology of acute mitral regurgitation (AMR) is compared with that of normal (N) competent mitral valve. The acute volume overload of MR increases the sarcomere length (SL) of existing sarcomeres toward maximum, producing a modest increase in end-diastolic volume (EDV) [8].

Simultaneously, the new pathway for left ventricular ejection into the left atrium (LA) effectively reduces the resistance to ejection (afterload), characterized as end-systolic stress (ESS) [9]. Reduced afterload allows the ventricle to eject more completely and thus end-systolic volume (ESV) is reduced.

Although contractile function (CF) has not changed, the changes in loading conditions increase total stroke volume in this example to 140 mL and increase ejection fraction (EF) to 82%. However, because 50% of the total stroke volume of the left ventricle is now entering the LA (regurgitant fraction [RF]= 0.5), LA pressure increases and forward stroke volume (FSV) decreases to 70 mL. At this point in the disease the patient will suffer from symptoms of congestive failure (fatigue and dyspnea) even though ventricular muscle function is normal.

B, If the patient in *panel A* tolerated the insult of AMR without the need for surgery and he were followed for several months, he might enter the chronic compensated mitral regurgitation (CCMR) phase, contrasted with the acute phase here. The major compensatory change is the development of eccentric cardiac hypertrophy in which the cardiocytes are elongated by the addition of sarcomeres in series [10]. The result is that EDV has increased from 170 mL during AMR to 240 mL in the CCMR. Total stroke volume is now 190 mL, allowing FSV to return nearly to normal. At the same time the LA has enlarged and can now better accommodate the volume overload and thus LA pressure has fallen significantly from the acute phase. CF is still relatively normal, which together with the compensatory hypertrophy and still favorable loading conditions, might allow the patient to be asymptomatic. (*continued*)

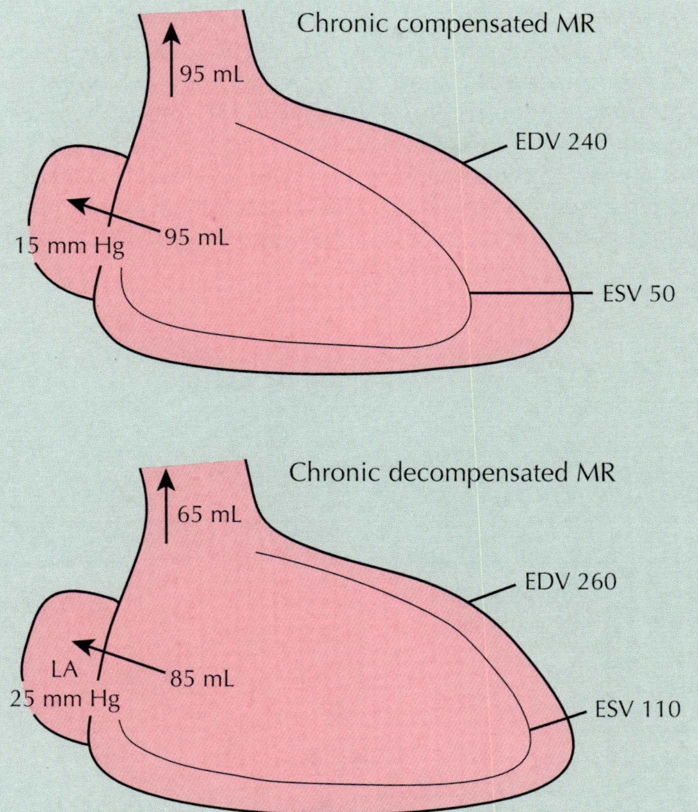

	Preload SL, μ	Afterload ESS, *Kdyne/cm²*	CF	EF	RF	FSV, *mL*
CCMR	2.19	90	N	0.79	0.50	95
CDMR	2.19	120	↓	0.58	0.57	65

C

FIGURE 9-4. (*continued*) **C,** Although the patient may tolerate CCMR for years, eventually left ventricular CF deteriorates and the patient enters a chronic decompensated MR (CDMR) phase, which is compared with the compensated phase. Contractile dysfunction impairs left ventricular ejection, resulting in a larger ESV, in turn leading to a further increase in EDV. The increase in EDV may cause greater annular dilatation and misalignment of the papillary muscles, making the MR worse. The result of worsened muscle function and increased regurgitation is that both forward and total stroke volume fall. Increased left ventricular diastolic volume causes elevation of left ventricular end-diastolic pressure and LA pressure. The patient may again notice fatigue and dyspnea. Despite the presence of contractile dysfunction, EF remains in the normal range as a result of the still favorable loading conditions, although it is lower than in the compensated phase. CC—chronic compensated. (*Adapted from* Carabello [7].)

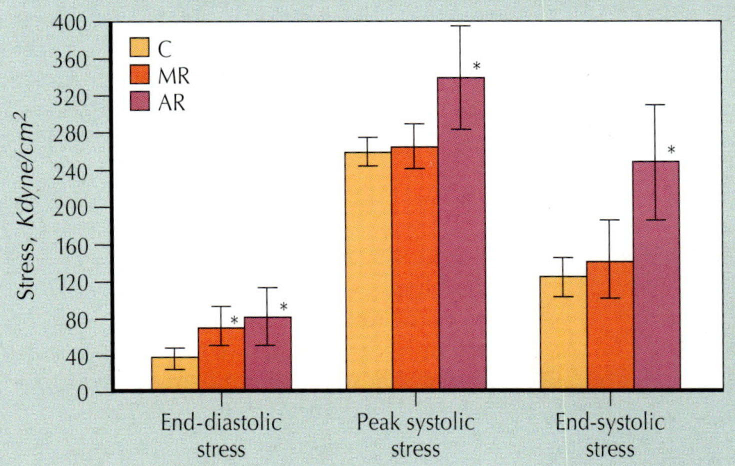

FIGURE 9-5. Loading conditions. The loading conditions of severe MR are contrasted with those in normal individuals (C) and are also compared with a group of patients with a similar amount of severe aortic regurgitation (AR) [1]. End-diastolic stress, an estimate of preload, is increased in both groups of patients with regurgitation as might be expected for volume overloading lesions that increase left ventricular filling. However, afterload characterized as either peak systolic stress or end-systolic stress was elevated in AR but not in MR. In MR the extra volume is delivered under normal pressure into the left atrium and thus afterload is reduced acutely (*see* Fig. 9-4*A*) or remains normal in chronic MR [11]. However, in AR the extra volume pumped into the aorta increases systolic pressure, causing pressure overload as well as volume overload reflected by the increase in left ventricular afterload. *Asterisks* indicate a significant difference ($P < 0.05$) from the control group. (*Adapted from* Wisenbaugh and coworkers [1].)

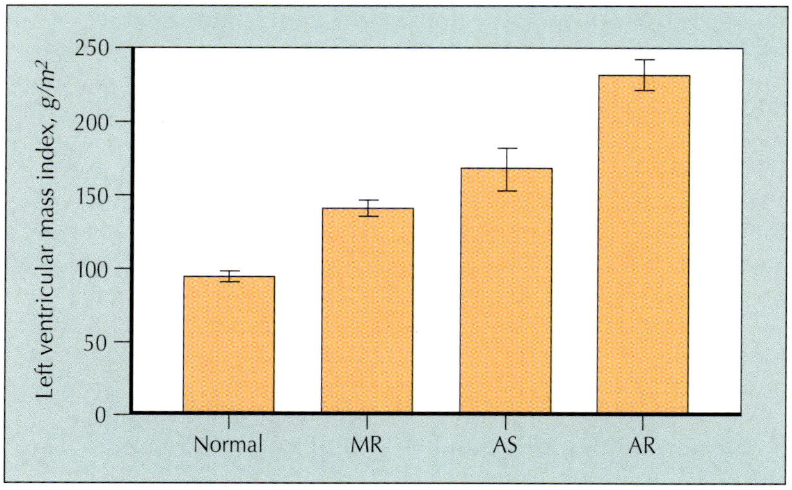

FIGURE 9-6. Left ventricular hypertrophy. The amount of left ventricular hypertrophy as reflected by left ventricular mass index is demonstrated for patients with MR, aortic stenosis (AS), or aortic regurgitation (AR) and contrasted to normal subjects [12]. The amount of hypertrophy is the least in MR, probably reflecting the loading conditions demonstrated in Fig. 9-5. The hypertrophy in MR is characterized by the lowest mass-to-volume ratio of the left-sided valve lesions. Thus, in MR there is the least amount of mass present to pump the additional volume, potentially overloading the existing myocardium.

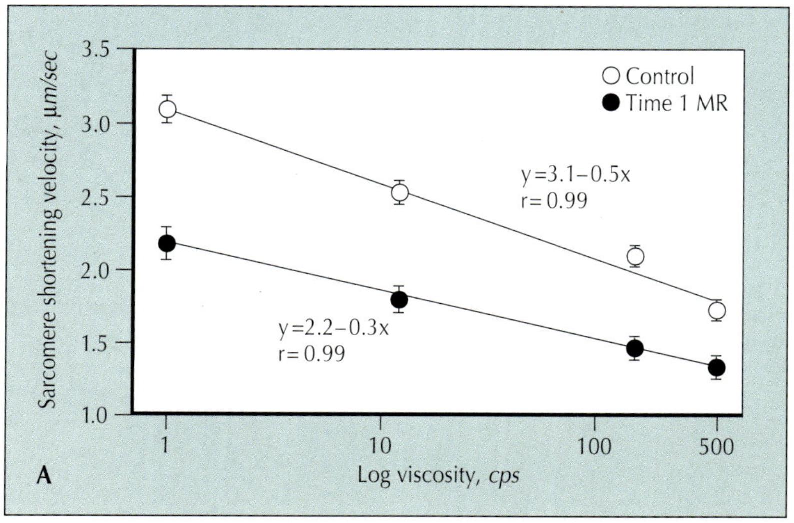

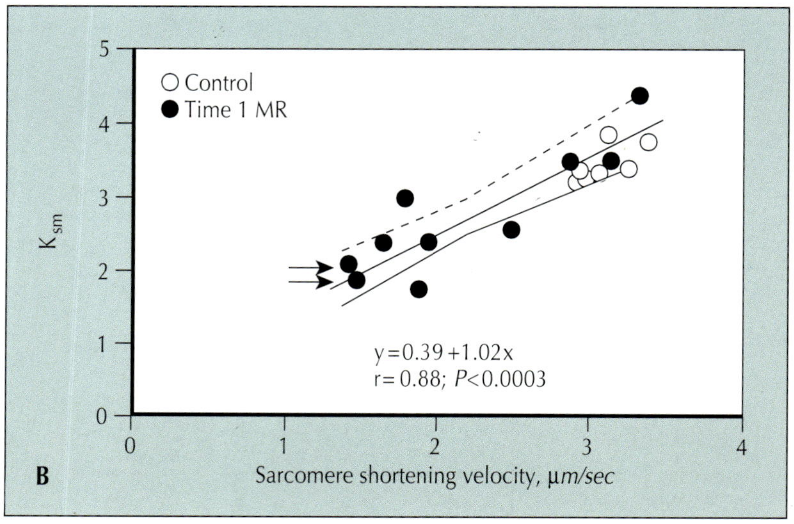

FIGURE 9-7. Canine model. Examining the mechanisms leading to the phase of decompensated muscle function (*see* Fig. 9-4C) has been difficult. However, insights into the nature of the muscle dysfunction have been gained from a canine model of MR. **A,** The sarcomere shortening velocity-viscosity relationship of isolated cardiocytes taken from control dogs and from dogs with chronic MR (Time 1 MR) is demonstrated [14]. As viscosity is increased by the inclusion of inert methylcellulose into the medium surrounding the cell, it imparts a viscous afterload on the cell. The sarcomere viscosity-velocity relationship is analogous to the force-velocity relationship of classic cardiac mechanics. This relationship is severely depressed for the myocytes taken from mitral regurgitant ventricles, indicating that contractile abnormalities of the cardiocytes comprising the ventricles underlie the contractile dysfunction of the whole ventricle.

B, End-systolic stiffness (K_{sm}), an index of *in vivo* ventricular contractile function, is plotted against sarcomere shortening velocity, a measure of myocyte contractile function. The two are well correlated, suggesting that the contractile abnormalities of the ventricle are well explained by abnormalities of the myocytes themselves. Dogs with abnormal left ventricular function fell at the left lower corner of the relationship (*arrows*) indicating both contractile dysfunction at the ventricular level and contractile dysfunction at the cellular level. cps—cycles per second. (*Adapted from* Urabe and coworkers [14].)

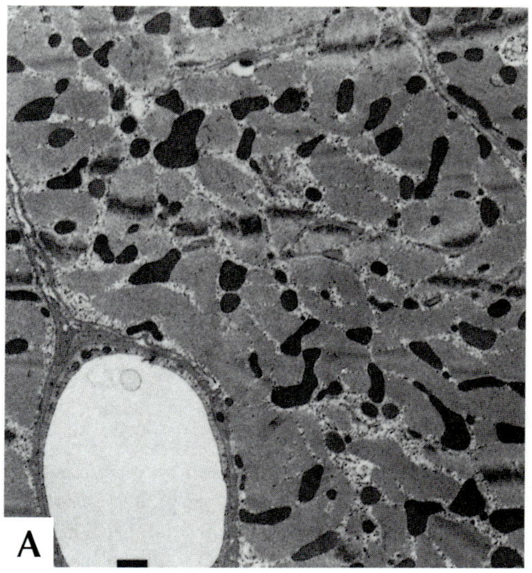

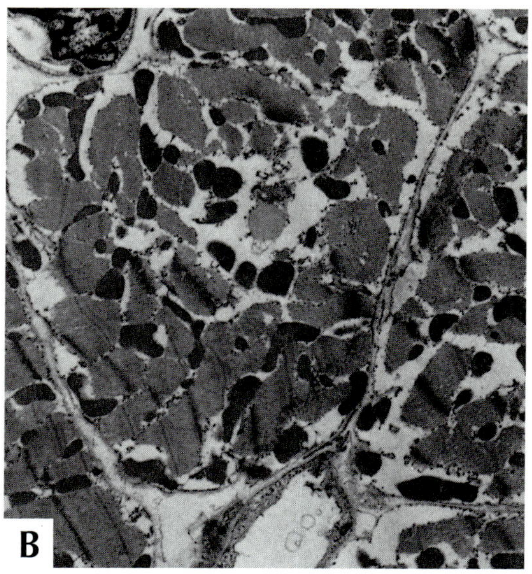

FIGURE 9-8. Myocardial histology. Histology of normal myocardium (**A**), myocardium from an animal with MR and mild dysfunction (**B**), and myocardium from a dog with MR and severe dysfunction (**C**) are demonstrated. (*continued*)

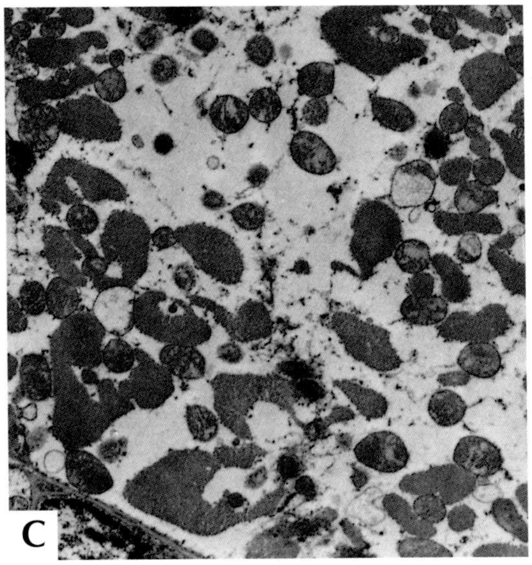

FIGURE 9-8. *(continued)* In *panel C*, there is a 35% loss of myofibrils, which accounts for the loss of contractility. In fact the correlation coefficient relating the loss of myofibrils to indexes of both *in vivo* ventricular function and *in vitro* cellular contractile function is 0.9. This disordered histology is virtually identical to that of human papillary muscles taken from patients with severe MR although the epicardium from such patients fails to show the myofibril loss [15]. Bar = 1 µm. (*Adapted from* Urabe and coworkers [14]; with permission.)

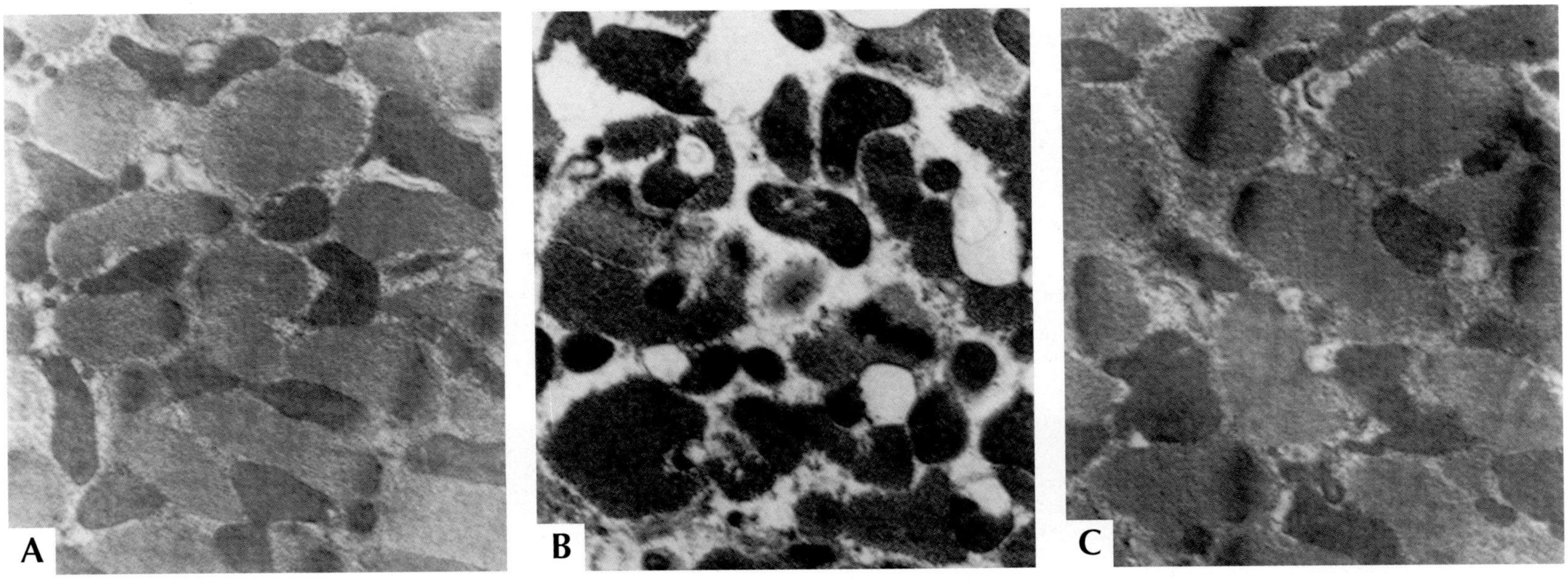

FIGURE 9-9. Myocardial histology after mitral valve replacement. To determine whether the contractile dysfunction of canine MR is reversible, seven dogs with MR underwent mitral valve replacement after dysfunction had developed and then were followed for 3 months [16]. Three indexes of ventricular contractile function were depressed after 3 months of MR. Three months after mitral valve replacement all indexes improved. Concordantly, the abnormal histology of the myocardium also improved as is shown here [17]. **A,** Photomicrograph of the myocardium of a normal dog. **B,** Myocardium taken from a dog with chronic severe MR shows severe myofibrillar loss similar to that seen in Fig. 9-8. **C,** Photomicrograph of the myocardium of a dog with severe chronic MR 3 months after mitral valve replacement shows myofibrillar restoration. These data demonstrate that the ventricular dysfunction of MR is reversible if the volume overload is corrected in a timely fashion. Importantly, studies in patients with MR also have demonstrated improvement in left ventricular dysfunction after surgery [18]. (*Adapted from* Spinale and coworkers [17]; with permission.)

DIAGNOSIS

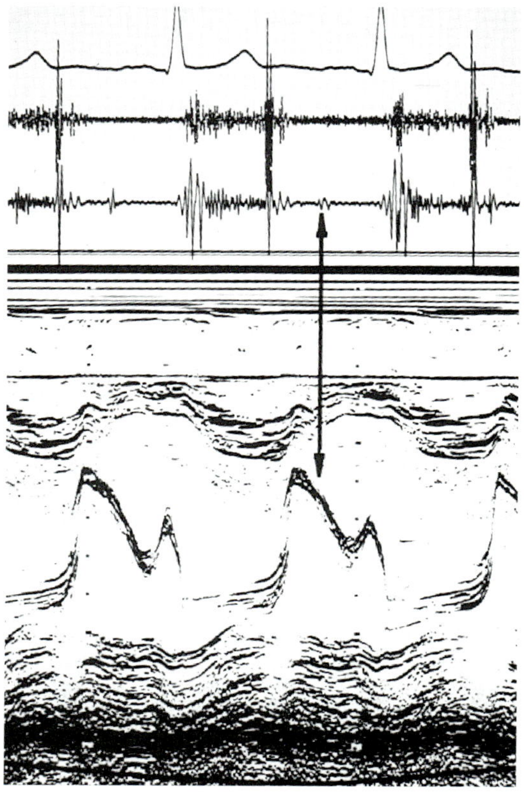

FIGURE 9-10. Phonocardiogram and echocardiogram of a patient with MR. The classic murmur of MR is demonstrated by the phonocardiogram (*second and third tracings from the top*). Because turbulent flow into the left atrium begins as soon as left ventricular pressure exceeds left atrial pressure, the murmur is virtually holosystolic. In early diastole, the volume overloaded left atrium discharges its contents rapidly into the left ventricle under high pressure usually producing a third heart sound (S_3) whether or not congestive heart failure is present. The *arrows* connect the S_3 recorded by the phonocardiogram to the rapid opening of the mitral valve on the echocardiogram.

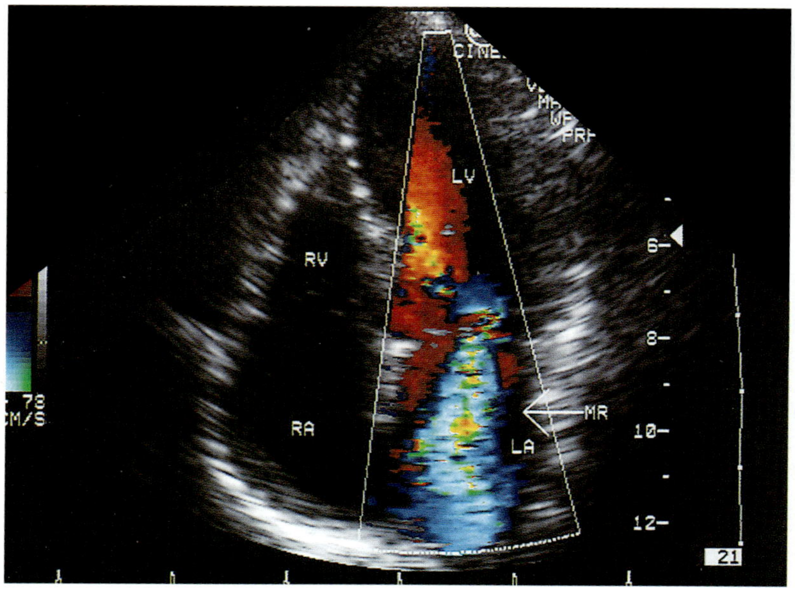

FIGURE 9-11. Doppler pattern. The color-flow Doppler pattern of disturbed flow produced by the mitral regurgitant jet (MR) is demonstrated in the left atrium (LA). The size of jet is usually proportional to the amount of regurgitation but because the Doppler pattern represents flow velocity not quantity, the jet size may over- or underestimate the amount of regurgitation. Jet velocity may also vary according to loading conditions altering estimation of the amount of MR present. LV—left ventricle; RA—right atrium; RV—right ventricle.

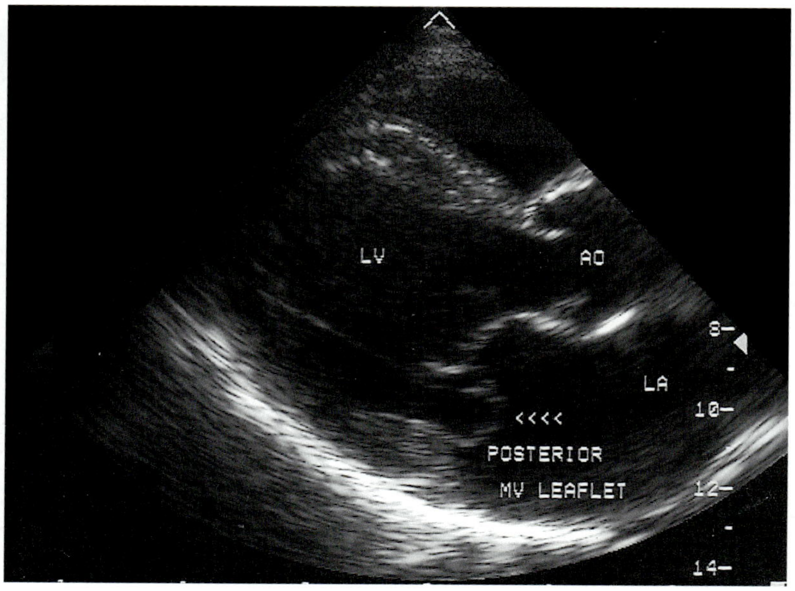

FIGURE 9-12. Echocardiography. The echocardiographic appearance of mitral valve prolapse (< posterior mitral valve [MV] leaflet) is demonstrated as is the utility of the two-dimensional echocardiogram in defining mitral valve anatomy. AO—aorta; LA—left atrium; LV—left ventricle.

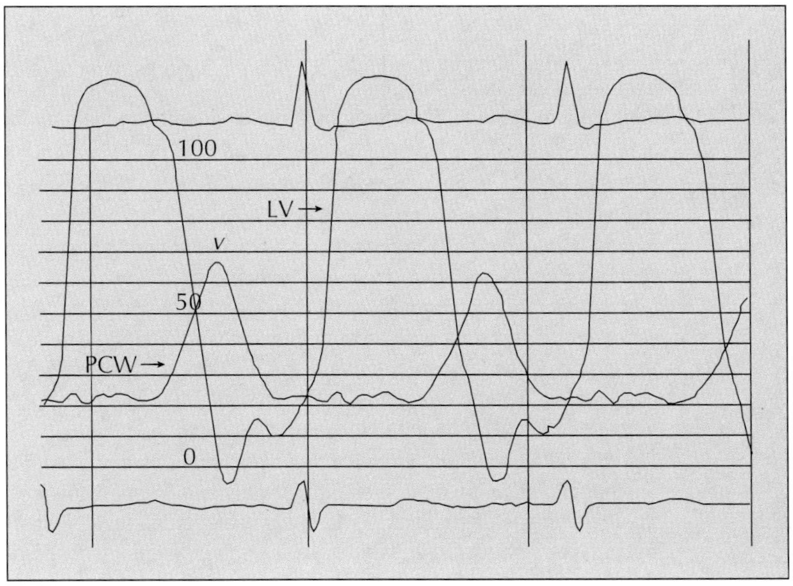

Figure 9-13. Pulmonary capillary wedge (PCW) pressure tracing (which reflects left atrial pressure) with characteristic large *v* wave in MR. The *v* wave is increased due to systolic transfer of both ventricular pressure and volume to the left atrium and also due to simultaneous left atrial filling occurring from pulmonary venous return. However, in long-standing chronic MR, increased left atrial size may allow the regurgitant volume to be accommodated without a large systolic increase in atrial pressure, reducing the amplitude of the *v* wave. Conversely, large *v* waves do not always indicate the presence of severe MR; they may also occur in ventricular septal defect and cardiomyopathy. LV—left ventricle.

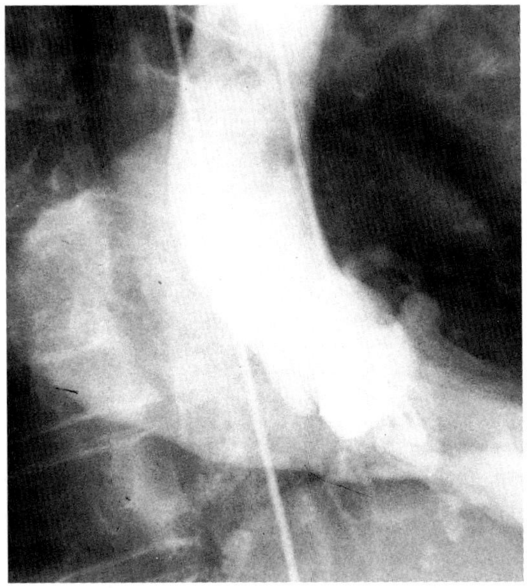

Figure 9-14. Cineangiography. A left ventricular cineangiogram of a patient with MR demonstrates opacification of the left atrium after a large quantity of contrast injected into the left ventricle was regurgitated into the left atrium.

Medical Therapy

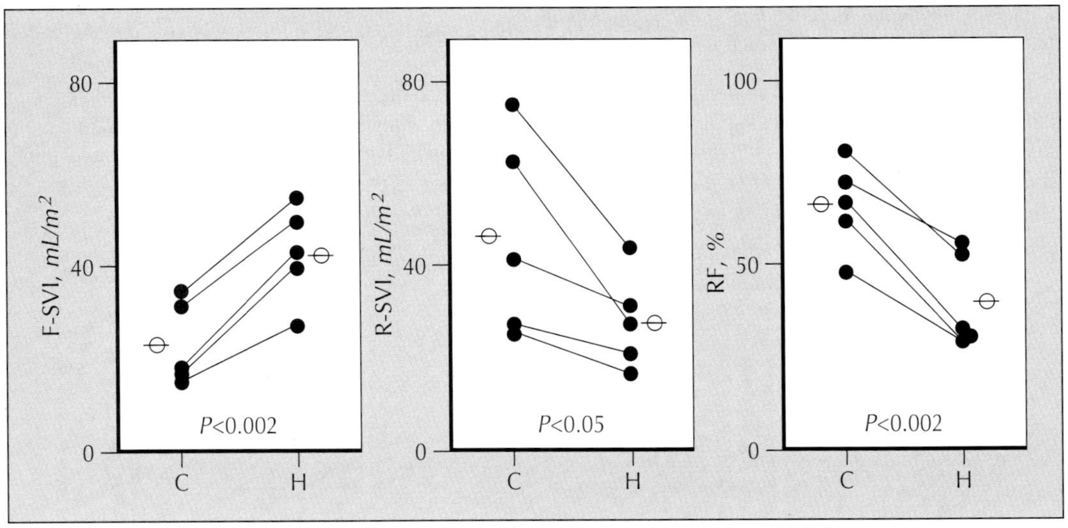

Figure 9-15. Vasodilators. Arterial vasodilators such as hydralazine (H) allow more flow to preferentially enter the aorta during systole, simultaneously increasing forward stroke volume (F-SVI) while reducing regurgitant flow (R-SVI) and regurgitant fraction (RF) [19]. Vasodilators are effective in improving the hemodynamics and reducing the symptoms of patients with acute MR. However, a role for these agents in the therapy of chronic MR is unproven. Other vasodilators that might be effective in chronic MR include angiotensin-converting enzyme inhibitors and dihydropyridine calcium channel blockers [20,21].C—control; Θ—mean value.(*Adapted from* Greenberg and coworkers [19].)

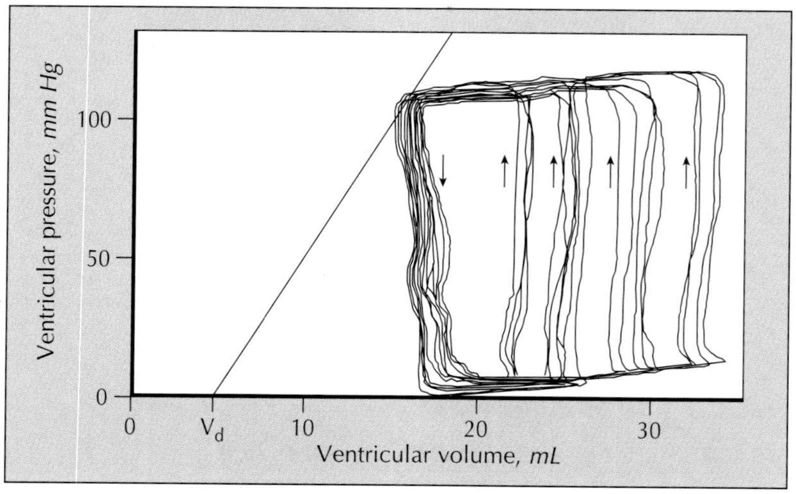

FIGURE 9-16. Pressure-volume loops. Mitral valve surgery should occur before irreversible left ventricular dysfunction has developed. Because preload is augmented and afterload is reduced in MR, it causes ejection fraction, a preload-dependent index, to overestimate contractile function. Ideally, load-independent indexes should be used to estimate contractile function. Pressure-volume loops from an isolated canine left ventricle demonstrate that regardless of the extent of left ventricular filling during diastole (preload), the ventricle ejects to the same end-systolic volume as long as end-systolic pressure, a measure of afterload, remains constant [22]. Thus, end-systolic volume (or dimension) is nearly independent of preload, which is why these end-systolic indexes have been used successfully in addition to ejection phase indexes to assess left ventricular function as a guide to the proper timing of surgery in MR. *Arrows* show the direction of movement of the pressure-volume curve. (*Adapted from* Suga and coworkers [22].)

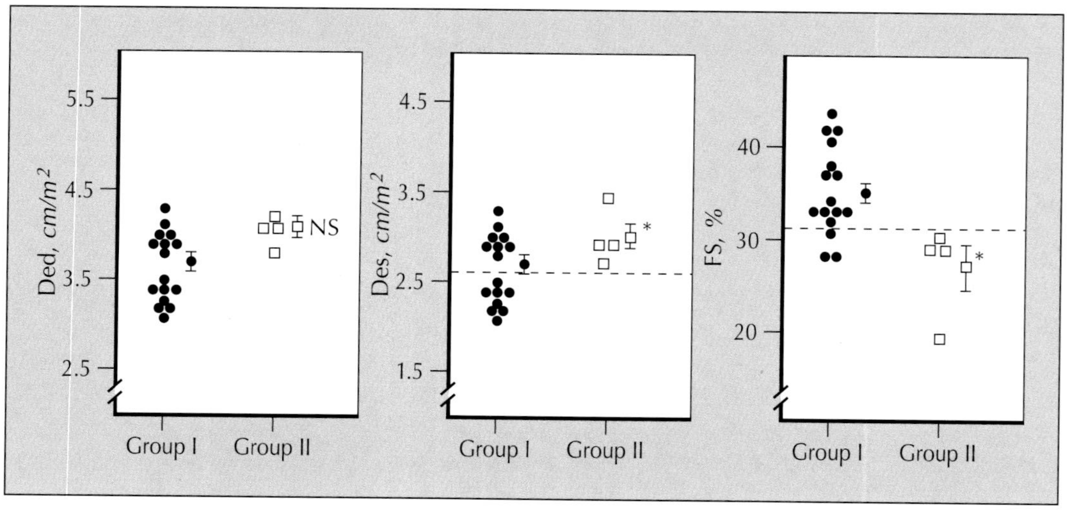

FIGURE 9-17. Postoperative symptomatic status. Patients with MR who became asymptomatic after mitral valve replacement (group I, *solid circles*) are compared with patients who remained symptomatic after surgery (group II, *open squares*) [23]. As might be predicted from Fig. 9-16, echocardiographic end-diastolic dimension (Ded) did not distinguish group I from group II, whereas end-systolic dimension (Des) was a useful predictor of outcome. Patients with MR whose Des indexed for body surface area exceeded 2.6 cm/m^2 did poorly, whereas patients whose left ventricles were able to contract to a smaller dimension had a good outcome. However, there were many patients who were asymptomatic even though Des exceeded 2.6 cm^2. Note that fractional shortening (FS) was higher than normal (35%) in group I because preserved contractile function in that group together with the favorable loading conditions of MR augmented ejection performance. Thus, in MR an ejection fraction in the low normal range may in fact indicate that significant muscle dysfunction exists. Indeed, Enriquez-Sarano *et al.* demonstrated that ejection fraction had to be greater than 60% preoperatively to ensure a normal life span after mitral valve surgery [24]. *Asterisk* indicates $P < 0.01$. (*Adapted from* Zile and coworkers [23].)

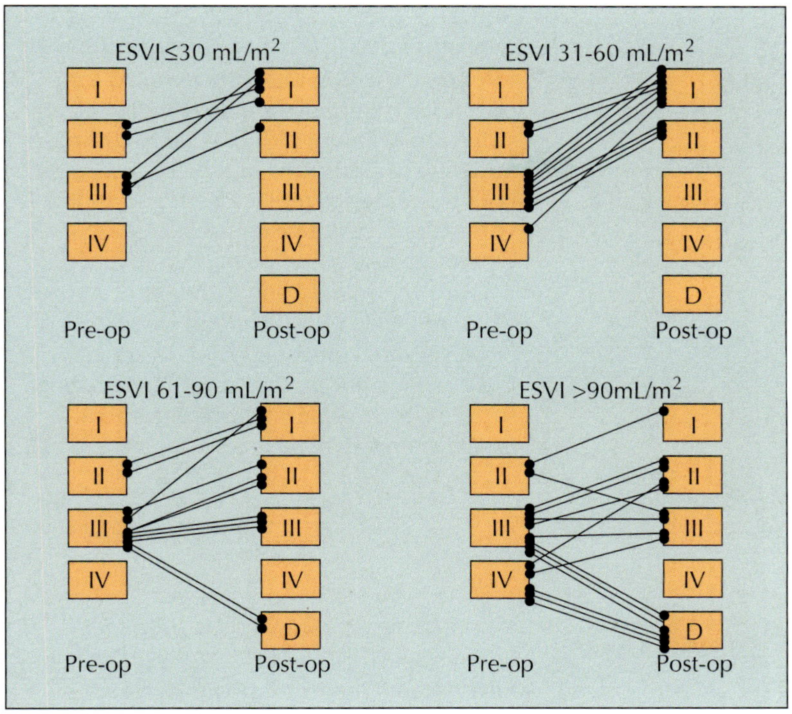

FIGURE 9-18. Angiographic data. When patients with mitral or aortic regurgitation develop left ventricular dysfunction such that end-systolic volume index (ESVI) exceeds 60 mL/m², postoperative (post-op) outcome may be unfavorable [25]. The indexed end-systolic dimension of 2.6 cm/m² from Fig. 9-17 equates approximately to 53 mL/m², very similar to the data in this figure. Both studies are consistent with the results of a large cooperative trial where a preoperative (pre-op) ESVI of 50 mL/m² was a good cutoff for separating good from suboptimal postoperative outcome [26]. Further, the predictive value of 2.6 mL/m² in Zile *et al.*'s study [23], when multiplied by the average body surface area of the patients studied, yields an end-systolic dimension of 45 mm. This value was also found to be predictive in a recent study by Wisenbaugh *et al.* [27]. I,II,II,IV—NewYork Heart Association classes; D—deaths. (*Adapted from* Borow and coworkers [25].)

OPERATIVE RESULTS

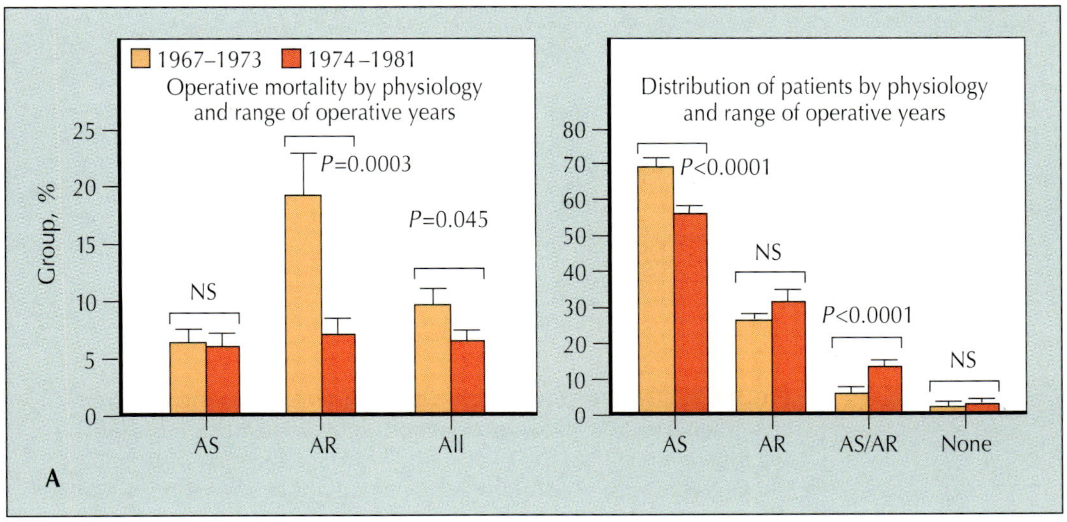

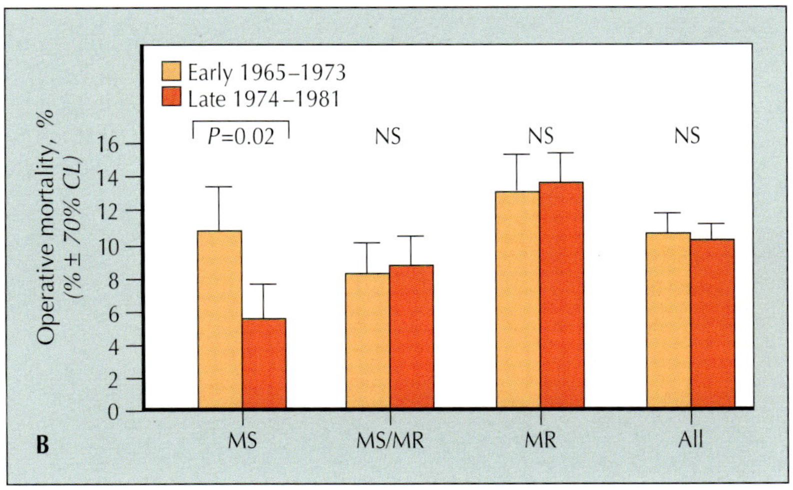

FIGURE 9-19. Operative mortality for aortic valve (**A**) and mitral valve (**B**) disease for a large tertiary care institution [28,29]. Operative mortality for correction of aortic stenosis (AS) was low both early and late in this experience. Operative mortality for both mitral stenosis (MS) and aortic regurgitation (AR) initially was high but improved dramatically with experience. However, mortality for mitral valve replacement for MR persisted in being higher than all other lesions. CL—confidence level; NS—not significant. (Part A *adapted from* Scott and coworkers [28]; part B *adapted from* Scott and coworkers [29].)

COMPARISON OF OPERATIVE MORTALITY RATES*

STUDY	REPAIR		REPLACEMENT	
	PATIENTS, *n*	MORTALITY, %	PATIENTS, *n*	MORTALITY, %
Oury *et al.* [31]	34	0	46	13.0
Duran *et al.* [32]	255	1.8	307	11.4
Yacoub *et al.* [33]	86	5.0	46	11.0
Oliveira *et al.* [34]	84	4.9	101	5.0
Adebo and Ross [35]	21	0	44	6.8
Total	480	1.9	544	10.3

**P*<0.0001 for the comparison between the repair and replacement groups.

FIGURE 9-20. Comparative operative mortality rates. The operative mortality rate for correction of MR is reduced for mitral valve repair compared with mitral valve replacement [30]. The table compares outcome from groups in which statistics for both mitral valve replacement and mitral valve repair could be compiled [31–35]. Operative mortality for mitral valve repair was approximately one fifth that of mitral valve replacement. Although these data do not represent controlled trials of replacement versus repair, they are suggestive of superiority of repair over replacement. (*Adapted from* Cosgrove and coworkers [30].)

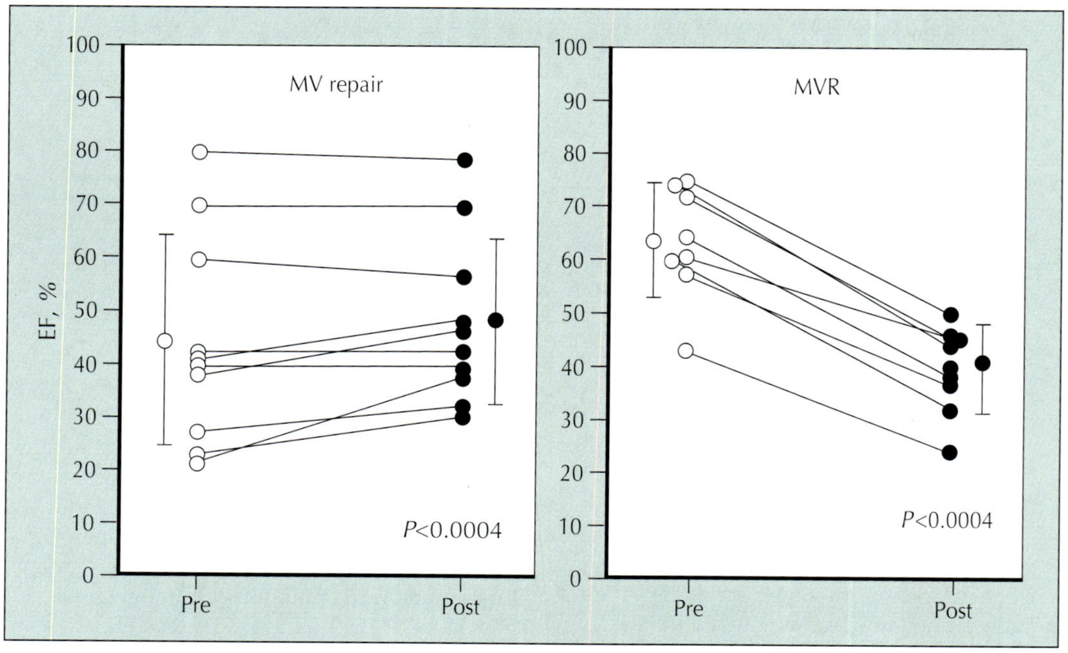

FIGURE 9-21. Reasons for mitral valve repair superiority over valve replacement. Mitral valve repair retains the patient's native mitral valve, which is more resistant to endocarditis than is a prosthetic valve. Additionally, the repaired native valve has a low risk for thromboembolism, obviating anticoagulation. Perhaps the most important reason for repair's superiority to replacement is shown in this figure that demonstrates preoperative (pre) and postoperative (post) ejection fraction for mitral valve replacement (MVR) and mitral valve repair (MV repair) [36]. Ejection fraction fell after replacement but was preserved at its preoperative level after repair. These findings have been confirmed by additional studies [37–39]. (*Adapted from* Goldman and coworkers [36].)

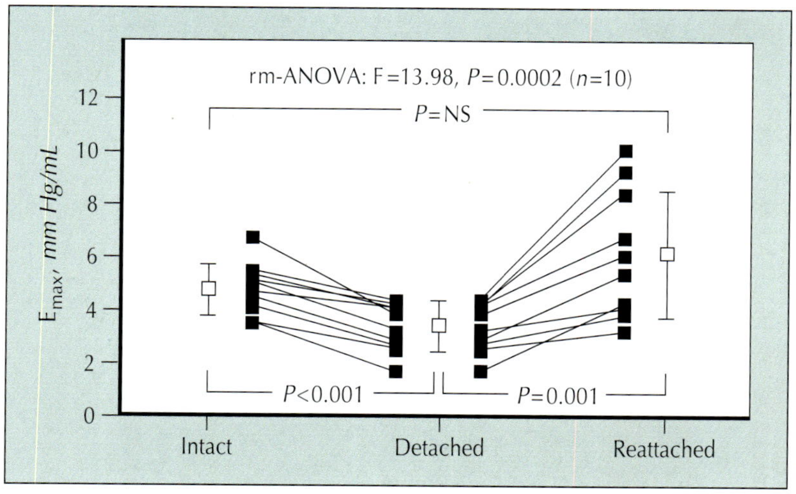

FIGURE 9-22. Chordal detachment and reattachment in swine in situ. One reason chordal preservation helps maintain ejection performance is that the mitral apparatus is important in maintaining chamber contractile efficiency. E_{max}, a measure of ventricular contractile function, was examined at baseline, after the chordae tendineae were detached and after the chordae tendineae were reattached in a swine in situ left ventricular isovolumic model [40]. Detachment of the chordae tendineae produced an acute fall in contractile function, which was restored when the chordae tendineae were reattached. rm-ANOVA—analysis of variance for repeated measurement. (*Adapted from* Sarris and coworkers [40].)

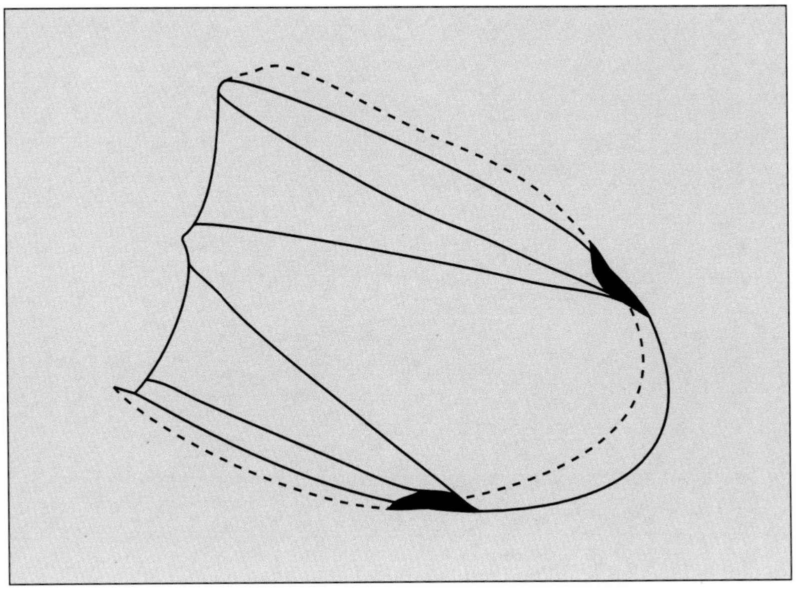

FIGURE 9-23. Mechanism whereby the chordae tendineae might influence left ventricular contractile function. The *solid outline* represents the left ventricular end-diastolic silhouette. The *dotted outline* represents the silhouette early in isovolumic systole. In early systole the papillary muscles pulling on the chordae tendineae against the mitral valve shorten the long axis of the heart. Because systole is in its isovolumetric phase, shortening of the long axis must be associated with lengthening of the short axis. Lengthening of the short axis in turn augments short axis preload preparing the short axis (where most of ejection is developed) for the ensuing systolic ejection [3]. Severing the chordae tendineae destroys this mechanism and reduces left ventricular function.

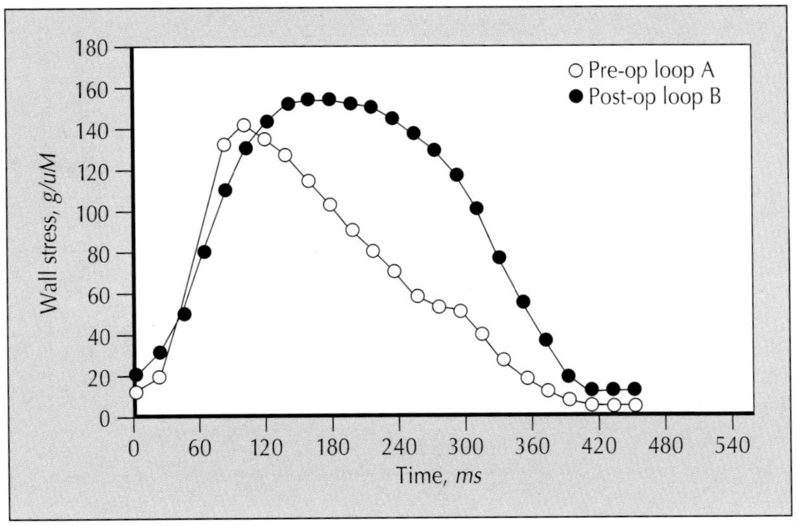

FIGURE 9-24. Left ventricular stress during systole before and after mitral valve replacement (MVR) in humans. Preoperative systolic wall stress (afterload) plotted over time (*loop A*) is compared with postoperative stress (*loop B*) [41]. Following MVR, afterload increased, presumably because surgery removed the low impedance pathway for ejection into the left atrium. However, this presents a paradox. If both MVR and repair remove the low impedance pathway for ejection, then both procedures should increase afterload and lower ejection performance postoperatively, but valve repair does not. (*Adapted from* Wong and Spotnitz [41].)

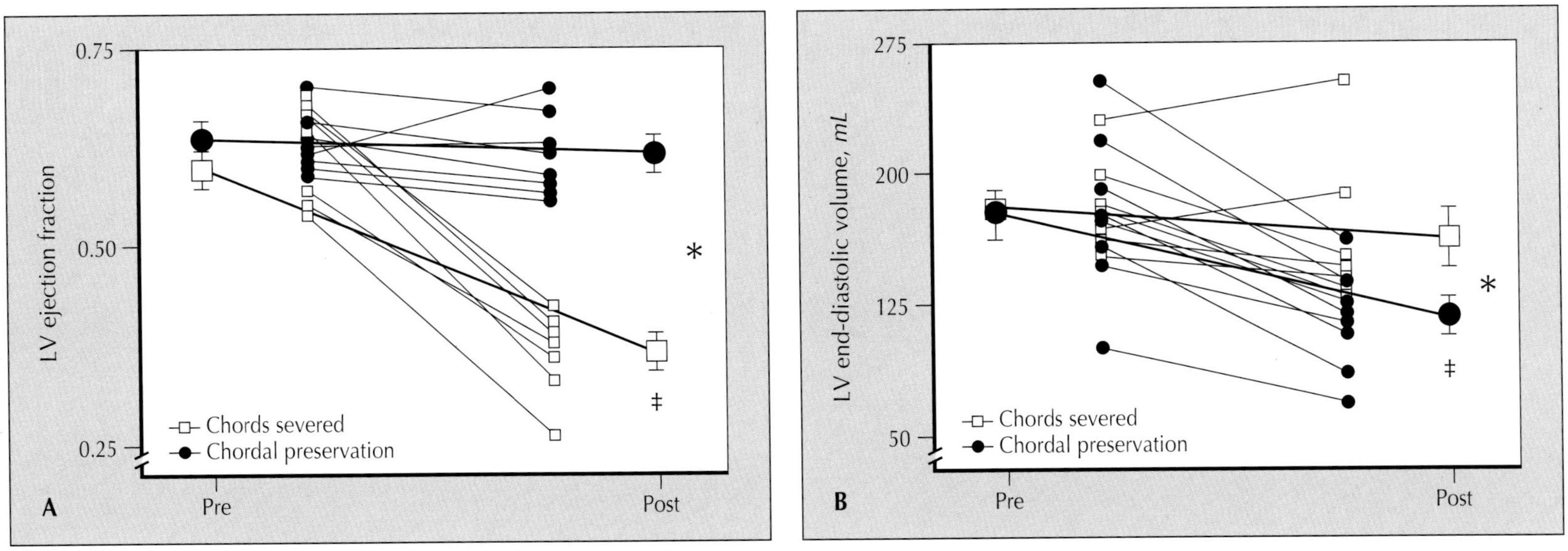

FIGURE 9-25. Interaction of chordinae tendineae. The interaction of the chordae tendineae with preoperative (pre) and postoperative (post) cardiac loading was examined to explain further the differences in postoperative performance between procedures that sever the chordae versus procedures that conserve them [42]. Two groups of patients with similar preoperative left ventricular (LV) function underwent mitral valve replacement. In one group the chordae tendineae were severed, whereas in the other group the chordae tendineae were preserved around the prosthetic valve using a procedure similar to that described by David *et al.* [43]. **A,** Postoperative ejection performance was preserved at its preoperative level when the chordae tendineae were preserved, whereas ejection fraction fell postoperatively if the chordae tendineae were severed, consistent with previous data [36–39](*see* Fig. 9-21). **B,** Postoperative end-diastolic volume decreased substantially when the chordae tendineae were preserved. Decreased end-diastolic volume should actually reduce ejection fraction rather than preserve it. Thus, these data do not directly explain the maintenance of ejection performance when the valve apparatus is preserved. (*continued*)

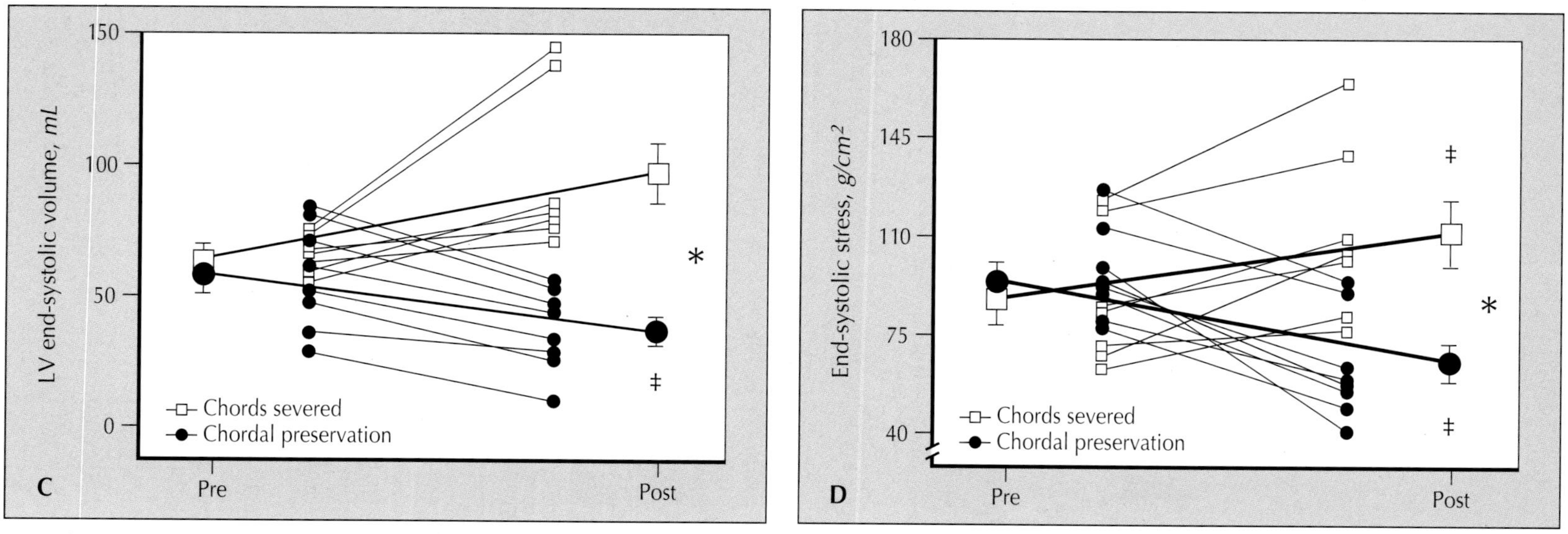

FIGURE 9-25. *(continued)* **C,** End-systolic volume, which is regulated by afterload and contractility, increased when the chordae tendineae were severed but fell when the chordae tendineae were preserved. It is this reduction in postoperative end-systolic volume that preserves ejection fraction when the mitral valve apparatus is preserved.

Consistent with observations in *panel C*, **D** demonstrates that end-systolic stress, a measure of afterload, increased when the chordae tendineae were severed but actually fell despite closure of the low impedance pathway when the chordae tendineae were preserved. *Asterisk* indicates $P < 0.05$ versus between patient groups; *double dagger* signifies $P < 0.05$ preoperative versus postoperative. (*Adapted from* Rozich and coworkers [42].)

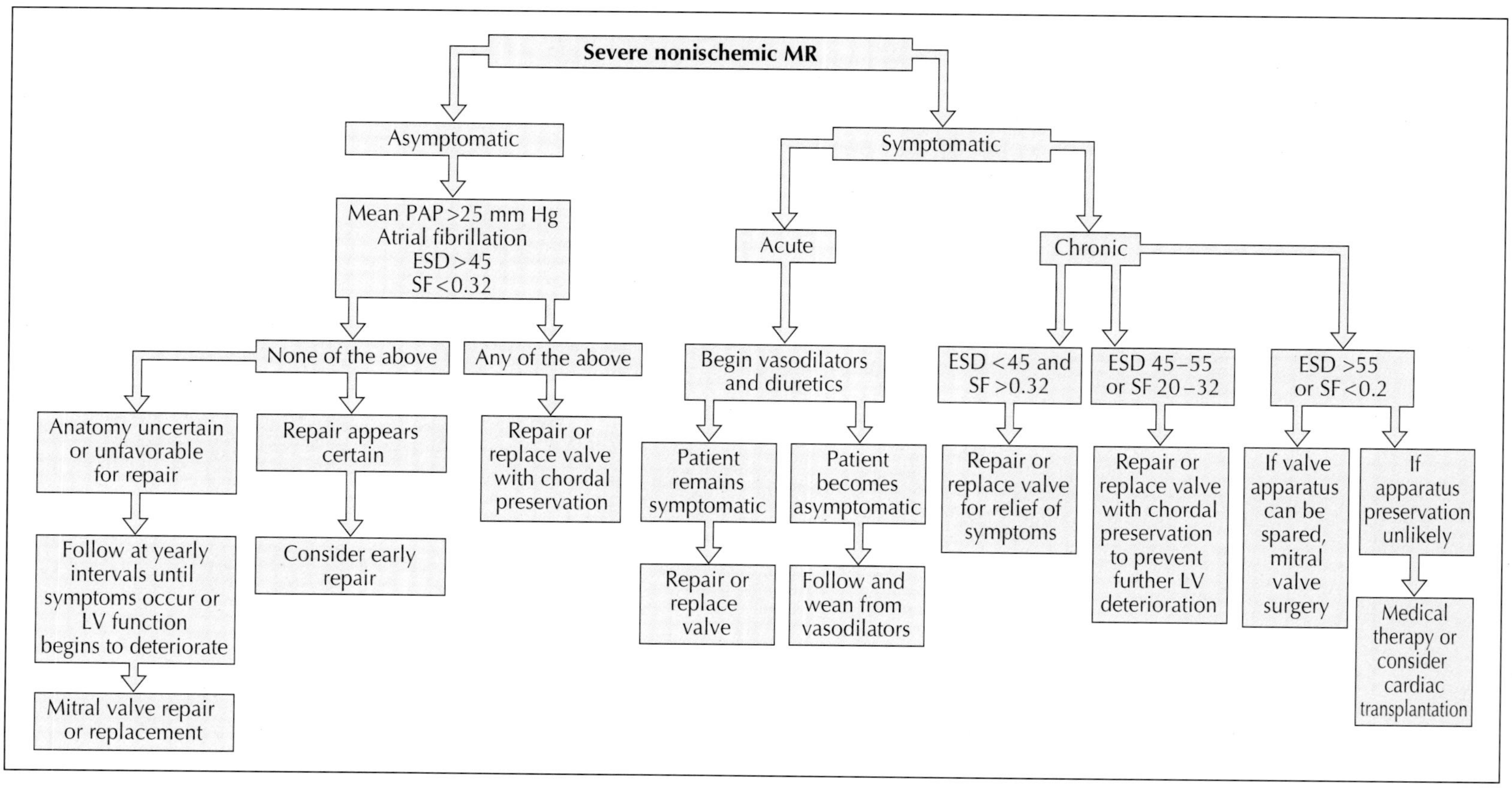

FIGURE 9-26. Algorithm for the management of patients with severe, nonischemic MR. It is likely that preservation of the chordae tendineae and their effects on contractile function [39] allowed the entire ventricle to decrease in size postoperatively, reducing the radius (r) term in the stress equation (stress = P x r/2h, where *P* = pressure and *h* = wall thickness). Thus, wall stress actually fell when the chordae were preserved. The data from Figs. 9-21 through 9-25 are consistent with the hypothesis that the chordae tendineae are an integral part of the left ventricle (LV) and its systolic function. When the chordae tendineae are severed, LV function worsens; this tendency is exaggerated if preoperative muscle dysfunction is already present. When the chordae tendineae are preserved, LV ejection fraction is maintained both because afterload is reduced and because ventricular contractile performance is maintained at its preoperative level. These factors combined with a lower incidence of thromboembolism, the avoidance of anticoagulation, and a lower risk of late postoperative valve failure all lead to a reduced operative mortality rate and better long-term outcome for repair than for replacement with valve ablation.

It is important to note that not all valves can be repaired. Abnormalities involving the anterior leaflet of the mitral valve are more difficult to repair than those involving the posterior leaflet and severe rheumatic deformity may prevent an adequate repair. ESD—end-systolic dimension; PAP—pulmonary artery pressure; SF—shortening fraction.

References

1. Wisenbaugh T, Spann JF, Carabello BA: Differences in myocardial performance and load between patients with similar amounts of chronic aortic versus chronic mitral regurgitation. *J Am Coll Cardiol* 1984, 3:916–923.
2. Spain MG, Smith MD, Grayburn PA, *et al.*: Quantitative assessment of mitral regurgitation by Doppler color flow imaging: angiographic and hemodynamic correlations. *J Am Coll Cardiol* 1989, 13:585–590.
3. Rushmer RF: Initial phase of ventricular systole: asynchronous contraction. *Am J Physiol* 1956, 184:188–194.
4. Wieting DW, Stripling TE: Dynamics and fluid dynamics of the mitral valve. In *Recent Progress in Mitral Valve Disease*. Edited by Duran C, Angell WW, Johnson AD, Oury JH. London: Butterworths; 1984:13–46.
5. Roberts WC: Morphologic features of the normal and abnormal mitral valve. *Am J Cardiol* 1983, 51:1005–1028.
6. Olson LJ, Subramanian R, Ackermann DM, *et al.*: Surgical pathology of the mitral valve: a study of 712 cases spanning 21 years. *Mayo Clin Proc* 1987, 62:22–34.
7. Carabello BA: Mitral regurgitation: basic pathophysiologic principles. Part 1. *Mod Concepts Cardiovasc Dis* 1988, 57:53–58.
8. Sonnenblick EH, Ross J Jr, Covell JW, *et al.*: Ultrastructure of the heart in systole and diastole: changes in sarcomere length. *Circ Res* 1967, 21:423–431.
9. Urschel CW, Covell JW, Sonnenblick EH, *et al.*: Myocardial mechanics in aortic and mitral valvular regurgitation: the concept of instantaneous impedance as a determinant of the performance of the intact heart. *J Clin Invest* 1968, 47:867–883.
10. Grossman W, Jones D, McLaurin LP: Wall stress and patterns of hypertrophy in the human left ventricle. *J Clin Invest* 1975; 56:56–64.
11. Corin WJ, Monrad ES, Murakami T, *et al.*: The relationship of afterload to ejection performance in chronic mitral regurgitation. *Circulation* 1987, 76:59–67.
12. Dodge HT, Kennedy JW, Peterson JL: Quantitative angiocardiographic methods in the evaluation of valvular heart disease. *Prog Cardiovasc Dis* 1973, 16:1–23.
13. Carabello BA, Nakano K, Corin W, *et al.*: Left ventricular function in experimental volume overload hypertrophy. *Am J Physiol* 1989, 256(*Heart Circ Physiol* 25):H974–H981.
14. Urabe Y, Mann DL, Kent RL, *et al.*: Cellular and ventricular contractile dysfunction in experimental canine mitral regurgitation. *Circ Res* 1992, 70:131–147.
15. Mulieri LA, Leavitt BJ, Ittleman FP, *et al.*: Forskolin reverses the force-frequency defect in left ventricular subepicardium (EPI) but not in papillary myocardium (PAP) in human mitral regurgitation heart failure [Abstract]. *Circulation* 1993, 88:I-406.
16. Nakano K, Swindle MM, Spinale F, *et al.*: Depressed contractile function due to canine mitral regurgitation improves after correction of the volume overload. *J Clin Invest* 1991, 87:2077–2086.
17. Spinale FG, Ishihara K, Zile M, *et al.*: Structural basis for changes in left ventricular function and geometry because of chronic mitral regurgitation and after correction of volume overload. *J Thorac Cardiovasc Surg* 1993, 106:1147–1157.
18. Starling MR: Effects of valve surgery on left ventricular contractile function in patients with long-term mitral regurgitation. *Circulation* 1995, 92:811–818.
19. Greenberg BH, Massie BM, Brundage BH, *et al.*: Beneficial effects of hydralazine in severe mitral regurgitation. *Circulation* 1978, 58:273–279.
20. Schön H-R, Schröter G, Blömer H, Schömig A: Beneficial effects of a single dose of quinapril on left ventricular performance in chronic mitral regurgitation. *Am J Cardiol* 1994, 73:785–791.
21. Röthlisberger C, Sareli P, Wisenbaugh T: Comparison of single dose nifedipine and captopril for chronic severe mitral regurgitation. *Am J Cardiol* 1994, 73:978–981.
22. Suga H, Sagawa K, Shoukas AA: Load independence of the instantaneous pressure-volume ratio of the canine left ventricle and effects of epinephrine and heart rate on the ratio. *Circ Res* 1973, 32:314–322.
23. Zile MR, Gaasch WH, Carroll JD, Levine HF: Chronic mitral regurgitation: predictive value of preoperative echocardiographic indexes of left ventricular function and wall stress. *J Am Coll Cardiol* 1984, 3:235–242.
24. Enriquez-Sarano M, Tajik AJ, Schaff HV, *et al.*: Echocardiographic prediction of survival after surgical correction of organic mitral regurgitation. *Circulation* 1994, 90:830–837.
25. Borow KM, Green LH, Mann T, *et al.*: End-systolic volume as a predictor of postoperative left ventricular performance in volume overload from valvular regurgitation. *Am J Med* 1980, 68:655–663.
26. Crawford MH, Souchek J, Oprian CA, *et al.*: Determinants of survival and left ventricular performance after mitral valve replacement. *Circulation* 1990, 81:1173–1181.
27. Wisenbaugh T, Skudicky D, Sareli P: Prediction of outcome after valve replacement for rheumatic mitral regurgitation in the era of chordal preservation. *Circulation* 1994, 89:191–197.
28. Scott WC, Miller DC, Haverich A, *et al.*: Determinants of operative mortality for patients undergoing aortic valve replacement. Discriminant analysis of 1479 operations. *J Thorac Cardiovasc Surg* 1985, 89:400–413.
29. Scott WC, Miller DC, Haverich A, *et al.*: Operative risk of mitral valve replacement: discriminant analysis of 1329 procedures. *Circulation* 1985, 72(suppl II):II-108–II-119.
30. Cosgrove DM, Chavez AM, Lytle BW, *et al.*: Results of mitral valve reconstruction. *Circulation* 1986, 74(suppl I):I-82–I-87.
31. Oury JH, Peterson KL, Folkerth TL, Daily PO: Mitral valve replacement versus reconstruction. An analysis of indications and results of mitral valve procedures in a consecutive series of 80 patients. *J Thorac Cardiovasc Surg* 1977, 73:825–835.
32. Duran CG, Pomar JL, Revuelta JM, *et al.*: Conservative operation for mitral insufficiency: critical analysis supported by postoperative hemodynamic studies in 72 patients. *J Thorac Cardiovasc Surg* 1980, 79:326–337.
33. Yacoub M, Halim M, Radley-Smith R, *et al.*: Surgical treatment of mitral regurgitation caused by floppy valves: repair versus replacement. *Circulation* 1981, 64(suppl II):II-210–II-216.
34. Oliveira DBG, Dawkins KD, Kay PH, Paneth M: Chordal rupture. II. Comparison between repair and replacement. *Br Heart J* 1983, 50:318–324.
35. Adebo OA, Ross JK: Surgical treatment of ruptured mitral valve chordae. A comparison between valve replacement and valve repair. *Thorac Cardiovasc Surg* 1984, 32:139–142.
36. Goldman ME, Mora F, Guarino T, *et al.*: Mitral valvuloplasty is superior to valve replacement for preservation of left ventricular function. An intraoperative two-dimensional echocardiographic study. *J Am Coll Cardiol* 1987, 10:568–575.
37. Bonchek LI, Olinger GN, Siegel R, *et al.*: Left ventricular performance after mitral reconstruction for mitral regurgitation. *J Thorac Cardiovasc Surg* 1984, 88:122–127.

38. Lessana A, Herreman F, Boffety C, *et al.*: Hemodynamic and cineangiographic study before and after mitral valvuloplasty (Carpentier's technique). *Circulation* 1981, 64(suppl II):II-195–II-202.
39. Straub U, Feindt P, Huwer, *et al.*: Mitral valve replacement with preservation of the subvalvular structures where possible: an echocardiographic and clinical comparison with cases where preservation was not possible. *Thorac Cardiovasc Surg* 1994, 42:2–8.
40. Sarris GE, Cahill PD, Hansen DE, *et al.*: Restoration of left ventricular systolic performance after reattachment of the mitral chordae tendineae. The importance of valvular-ventricular interaction. *J Thorac Cardiovasc Surg* 1988, 95:969–979.
41. Wong CYH, Spotnitz HM: Systolic and diastolic properties of the human left ventricle during valve replacement for chronic mitral regurgitation. *Am J Cardiol* 1981, 47:40–50.
42. Rozich JD, Carabello BA, Usher BW, *et al.*: Mitral valve replacement with and without chordal preservation in patients with chronic mitral regurgitation: mechanism for differences in postoperative ejection performance. *Circulation* 1992, 86:1718–1727.
43. David TE, Burns RJ, Bacchus CM, Druck MN: Mitral valve replacement for mitral regurgitation with and without preservation of chordae tendineae. *J Thorac Cardiovasc Surg* 1984, 88:718–725.

Mitral Valve Prolapse

10

CHAPTER

Sumanth D. Prabhu and Robert A. O'Rourke

Mitral valve prolapse (MVP) is defined as the systolic billowing or displacement of the mitral valve into the left atrium. This may involve one or both mitral valve leaflets and may result in mitral regurgitation. The most common mechanism underlying MVP is valvular collagen disruption and myxomatous proliferation producing an enlarged, redundant mitral valve (*primary MVP;* floppy mitral valve). Primary MVP can occur alone or in association with connective tissue diseases such as Marfan's syndrome and thoracic skeletal abnormalities such as pectus excavatum. It may also occur in association with other cardiac disorders such as tricuspid valve prolapse, ostium secundum atrial septal defect, and the Wolff-Parkinson-White syndrome. *Secondary MVP* occurs without valvular myxomatous proliferation and is related to structural factors such as reduced left ventricular (LV) size relative to the mitral valve, altered papillary muscle alignment, and postinflammatory valvular changes. MVP is a common disorder, occurring in approximately 4% to 8% of the general population [1–4].

Patients with MVP are often asymptomatic. Commonly, the diagnosis is made during cardiac auscultation or echocardiographic examination performed for other reasons. Symptoms associated with MVP include chest pain, palpitations, dyspnea, fatigue, light-headedness, and syncope. These symptoms can be associated with autonomic dysfunction and orthostatic signs. The frequency of transient ischemic attacks increases slightly; these may be secondary to platelet-fibrin emboli arising from the mitral valve-left atrial junction. The key to the diagnosis of MVP is dynamic cardiac auscultation that reveals a mid-systolic click with or without a late systolic murmur. The click and murmur change their systolic timing in response to maneuvers that alter LV chamber size. The auscultatory findings can vary significantly among different examinations, ranging from normal to an isolated click (or clicks), an isolated murmur, or both. Thus, serial auscultatory examinations are often required for diagnosis.

The most useful diagnostic test is echocardiography. It provides confirmatory evidence for the clinical diagnosis and helps to define prognosis, risk of endocarditis, and degree of mitral regurgitation. Electrocardiography can reveal inferior ST-and T-wave abnormalities and evidence for preexcitation; these occur with increased frequency in patients with MVP.

Ancillary testing, including ambulatory electrocardiographic monitoring, exercise thallium scintigraphy, cardiac catheterization, and electrophysiologic studies, are performed in selected patient subsets with significant symptoms or complications related to MVP.

The prognosis in MVP is generally favorable, with most patients following a benign course. Factors that confer higher risk include male gender, older age (over 45 years), mitral regurgitation, thickened mitral valve leaflets, and increased LV size. These subgroups are more likely to develop the complications associated with MVP, which include infective endocarditis, chordal rupture, progressive mitral regurgitation and LV dysfunction, and sudden death. The frequency of embolic events, however, is not influenced by this risk profile.

Management of patients with MVP includes prophylaxis for bacterial endocarditis, especially in patients with mitral regurgitation or thickened mitral valve leaflets. β-Blockers are often useful in patients with increased adrenergic activity and symptoms such as palpitations and chest pain. Aspirin is recommended for patients with transient embolic events. Postural symptoms are treated by liberalizing salt and fluid intake; refractory cases require mineralocorticoid therapy. Regular clinical and echocardiographic follow-up is warranted, with the follow-up interval ranging from yearly to every 5 years depending on the patient's risk profile and degree of mitral regurgitation. As in patients with severe mitral regurgitation from other etiologies, patients with MVP and severe regurgitation associated with symptoms of dyspnea (New York Heart Association class II or greater) or LV systolic dysfunction should undergo cardiac catheterization and consideration for valve surgery. Mitral valve repair can often be performed instead of valve replacement; the former is associated with less morbidity and mortality.

Background and Classification

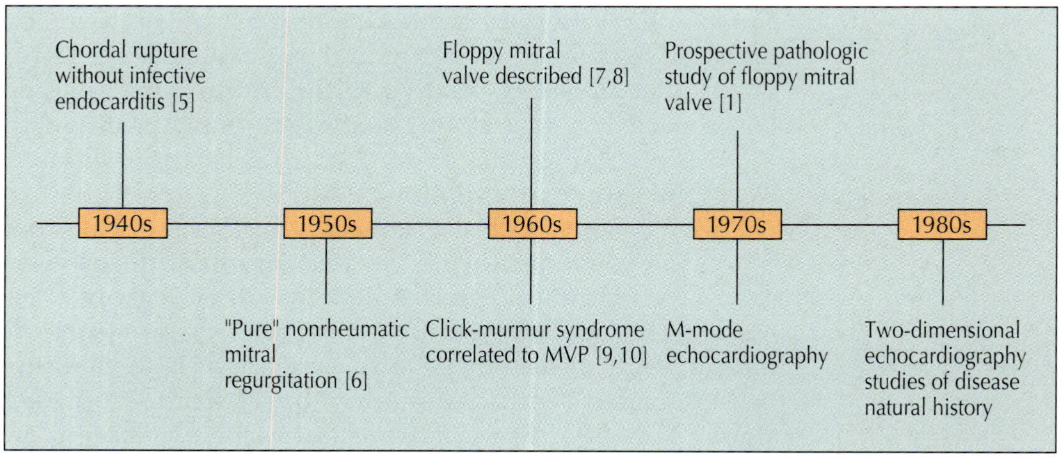

FIGURE 10-1. Modern historical overview of mitral valve prolapse (MVP). Given the prevalence of rheumatic heart disease in the early and mid-1900s, the recognition of nonrheumatic mitral regurgitation occurred relatively late. In 1944, Bailey and Hickam [5] described thickened, ballooning mitral valves and chordal rupture without associated endocarditis or rheumatic fever. Subsequent clinicopathologic, auscultatory, phonocardiographic, and cineangiographic studies defined MVP as a discrete disease entity and established MVP as the pathologic substrate for certain auscultatory (nonejection clicks, late systolic murmurs) and hemodynamic (mitral regurgitation) events [1,6–10]. M-mode, two-dimensional, and Doppler ultrasound came into prominence in the 1970s and 1980s, improving the definition of morphologic and functional abnormalities in MVP. Natural history studies combining clinical and echocardiographic variables followed, providing a framework for identifying higher-risk patients.

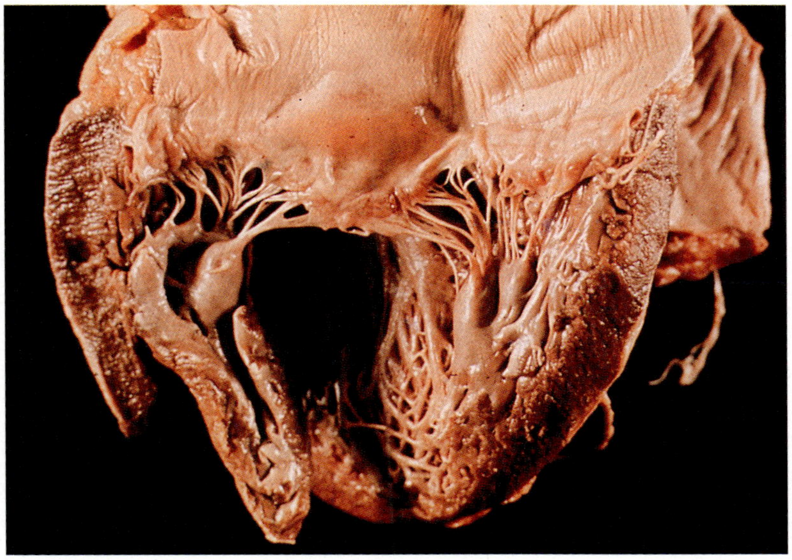

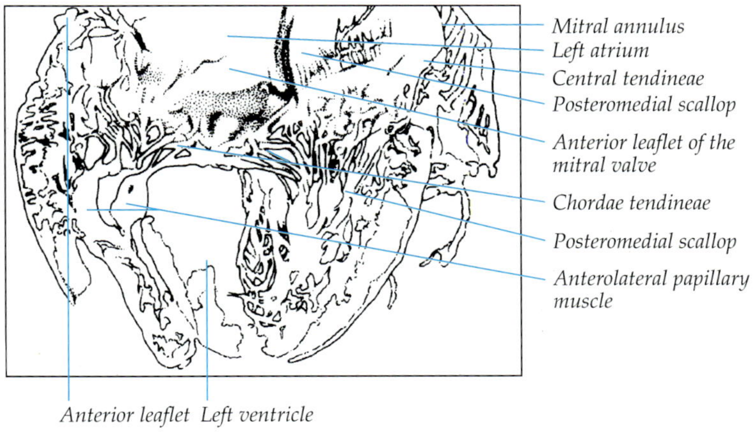

FIGURE 10-2. Normal mitral valve apparatus. The mitral valve apparatus consists of the valve leaflets, mitral annulus (MA), chordae tendineae (CT), papillary muscles, and the walls of the adjacent left atrium (LA), left ventricle (LV), and aorta. Pathologic changes in any of these components can result in valvular dysfunction. In this view, the LA and LV free wall have been cut and opened. The mitral valve is composed of the anterior leaflet, and posteromedial, central, and anterolateral scallops of the posterior leaflet. The anterolateral and posteromedial papillary muscles are shown (ALPM and PMPM, respectively). The CT are seen joining the ALPM and PLPM to the valve leaflets.

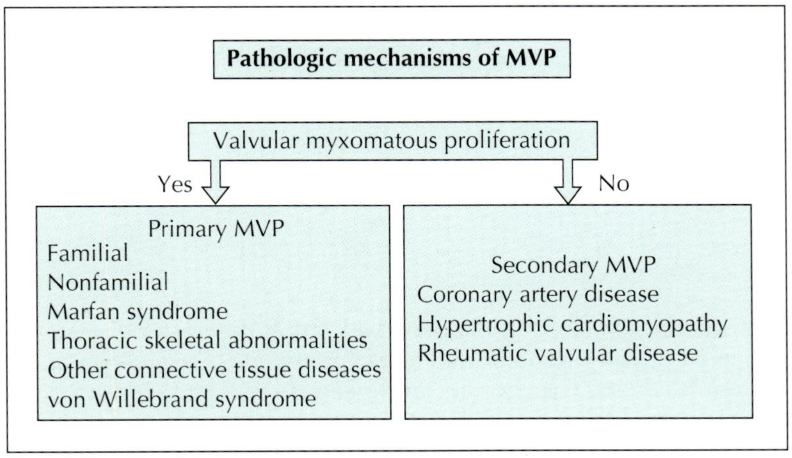

FIGURE 10-3. Causes of MVP. A variety of pathologic mechanisms involving any of the functional components of the mitral valve apparatus can result in MVP. Prominent among these is valvular collagen disruption and myxomatous infiltration, termed *primary MVP*. In most cases, primary MVP is an inherited disorder [11,12]; it can also occur in a nonfamilial, isolated form [2,3]. Less commonly, primary MVP is associated with connective tissue diseases. The most important of these is Marfan syndrome, where it can be detected echocardiographically in greater than 90% of affected patients [13]. Thoracic skeletal abnormalities (pectus excavatum, pectus carinatum, straight back syndrome, scoliosis) are also associated with primary MVP [14]. Primary MVP may be a manifestation of a generalized disorder of connective tissue, with a variable range of phenotypic expression within and outside of the cardiovascular system. For example, it can also be associated with myxomatous changes and prolapse of the tricuspid (40%), pulmonic (10%), and aortic valves (2%) [4]. The histologic changes are similar to those seen in the mitral valve. Other associated conditions include ostium secundum atrial septal defect [4,15] and Wolff-Parkinson-White syndrome [16]. *Secondary MVP* occurs in the absence of myxomatous valvular proliferation and can occur in patients with hypertrophic cardiomyopathy [17] and occasionally as a result of coronary artery disease [18]. Prior rheumatic fever may result in secondary MVP, especially of the anterior leaflet [19].

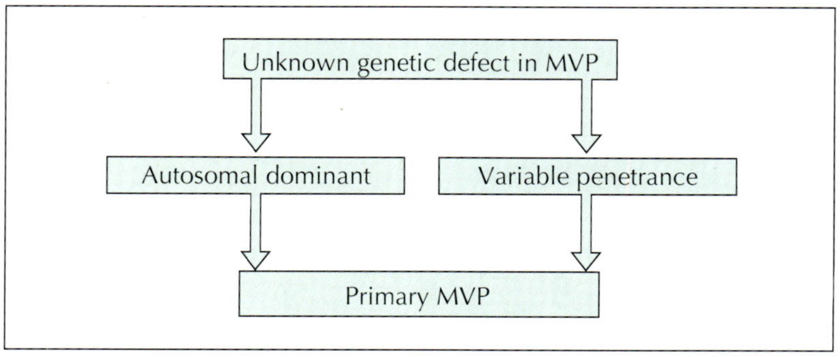

FIGURE 10-4. Genetics of primary MVP. Familial studies have revealed an autosomal dominant mode of transmission with variable penetrance affected by age and gender [11,12]. Expression is reduced in adult men, older women (over 50 years), and children of either gender. Expression approaches pure autosomal dominant transmission (*ie*, 50%) in adult women less than 50 years of age. Gender-related differences may also be associated with structural factors because the mitral valve and annulus are larger in size relative to the left ventricular cavity in normal women than in men [20]. The underlying genetic defect is unknown. There is disruption of valvular collagen primarily; however, there is no linkage of MVP to the genes for types I, III, and V collagen [21].

PATHOLOGY AND PATHOGENESIS

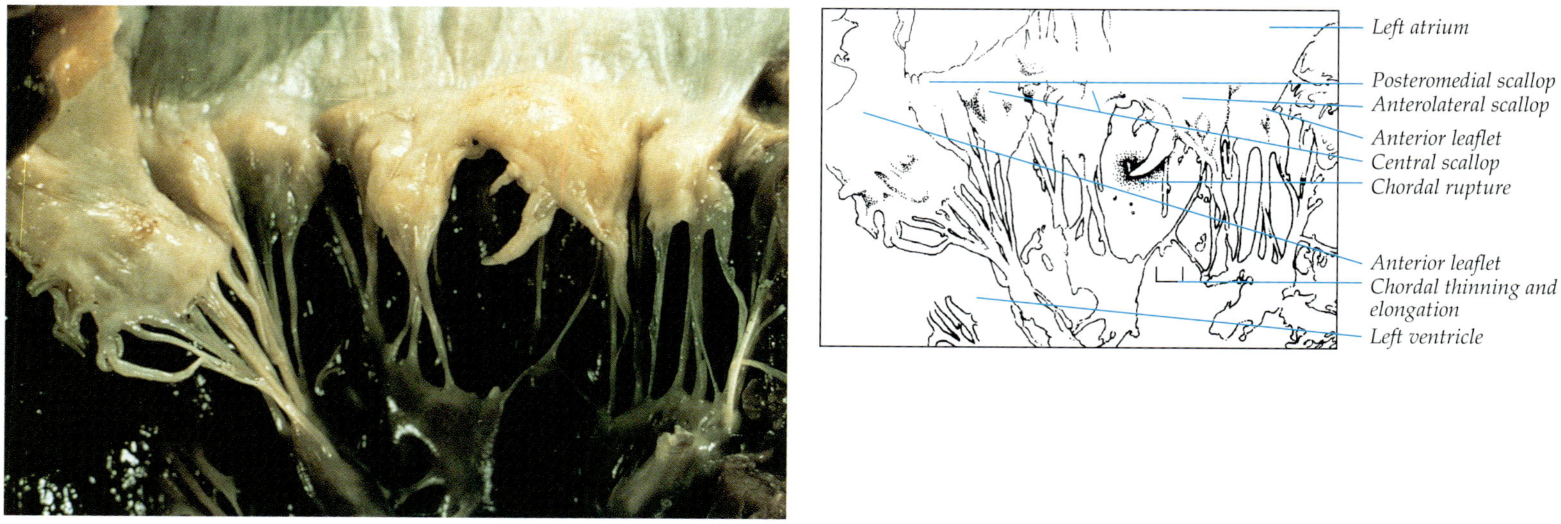

FIGURE 10-5. Pathologic specimen of a prolapsing mitral valve. The gross pathologic changes in primary MVP are leaflet redundancy and interchordal hooding, increased valve surface area, thinning and elongation (and rupture) of the chordae tendineae, and ventricular friction lesions secondary to excess leaflet and chordal mobility [4]. In this specimen, the left atrium and left ventricle have been cut and opened such that the posterior leaflet is viewed directly. Interchordal hooding involves the anterior and posterior leaflets. The chordae tendineae are thin and elongated. Chordal rupture involves the anterolateral scallop of the posterior leaflet. (Courtesy of Dr. Steven Bailey, University of Texas Health Science Center, San Antonio TX.)

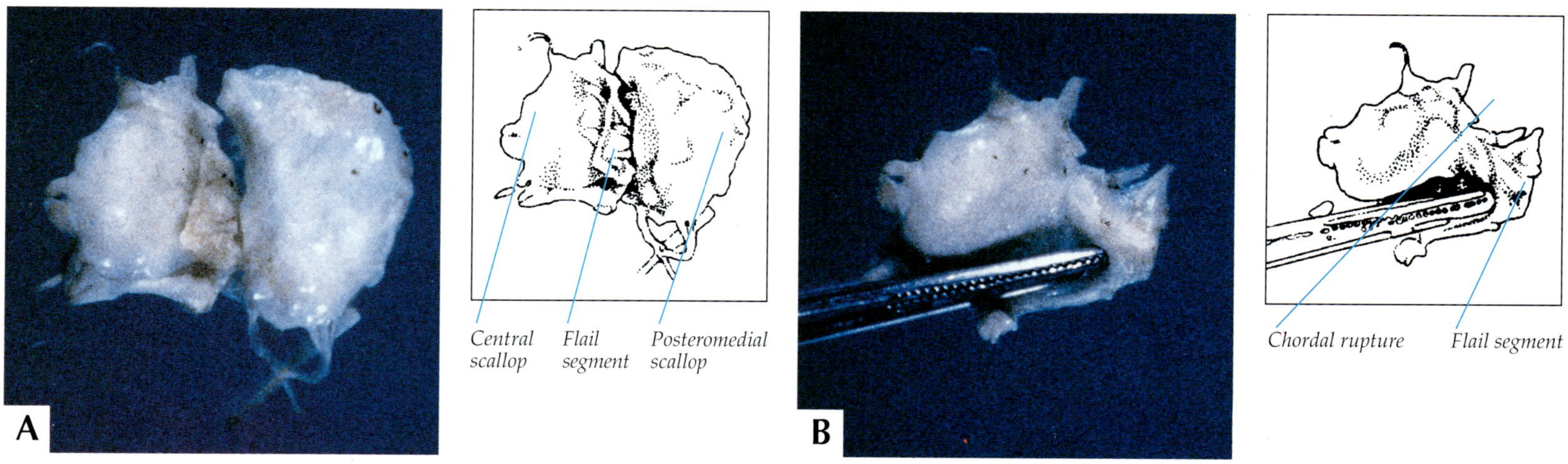

FIGURE 10-6. Resected posteromedial and central scallops of a myxomatous, prolapsing mitral valve (posterior leaflet). This specimen is from a 71-year-old man who had successful mitral valve repair. **A,** The leaflets are viewed from the atrial aspect and are enlarged and balloon toward the left atrial chamber. The leaflet surface area is markedly increased. **B,** There is a flail portion of the central scallop associated with chordal rupture.

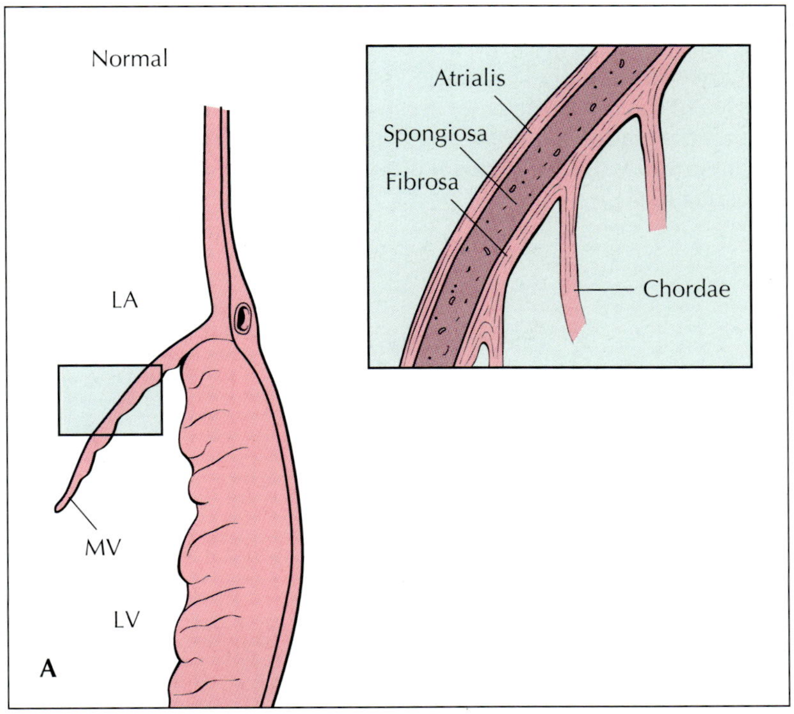

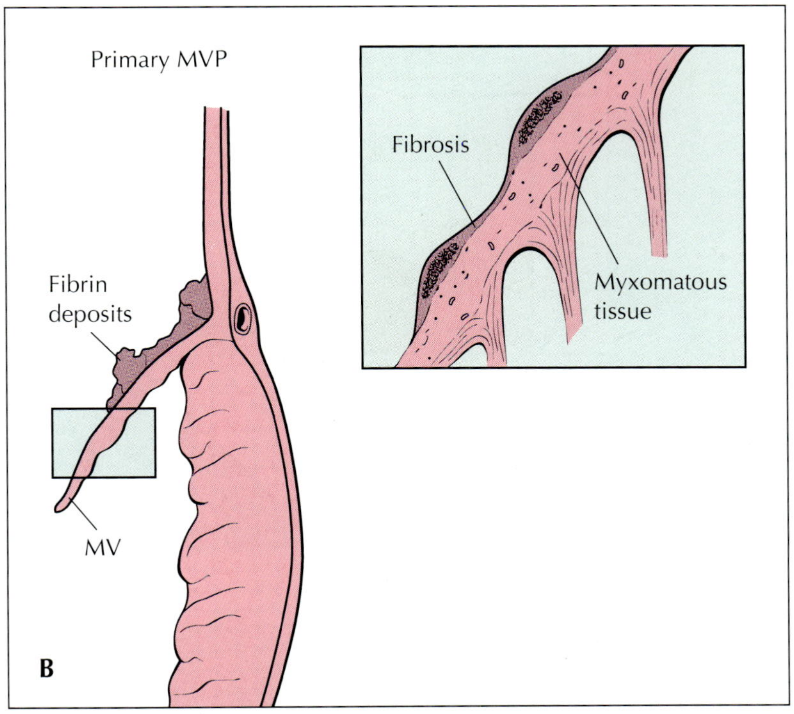

Figure 10-7. Histopathology of primary MVP. **A,** The normal mitral valve (MV) is composed of three layers: 1) the atrialis, a thin layer of collagen and elastic tissue along the atrial aspect of the leaflet; 2) the fibrosa (ventricularis), a denser layer of collagen along the ventricular aspect; and 3) the spongiosa, the fine myxomatous connective tissue layer between the two [4]. **B,** In primary MVP, dissolution of collagen bundles occurs primarily with secondary myxomatous proliferation of the spongiosa and interruption of the fibrosa and fibrosis of the atrial and ventricular surfaces of the valve [4,22]. These secondary effects appear to occur as a response to repeated stress on the valve apparatus. Focal endothelial disruption occurs commonly and may provide a site for thrombus formation [23]. Fibrin deposits often form at the mitral valve–left atrial (LA) angle. Similar histologic changes can occur in the chordae tendineae and result in chordal thinning and rupture. Myxomatous degeneration of the annulus can occur as well, especially in patients with connective tissue disorders, resulting in annular dilation and calcification and worsening of mitral regurgitation. LV—left ventricle.

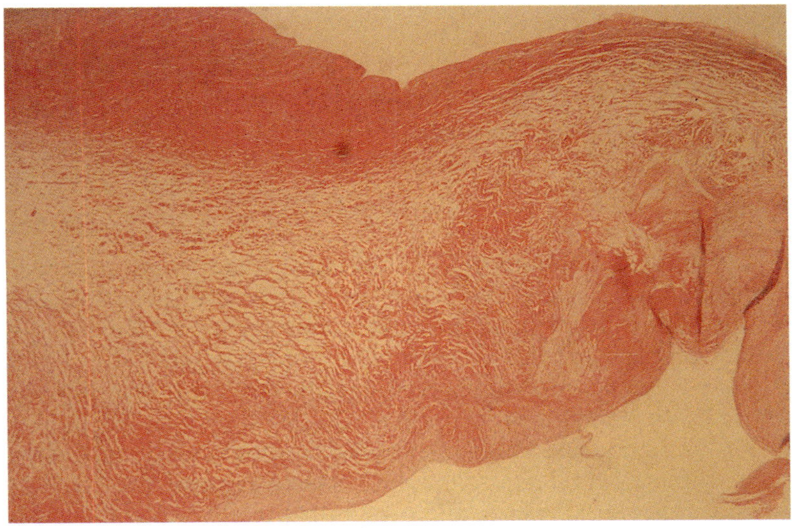

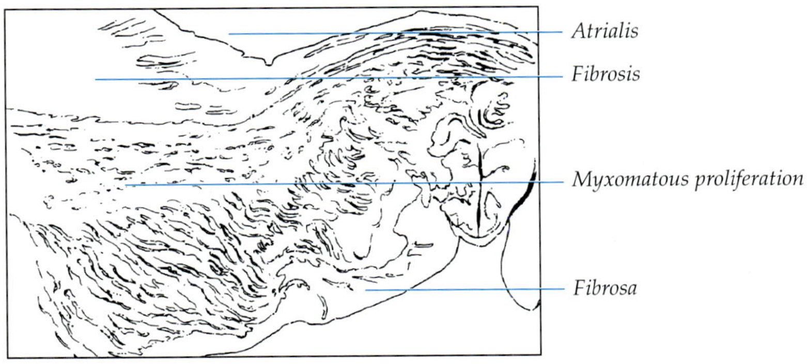

Figure 10-8. Photomicrograph of posterior mitral valve leaflet shown in Fig. 10-7. The valve is thickened with marked myxomatous proliferation and interruption of the fibrosa and atrialis by the spongiosa tissue. Focal areas of fibrosis are seen on the ventricular and atrial aspects of the valve.

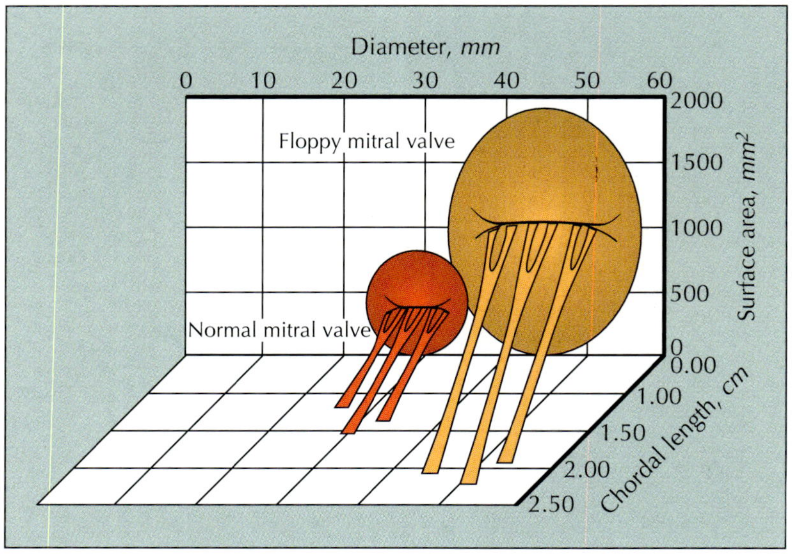

FIGURE 10-9. Relationship of valve morphology to valve dysfunction. Valve surface area, valve diameter, and chordal length are all increased in MVP. The mitral valve is thus inordinately large relative to the left ventricular chamber and does not maintain normal coaptation/apposition during systole. This results in prolapse and valvular regurgitation. (*Adapted from* Fontana and coworkers [24].)

CLINICAL FEATURES

SYMPTOMS

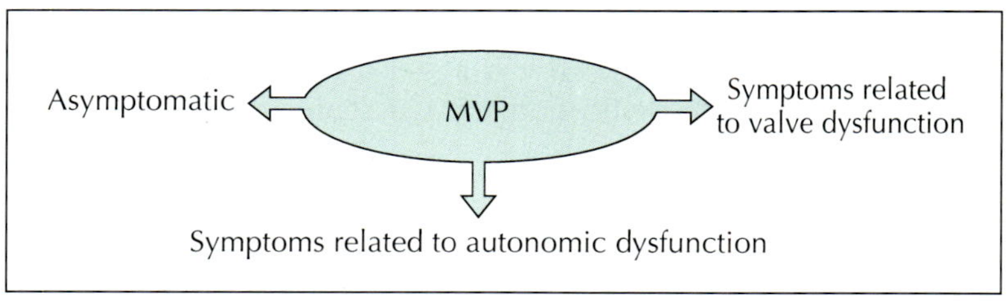

FIGURE 10-10. Symptom complexes in MVP. The vast majority of patients with MVP are asymptomatic [25]. Some patients with MVP have symptoms secondary to valve dysfunction, that is, progressive mitral regurgitation, left atrial enlargement, atrial fibrillation, left ventricular enlargement and dysfunction, and congestive heart failure. Other patients may have symptoms without objective hemodynamic valvular dysfunction. Often these patients show evidence for autonomic dysfunction; this constellation has been termed the "MVP syndrome" by Fontana and coworkers [24] and Boudoulas and coworkers [25].

SYMPTOMS IN MVP

Palpitations
Chest pain
Dyspnea
Fatigue
Syncope and lightheadedness
Focal neurologic events
Anxiety

FIGURE 10-11. Symptoms in MVP. The most common symptom is palpitations [26], which often correlates poorly with arrhythmias on ambulatory electrocardiographic monitoring. Chest pain is usually atypical and does not resemble angina pectoris. The etiology is unknown. It has been suggested that the prolapsing mitral valve places undue tension on the papillary muscles and results in subendocardial ischemia [24]. Dyspnea and fatigue may occur without mitral regurgitation or objective impairment of exercise tolerance. Syncope and presyncope may occur in association with postural hypotension and arrhythmias but often are present without any clinical correlates. Transient neurologic events occur with greater frequency in patients with MVP, although the overall incidence is quite low [24,27–29]. These may be the result of platelet and fibrin emboli occurring at sites of endothelial disruption and at the mitral valve–left atrial junction. The true association of MVP and neuropsychiatric syndromes remains controversial [30,31].

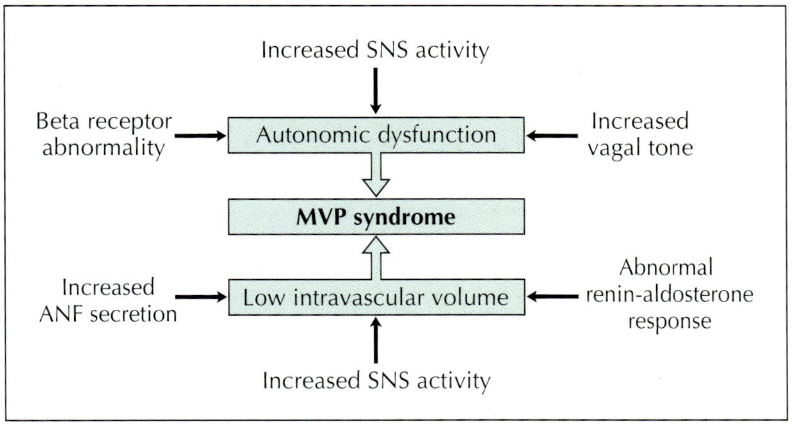

FIGURE 10-12. MVP syndrome—neuroendocrine and autonomic dysfunction. Several studies have reported autonomic and neuroendocrine abnormalities in patients with MVP (*see* [24] for review). These include increased adrenergic tone, adrenergic hyperresponsiveness, β-receptor abnormalities, increased vagal tone, and low intravascular volume with abnormalities in atrial natriuretic factor (ANF) secretion and in the renin-aldosterone axis. These abnormalities may play a role in the pathogenesis of symptoms in the MVP syndrome that cannot be explained on the basis of valvular abnormalities alone. A possible schema of interaction among these abnormalities is depicted. SNS—sympathetic nervous system.

PHYSICAL EXAMINATION

GENERAL PHYSICAL FINDINGS

Thoracic skeletal abnormalities
Arachnodactyly
High-arched palate
Low body weight (< 90% ideal)
Low blood pressure (< 120 mm Hg systolic)
Orthostatic hypotension and tachycardia

FIGURE 10-13. General physical findings in MVP. Thoracic skeletal abnormalities can be seen in association with MVP [14,26]. Arachnodactyly may be seen without other evidence for Marfan syndrome and these cases may represent formes frustes of this disorder. Patients with MVP tend to have low body weight, low systolic blood pressure, and postural hypotension and tachycardia [24,26]. These signs may be related to a combination of autonomic dysfunction and reduced intravascular volume in these patients.

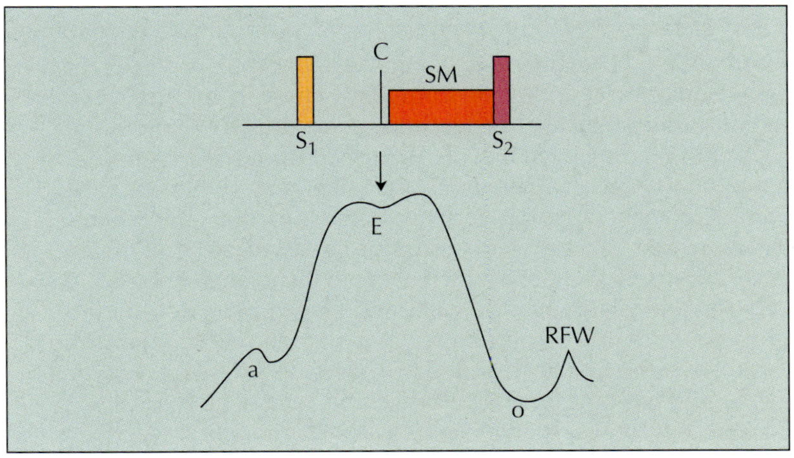

FIGURE 10-14. Cardiac examination. The auscultatory hallmark of MVP is the mid-systolic click, which varies in timing during systole according to changes in ventricular loading conditions and contractility [9,10,24,32]. The click(s) may be single or multiple, may vary in intensity, and may be associated with a late systolic murmur of mitral regurgitation. This figure depicts a typical phonocardiogram (*top*) and apex cardiogram (*bottom*) from a patient with MVP. The mid-systolic click (C) occurs *after* the beginning of ejection into the aorta (E) (hence the term nonejection click), is associated with mild apical systolic retraction (*arrow*), and is followed by a late systolic murmur (SM). The click is caused by the sudden tensing of the mitral valve apparatus at the time of leaflet prolapse; multiple clicks suggest asynchronous prolapse of different portions of the mitral valve leaflet. It must be emphasized that the auscultatory findings can be highly variable in the same patient at different times. On different occasions, the examination may reveal only a click, only a murmur, both a click and a murmur, or neither. (*a*—presystolic *a* wave; o—mitral valve opening, RFW—rapid filling wave; S_1—first heart sound; S_2—second heart sound.

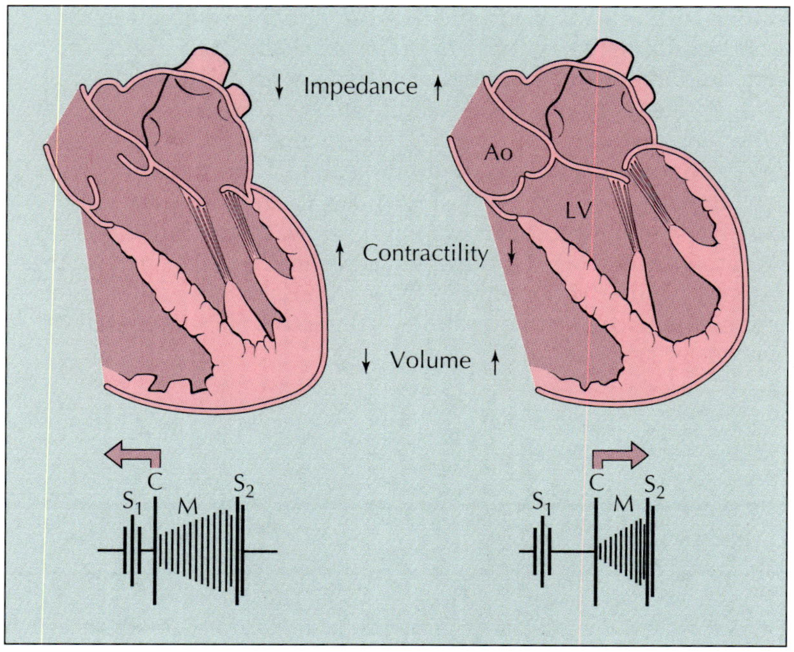

FIGURE 10-15. Dynamic auscultation. Mid-systolic clicks (C) may be secondary to factors aside from MVP. These include extracardiac causes, atrial septal aneurysms, and pericarditis. The mid-systolic click of MVP can be reliably distinguished from these by its temporal response to maneuvers that alter hemodynamic conditions. Any maneuver that decreases left ventricular (LV) volume (*eg*, decreased venous return, tachycardia, decreased outflow impedance, increased contractility) will worsen the mismatch in size between the enlarged mitral valve and LV chamber, resulting in prolapse earlier in systole and movement of the click and murmur (M) toward the first heart sound (S_1). Conversely, maneuvers that increase LV volume (*eg*, increased venous return, bradycardia, increased outflow impedance, decreased contractility) will delay the occurrence of prolapse, resulting in movement of the click and murmur toward the second heart sound (S_2). Ao—aorta. (*Adapted from* O'Rourke and Crawford [32].)

EFFECT OF VARIOUS MANEUVERS ON THE CLICK AND MURMUR OF MVP

MANEUVER	TIMING	MURMUR INTENSITY	MECHANISM
Standing	←	↑	↓VR
Squatting	→	↑↓	↑VR, ↓HR
Valsalva	←	↑↓	↓VR, ↑HR
Maximal handgrip	→	↑	↑AL, ↓HR
Amyl nitrite	←	↓	↓VR, ↓AL
β-blockers	→	↓	↓HR, ↓C

FIGURE 10-16. Effect of various maneuvers on the click and murmur of MVP. Although maneuvers that change left ventricular volume have consistent effects on the timing of the click and duration of the murmur, there may be divergent effects on the intensity of the murmur. For example, although amyl nitrite results in an earlier click and murmur, the decrease in systolic pressure results in less regurgitation and a softer murmur. Thus in diagnosing MVP, changes in the timing of the click are usually more helpful than changes in the intensity of the murmur. ←—earlier; →—later; ↑—increase; ↓—decrease; ↑-↓—variable; AL—afterload; C—contractility; HR—heart rate; VR—venous return.

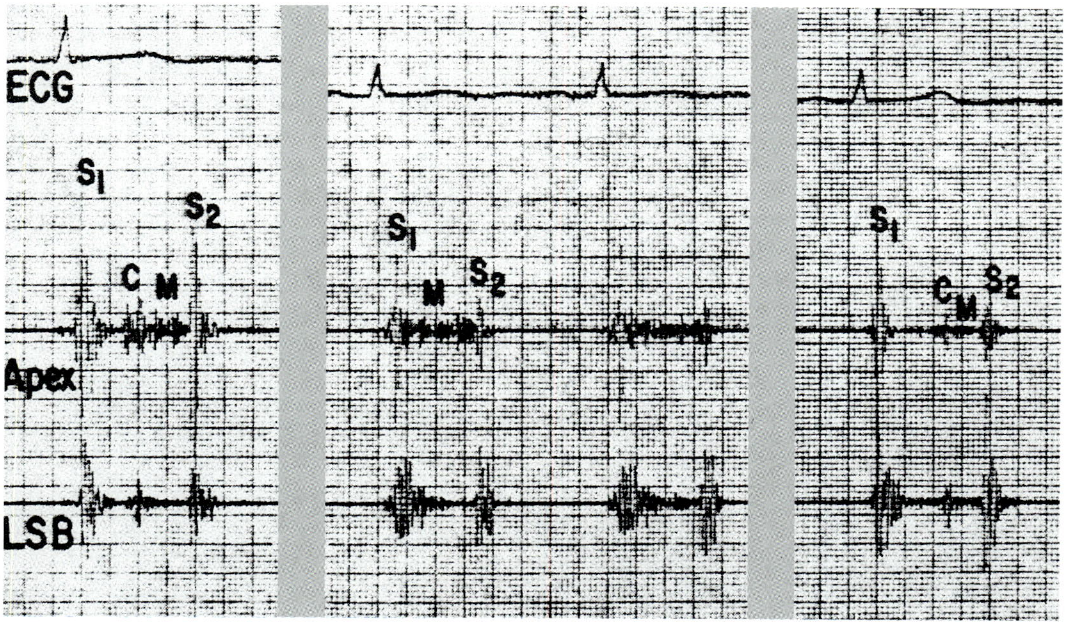

FIGURE 10-17. Response of the MVP click-murmur to postural changes. The electrocardiogram (ECG), apex phonocardiogram, and lower left sternal border (LSB) phonocardiogram from a 23-year-old man with MVP are shown. In the tracing obtained in the supine position (*left*), a mid-systolic click (C) and a late systolic murmur (M) are evident. With standing (*center*), the click-murmur complex moves toward the first heart sound (S_1) such that the click has merged with S_1 and the murmur is holosystolic. With prompt squatting (*right*), the click and murmur move back toward the second heart sound (S_2). (*Adapted from* O'Rourke and Crawford [32]; with permission.)

Diagnostic Testing

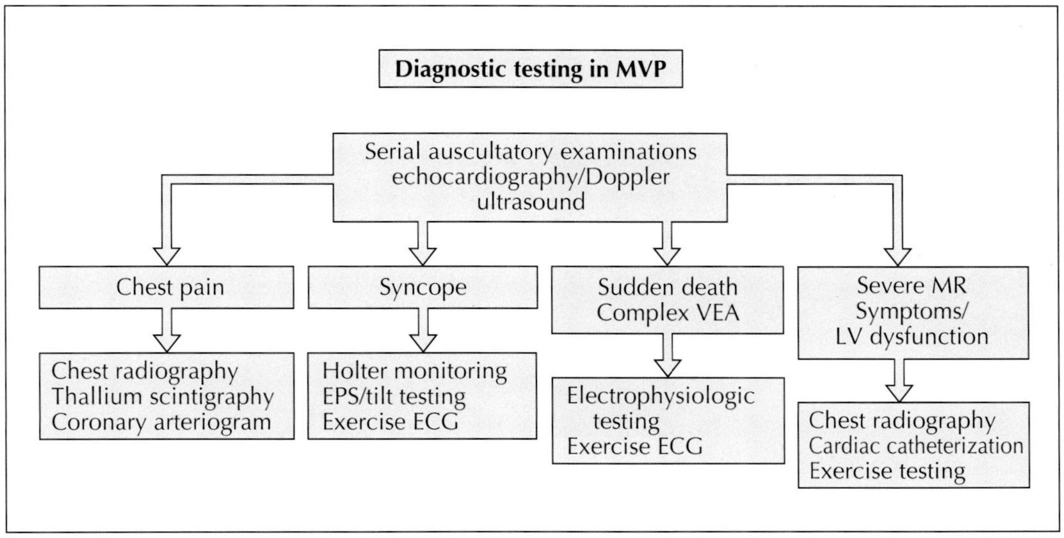

FIGURE 10-18. Diagnostic testing in MVP. The diagnosis of MVP is based on the presence of typical auscultatory findings detected during carefully performed serial examinations. Echocardiography (M-mode, two-dimensional, and Doppler) is the single most useful test in the definition of MVP. It is used to assess natural history and prognosis, the presence of associated conditions (*eg*, atrial septal defect, hypertrophic cardiomyopathy), the need for antibiotic prophylaxis, and the degree of mitral regurgitation (MR). Echocardiography should *not* supplant the physical examination in the diagnosis of MVP; up to 10% of patients diagnosed with MVP by typical auscultatory findings will have a nondiagnostic two-dimensional echocardiogram [33]. Electrocardiography (ECG) is routinely performed to assess for ventricular preexcitation and resting ST- and T-wave abnormalities (*see* Fig. 10-19). The tests listed in the lowest level of the flow diagram are not required for the diagnosis of MVP, but they are useful in assessing certain symptoms and complications that can occur in this disorder. EPS—electrophysiology; LV—left ventricular; MR—mitral regurgitation; VEA—ventricular ectopic arrhythmia.

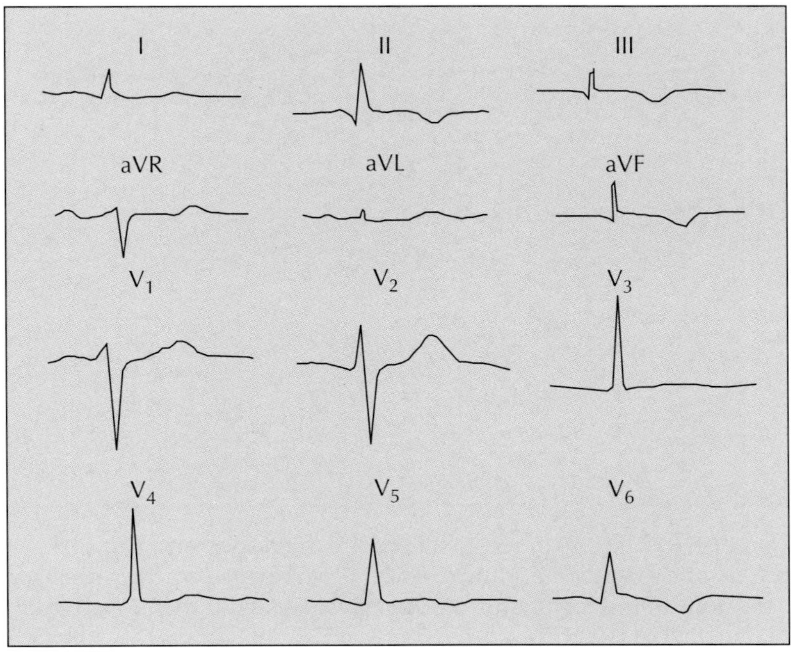

FIGURE 10-19. Electrocardiography (ECG). The ECG in patients with MVP is usually normal. As shown here, in some patients there may be T-wave inversion and nonspecific ST-segment changes in the inferior leads (II, III, aVF) and anterolateral leads (V_5, V_6) [34]. The genesis of these ECG abnormalities is unclear. They may be related to papillary muscle ischemia secondary to traction from the prolapsing mitral apparatus. These changes can become more accentuated with interventions that cause earlier prolapse of the mitral valve. Other less frequent ECG findings include prominent U waves and QT-interval prolongation. Continuous ambulatory ECG monitoring can detect a variety of arrhythmias including premature ventricular and supraventricular beats, supraventricular tachycardia (SVT), ventricular tachycardia, and atrioventricular block [24,35]. The most common sustained tachycardia is paroxysmal macroreentrant SVT due to macroreentry using a left-sided bypass tract [19]. The incidence of atrioventricular bypass tracts is increased in patients with MVP. The incidence of significant ventricular arrhythmias is greater in patients with ECG ST- and T-wave abnormalities and in those with QT-interval prolongation [36].

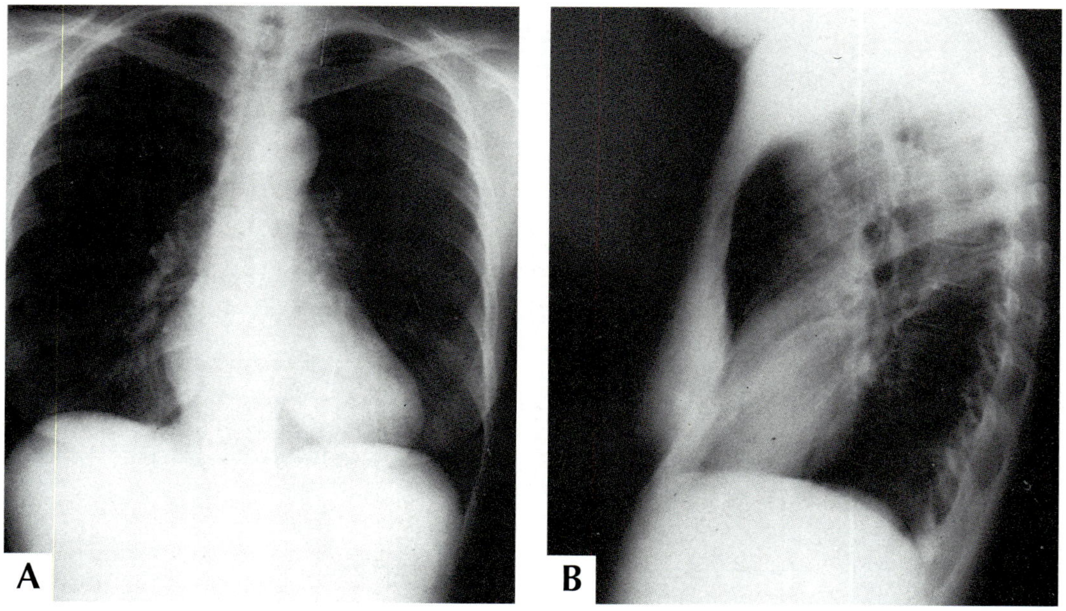

FIGURE 10-20. Chest roentgenography. The chest radiograph is usually normal. Thoracic skeletal abnormalities may be visualized. This radiograph is from a 26-year-old woman with MVP and reveals mild scoliosis on the posteroanterior view (**A**) and pectus excavatum on the lateral view (**B**). The mitral annulus may be calcified, especially in adult patients with Marfan's syndrome. In patients with progressive mitral regurgitation, left atrial and left ventricular enlargement can be seen. Pulmonary venous congestion and pulmonary edema are present in patients with heart failure. (*Adapted from* O'Rourke and Crawford [32]; with permission.)

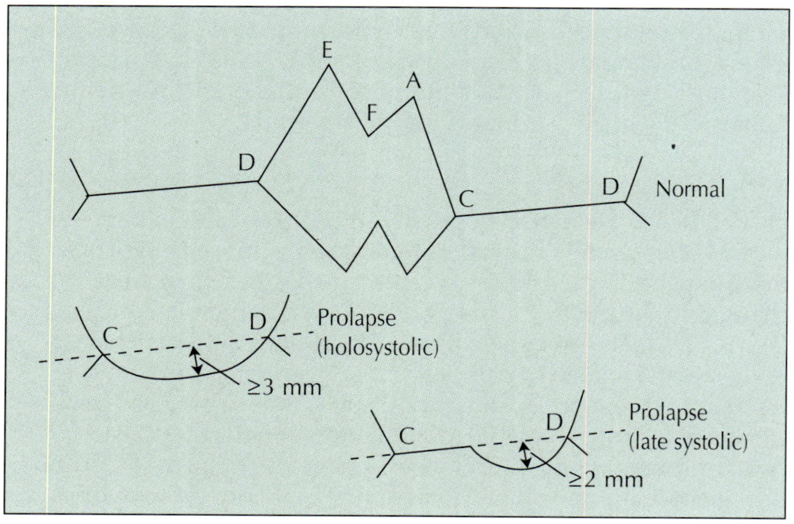

FIGURE 10-21. M-mode echocardiography. A normal mitral valve M-mode tracing is shown in the top of the figure. The points labeled are *D*, end-systole just prior to valve opening; *E*, peak initial opening of the anterior leaflet; *F*, nadir of the initial closing of the anterior leaflet; *A*, peak opening of the anterior leaflet with atrial systole; *C*, complete valve closure with the onset of ventricular systole. The posterior leaflet moves similiary but in the opposite direction and with reduced amplitude. Generally accepted M-mode criteria for the diagnosis of MVP are posterior displacement of one or both leaflets beyond the C–D line of the valve closure by at least 3 mm for holosystolic prolapse or by at least 2 mm for late systolic prolapse [24,37,38].

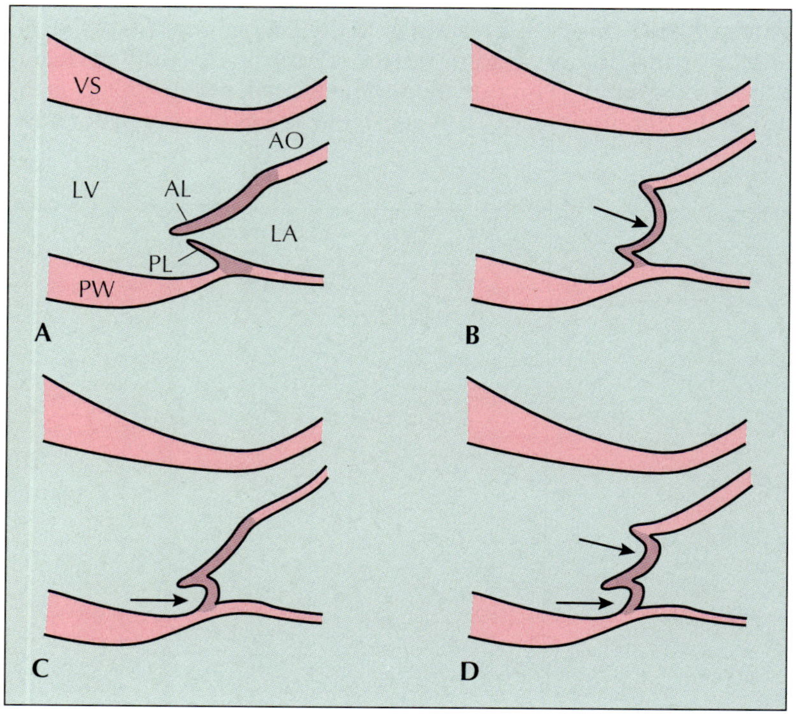

FIGURE 10-22. Two-dimensional echocardiography and Doppler ultrasound. M-mode findings should be confirmed by the presence of systolic billowing of one or both leaflets across the mitral annular plane into the left atrium (LA) in the parasternal (or apical), long-axis, two-dimensional view [24,38,39]. **A,** A parasternal long-axis view at end-diastole immediately preceding mitral valve closure. Labeled are the anterior leaflet (AL), posterior leaflet (PL), ventricular septum (VS), posterior wall (PW), aorta (AO), LA, and left ventricle (LV). Systolic prolapse may be predominantly anterior leaflet, (**B,** *arrow*), predominantly posterior (**C**, *arrow*), or both (**D**, *arrows*) The presence of leaflet thickening, leaflet redundancy, chordal elongation, and annular dilation should also be assessed on the two-dimensional study. Color-flow and pulsed-wave Doppler studies are used to determine the presence and extent of mitral regurgitation, an important supporting finding in borderline cases.

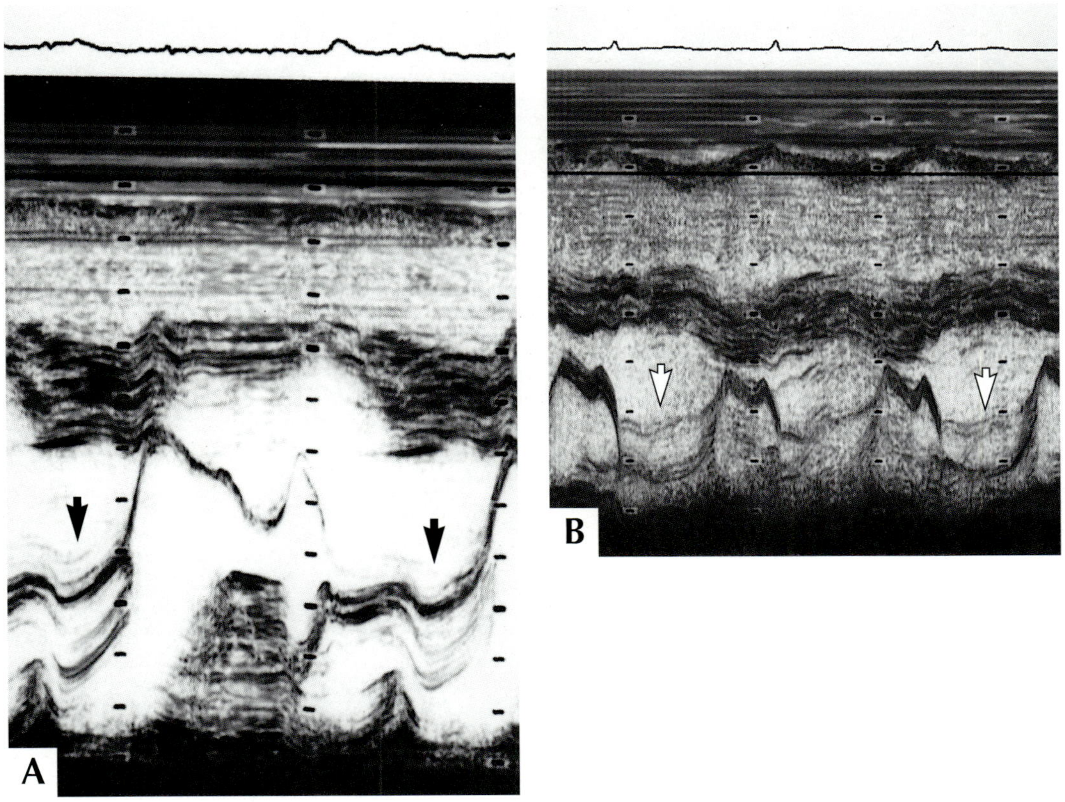

FIGURE 10-23. M-mode echocardiographic studies. **A,** This tracing is from a 41-year-old man with MVP. There is late systolic posterior displacement of both mitral valve leaflets (*arrows*). **B,** This tracing is from a 56-year-old woman with predominantly anterior leaflet prolapse. Significant holosystolic hammocking is seen (*arrows*). Both patients had evidence of leaflet thickening. Each division is 1 cm.

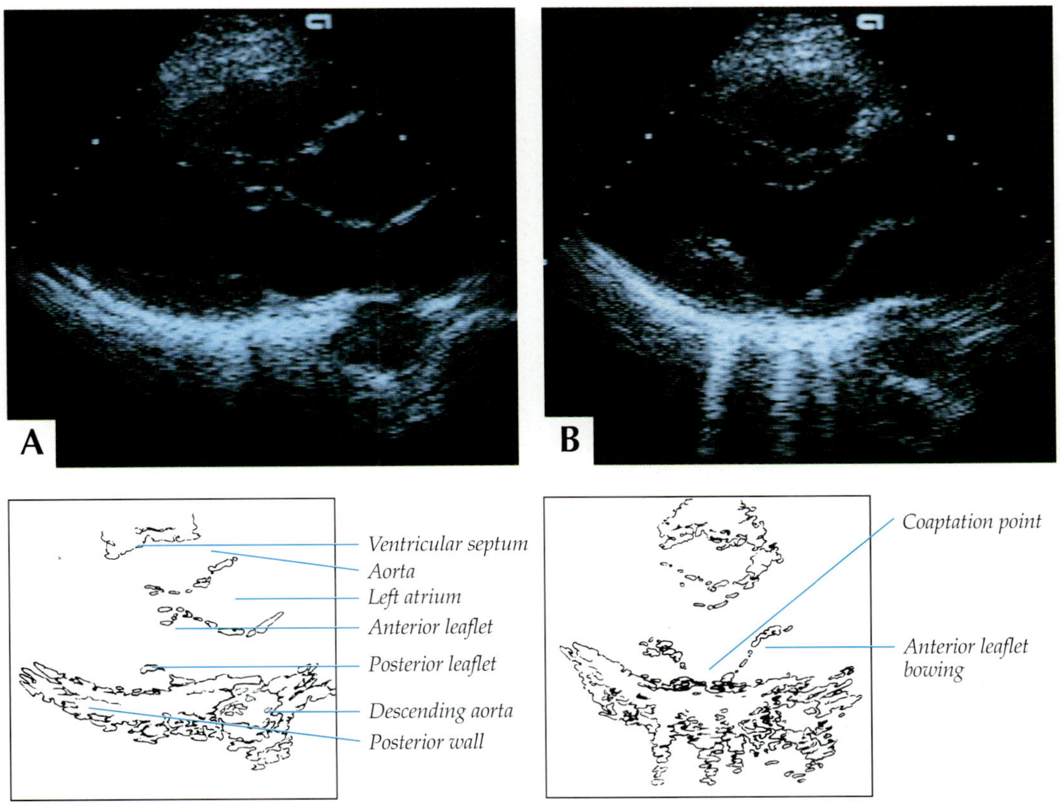

FIGURE 10-24. Two-dimensional echocardiographic and Doppler ultrasound studies. **A and B,** Two-dimensional study from a 51-year-old man with predominantly anterior mitral leaflet prolapse. The diastolic frame in *panel A* reveals a large, thickened anterior leaflet in the parasternal long axis (PLAX) view. The systolic frame in *panel B* shows billowing of the anterior leaflet beyond the annular plane and excessive posterior displacement of the coaptation point. (*continued*)

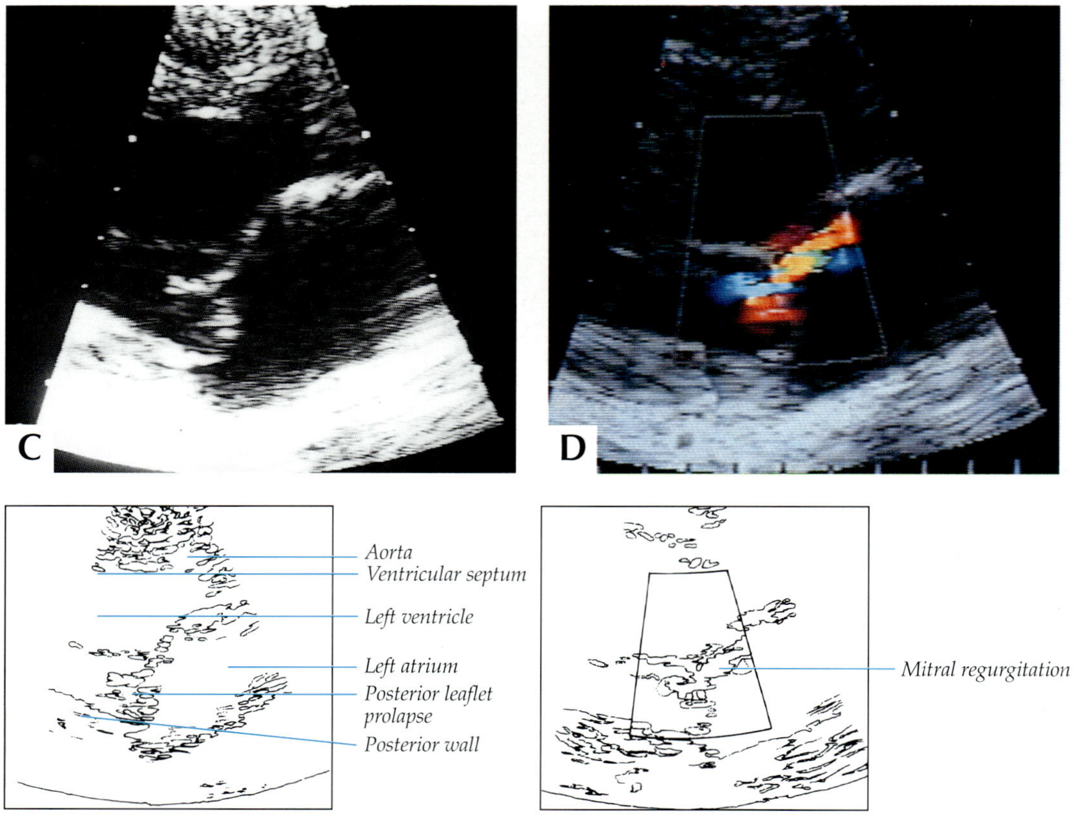

Figure 10-24. (*continued*) **C** and **D,** Two-dimensional and Doppler ultrasound study from a 25-year-old woman with predominantly posterior mitral leaflet prolapse. In *panel C,* the posterior leaflet is displaced beyond the annular plane in the PLAX view. Color Doppler imaging in *panel D* reveals an eccentric jet of mitral regurgitation directed anteriorly and toward the interatrial septum.

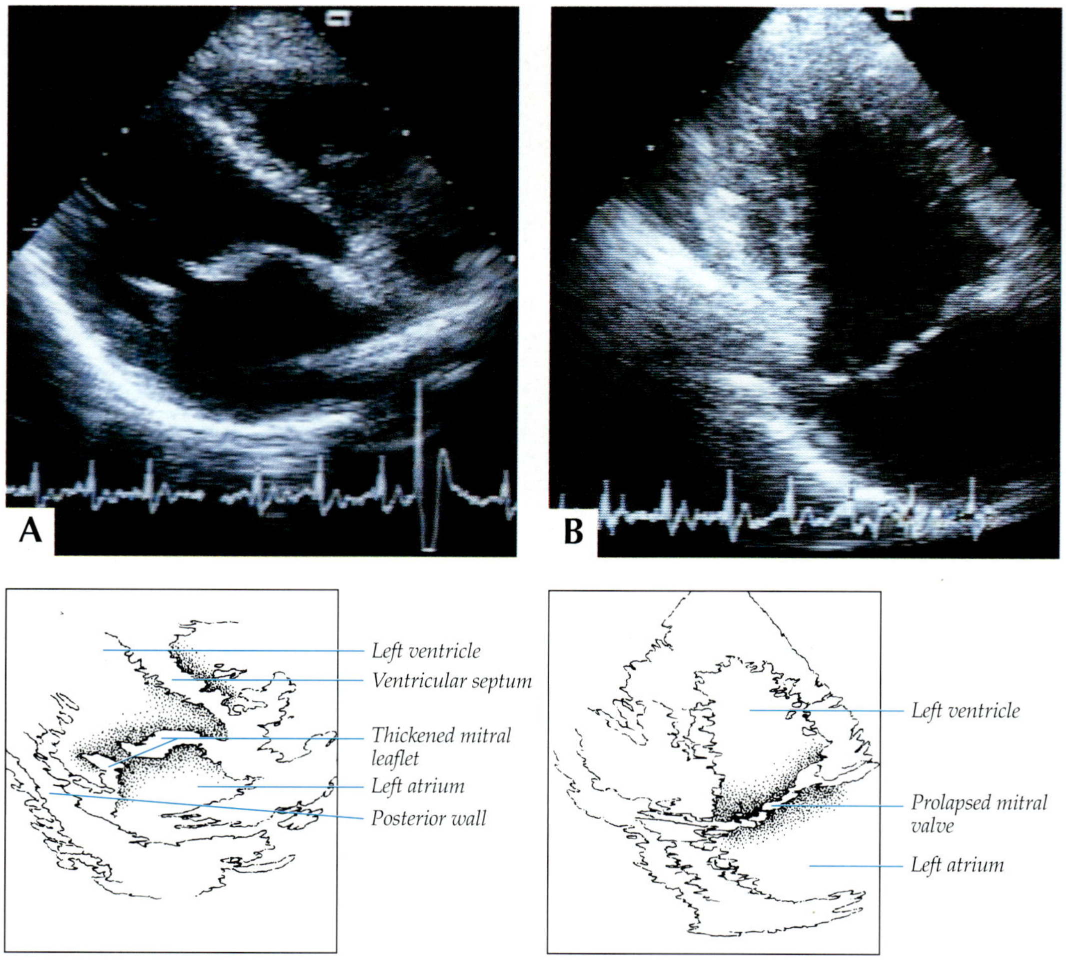

Figure 10-25. Two-dimensional echocardiographic and Doppler ultrasound images from a 55-year-old man with classic MVP and associated tricuspid valve prolapse. The parasternal long axis view shows significant leaflet thickening of both mitral leaflets (**A**). The apical long axis view shows prolapse of both leaflets and the coaptation point beyond the annular plane (**B**). (*continued*)

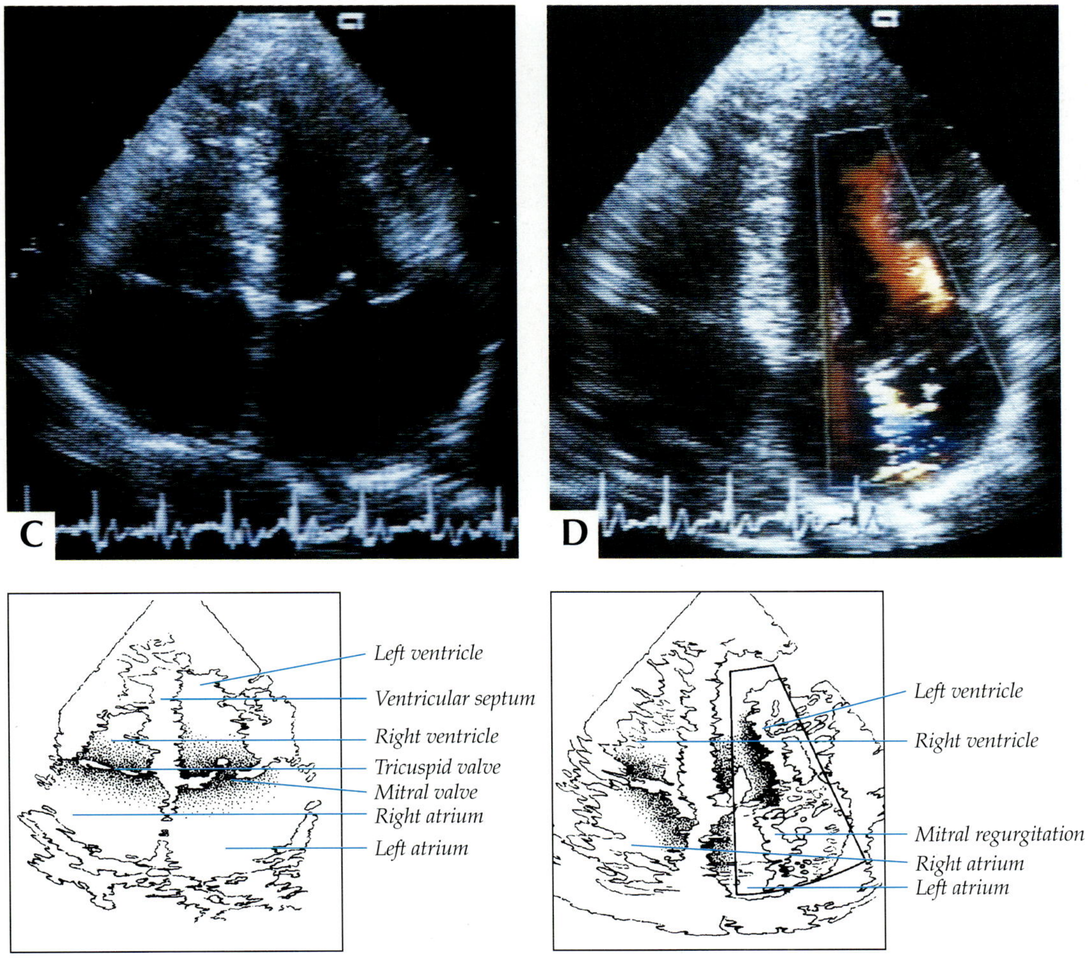

Figure 10-25. (*continued*) The apical four-chamber view displays a systolic prolapse of both the mitral and tricuspid valves (**C**). Color flow Doppler mapping in the left atrium demonstrates central mitral regurgitation (**D**). Tricuspid regurgitation was noted as well (not shown).

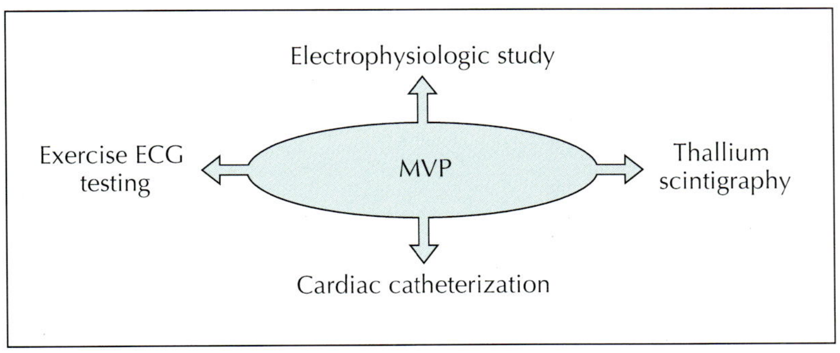

Figure 10-26. Additional testing in MVP. There is an increased incidence of false-positive exercise electrocardiographic (ECG) responses in patients with MVP [40], and the use of thallium scintigraphy with exercise is more helpful in excluding coronary artery disease (CAD) in patients with chest pain. Although a negative thallium scan essentially excludes significant CAD, the converse is not always true and patients with thallium perfusion defects may not have coexisting CAD [41]. Cardiac catheterization is not required for diagnosis of MVP. It is helpful in evaluating associated conditions (*eg*, CAD, atrial septal defect) and is needed to assess the hemodynamic effects of severe mitral regurgitation (as well as coronary anatomy) before consideration for valve repair or replacement. The indications for electrophysiologic testing are similar to those in the general population (*eg*, aborted sudden death, recurrent syncope of unknown cause, symptomatic or sustained ventricular tachycardia) [36].

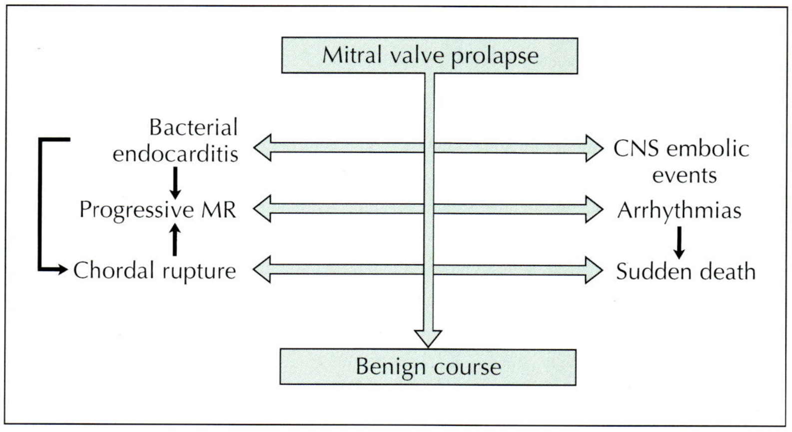

FIGURE 10-27. Overview of the clinical course in MVP. The majority of patients with MVP follow a benign course and their age-adjusted survival is similar to persons without MVP. However, serious complications can occur in 10% to 20% of patients [4,39,42–44]. These include infective endocarditis, chordal rupture, progressive mitral regurgitation (MR), life-threatening arrhythmias, neurologic and embolic events, and sudden death. The risk of infective endocarditis is five to eight times greater in patients with MVP than in the general population [45,46] and MVP is the leading underlying diagnosis in patients with endocarditis [24]. Progressive MR is often accelerated by infective endocarditis or chordal rupture. The overall incidence of ophthalmologic and central nervous system (CNS) embolic events is generally low [29]. An increase in risk for CNS events associated with MVP is detectable in patients who do not have other cerebrovascular risk factors, especially young women [27,28]. Sudden death is the least common complication of MVP and occurs mainly in patients with significant MR, reduced ventricular function, and malignant ventricular arrhythmias [35,38].

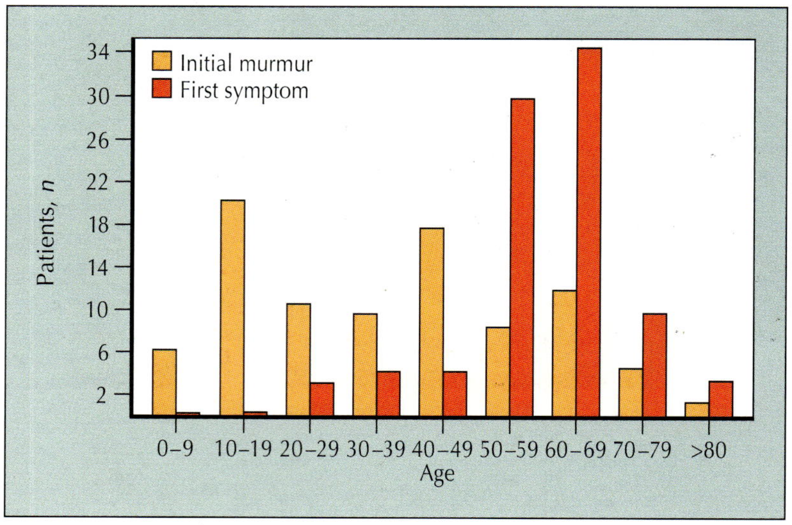

FIGURE 10-28. Natural history of severe mitral regurgitation in MVP. Approximately 5% to 6% of men and 1% to 2% of women with MVP will require mitral valve surgery during their lifetime [38]. In patients with progressive mitral regurgitation, there is often a prolonged asymptomatic interval with an accelerated phase of decompensation due to factors such as left atrial and left ventricular dysfunction, atrial fibrillation, chordae tendineae rupture, infective endocarditis, and arrhythmias. This figure depicts natural history data from 86 patients with MVP and progressive mitral regurgitation [47]. The average time between initial detection of the murmur and the onset of symptoms was 24 years. The average age at onset of symptoms was 59 years. The time interval between onset of symptoms and referral for valve surgery was brief, usually within 1 year. (*Adapted from* Kolibash and coworkers [47].)

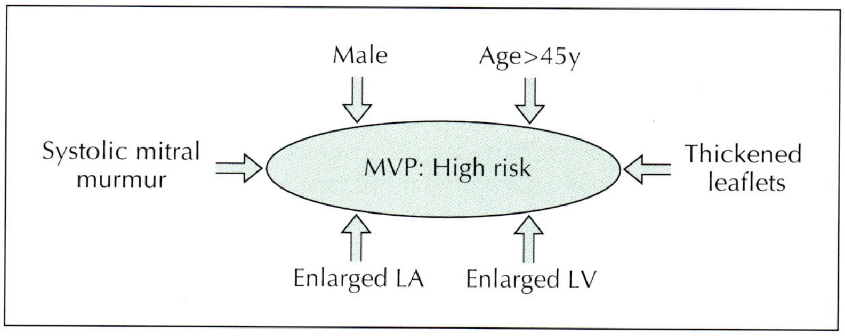

FIGURE 10-29. Identification of the high-risk patient. Several studies [39,42,46,48,49] have established that the incidence of most complications increases with male gender, age greater than 45 years, thickened and redundant mitral valve leaflets, the presence of at least mild mitral regurgitation, and increased left ventricular (LV) and left atrial (LA) size. Patients with these characteristics are more likely to develop infective endocarditis, require mitral valve surgery, and suffer sudden death. However, thromboembolic complications do not appear to depend on these risk factors [39]. Patients without this risk profile generally have an excellent prognosis.

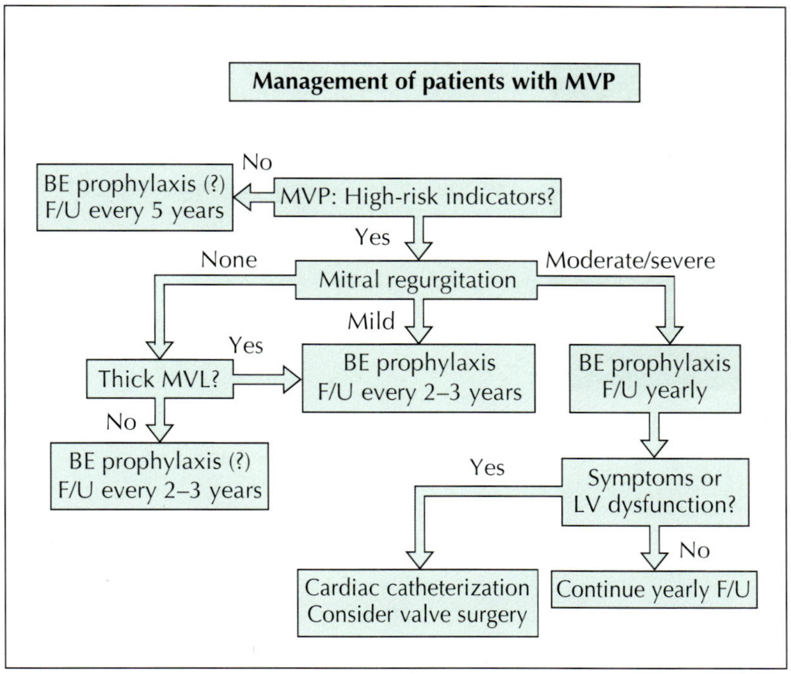

FIGURE 10-30. Management of patients with MVP. High-risk characteristics in MVP patients are additive, that is, the more indicators present, the greater the total risk. The majority of patients with MVP are asymptomatic and have no or minimal high-risk indicators. They are treated with reassurance and can lead a normal life [24,38]. Clinical and echocardiographic assessment every 5 years is reasonable to determine passage into a higher-risk group. If any high-risk indicators are present, patients can be further stratified based on the presence of mitral regurgitation (MR). Some authorities advocate prophylaxis for bacterial endocarditis (BE) only if MVP is associated with MR or thickened mitral valve leaflets (MVL). However, given the variability of physical findings and the dynamic nature of MR in MVP, prophylaxis may be reasonable in all patients with MVP. Patients with MVP and severe MR should be managed in the same manner as patients with severe MR due to other causes. The decision to proceed with valve surgery is based on the presence of symptoms or impairment of left ventricular (LV) systolic function. Mitral valve reconstructive surgery can often be used in lieu of valve replacement to correct regurgitant floppy valves [50–52]. Compared to valve replacement, valve repair is associated with a lower operative and late mortality, lower long-term thromboembolic risk, and lower BE risk [50,52]. F/U—follow-up.

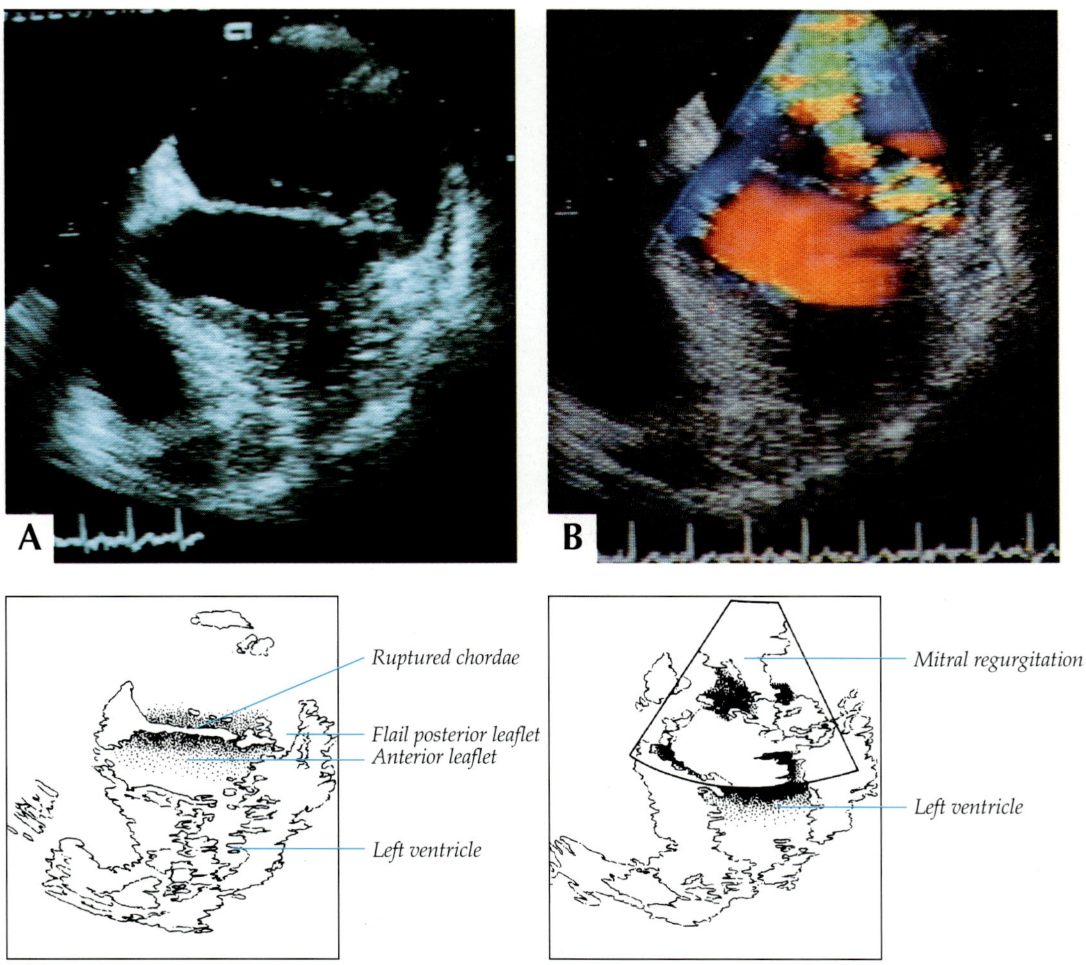

FIGURE 10-31. Chordal rupture and flail posterior leaflet in a 71-year-old man before and after mitral valve repair. **A,** Transesophageal echocardiographic image of a floppy mitral valve showed ruptured chordae tendineae and flail posterior leaflet. **B,** Color-flow Doppler study revealed severe mitral regurgitation. *(continued)*

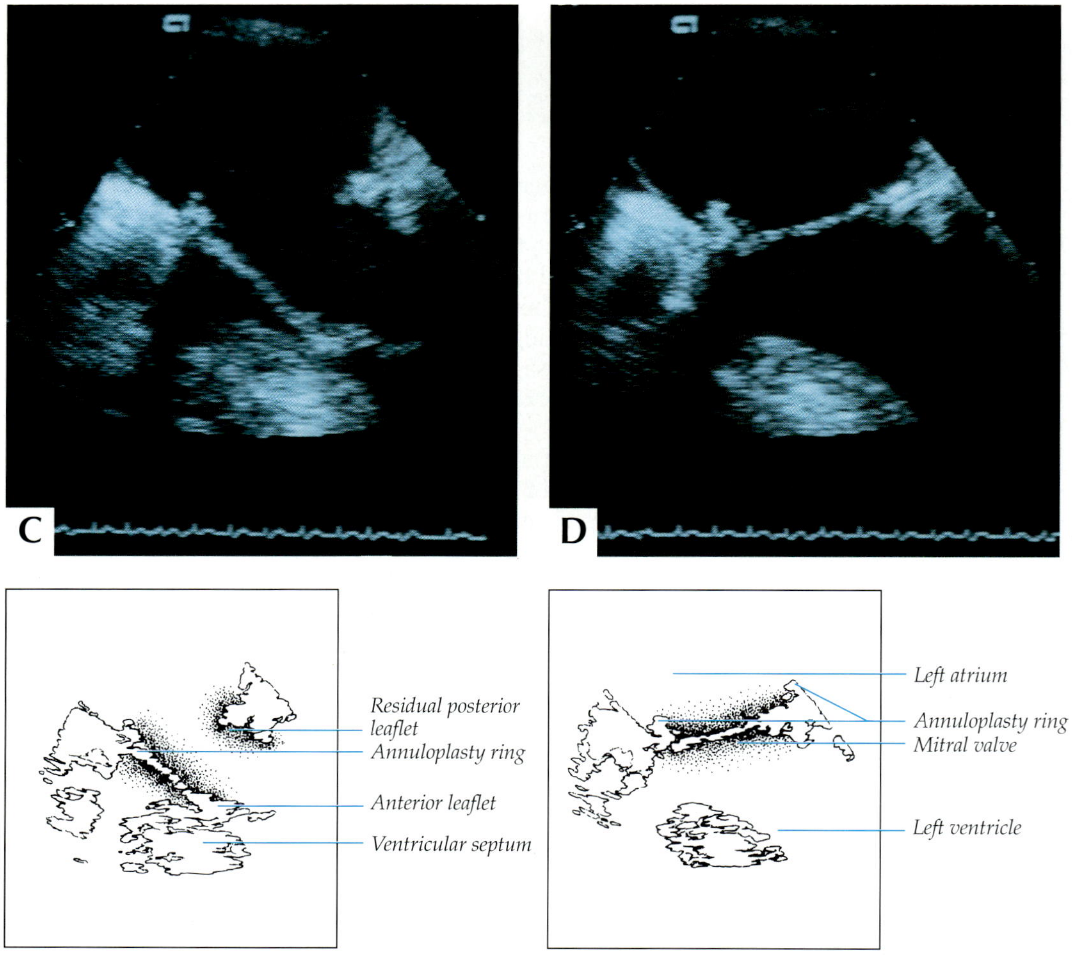

FIGURE 10-31. (*continued*) **C** and **D**, Intraoperative study from the same patient after valve repair (quadrangular resection of the posterior leaflet, annular reduction with annuloplasty ring, and primary leaflet resuture). A diastolic frame is shown in *panel C*; a systolic frame is shown in *panel D*. There is excellent coaptation without prolapse or systolic anterior motion. Color-flow Doppler study revealed no mitral regurgitation (not shown). The gross pathology and histopathology from the same patient are shown in Figs. 10-7 and 10-9.

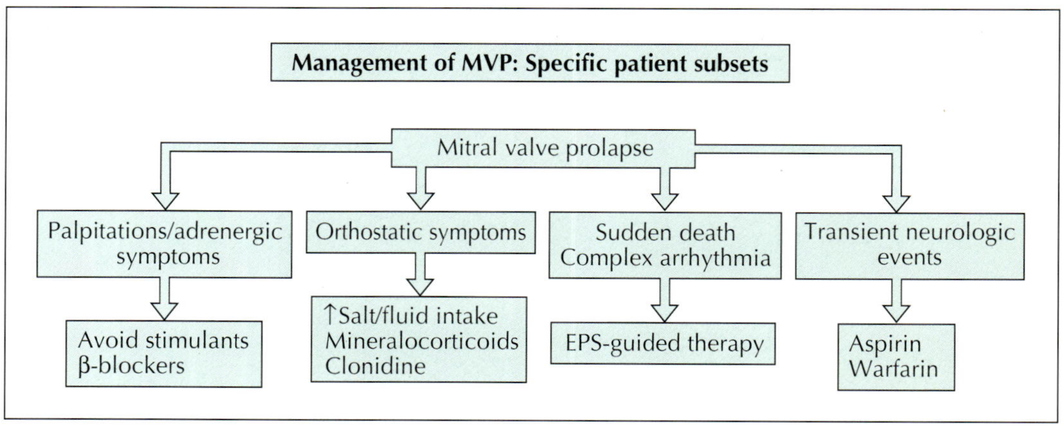

FIGURE 10-32. Management of specific patient subsets. Patients with palpitations and mild tachyarrhythmias or increased adrenergic symptoms often respond to cessation of stimulants (*eg*, caffeine) or β-blockers [24]. Postural hypotension and tachycardia are treated by liberalizing salt and fluid intake. Mineralocorticoid therapy or clonidine may be required for refractory cases. Embolic episodes and transient ischemic attacks are treated with daily aspirin and cessation of cigarette and oral contraceptive use. Warfarin is recommended for symptoms occurring despite aspirin therapy. Therapy for symptomatic complex arrhythmias and sudden death should be guided by electrophysiologic (EPS) testing.

References

1. Davies MJ, Moore BP, Braimbridge MW: The floppy mitral valve: study of incidence, pathology, and complications in surgical, necropsy, and forensic material. *Br Heart J* 1978, 40:468–481.
2. Procacci PM, Savran SV, Schreiter SL, *et al.*: Prevalence of clinical mitral valve prolapse in 1169 young women. *N Engl J Med* 1976, 294:1086–1088.
3. Savage DD, Garrison RJ, Devereux RB, *et al.*: Mitral valve prolapse in the general population. I. Epidemiologic features: the Framingham study. *Am Heart J* 1983, 106:571–576.
4. Lucas RV Jr, Edwards JB: The floppy mitral valve. *Curr Probl Cardiol* 1982, 7:1–48.
5. Bailey OT, Hickam JB: Rupture of mitral chordae tendineae. *Am Heart J* 1944, 28:578–600.
6. Brigden W, Leatham A: Mitral incompetence. *Br Heart J* 1953, 15:55–73.
7. Read RC, Thal AP, Wendt VE: Symptomatic valvular myxomatous transformation (the floppy valve syndrome). *Circulation* 1965, 32:897–910.
8. Pomerance A: Ballooning deformity (mucoid degeneration) of atrioventricular valves. *Br Heart J* 1969, 31:343–351.
9. Barlow JB, Bosman CK, Pocock WA, *et al.*: Late systolic murmurs and non-ejection ("mid-late") systolic clicks: an analysis of 90 patients. *Br Heart J* 1968, 30:203–218.
10. Criley JM, Lewis KB, Humphries JO, *et al.*: Prolapse of the mitral valve: clinical and cineangiocardiographic findings. *Br Heart J* 1966, 28:488–496.
11. Devereux RB, Brown WT, Kramer-Fox R, *et al.*: Inheritance of mitral valve prolapse: effect of age and sex on gene expression. *Ann Intern Med* 1982, 97:826–832.
12. Hickey AJ, Wilcken DE: Age and the clinical profile of idiopathic mitral valve prolapse. *Br Heart J* 1986, 55:582–586.
13. Pan CW, Chen CC, Wang SP, *et al.*: Echocardiographic study of cardiac abnormalities in families of patients with Marfan's syndrome. *J Am Coll Cardiol* 1985, 6:1016–1020.
14. Udoshi MB, Shah A, Fisher VJ, *et al.*: Incidence of mitral valve prolapse in subjects with thoracic skeletal abnormalities—a prospective study. *Am Heart J* 1979, 97:303–311.
15. Betriu A, Wigle ED, Felderhof CH, *et al.*: Prolapse of the posterior leaflet of the mitral valve associated with secundum atrial septal defect. *Am J Cardiol* 1975, 35:363–369.
16. Josephson ME, Horowitz LM, Kastor JA: Paroxysmal supraventricular tachycardia in patients with mitral valve prolapse. *Circulation* 1978, 57:111–119.
17. Crawford MH, O'Rourke RA: Mitral valve prolapse: a cardiomyopathic state? *Prog Cardiovasc Dis* 1984, 27:133–139.
18. Crawford MH: Mitral valve prolapse due to coronary artery disease. *Am J Med* 1977, 62:447–451.
19. Lembo NJ, Dell'Italia LJ, Crawford MH, *et al.*: Mitral valve prolapse in patients with prior rheumatic fever. *Circulation* 1988, 77:830–836.
20. Pini R, Greppi B, Kramer-Fox R, *et al.*: Mitral valve dimensions and motion and familial transmission of mitral valve prolapse with and without mitral leaflet billowing. *J Am Coll Cardiol* 1988, 12:1423–1431.
21. Henney AM, Tsipouras P, Schwartz RC, *et al.*: Genetic evidence that mutations in the COL1A2, COL3A1, or COL5A2 collagen genes are not responsible for mitral valve prolapse. *Br Heart J* 1989, 61:292–299.
22. King BD, Clark MA, Baba N, *et al.*: "Myxomatous" mitral valves: collagen dissolution as the primary defect. *Circulation* 1982, 66:288–296.
23. Stein PD, Wang CH, Riddle JM, *et al.*: Scanning electron microscopy of operatively excised severely regurgitant floppy mitral valves. *Am J Cardiol* 1989, 64:392–394.
24. Fontana ME, Sparks EA, Boudoulas H, *et al.*: Mitral valve prolapse and the mitral valve prolapse syndrome. *Curr Probl Cardiol* 1991, 16:315–375.
25. Boudoulas H, Kolibash AJ, Baker P, *et al.*: Mitral valve prolapse and the mitral valve prolapse syndrome: a diagnostic classification and pathogenesis of symptoms. *Am Heart J* 1989, 118:796–818.
26. Devereux RB, Kramer-Fox R, Brown WT, *et al.*: Relation between clinical features of the mitral prolapse syndrome and echocardiographically documented mitral valve prolapse. *J Am Coll Cardiol* 1986, 8:763–772.
27. Barnett HJ, Boughner DR, Taylor DW, *et al.*: Further evidence relating mitral valve prolapse to cerebral ischemic events. *N Engl J Med* 1980, 302:139–144.
28. Kelley RE, Pina I, Lee SC: Cerebral ischemia and mitral valve prolapse: case control study of associated factors. *Stroke* 1988, 19:443–446.
29. Orencia AJ, Petty GW, Khanderia BK, *et al.*: Risk of stroke with mitral valve prolapse in population-based cohort study. *Stroke* 1995, 26:7–13.
30. Hickey AJ, Andrew G, Wilcken DE: Independence of mitral valve prolapse and neurosis. *Br Heart J* 1983, 50:333–336.
31. Katerndahl DA: Panic and prolapse: meta-analysis. *J Nerv Ment Dis* 1993, 181:539–544.
32. O'Rourke RA, Crawford MH: The systolic click-murmur syndrome: clinical recognition and management. *Curr Probl Cardiol* 1976, 1:9–60.
33. Alpert MA, Cardney RJ, Flaker GC, *et al.*: Sensitivity and specificity of two-dimensional echocardiographic signs of mitral valve prolapse. *Am J Cardiol* 1984, 54:792–796.
34. Bhutto ZR, Barron JT, Liebson PR, *et al.*: Electrocardiographic abnormalities in mitral valve prolapse. *Am J Cardiol* 1992, 70:265–266.
35. Kligfield P, Levy D, Devereux RB, *et al.*: Arrhythmias and sudden death in mitral valve prolapse. *Am Heart* 1987, 113:1298–1307.
36. Schaal SF: Ventricular arrhythmias in patients with mitral valve prolapse. *Cardiovasc Clin* 1992, 22:307–316.
37. Abbasi AS, DeCristofaro D, Anabtawi J, *et al.*: Mitral valve prolapse: comparative value of M-mode, two-dimensional, and Doppler echocardiography. *J Am Coll Cardiol* 1983, 2:1219–1223.
38. Devereux RB, Kramer-Fox R, Kligfield P: Mitral valve prolapse: causes, clinical manifestations, and management. *Ann Intern Med* 1989, 111:305–317.
39. Marks AR, Choong CY, Chir MBB, *et al.*: Identification of high-risk and low-risk subgroups of patients with mitral valve prolapse. *N Engl J Med* 1989, 320:1031–1036.
40. Engel PJ, Alpert BL, Hickman JR Jr: The nature and prevalence of the abnormal exercise electrocardiogram in mitral valve prolapse. *Am Heart J* 1979, 98:716–724.
41. Butman S, Chandraratna PAN, Milne N, *et al.*: Stress myocardial imaging in patients with mitral valve prolapse: evidence of a perfusion abnormality. *Cathet Cardiovasc Diagn* 1982, 8:243–252.
42. Nishimura RA, McGoon MD, Shub C, *et al.*: Echocardiographically documented mitral-valve prolapse: long term followup of 237 patients. *N Engl J Med* 1985, 313:1305–1309.
43. Mills P, Rose J, Hollingsworth J, *et al.*: Long-term prognosis of mitral valve prolapse. *N Engl J Med* 1977, 297:13–18.

44. Allen H, Harris A, Leatham A: Significance and prognosis of an isolated late systolic murmur: a 9- to 22-year followup. *Br Heart J* 1974, 36:525–532.

45. Clemens JD, Horwitz RI, Jaffe CC, *et al.*: A controlled evaluation of the risk of bacterial endocarditis in persons with mitral valve prolapse. *N Engl J Med* 1982, 307:776–781.

46. Devereaux RB, Hawkins I, Kramer-Fox R, *et al.*: Complications of mitral valve prolapse: disproportionate occurrence in men and older patients. *Am J Med* 1986, 81:751–758.

47. Kolibash AJ, Kilman JW, Bush CA, *et al.*: Evidence for progression from mild to severe mitral regurgitation in mitral valve prolapse. *Am J Cardiol* 1986, 58:762–767.

48. You-Bing D, Takenaka K, Sakamoto T: Followup in mitral valve prolapse by phonocardiography, M-mode and two-dimensional echocardiography, and Doppler echocardiography. *Am J Cardiol* 1990, 65:349–354.

49. Stoddard MF, Prince CR, Dillon S, *et al.*: Exercise-induced mitral regurgitation is a predictor of morbid events in subjects with mitral valve prolapse. *J Am Coll Cardiol* 1995, 25:693–699.

50. Cosgrove DM, Altagracia M, Chavez MD, *et al.*: Results of mitral valve reconstruction. *Circulation* 1986, 74(suppl 1):82–87.

51. Salati M, Scrofani R, Fundaro P, *et al.*: Correction of anterior mitral prolapse: results of chordal transposition. *J Thorac Cardiovasc Surg* 1992, 104:1268–1273.

52. Cohn LH, Couper GS, Aranki SF, *et al.*: Long-term results of mitral valve reconstruction for regurgitation of the myxomatous mitral valve. *J Thorac Cardiovasc Surg* 1994, 107:143–151.

Acquired Tricuspid and Pulmonic Valve Disease

11

CHAPTER

Melvin D. Cheitlin and
John S. MacGregor

The frequency of acquired diseases of the cardiac valves seems to be related to the hemodynamic stress to which the valves are exposed. In rheumatic fever and infective endocarditis the mitral valve is most commonly affected followed by the aortic, tricuspid, and pulmonic valves in order of descending frequency.

Diseases causing tricuspid regurgitation are more numerous than those causing tricuspid stenosis. The normal tricuspid valve frequently does not completely coapt in systole, as is shown by the high frequency of tricuspid regurgitation jets on Doppler ultrasound. Most often the volume of regurgitant blood is so small that the tricuspid regurgitation is silent, and because it is found in from 24% to 96% of normal people, this finding must be considered a variant of normal by Doppler ultrasound [1].

The two major categories of diseases causing acquired tricuspid regurgitation are diseases causing right ventricular dilatation and primary diseases of the tricuspid valve apparatus, which include the tricuspid annulus, the leaflets, the chordae, the papillary muscles, and the right ventricular wall. Tricuspid regurgitation is usually well tolerated in patients who do not have coexistent pulmonary hypertension. The combination of significant tricuspid regurgitation and pulmonary hypertension, however, results in decreased cardiac output and clinical findings that may include fatigue, weakness, ascites, hepatomegaly, edema, and elevated jugular venous pressure.

The most common cause of tricuspid stenosis is rheumatic heart disease. Coexistent involvement of the mitral valve is almost always present in this condition. Tricuspid stenosis must be distinguished from other conditions that interfere with right atrial emptying. These conditions include right atrial myxoma prolapsing across the tricuspid valve; tumors such as renal cell carcinoma and lymphoma, which can grow in the inferior vena cava and right atrium resulting in tricuspid valve obstruction; and massive vegetations on the tricuspid valve.

Clinical features of tricuspid stenosis include symptoms of fatigue, abdominal pain localized to the right upper quadrant due to congestive hepatomegaly, abdominal swelling due to ascites, edema, and elevated neck veins with a large *a* wave. The lung fields are clear in patients without coexistent left heart failure. Patients who also have mitral valve disease may exhibit symptoms of left heart failure. Findings on auscultation may include a diastolic murmur that is usually heard best in the fourth intercostal space on the left sternal border.

Acquired pulmonic regurgitation is most commonly due to conditions that result in dilatation of the pulmonary annulus as a result of pulmonary hypertension or to conditions that lead to dilatation of the pulmonary artery. Conditions that produce pulmonic regurgitation by primarily affecting the valve leaflets include infective endocarditis, rheumatic disease, penetrating trauma, postrepair of congenital heart disease, and carcinoid heart disease. Pulmonic regurgitation is usually asymptomatic unless it is severe enough to produce right ventricular dilatation and failure, in which case symptoms are similar to those of severe tricuspid regurgitation, including fatigue, exertional dyspnea, and right upper quadrant pain.

In severe cases the right ventricular impulse may be hyperdynamic.

Pulmonic stenosis is most often congenital in origin, but it may be acquired, for example, in cases of rheumatic and carcinoid heart disease. It is only symptomatic in severe cases, in which patients may experience fatigue, dyspnea, syncope, and other symptoms of right heart failure. Physical examination may reveal a prominent *a* wave in the jugular venous pulse or a *v* wave if tricuspid regurgitation is present, a right ventricular heave, and wide splitting of S_2 with a soft P_2. A harsh systolic murmur is loudest at the upper left sternal border. An ejection click preceding the murmur suggests valvular rather than subvalvular stenosis.

This chapter summarizes the radiographic, echocardiographic, and gross pathologic findings in these tricuspid and pulmonary valve diseases.

TRICUSPID VALVE

DISEASES CAUSING ACQUIRED TRICUSPID VALVE STENOSIS

- Rheumatic heart disease, almost always in association with mitral stenosis, rarely as an isolated finding
- Carcinoid heart disease
- Löffler's (eosinophilic) myocarditis with right ventricular plaques and thrombus
- Prosthetic valve thrombosis
- Prosthetic valve infective endocarditis
- Paraprosthetic valve degeneration and calcification

FIGURE 11-1. Diseases causing acquired tricuspid valve stenosis.

DISEASES CAUSING ACQUIRED TRICUSPID VALVE REGURGITATION

DISEASES CAUSING PULMONARY HYPERTENSION

- All left ventricular diseases with left ventricular failure
- Mitral stenosis/mitral regurgitation
- Pulmonary venous obstruction
- Diseases causing an increase in pulmonary vascular resistance
  - Primary pulmonary hypertension
  - Acquired pulmonary vascular disease (atrial septal defects, ventricular septal defects, patent ductus arteriosus)
  - Intrinsic pulmonary disease (chronic obstructive pulmonary disease, pulmonary fibrosis, and pulmonary resection)
  - Collagen vascular diseases
- Pulmonary emboli, acute and chronic

PRIMARY DISEASES OF THE TRICUSPID VALVE APPARATUS

- Rheumatic heart disease
- Trauma, penetrating and nonpenetrating
- Carcinoid heart disease
- Right atrial myxoma
- Infective endocarditis
- Eosinophilic myocarditis
- Prosthetic and bioprosthetic valve malfunction, including thrombosis and calcification
- Right ventricular myocardial infarction, almost always in association in diaphragmatic wall myocardial infarction
- Myxomatous tricuspid valve (tricuspid valve prolapse)

FIGURE 11-2. Diseases causing acquired tricuspid valvular regurgitation.

ETIOLOGY OF ACQUIRED TRICUSPID AND PULMONIC VALVE DISEASE

RHEUMATIC HEART DISEASE

Frequent pathologic involvement at autopsy in patients with rheumatic heart disease

Functional abnormality much less frequent than pathologic involvement

Most common cause of acquired tricuspid stenosis

Most often causes tricuspid stenosis or stenosis and regurgitation. Pure tricuspid regurgitation is rare.

CARCINOID HEART DISEASE

Primary sites of malignant carcinoid are appendix, ileum, small intestine, rectum

Symptoms of carcinoid, including flushing, diarrhea, and bronchospasm are caused by vasoactive substances (bradykinin, serotonin, and histamines) secreted by the tumor. Endothelial damage on the right side of the heart is also caused by these substances. Endothelial plaque is a reaction to this injury.

Carcinoid heart disease is seen in 19% to 53% of patients with carcinoid syndrome.

Usually causes tricuspid regurgitation and stenosis; pulmonic stenosis and less often pulmonic regurgitation

Vasoactive substances are metabolized by the lung. If there is pulmonary metastasis or patent foramen ovale, then the lung is bypassed and left-sided valvular lesions can develop.

The carcinoid plaque is free of elastic fibers and contains smooth muscle cells with thickened, reduplicated basement membranes, reticular fibers, and acid mucopolysaccharides. The normal valve and myocardium are not destroyed and can be seen to be intact under the plaque.

INFECTIVE ENDOCARDITIS

Triscuspid endocarditis is seen almost exclusively in intravenous drug users.

Staphylococcus aureus is the most frequent organsims, seen in 50% to 80% of cases. Other organisms are *Pseudomonas aeruginosa*, α-hemolytic streptococci, and *Candida albicans*.

Since right-sided endothelial lesions are seen in 50% of patients having indwelling Swan-Ganz catheters, there is a small incidence of infective endocarditis in patients with long-standing hemodynamic monitoring.

TRICUSPID VALVE PROLAPSE

Prevalence is 0.1% to 5.5% in the general population and 3% to 54% in patients with mitral valve prolapse.

Pathology is similar to that of mitral valve prolapse, that is, ballooning and redundant leaflets, and increase in both mucopolysaccharides in the spongiosa, and infiltration of the fibrosa of the valve. The attachment of the chordae can be weakened.

FIGURE 11-3. Etiology of acquired tricuspid and pulmonic valve disease.

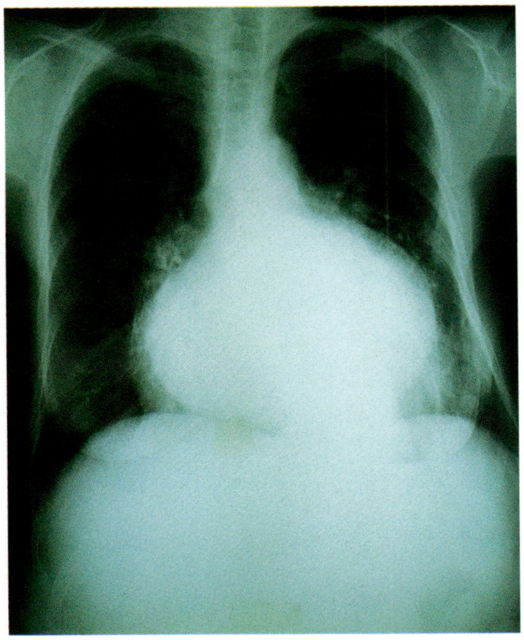

FIGURE 11-4. Chest roentgenogram, posteroanterior view, in a 42-year-old woman with rheumatic heart disease, severe mitral stenosis, and rheumatic involvement of the tricuspid valve causing severe tricuspid regurgitation. Note longer double-density of left atrium extending to the right beyond the large left atrium. There is vascular redistribution as well as the presence of Kerley B lines in the right costophrenic angle. Tricuspid regurgitation in the patient with mitral stenosis can be secondary to right ventricular dilatation secondary to pulmonary hypertension or because of rheumatic involvement of the tricuspid valve. The clinical differentiation of functional versus pathologic tricuspid regurgitation in the presence of mitral stenosis depends on demonstrating thickening of the valve and possibly right-sided subvalvular chordal fusion and obstruction by echocardiography. (*Adapted from* Virmani [2]; with permission.)

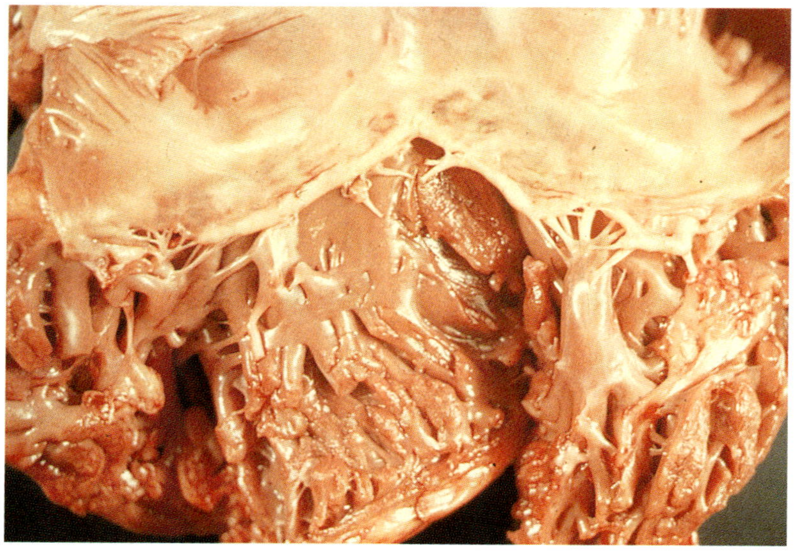

FIGURE 11-5. Heart displaying tricuspid valve with fused shortened chordae and rolled thickened, fibrotic edge, consistent with chronic rheumatic heart disease. Isolated rheumatic tricuspid regurgitation or stenosis is very rare; it occurs almost always in the presence of concomitant mitral stenosis. (*Adapted from* Farb and coworkers [3]; with permission.)

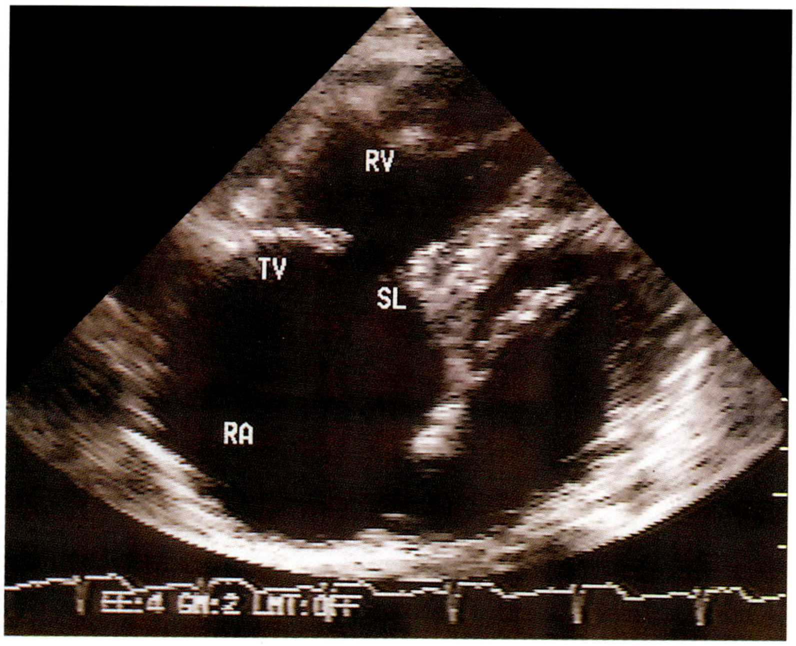

FIGURE 11-6. Two-dimensional echocardiogram of a 40-year-old patient, with carcinoid tumor of the testes without metastases. He presented with a testicular mass and was found to have a grade III/VI pansystolic murmur and grade III/VI diastolic murmur; both increased with inspiration.

This four-chamber view shows a thickened stenotic tricuspid valve (TV) in diastole. The right atrium (RA) is enlarged, and the atrial septum bulges to the left, indicating a higher RA than left atrial pressure, which is consistent with tricuspid stenosis. The liver was normal because the humoral products of the carcinoid tumor bypassed the liver by the testicular venous drainage flowing directly to the inferior vena cava and renal veins. Carcinoid tumors arise from neuroendocrine cells known as enterochromaffin cells, which are found in organs derived from the embryonic gut. Because the liver detoxifies the humoral products of the carcinoid tumor, which most often arises in the ileum, it is extremely rare to see carcinoid heart disease in the absence of liver metastases, making this case extremely unusual [4,5]. Only about 20% of patients with carcinoid tumors develop cardiovascular symptoms. RV—right ventricle; SL—septal leaflet.

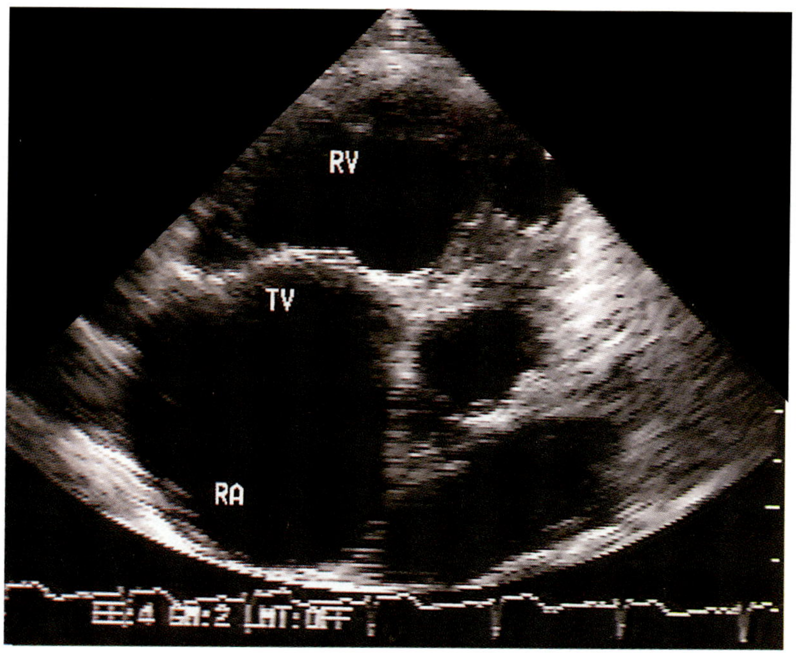

FIGURE 11-7. Two-dimensional echocardiogram in diastole. This is from the same patient as in Fig. 11-6. Note the thickened tricuspid valve (TV) and the lack of excursion of the TV from diastole to systole. This washer-like thickened TV is characteristic of carcinoid heart disease. It is common for a carcinoid TV to be both stenotic and insufficient. With carcinoid TV disease the valve becomes thickened and its mobility and flexibility are reduced [5]. RA—right atrium; RV—right ventricle.

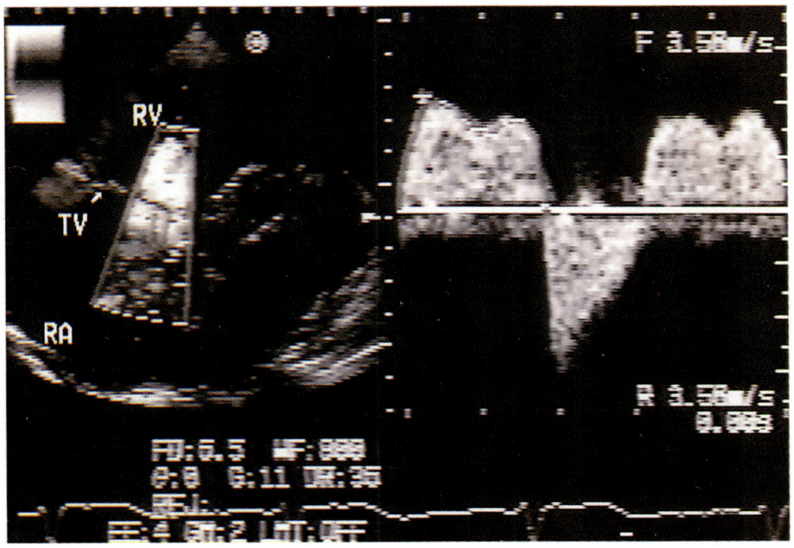

FIGURE 11-8. Doppler signal across the tricuspid valve (TV). This echocardiogram from the same patient as in Figs. 11-6 and 11-7 demonstrates the increased velocity in diastole across the tricuspid valve, calculating to a 17.8-mm Hg peak gradient with a 10-mm Hg mean gradient.

In systole there is a peak gradient of 30 mm Hg that rapidly decays in a manner consistent with severe tricuspid regurgitation. The hemodynamics of combined tricuspid stenosis and insufficiency are worse than with either lesion alone. The mean right atrial (RA) pressure is increased in tricuspid stenosis by the increase in RA volume in systole caused by the regurgitant volume due to the tricuspid insufficiency. With tricuspid regurgitation the mean RA pressure is increased by the presence of some degree of tricuspid stenosis because of the increase in RA pressure during diastole. Because the regurgitant volume increases the diastolic blood flow in the combined tricuspid stenosis and insufficiency lesion, the diastolic rumble of tricuspid stenosis is frequently very loud [4]. RV—right ventricle.

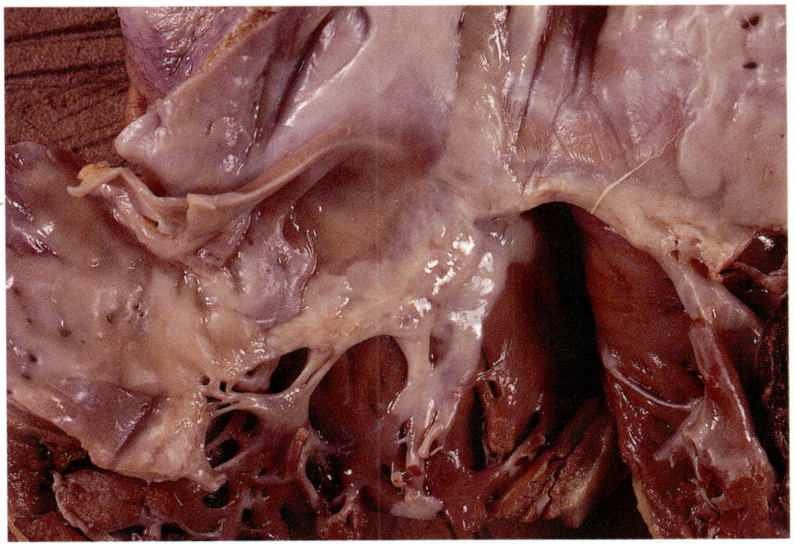

FIGURE 11-9. Tricuspid valve. Note thickened leaflets and fused thickened chordae. This patient had carcinoid heart disease with severe tricuspid regurgitation, tricuspid stenosis, and pulmonic valve stenosis. In carcinoid, the serotonin, histamine bradykinin, their metabolites, and possibly other humoral agents that cause the fibrotic changes seen in the right heart affect the endocardium and both tricuspid and pulmonic valves (*see* Fig. 11-8). Thus, there is fusion of the chordae, shortening of the width of the tricuspid and pulmonic leaflets, and marked thickening of the valves, which result in a combined tricuspid and pulmonic stenosis and regurgitation [4].

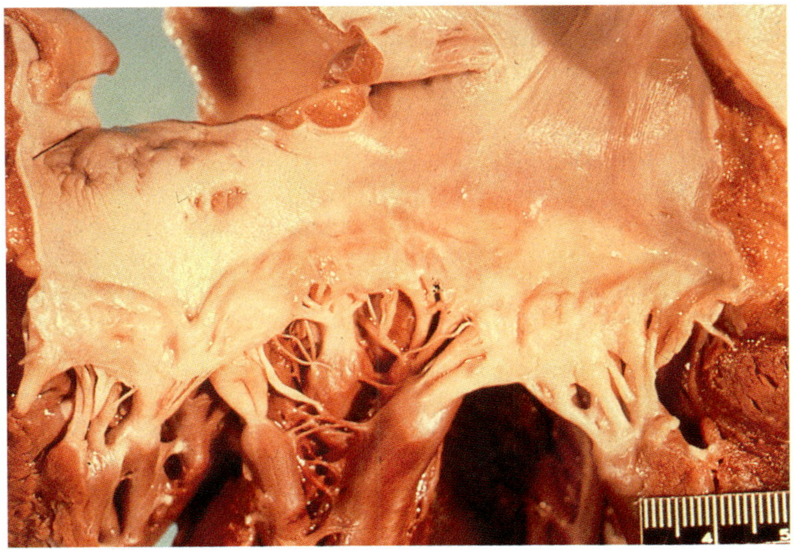

FIGURE 11-10. Tricuspid valve (TV) from a patient with carcinoid heart disease who had severe tricuspid regurgitation. Note thickened opaque TV with chordal fusion. Pathologically the normal valve and endocardium are thickened by the deposition of plaques composed of a collagenous stroma rich in glycosaminoglycans devoid of elastic fibers. (*Adapted from* Farb and coworkers [3]; with permission.)

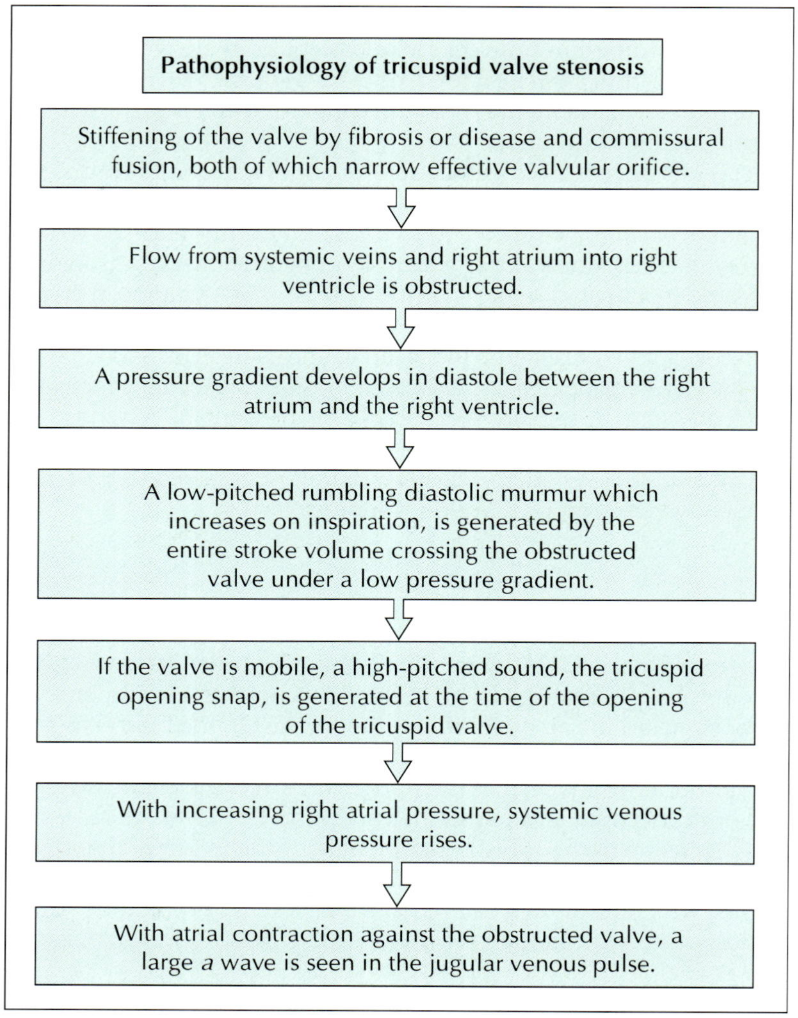

FIGURE 11-11. Pathophysiology of tricuspid valve stenosis.

CLINICAL FINDINGS IN TRICUSPID VALVE STENOSIS

A large *a* wave in the jugular venous pulse
Elevated central venous pressure
Findings of right heart failure with hepatomegaly, edema, and ascites
Tricuspid opening snap (mobile valves)
Loud S_1 heart sound (mobile valves)
Tricuspid rumbling diastolic murmur in the third and fourth intercostal space, left sternal border
Murmur and opening snap are increased with inspiration as more blood is drawn back into the right atrium (the Rivera-Carvallo's sign)
Occurrence of atrial arrhythmias, including flutter and atrial fibrillation

FIGURE 11-12. Clinical findings in tricuspid valve stenosis.

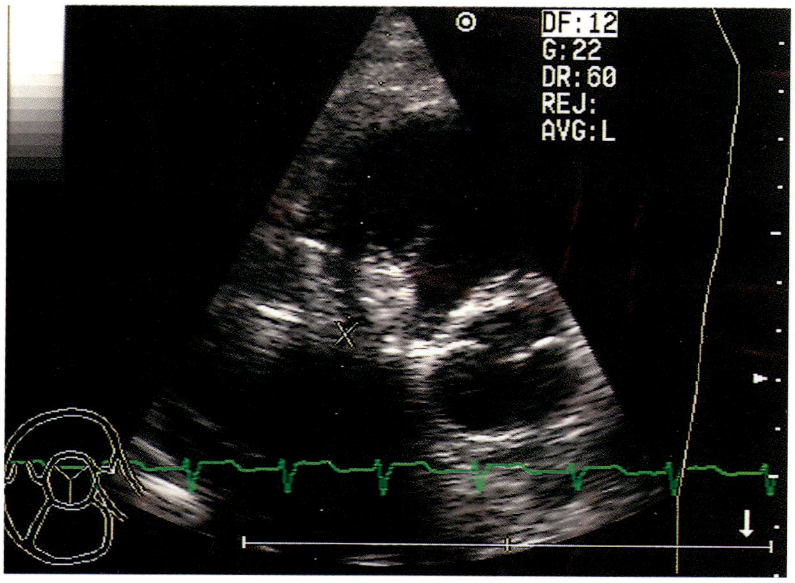

FIGURE 11-13. Short-axis view at the aortic level of a two-dimensional echocardiogram in a 30-year-old woman who was an intravenous drug-user and who had fever, multiple septic pulmonary emboli, and a large vegetation on a bioprosthetic valve (*X*). The picture was taken at the onset of systole. The patient had a grade III/VI harsh diastolic murmur along the left sternal border markedly increased in intensity by inspiration. Jugular venous pressure was elevated to 16 cm with a prominent *a* wave. It is frequently difficult to distinguish a vegetation due to infective endocarditis from a thrombus developing on the valve. Differentiation depends on the clinical picture and the results of blood cultures. With prosthetic valves, transesophageal echocardiography is more sensitive in detecting ring abscesses than transthoracic echocardiography [6].

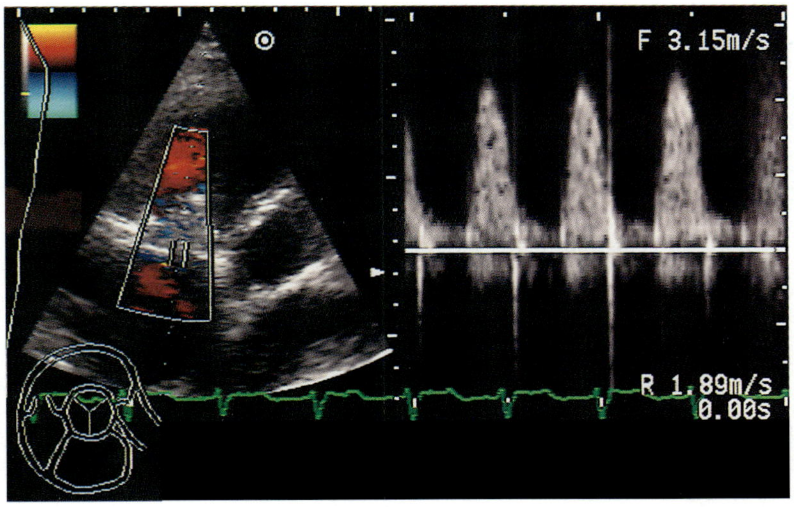

FIGURE 11-14. Color Doppler ultrasound across the bioprosthetic tricuspid valve in the short-axis view at the aortic level. This is from the same patient as in Fig. 11-13. Notice the 2.4 m/sec peak velocity in diastole, calculating to a 23-mm peak gradient across the obstructed and infected prosthesis. The patient was in extremis with a cardiac output of less than 1 L/min. An emergency balloon valvuloplasty was performed with improvement of cardiac output and reduction in central venous pressure, but several days later the patient died of the pulmonary infection.

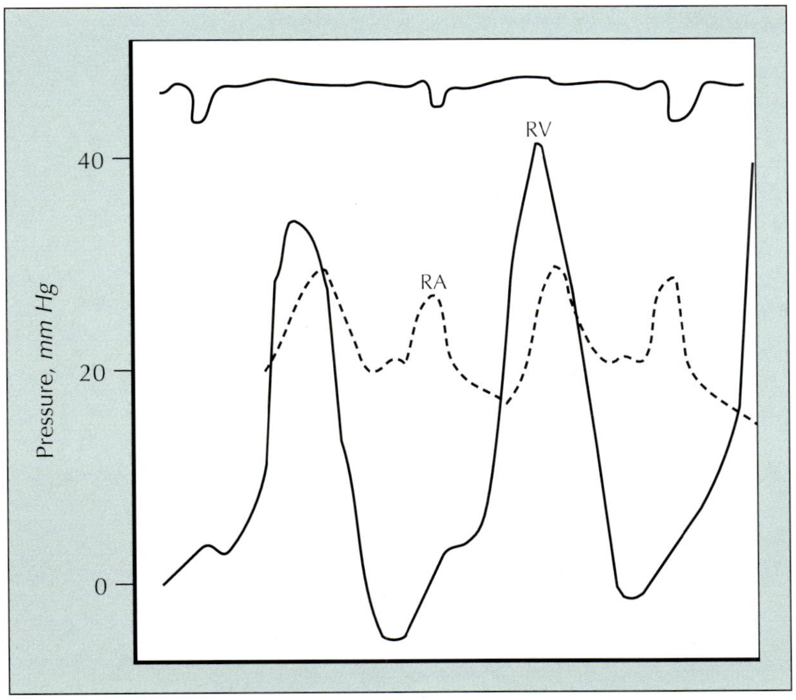

FIGURE 11-15. Simultaneous right ventricular (RV) and right atrial (RA) pressure before valvuloplasty. Note the large diastolic gradient across the tricuspid valve. Hemodynamics were done prior to the balloon valvuloplasty. This is from the same patient as in Fig. 11-13.

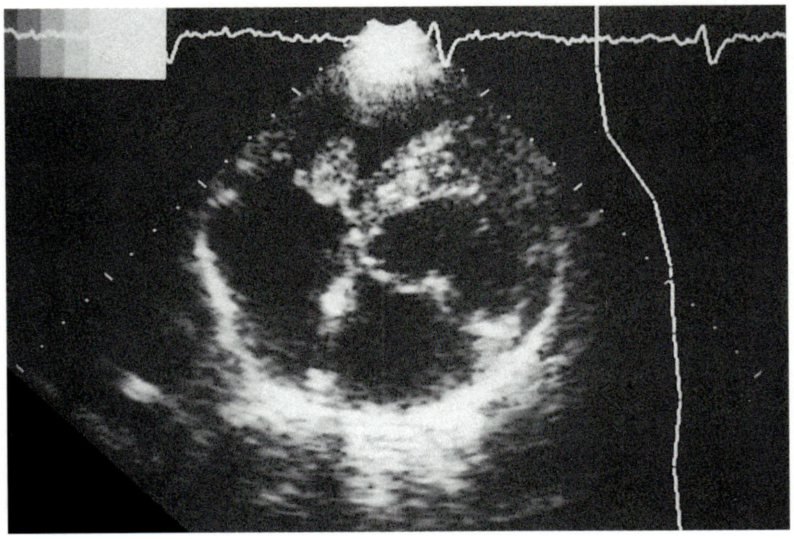

FIGURE 11-16. Infective endocarditis on the native tricuspid valve in a 23-year-old female intravenous drug user. Note in the four-chamber view of this two-dimensional echocardiogram the large vegetation on the septal leaflet of the tricuspid valve and the large right atrium caused by the severe tricuspid insufficiency. The organism seen in infective endocarditis involving the tricuspid valve is *Staphylococcus aureus* in 90% of cases [7]. Even with severe tricuspid regurgitation these patients usually do well at least for the short-term with control of the infection. Patients with drug-resistant organisms such as *Pseudomonas aeruginosa* causing tricuspid endocarditis have been treated by excising the tricuspid valve without prosthetic valve replacement, with the result that patients do well for several years with severe tricuspid regurgitation [8,9].

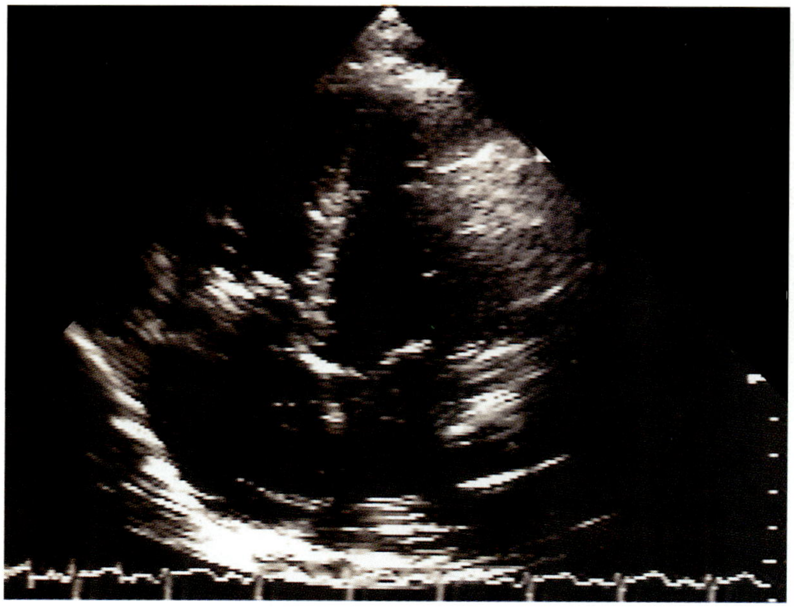

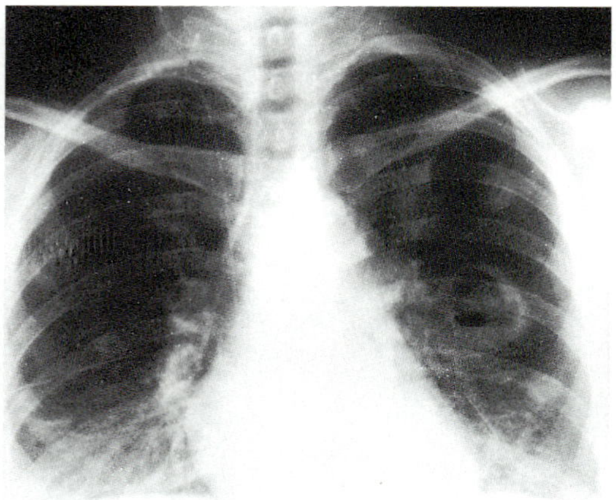

Figure 11-17. Four-chamber echocardiogram of a 25-year-old female intravenous drug user, who is febrile with multiple infiltrations in both lungs on chest roentgenogram. There is a large 2-cm long vegetation on the tricuspid valve and an enlarged right atrium. Large vegetations are more likely than small ones to embolize to the lung. Extremely large vegetations can cause massive pulmonary emboli that are hemodynamically significant [7]. With severe tricuspid insufficiency the high right atrial pressure can blow open a patent foramen ovale and cause arterial desaturation by a right-to-left shunt. Occasionally even paradoxical systemic emboli can be seen.

Figure 11-18. Chest roentgenogram, posteroanterior view of the same patient as in Fig. 11-17. Note the multiple pulmonary infiltrates caused by septic emboli in both lung fields. There is an abscess with an air-fluid level in the left lung. This patient had hemoptysis and eventually respiratory failure due to the extensive septic pulmonary emboli [7].

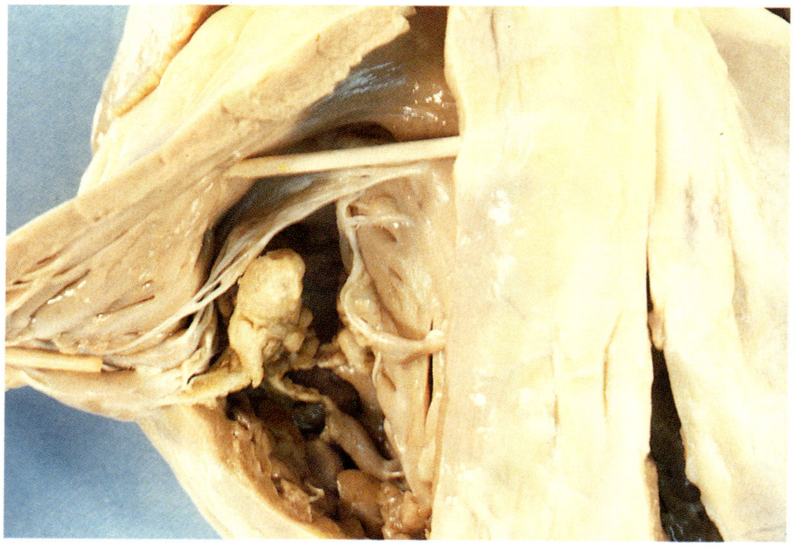

Figure 11-19. Heart at autopsy. Right ventricle is opened with large vegetation on the posterior leaflet of the tricuspid valve. The patient was a 30-year-old intravenous drug user who developed β-hemolytic streptococcal infective endocarditis involving the tricuspid, aortic, and mitral valves. The tricuspid valve is viewed from the ventricular surface. Note the opened and retracted right ventricle with chordae.

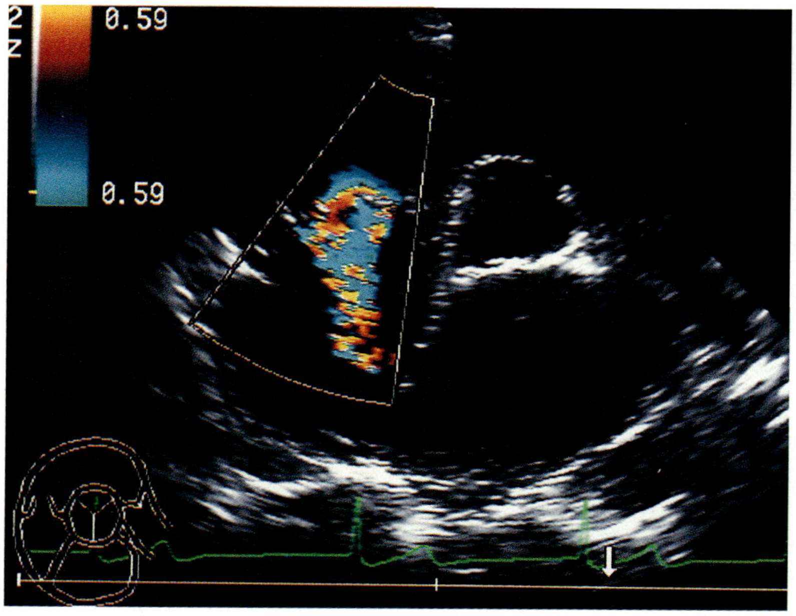

Figure 11-20. Two-dimensional Doppler ultrasound in a short-axis view at the level of the aortic root. Continuous Doppler across the tricuspid valve shows high-velocity jet regurgitation of tricuspid regurgitation. The patient had tricuspid endocarditis. Note the regurgitant jet fans out into the right atrium from a narrow origin of the atrial surface of the tricuspid valve. The right ventricular (and pulmonary artery) systolic pressure can be estimated by adding the systolic gradient of the regurgitant jet to the estimated central venous pressure [10].

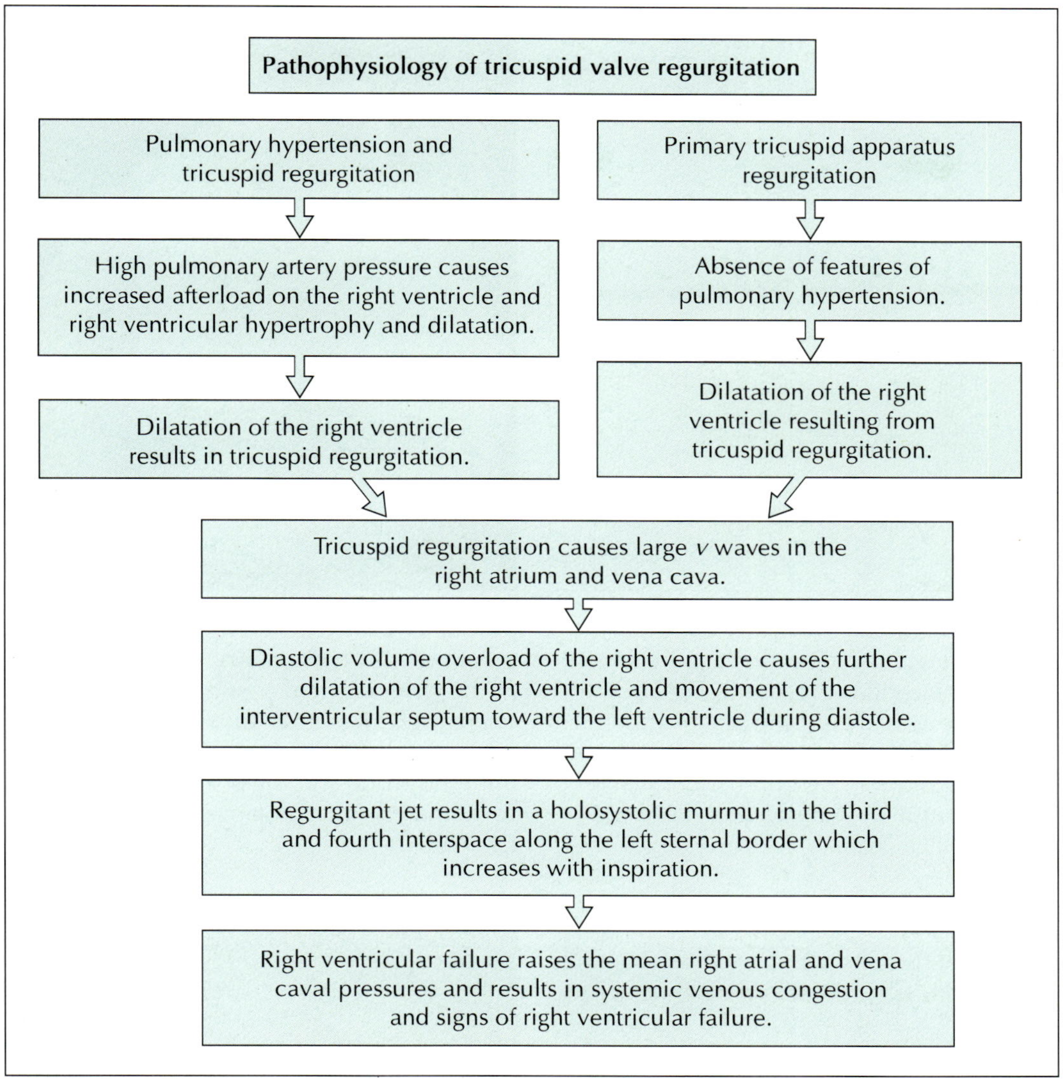

FIGURE 11-21. Pathophysiology of tricuspid regurgitation.

CLINICAL FEATURES OF TRICUSPID VALVE REGURGITATION

WITH PULMONARY HYPERTENSION

Accentuated pulmonic component of S_2.

High-frequency diastolic murmur of pulmonic valve regurgitation in the second and third interspace along the left sternal border.

Plus other features below.

WITH PRIMARY TRICUSPID APPARATUS REGURGITATION

Dilated right ventricle with precordial heave.

Right-sided S_3 and S_4.

Holosystolic murmur of tricuspid regurgitation in the third and fourth interspace at the left sternal border. With a small gradient and large regurgitant orifice, you can have severe tricuspid regurgitation with only an ejection-type murmur or with no murmur at all.

With a large amount of blood returning to the right ventricle in diastole, a short diastolic rumble along the left sternal border is common.

All of these findings are increased with inspiration (Rivera-Carvallo'a sign).

Large *v* wave in the jugular venous pulse.

With right ventricular failure, the mean central venous pulse is elevated and the external jugular veins are also pulsatile and engorged.

FIGURE 11-22. Clinical features of tricuspid regurgitation.

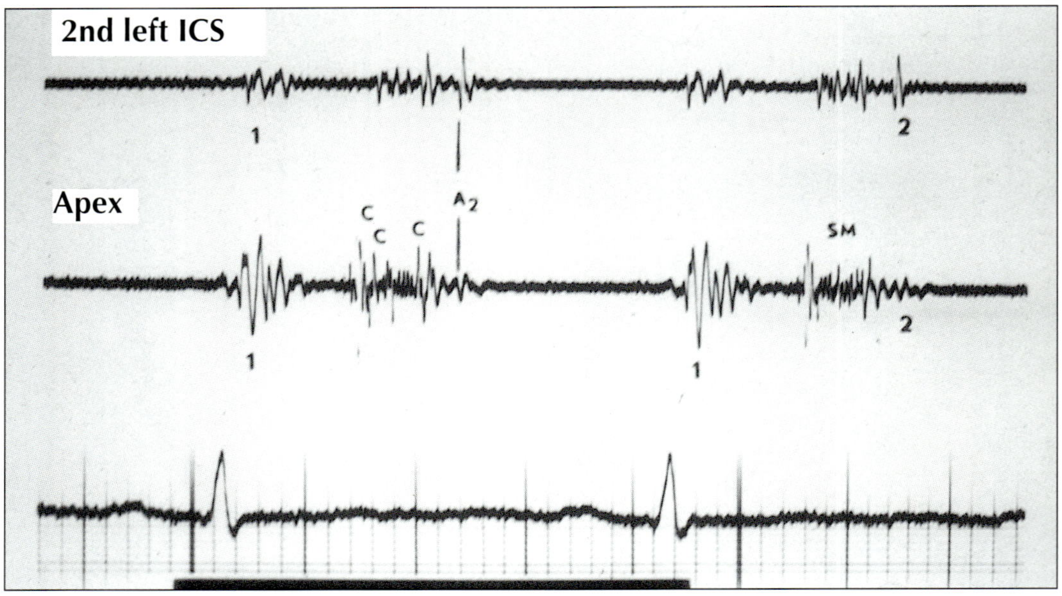

FIGURE 11-23. Phonocardiogram at the second left intercostal space (ICS) and at the apex in a patient with mitral valve prolapse. The number *1* is the mitral component of the first heart sound. The number *2* is the aortic component of the second heart sound. The *black bar* indicates inspiration. The nonejection clicks are probably due to the slipping and sudden checking of the valve leaflet as the systolic pressure in the left ventricle rises and the volume of the left ventricle decreases. When the mitral leaflets fail to coapt, a regurgitant orifice is formed and the regurgitant jet causes the late systolic murmur. C—nonejection clicks. SM—late systolic murmur of mitral valve prolapse. (Courtesy of Dr. William Nelson.)

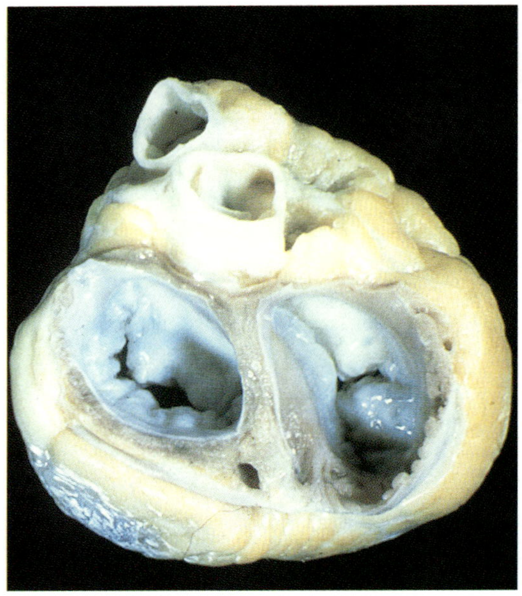

FIGURE 11-24. Heart viewed from above, great vessels anterior, atria removed down to the atrioventricular rings. The tricuspid valve (*right*) has three myxomatous, prolapsed leaflets. In the mitral valve (*left*), both the aortic and the posterior leaflets are myxomatous and prolapsed. (Courtesy of Dr. William Nelson.)

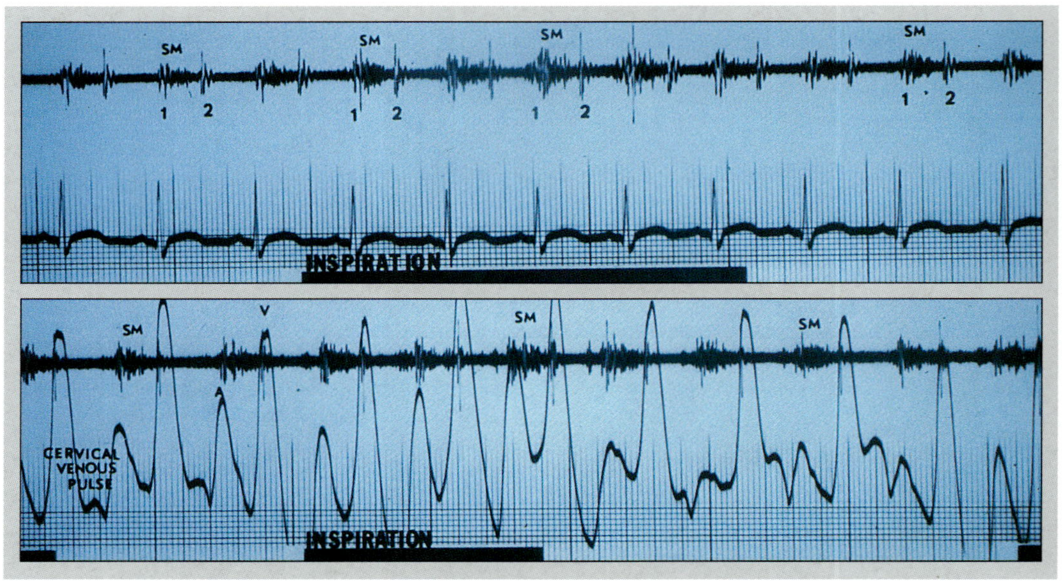

FIGURE 11-25. Phonocardiogram of a 24-year-old man with a severe tricuspid regurgitation following an automobile accident. **Top,** Phonocardiogram taken at lower left sternal border (LLSB) with electrocardiogram. **Bottom,** Phonocardiogram at same place with cervical venous pulse. The *black bar* is inspiration. The numbers *1* and *2* are the first and second heart sounds. Note the systolic regurgitant murmur, which increases in amplitude (loudness) with inspiration. Note the *v* wave is higher than the *a* wave in the cervical venous pulse. Tricuspid regurgitation after nonpenetrating trauma can result from either tearing of chordal structures or rupture of the papillary muscles. With right ventricular contusion, dilatation of the right ventricle and tricuspid annulus can cause tricuspid regurgitation [11]. (Courtesy of Dr. William Nelson.)

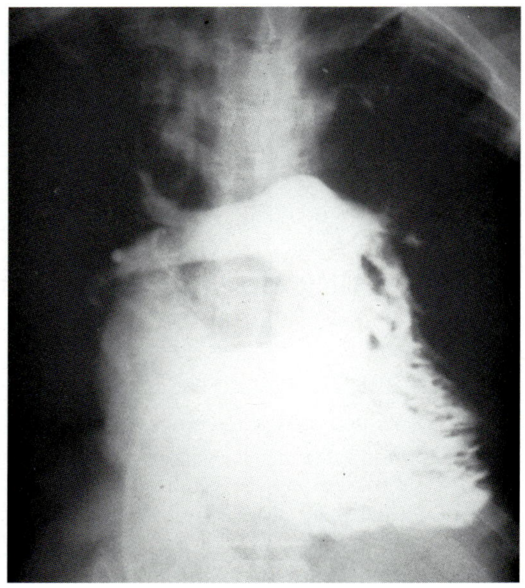

FIGURE 11-26. Posteroanterior angiocardiogram with injection into the right ventricle. Patient is a 25-year-old man with rupture of tricuspid papillary muscle after an automobile accident. Note the trabeculated right ventricle with complete opacification of the right atrium due to severe tricuspid regurgitation [11].

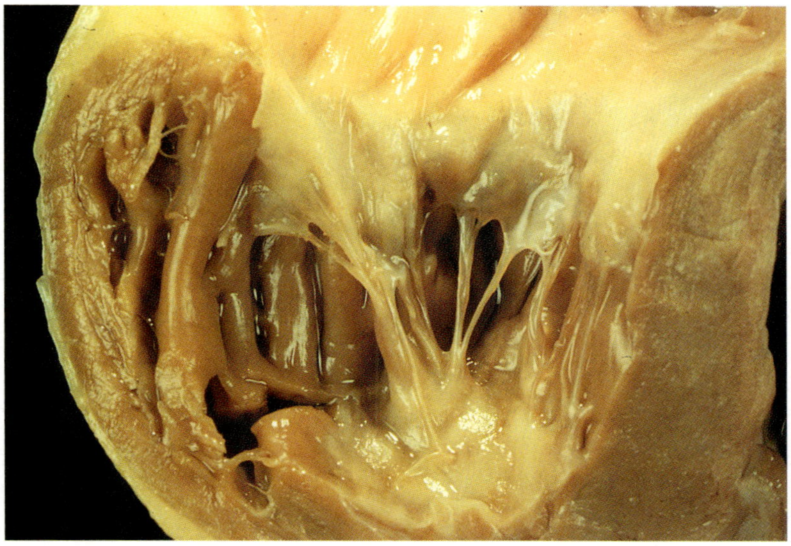

Figure 11-27. Right ventricle and tricuspid valve of a patient with Löffler's myocarditis. Note fibrous opaque mass at the apex of the right ventricle involving the chordae tendineae and portions of the tricuspid valve. The patient had severe tricuspid regurgitation. Löffler's myocarditis is one manifestation of endomyocardial disease caused by abnormal activity of eosinophils. Abnormal eosinophils produce a thrombogenic cationic protein that damages the endocardium and myocardium. Thrombus and fibrosis form almost invariably in the inflow tract of the right or left ventricle, usually sparing the ventricular outflow tracts. Because of involvement of the papillary muscles and chordae, tricuspid and/or mitral regurgitation is a prominent feature. The dominant pathophysiologic effect of the endocardial fibrosis and thrombosis is ventricular diastolic dysfunction [12,13]. (Courtesy of Renu Virmani, MD.)

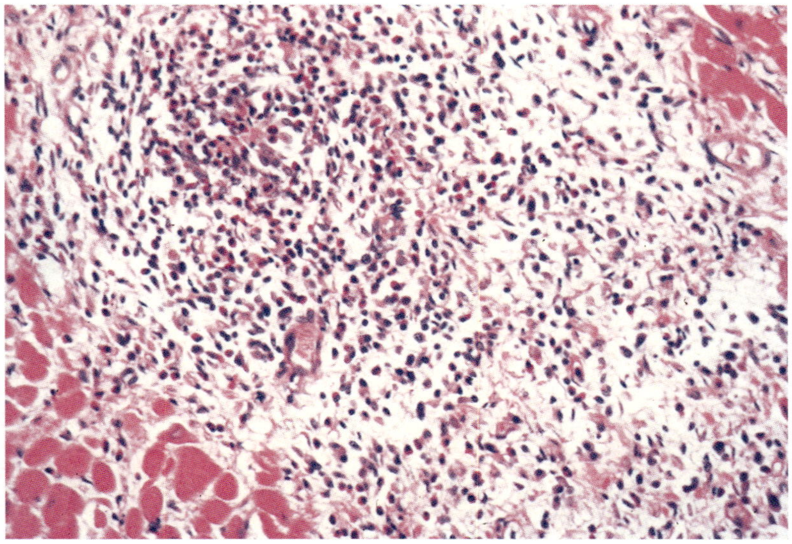

Figure 11-28. Microscopic section of myocardium from 34-year-old man with Löffler's syndrome. Note granuloma with masses of eosinophils. An early stage of the eosinophilic endomyocardial disease is that of acute inflammatory activity in the endomyocardium with eosinophilic infiltration of the endocardium and myocardium. Later there is organization with endomyocardial fibrosis and endarteritis obliterans of myocardial arterioles. Eosinophils become progressively less apparent. The final stage is that of layers of thrombus over the fibrotic endocardium [12]. (Courtesy of Renu Vermani, MD.)

Pulmonic Valve

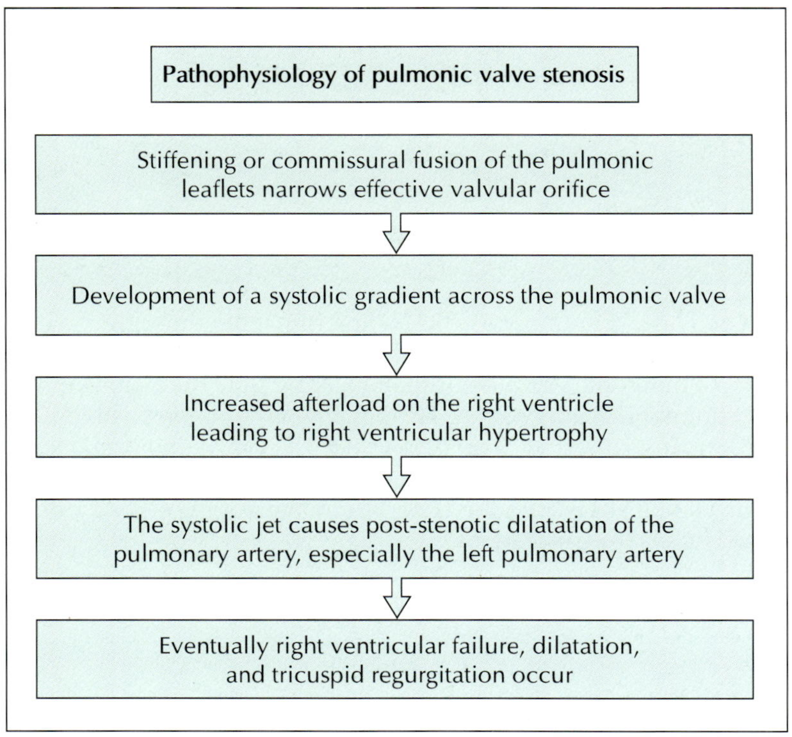

Figure 11-29. Pathophysiology of pulmonic valve stenosis.

CLINICAL FINDINGS IN PULMONIC VALVE STENOSIS

A systolic ejection murmur at the second interspace of the left sternal border generated by the entire right ventricular stroke volume. When stenosis is severe this murmur is loud, at least grade III or IV/VI.

In the absence of calcification there is a pulmonic valve ejection click that increases with expiration and decreases with inspiration.

Precordial parasternal heave from the hyperthrophied right ventricle.

Right-sided S_4 gallop.

Prominent *a* wave in the jugular venous pulse.

Figure 11-30. Clinical findings in pulmonic valve stenosis.

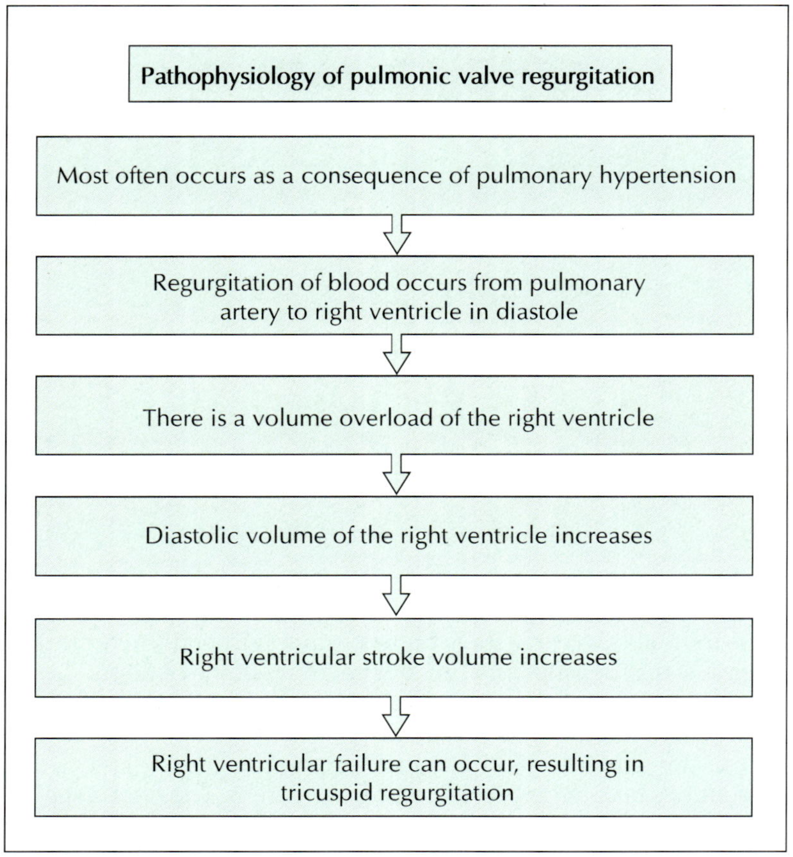

FIGURE 11-31. Pathophysiology of pulmonic valve regurgitation.

CLINICAL FINDINGS IN PULMONIC VALVE REGURGITATION

If pulmonary hypertension exists, there is an increased pulmonic component of the S_2.

There is a precordial heave of the right ventricle because of the volume overload.

There is a precordial lift due to right ventricular dilatation.

Diastolic murmur along the left sternal border. The pitch of the murmur depends on the pulmonary artery diastolic pressure. If the pulmonary artery pressure is high, the murmur is high frequency. In patients with pulmonic regurgitation with normal pulmonary artery pressure, the murmur is low-pitched and begins after the pulmonic component of the second heart sound.

Right-sided S_3 and S_4 gallops.

FIGURE 11-32. Clinical findings in pulmonic valve regurgitation.

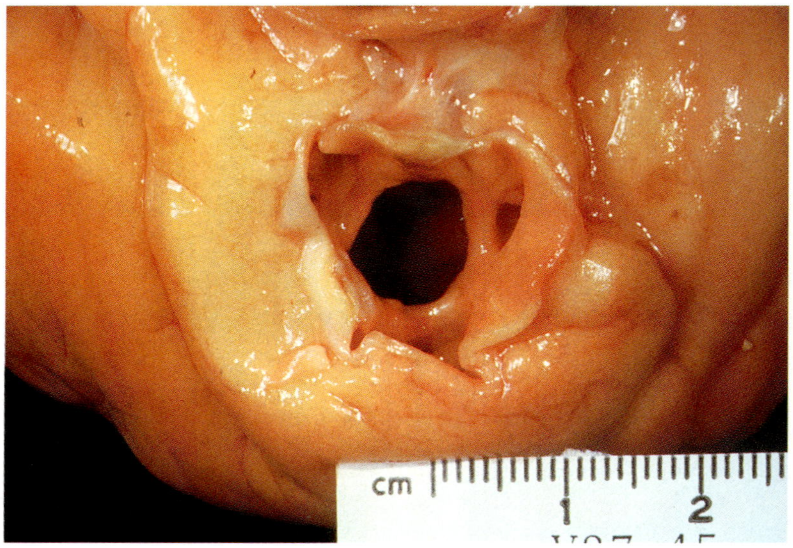

FIGURE 11-33. Pulmonic valve from a patient with carcinoid heart disease. The pulmonary artery is opened and the stenotic and insufficient pulmonic valve is visible. Note the thickened rigid cusps of the pulmonic valve [4,5]. (*Adapted from* Farb and coworkers [3]; with permission.)

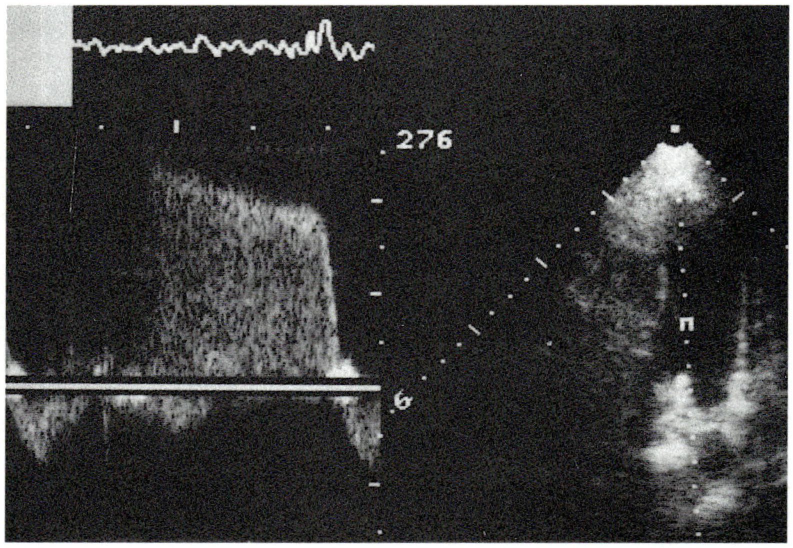

FIGURE 11-34. Continuous echo-Doppler imaging through pulmonic valve. Notice regurgitant jet in diastole across pulmonic valve of pulmonic valve regurgitation. Note slow decay indicating mild pulmonic regurgitation. The patient had pulmonic valve endocarditis caused by *Streptococcus pneumoniae*. With normal low pulmonary artery diastolic pressure, the murmur of pulmonic regurgitation starts after the aortic component of the second heart sound and is low pitched.

DISEASES CAUSING ACQUIRED PULMONIC VALVE STENOSIS

Carcinoid heart disease
Infective endocarditis with fungal ball
Calcification of a congenitally bicuspid pulmonic valve
Rheumatic heart disease

FIGURE 11-35. Diseases causing acquired pulmonic valvular stenosis.

DISEASES CAUSING ACQUIRED PULMONIC VALVE REGURGITATION

Rheumatic heart disease
Infective endocarditis, frequently from jet trauma from a ventricular septal defect
Carcinoid heart disease
Trauma, almost always penetrating
Disease causing pulmonary hypertension

FIGURE 11-36. Diseases causing acquired pulmonic valvular regurgitation.

REFERENCES

1. Kostucki W, Vandenbossche JL, Friart A, Engbert H: Pulsed Doppler regurgitant flow patterns of normal values. *Am J Cardiol* 1986, 58:309–313.
2. Virmani R: The tricuspid valve. *Mayo Clin Proc* 1988, 63:943-946.
3. Farb A, Burke AP, Virmani R: Anatomy and pathology of the right ventricle (including acquired tricuspid and pulmonic valve disease). *Cardiol Clin North Am* 1992, 10:1-21.
4. Pellikka PA, Tajik AJ, Khandheria BK, *et al*.: Carcinoid heart disease. Clinical and echocardiographic spectrum in 74 patients. *Circulation* 1993, 87:1188–1196.
5. Himelman RB, Schiller NB: Clinical and echocardiographic comparison of patients with the carcinoid syndrome with and without carcinoid heart disease. *Am J Cardiol* 1989, 63:347–352.
6. Daniel WG, Mugge A, Martin P, *et al*.: Improvement in the diagnosis of abscesses associated with endocarditis by transesophageal echocardiography. *N Engl J Med* 1991, 324:795–800.
7. Chambers HF, Korzeniowski OM, Sande MA: *Staphylococcus aureus* endocarditis: clinical manifestations in addicts and nonaddicts. *Medicine* 1983, 62:170-177.
8. Arbulu A, Thoms NW, Wilson RF: Valvulectomy without prosthetic replacement. A lifesaving operation for tricuspid pseudomonas endocarditis. *J Thorac Cardiovasc Surg* 1972, 64:103-107.
9. Robin E, Belamaric J, Thoms NW, *et al*.: Consequences of total tricuspid valvulectomy without prosthetic replacement in treatment of Pseudomonas endocarditis. *J Thorac Cardiovasc Surg* 1974, 68:461-465.
10. Yock PG, Popp RL: Noninvasive estimation of right ventricular systolic pressure by Doppler ultrasound in patients with tricuspid regurgitation. *Circulation* 1984, 70:657-662.
11. Cheitlin MD: The internist's role in the management of the patient with traumatic heart disease. *Cardiol Clin* 1991, 9:675-688.
12. Davies J, Spry CJ, Sapsford R, *et al*.: Cardiovascular features of 11 patients with eosinophilic endomyocardial disease. *Q J Med* 1983, 52:23-39.
13. Harley JB, McIntosh CL, Kirklin JJ, *et al*.: Atrioventricular valve replacement in the idiopathic hypereosinophilic syndrome. *Am J Med* 1982, 73:77-81.

Repair for Acquired Valvular Heart Disease

12

CHAPTER

Manuel J. Antunes

Cardiac valve replacement exchanges one disease with another. Mechanical valves are prone to thromboembolic phenomena that require lifelong anticoagulation, in turn complicated by hemorrhagic episodes. Both thromboembolism and hemorrhage are life-threatening complications. Bioprostheses, once hailed as the solution to the problem of prosthetic valve replacement, are subjected to biodegradation and ultimately to calcification, which are accelerated in younger patients and in pregnant women. Long-term comparative studies and randomized trials have failed to demonstrate a significant advantage of one type of prosthesis over the other. Within 10 years only about half the patients are free from prosthetic-related mortality and morbidity. Hence, valve conservation remains an appealing alternative, especially in the young and in the populations of the developing countries.

Mitral valvuloplasty is now widely accepted and performed by most surgical teams throughout the world [1–7]. Most will agree that mitral commissurotomy is the best option in the treatment of rheumatic mitral stenosis [8], but the indications for valvuloplasty for mitral regurgitation are much less consensual. Although patients with rheumatic heart disease would benefit theoretically the most from these procedures, early and late failures resulting from technical problems because of the usually difficult anatomy, or from persistent or recurrent rheumatic carditis, are not uncommon [4,9]. By contrast, valvuloplasty for degenerative, myxomatous-type mitral regurgitation has consistently yielded very good and durable results, despite the generalized involvement of all components of the valve apparatus [10]. Ischemic regurgitation often defies the surgeon's efforts to preserve the valve, except in the cases of isolated annular dilatation secondary to left ventricular enlargement and dysfunction.

Reoperation for persistent or recurrent regurgitations is by far the most common serious complication after mitral valvuloplasty. The incidence is much higher in rheumatic than in nonrheumatic cases. Nonetheless, more than 80% of the patients remain free from reoperation after 10 years. Also, reoperative mortality is much lower after valvuloplasty than after valve replacement. Hence, valvuloplasty is superior [11].

Tricuspid valve disease is commonly associated with left-sided valve disease, and intervention on the tricuspid valve is required in 10% to 15% of patients undergoing mitral or aortic valve surgery, but fewer than 1% require tricuspid valve replacement. Patients who require tricuspid valve surgery have a lower long-term survival than those who do not, presumably because of the more advanced stage of their disease. However, survival is probably better in those with significant regurgitation that is treated concomitantly with mitral or aortic surgery than in those in whom the tricuspid valve is left untouched [12].

The De Vega [13] and other suture annuloplasties remain the cornerstone of treatment of "functional" tricuspid regurgitation, but organic regurgitation, usually associated with stenosis, is probably better treated by a more comprehensive valvuloplasty, including the implantation of a preshaped (Carpentier) annuloplasty ring [2].

Finally, the aortic valve has been particularly refractory to conservation efforts. Decalcification of stenotic valves either by mechanical methods or by ultrasonic vibration (CUSA [cavitron ultrasonic surgical aspirator], Cooper Laser Sonics, Santa Clara, CA) has largely yielded poor results. On the other hand, attempts have been made at surgical centers to repair regurgitating aortic valves; however, long-term follow-up studies are not available. Nonetheless, some recent reports [14–16] and our own experience, appear to demonstrate that aortic valvuloplasty is indicated in selected areas and has good results in some patients with moderate aortic stenosis or regurgitation in whom surgery is required for severe mitral valve or coronary artery disease.

MITRAL VALVE

ANATOMY AND FUNCTION

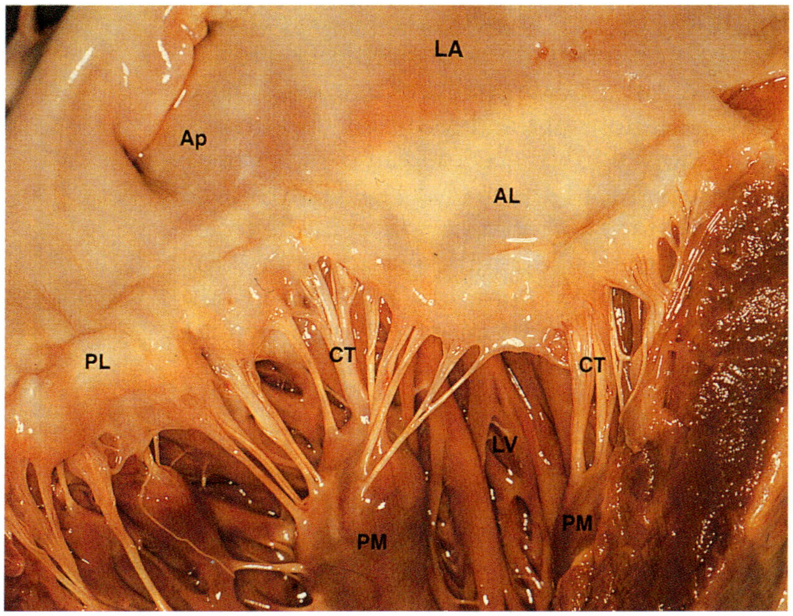

FIGURE 12-1. Mitral valve structure. The mitral valve, located between the left atrium (LA) and the left ventricle (LV), is a complex structure [17,18]. It has two leaflets, anterior (AL) and posterior (PL), which are attached to the annulus at the level of the junction of the atrial and ventricular walls, and are constituted by a layer of connective tissue covered by endocardium on both sides. Muscle fibers of atrial and ventricular origin may be present. The free edge and the body of the leaflets are attached to the chordae tendineae (CT), which in turn are connected to the heads of the papillary muscles (PM), digital extensions of the ventricular myocardium. The AL, triangular in shape, has a shorter insertion in the annulus but a greater width than the PL. The PL, which is rectangular, has a greater annular attachment but is much narrower. The AL has a surface similar to the area of the annulus and is, thus, sufficient to close the valvular orifice. Mitral regurgitation most often results from the pathologic involvement of more than one component of the valve apparatus. AP—atrial appendage.

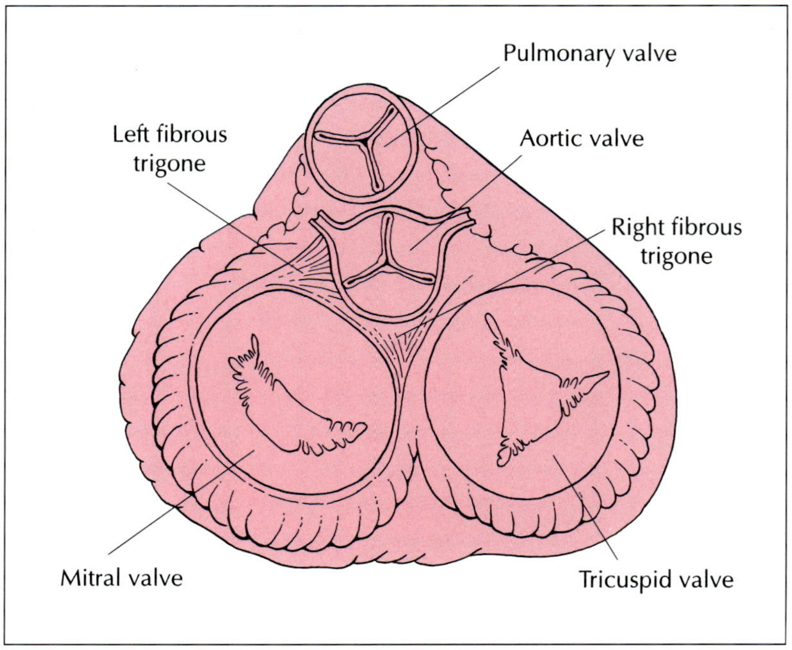

FIGURE 12-2. Fibrous skeleton of the heart. The mitral valve annulus, an incomplete fibrous ring, is part of the fibrous skeleton of the heart. Its main components are the left and right fibrous trigones, which are wedged between the mitral and aortic valves and are part of the mitroaortic curtain. This fibrous structure prevents dilatation of the anterior portion of the mitral annulus [19]. By contrast, the posterior one third to one half of the annulus is devoid of fibrous tissue, which facilitates dilatation, especially evident in some pathologic conditions such as the rheumatic and myxomatous diseases. Similarly, in the tricuspid valve, only the septal portion of the annulus is protected by the fibrous skeleton. The posterior and anterior segments are devoid of fibrous tissue and, therefore, prone to dilatation. The position of the fibrous trigones, especially the left, is usually recognizable from inside the left atrium, and they are used to anchor suture annuloplasties.

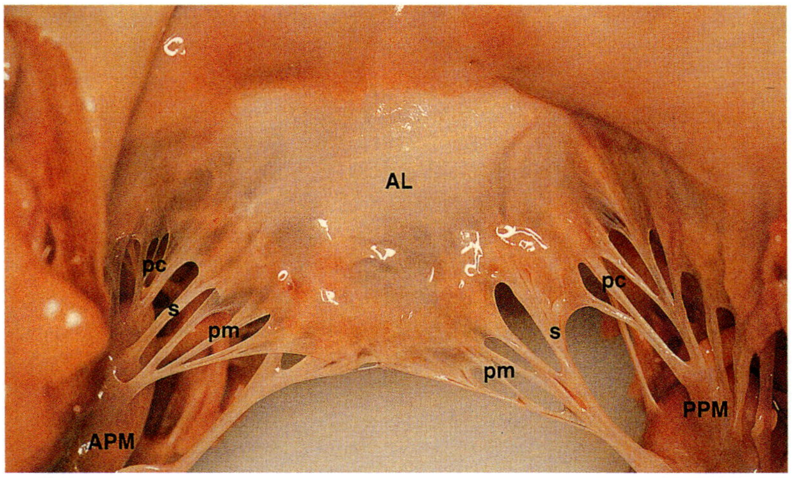

FIGURE 12-3. Chordae tendineae (CT) insertion. The insertions of the CT in the posterior leaflet occupy the whole of the ventricular surface, from free edge to annular attachment. By contrast, the CTs of the anterior leaflet (AL) insert exclusively in the free edge and adjacent area (rough zone) of the leaflet. These CTs may be grouped into paracommissural (pc), strut (s), and paramedial (pm) [17]. The strut chordae arise at the summit of the papillary muscle and constitute the "pillars" of the closing motion of the valve. Loss of the integrity of these chordae results in mitral valve regurgitation and often precludes repair. The paramedial and paracommissural chordae play an accessory role in the support of the AL. Finally, the fan-shaped commissural chordae insert in the free edges of the commissural portions of both the AL and the posterior leaflet. APM—anterior papillary muscle; PPM—posterior papillary muscle.

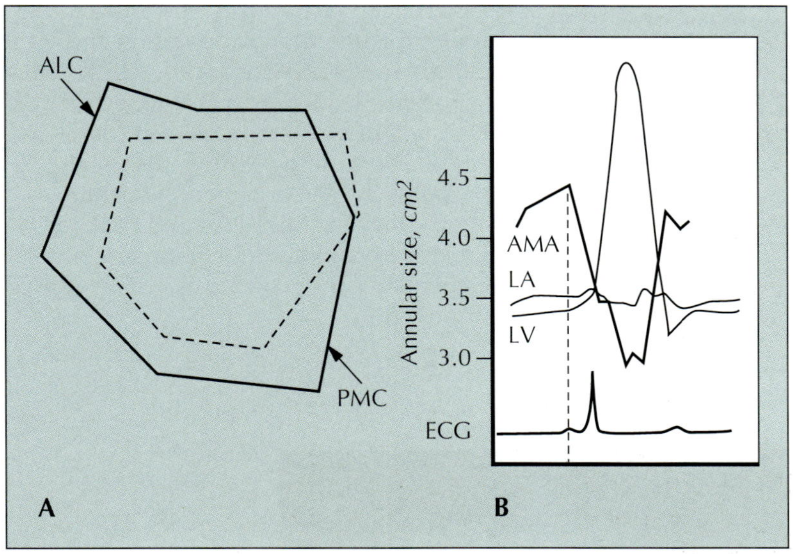

FIGURE 12-4. Mitral valve annulus movement. **A,** The movements of the mitral valve annulus during the cardiac cycle result in a reduction of approximately one third of the annulus area between diastole and systole. The nonhomogeneous structure of the annulus results in eccentric narrowing with a predominant anterior movement of its posterior segment, which approximates the posterior leaflet to the anterior leaflet, thus increasing the surface area of the leaflets available for coaption. **B,** The superimposition of the curve of variation of the area of the mitral annulus (AMA) to those of the left atrial (LA) and left ventricular (LV) pressures clearly demonstrates its relationship during the cardiac cycle. Maximal annular size occurs in late diastole, immediately before the onset of the atrial systole, simultaneous with the P wave of the electrocardiogram (ECG). One half to two thirds of the total narrowing of the annulus occurs during atrial systole and the remainder occurs during ventricular systole. ALC—anterolateral commissure; PMC—posteromedial commissure. (*Adapted from* Tsakiris and coworkers [20].)

PATHOLOGY

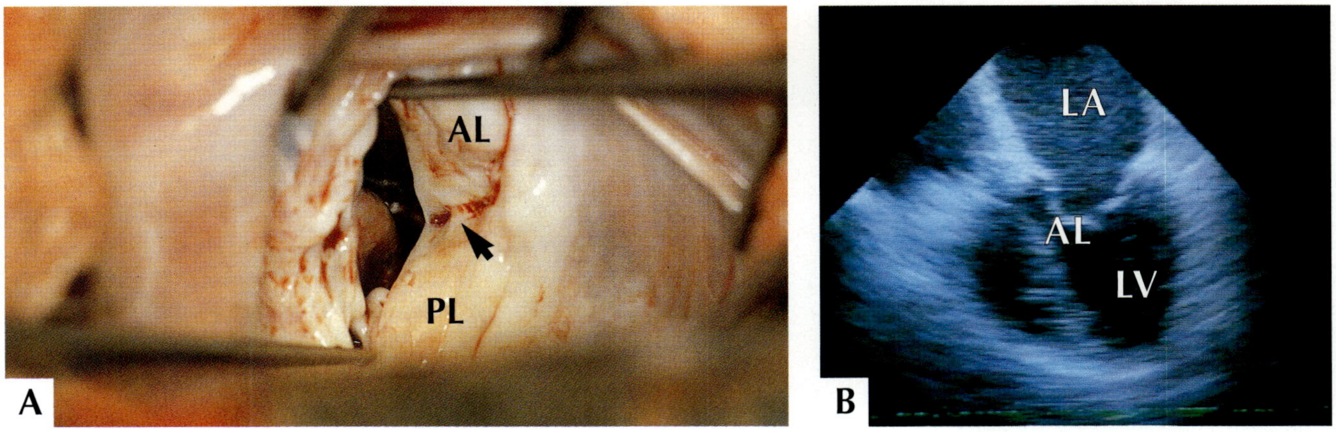

FIGURE 12-5. Rheumatic mitral valve stenosis. In rheumatic mitral valve stenosis there is fusion of the commissural edges of the leaflets. In the early stages, the fusion line is usually well demarcated (*arrow* in **A**). Later on, deposition and organization of fibrin and other blood elements in the immobile areas of the valve will result in scarring and contraction. Calcification may occur at an even later stage. Also, turbulent blood flow through the narrow orifice of the valve probably causes further fibrosis of the valve. Hence, early and complete relief of the obstruction is essential to break this vicious cycle [8]. Incomplete commissurotomy, which often results from closed methods (surgical or percutaneous balloon), may lead to early restenosis and accelerated fibrosis of the valve. In the author's experience open commissurotomy is feasible in over 80% of the cases. The most important preoperative predictor of the feasibility of a commissurotomy is the echocardiographic evidence of a mobile anterior leaflet (AL) demonstrated by the characteristic elbow during diastolic motion, as seen in this transesophageal echocardiogram (**B**). LA—left atrium; LV—left ventricle; PL—posterior leaflet.

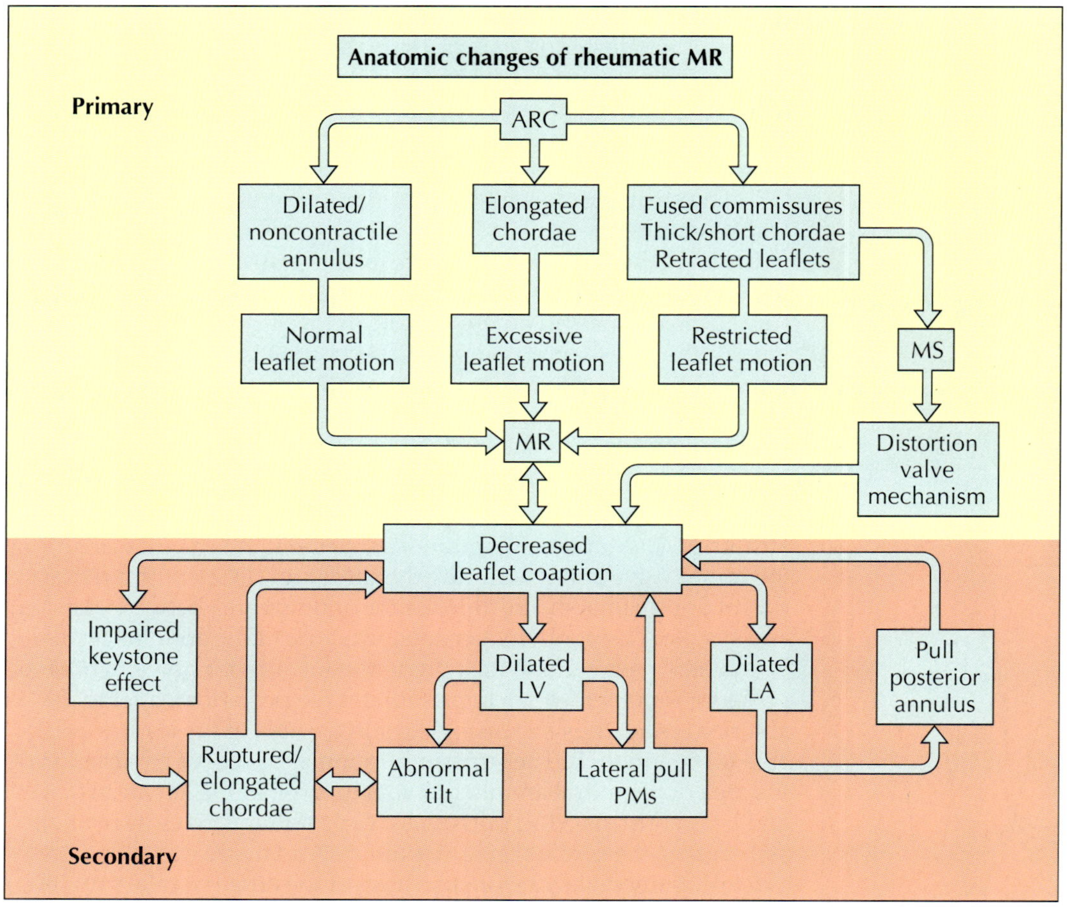

FIGURE 12-6. Pathophysiology of rheumatic mitral regurgitation (MR). Primary involvement of the valve by the rheumatic disease may result in restrictive or excessive leaflet motion. The arrangement of the mitral apparatus is such that a vicious cycle may be created by dysfunction of any of its elements. As a result, the valve is stressed further and other components of its mechanism may eventually be affected. Annular dilatation, which is one of the primary consequences of acute rheumatic carditis (ARC), reduces the keystone protection afforded by proper coaption and increases the stress on the leaflets and chordae tendineae. Papillary muscle (PM) dysfunction may also result from the increased stress. The left atrium (LA) responds to the valvular dysfunction by dilatation and expansion of its posterior wall, which pulls the posterior leaflet away from the anterior and results in further impairment of the coaption. Continuing MR results in left ventricular (LV) enlargement, which in turn modifies the mitral tilt and changes the relative position of the papillary muscles. MS—mitral stenosis. (*Adapted from* Antunes [21].)

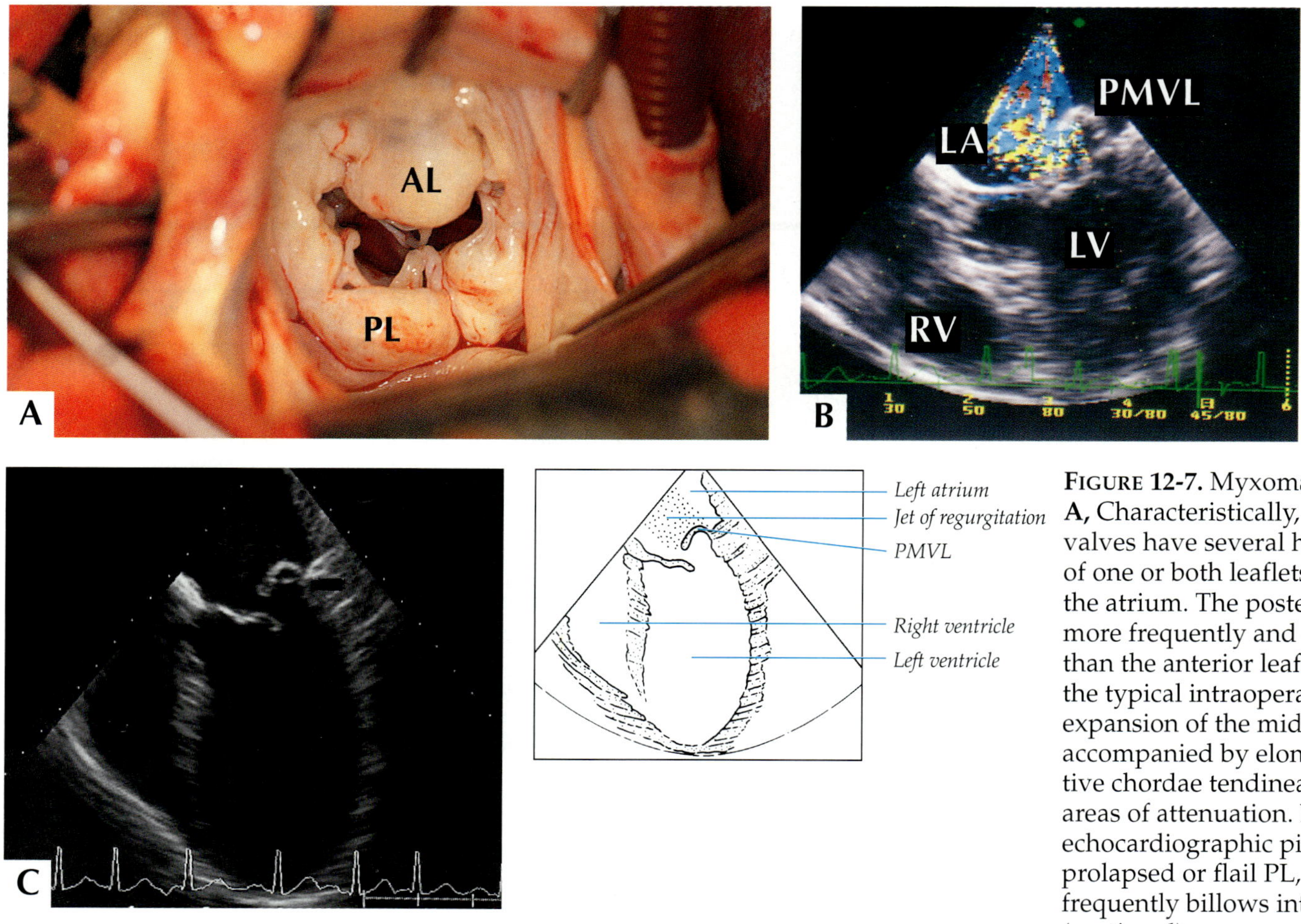

FIGURE 12-7. Myxomatous mitral valves. **A,** Characteristically, myxomatous mitral valves have several hoodlike deformities of one or both leaflets, which prolapse into the atrium. The posterior leaflet (PL) is more frequently and diffusely involved than the anterior leaflet (AL). In this case, the typical intraoperative finding is gross expansion of the middle scallop, invariably accompanied by elongation of the respective chordae tendineae, often with localized areas of attenuation. **B** and **C,** The typical echocardiographic picture is that of a prolapsed or flail PL, while the AL also frequently billows into the left atrium. (*continued*)

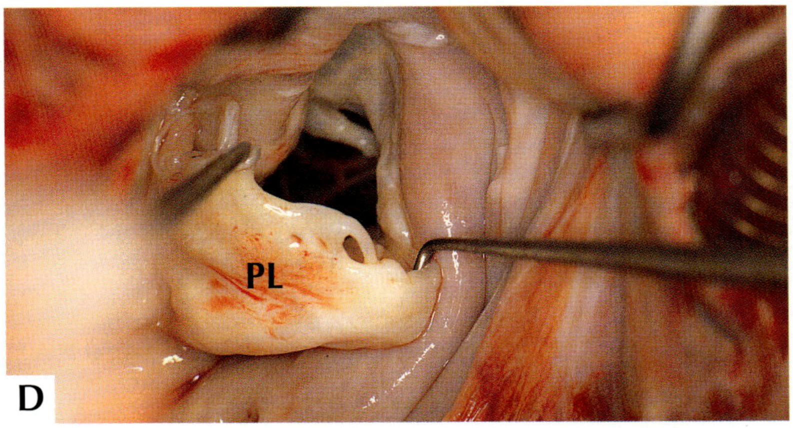

Figure 12-7. *(continued)* **D,** As the disease progresses, stress increases and results in rupture of the chordae, and the leaflet fails. The chordae tendineae of the adjacent scallops are also abnormal as are those of the AL. Nonetheless, these chordae tendineae usually hold very well after valvuloplasty. LA—left atrium; LV—left ventricle; PMVL—posterior mitral valve leaflet; RV—right ventricle.

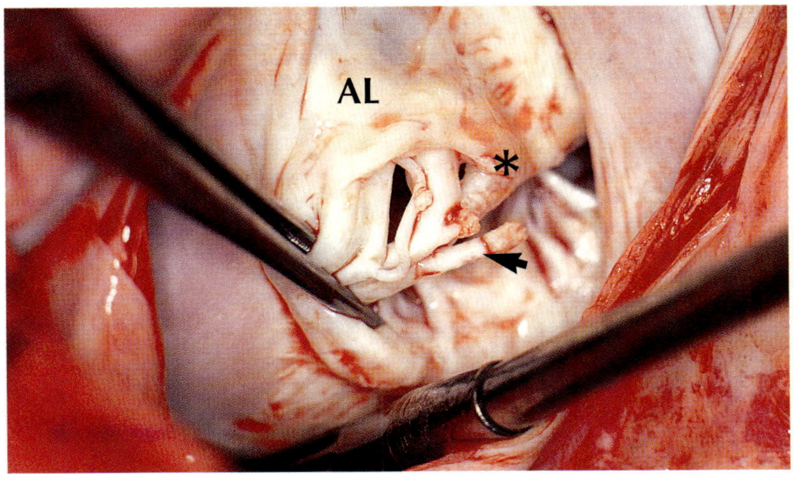

Figure 12-8. Infective endocarditis. Other common causes of mitral regurgitation (MR) are ischemic disease and infective endocarditis. Acute ischemic MR is caused by either papillary muscle rupture or dysfunction. By contrast, chronic ischemic MR is usually due to annular dilatation secondary to left ventricular enlargement with or without papillary muscle dysfunction and leaflet prolapse. Valvuloplasty is feasible in both acute and chronic cases, but the best results are obtained in the latter where an annuloplasty is usually sufficient to achieve valve competence [22].

Infective endocarditis was, for a long time, regarded as a contraindication to mitral valvuloplasty. Extensive infection of the mitral valve still requires valve replacement. However, valvuloplasty has been successful recently in many patients with localized infection (*asterisk*) and limited destruction of either leaflets or chordae tendineae (*arrow*), as seen in this intraoperative photograph, especially in patients with predominant infective endocarditis of the aortic valve [23]. In these cases, the leaflets may be repaired with patches of glutaraldehyde-treated autologous or bovine pericardium and new chordae tendineae may be created from polytetrafluoroethylene (Goretex, WL Gore and associates, Inc., Flagstaff, AZ) sutures (*see* Fig. 12-12). AL—anterior leaflet.

REPAIR TECHNIQUES

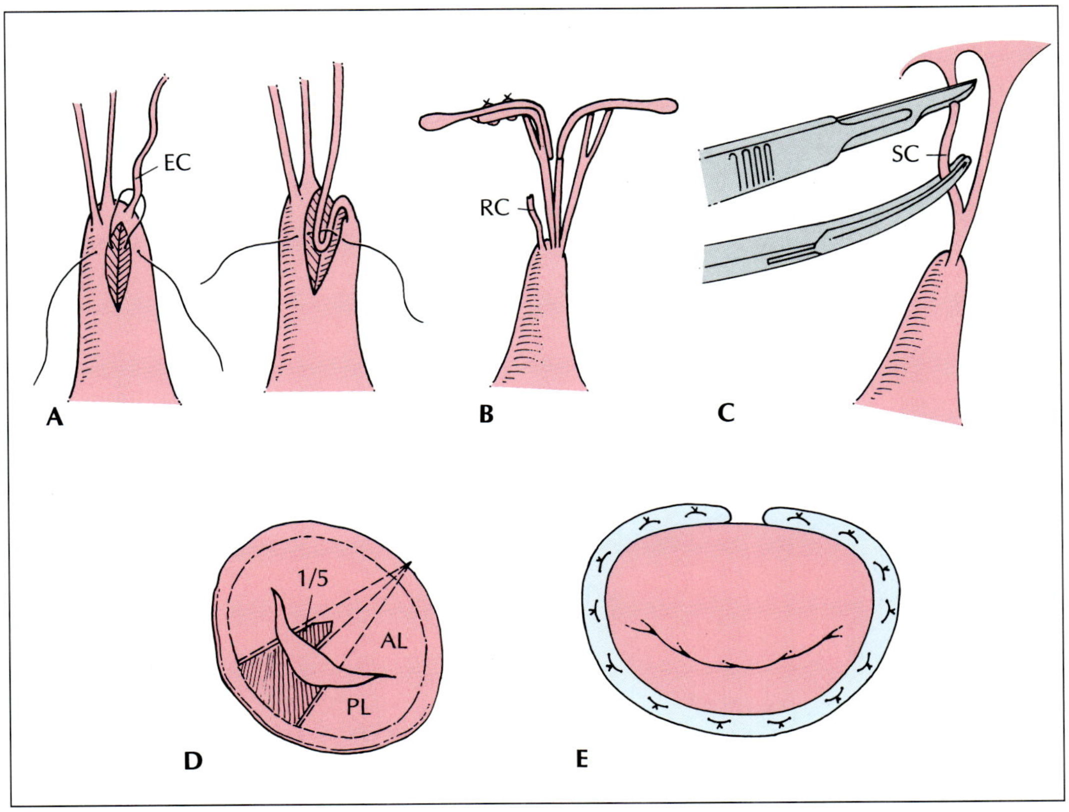

Figure 12-9. Reconstructive techniques. Because mitral valve disease, especially regurgitation, is usually multifactorial, that is, with simultaneous involvement of two or more components of the valve apparatus, several techniques of reconstruction must be applied, depending on the affected components, if a satisfactory result is to be achieved. **A,** Elongated chordae tendineae (EC) may be shortened by (among other techniques) burying the excessive length in the respective papillary muscle head. **B,** Ruptured chordae (RC) of the anterior leaflet (AL) may be replaced by transposing wormed chordae from the posterior leaflet (PL). **C,** Shortened chordae (SC), which retract the PL, may be excised. **D,** Flail segments of the PL, up to one third, may be resected; small triangular segments may very rarely be excised from the AL. **E,** In the last step, the dilated annulus is shortened and reshaped by implantation of a prosthetic ring. The mitral valve is seen as a functional unit and reconstructed accordingly.

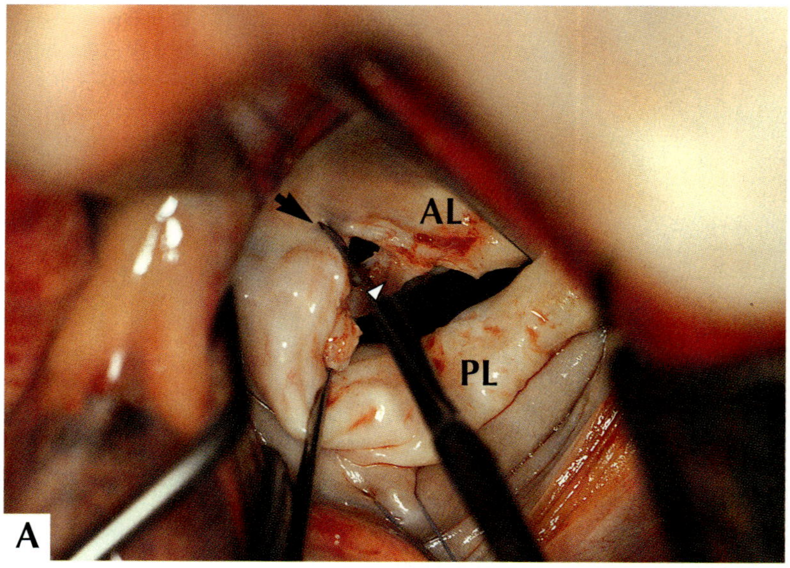

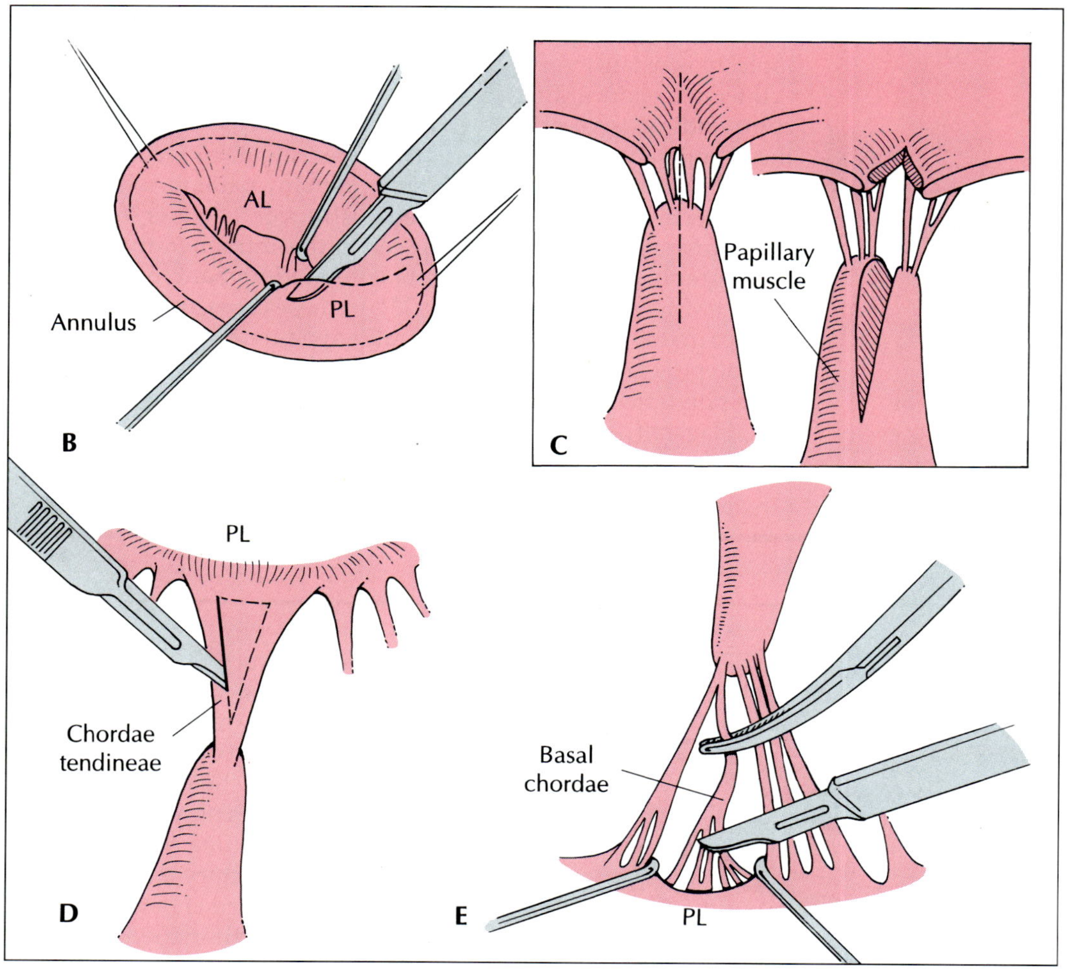

FIGURE 12-10. Technique of open mitral commissurotomy. **A,** Intraoperative image demonstrating incision of the anterolateral commissure (*arrow*) and of fused papillary muscle (*arrowhead*). **B,** The fused commissures are incised with a scalpel, commencing in the central orifice and progressing toward the annulus in a gentle upward curve. The direction of the incision is adjusted in accordance with the position of the commissural chordae. **C,** Incision of the papillary muscles at commissural level is often necessary to open the lateral portions of the mitral orifice. **D,** When several chordae tendineae are fused and constitute a significant obstruction to flow, a fenestration is performed by excising a triangular segment of fibrous tissue. **E,** Finally, resection of thickened secondary and basal chordae, causing retraction of the posterior leaflet, may help significantly in mobilizing this leaflet. Although dilatation of the annulus is often present in mitral stenosis, annuloplasty is usually not necessary. However, the author has recently found that annular plication at the commissural level improves coaption and may contribute to preventing occurrence of late regurgitation in the commissural regions. AL—anterior leaflet; PL—posterior leaflet.

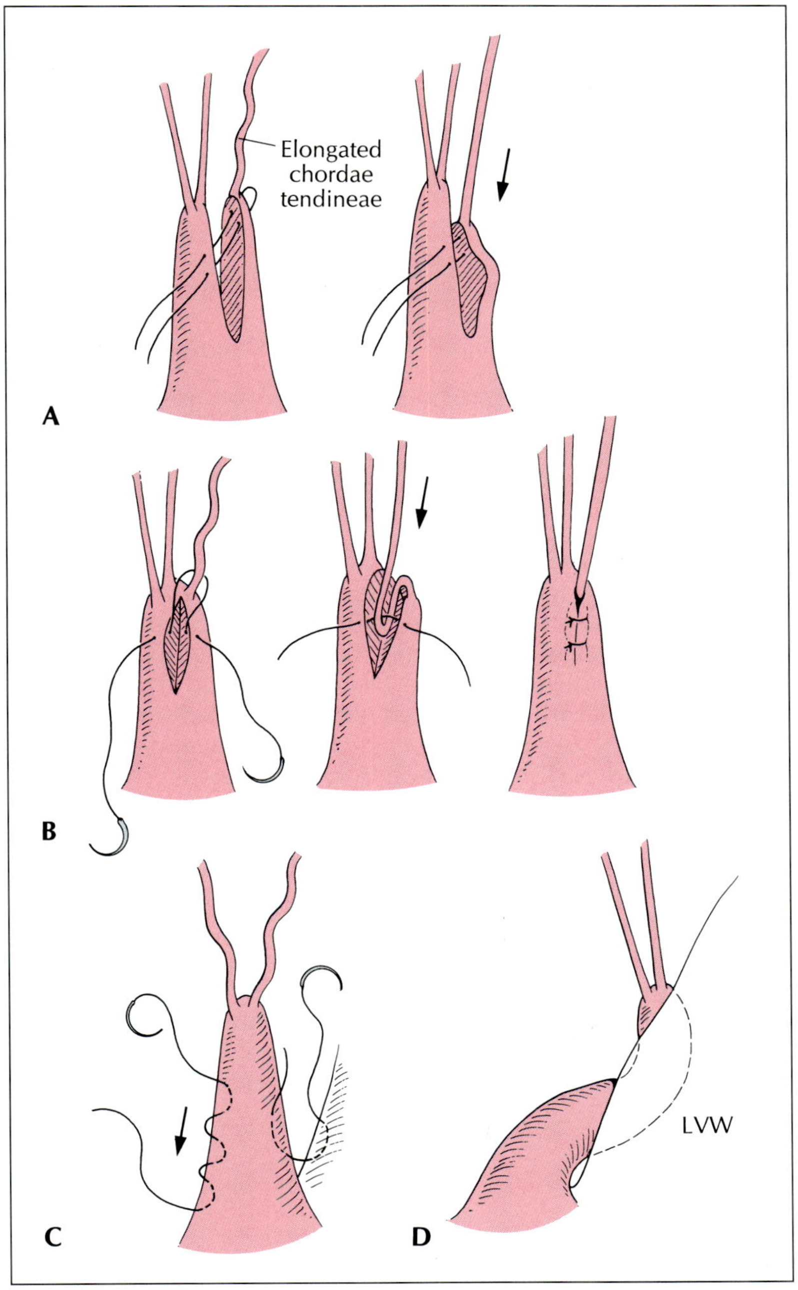

Figure 12-11. Methods of treatment of elongated chordae tendineae of the anterior leaflet. In rheumatic cases, the chordae tendineae of the posterior leaflet are usually normal. Hence, the degree of elongation is estimated by the relative degree of prolapse of the free edge of the anterior leaflet when matched to that of the posterior leaflet. Shortening of the elongated chordae tendineae may be activated by sliding the papillary muscle head (**A**), by chordal plasty (**B**), or by shortening of the papillary muscle (**C** and **D**). In chordal plasty, the most effective and stable technique, a longitudinal incision in the papillary muscle is made, which creates a trench where the elongated chorda is folded and buried. Several chordae may be buried simultaneously within the same trench or separate ones may be created if the thickness of the papillary muscle permits. When the chordae tendineae are very thin and threaten rupture, they may be reinforced by artificial chordae or natural chordae transferred from the posterior leaflet or from adjacent positions of the anterior leaflet (*see* Fig. 12-12). Sutures are 5–0 polypropylene. LVW—left ventricular wall.

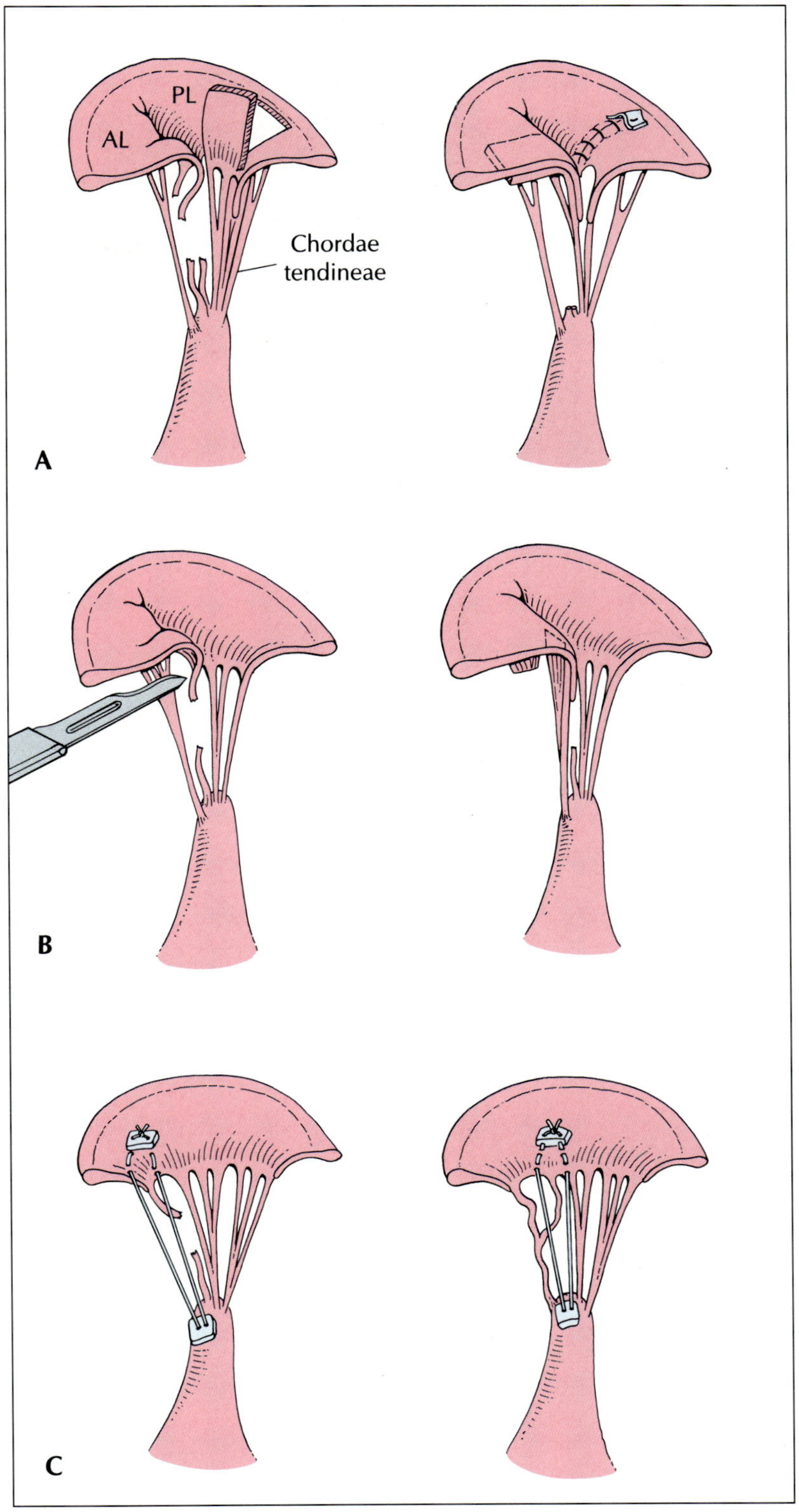

Figure 12-12. Ruptured chordae tendineae. **A,** To treat ruptured chordae tendineae of the anterior mitral leaflet a group of chordae tendineae may be transposed from the posterior leaflet (PL) with a portion of leaflet tissue to facilitate resuture. **B,** Secondary or rough zone chordae of the anterior leaflet (AL) may also be transferred to the adjacent free edge. **C,** Alternatively, ruptured chordae may be substituted by new chordae made of natural or artificial materials. This technique may also be used for reinforcement of very thin and elongated chordae. Polytetrafluoroethylene suture material (Goretex) has yielded the best results because it appears to remain unaltered with time [25]. (*Adapted from* Cosgrove and coworkers [10].)

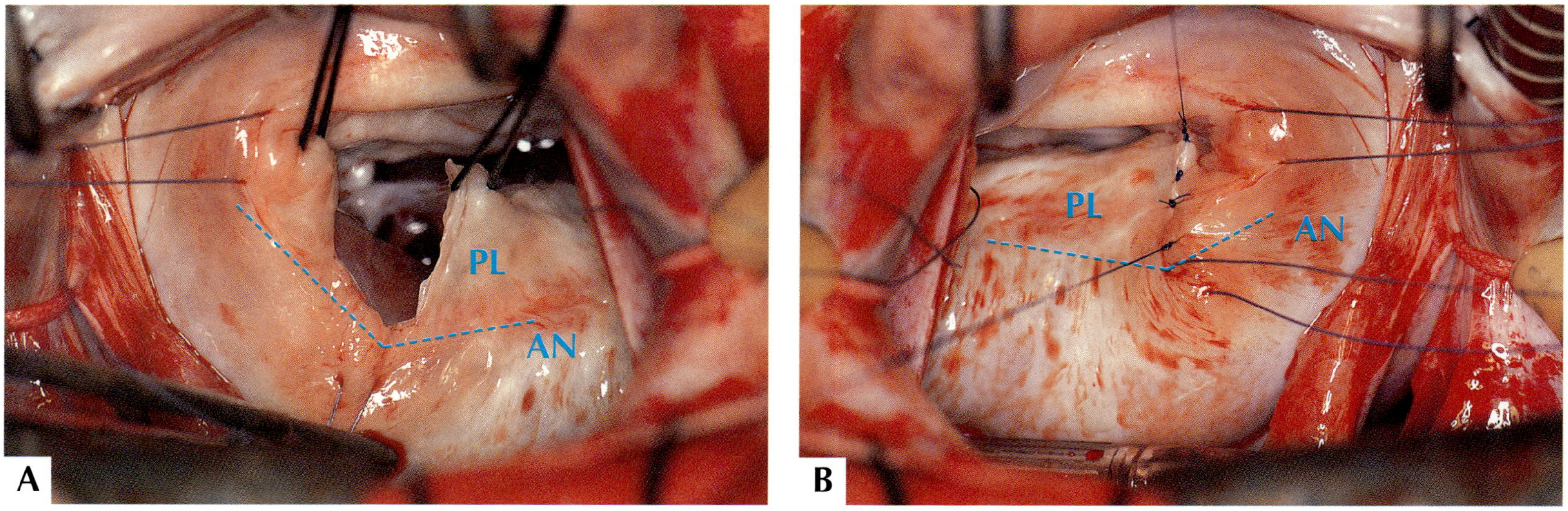

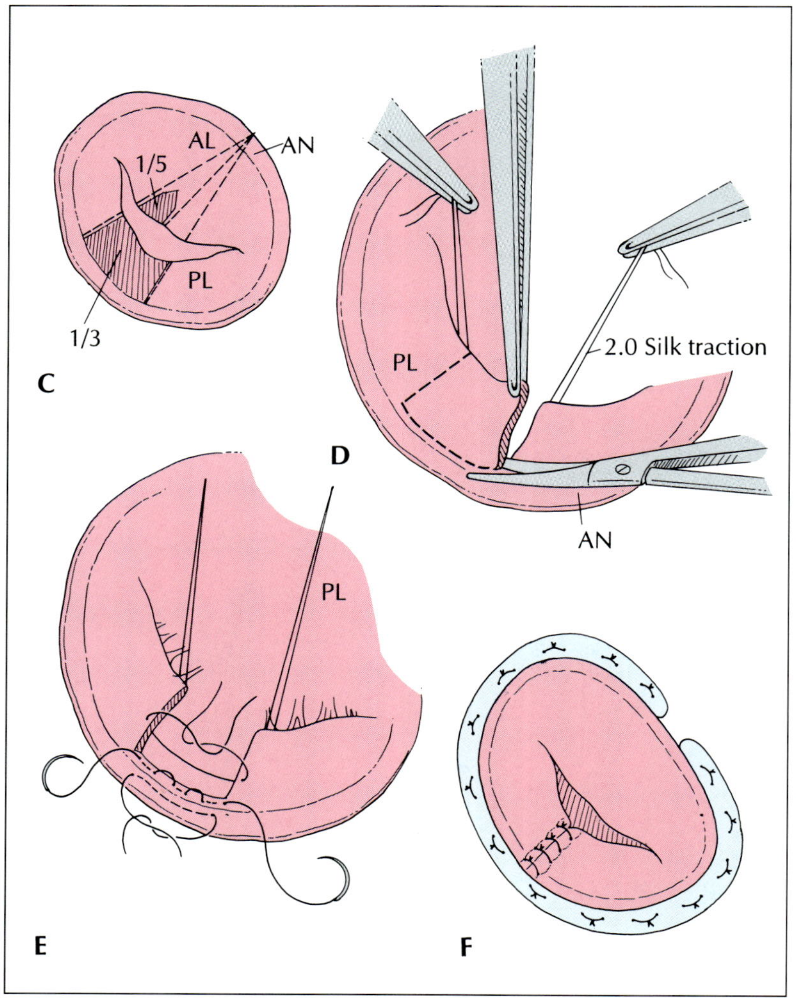

FIGURE 12-13. Posterior leaflet (PL) prolapse. When mitral regurgitation is caused by localized prolapse of the PL, as in myxomatous disease, a quadrangular resection of this leaflet is performed (**A** and **B**). A segment of one third to one half of the length of the leaflet, and the whole width, may be excised (**C** and **D**). The continuity of the leaflet is re-established with interrupted sutures, and the annulus (AN) (*dotted line* in *panels A and B*) is reinforced with one or two sutures (**E** and **F**). Exceptionally, elongated chordae tendineae of adjacent segments of the PL or of the anterior leaflet (AL) may be shortened or replaced. Finally, an annuloplasty ring, either flexible or rigid, is usually implanted to protect the annulus from disruption or further dilatation (*see* Figs. 12-14 and 12-15). The AL does not tolerate partial resection well because it is essential to the closure of the orifice. When absolutely necessary, a small triangular segment, involving no more than one fifth of the free edge, may be resected (*panel C*). Hence, when the degenerative process affects both leaflets significantly, the valve should probably be replaced, but this circumstance is the exception rather than the rule.

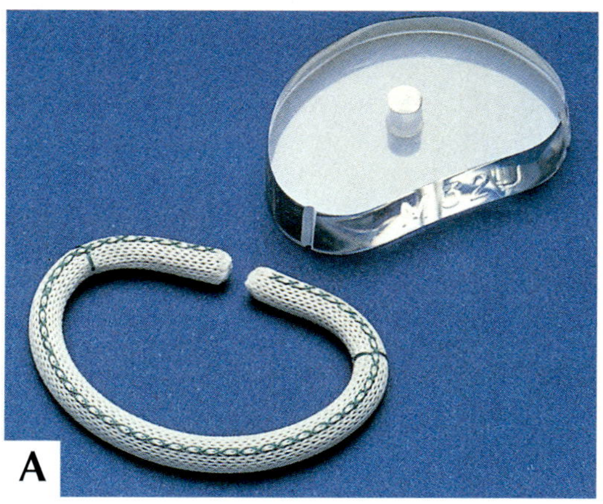

FIGURE 12-14. Annuloplasty ring implantation. In the majority of cases of mitral regurgitation, an annuloplasty ring is implanted once repair of the affected chordae tendineae and leaflets is completed. Besides reduction and reshaping of the dilated and often noncontractile annulus, the ring protects the annulus from disruption in areas where leaflet resection may threaten annular integrity. Annuloplasty rings are of one of two types: preshaped (rigid or semirigid) and flexible. **A,** The Carpentier-Edwards ring (Baxter Healthcare Co., Inc., Irvine, CA) is semirigid, presized, and preshaped with the normal systolic configuration of the mitral valve annulus. (*continued*)

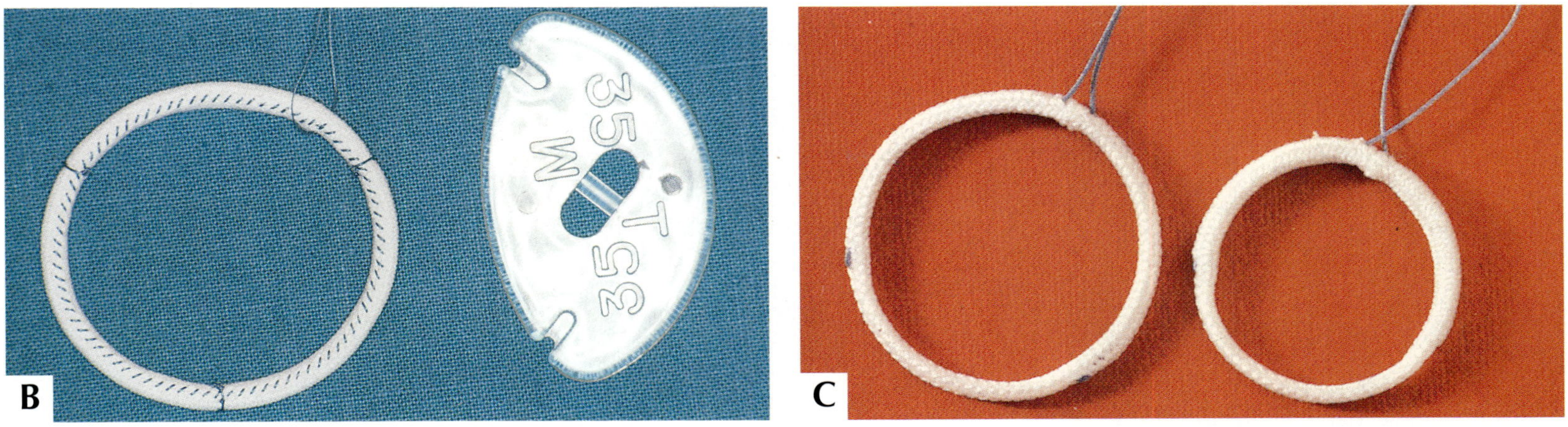

Figure 12-14. *(continued)* **B,** The Duran ring (Medtronic Inc, Minneapolis, MN) is flexible and presized. **C,** The Puig-Massana (Sorin Biomedical, Inc, Irvine, CA) and the St. Jude (St. Jude Medical, Inc., St. Paul, MN, not shown) rings are flexible and of variable size.

Arguments for and against one or the other type have been widely expressed [26]. Theoretically, flexible rings permit normal motion of the annulus during the cardiac cycle. However, this natural motion may have been lost in some types of pathology such as rheumatic disease. In these cases the annulus needs reshaping, which can only be achieved by preshaped rings. Several authors have demonstrated impairment of the left ventricular function immediately after implantation of rigid rings as a result of the fixation of the basal segments of the left ventricular free wall, but this adverse effect may attenuate or even disappear with time. Other authors, however, have been unable to demonstrate any difference between various types of rings and between cases with and without rings.

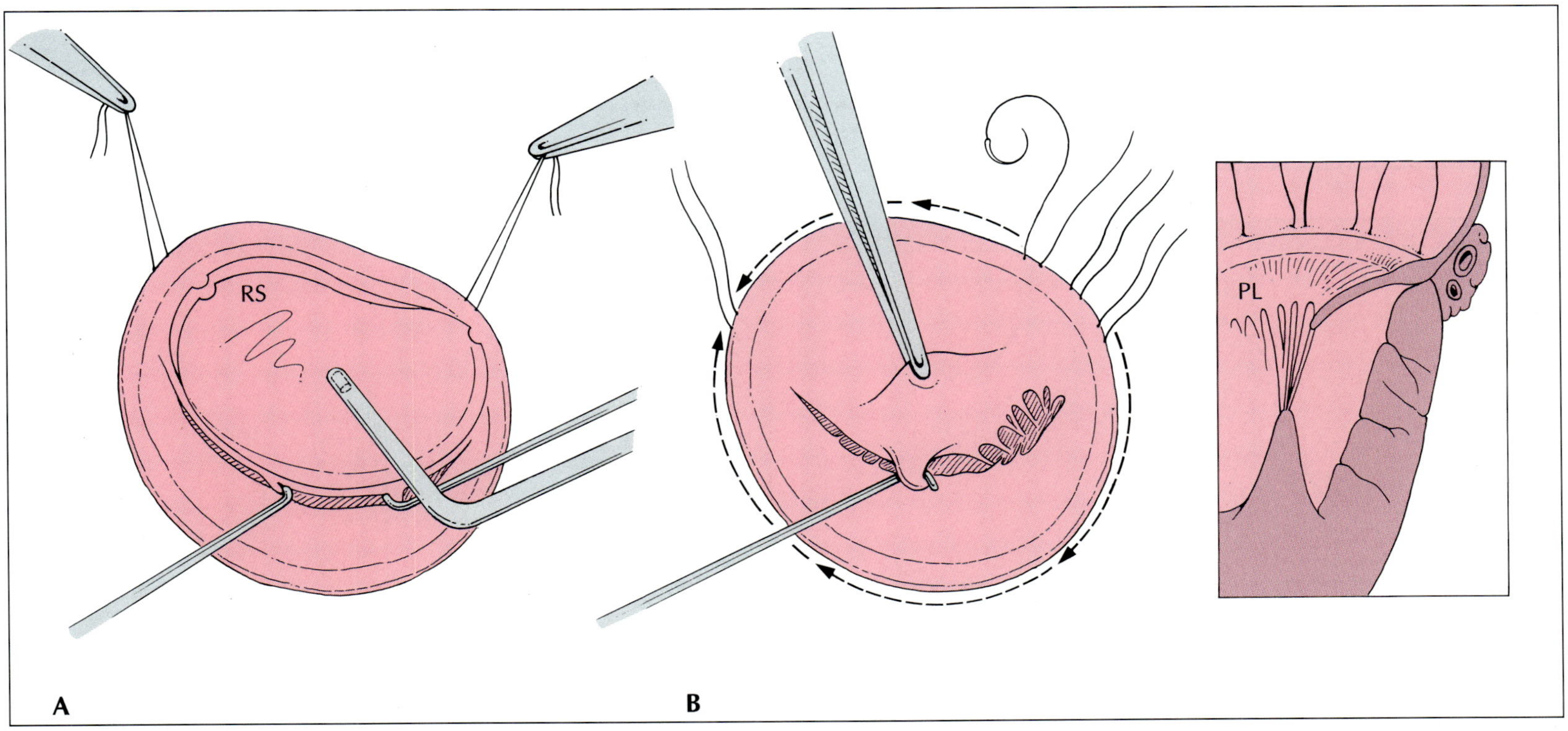

Figure 12-15. Annulus reshaping. Reduction of the size of the annulus and protection from disruption are obtained by all types of rings, but reshaping can only be achieved by preshaped rings. Because the shape of these rings approximates the systolic shape of the normal mitral valve, accurate sizing and positioning of the ring are essential. Otherwise, distortion with regurgitation may occur. **A,** The ring sizer (RS) is chosen appropriately to match the size of the anterior leaflet. **B,** The sutures (3–0 Ticron) must be precisely placed and distributed in the annulus, just outside the leaflet hinge to avoid interference with leaflet motion (**inset**). Similarly, precise distribution of the sutures through the ring is essential. Left ventricular outflow tract obstruction has been demonstrated after mitral valve repair, especially when a Carpentier ring has been implanted (although it has also occurred after repair with a flexible ring and without a ring). This is due to systolic anterior motion of the anterior leaflet, presumably due to excessive leaflet tissue. The prevalence of this complication is low and the obstruction decreases and may even disappear with time [27,28]. PL—posterior leaflet.

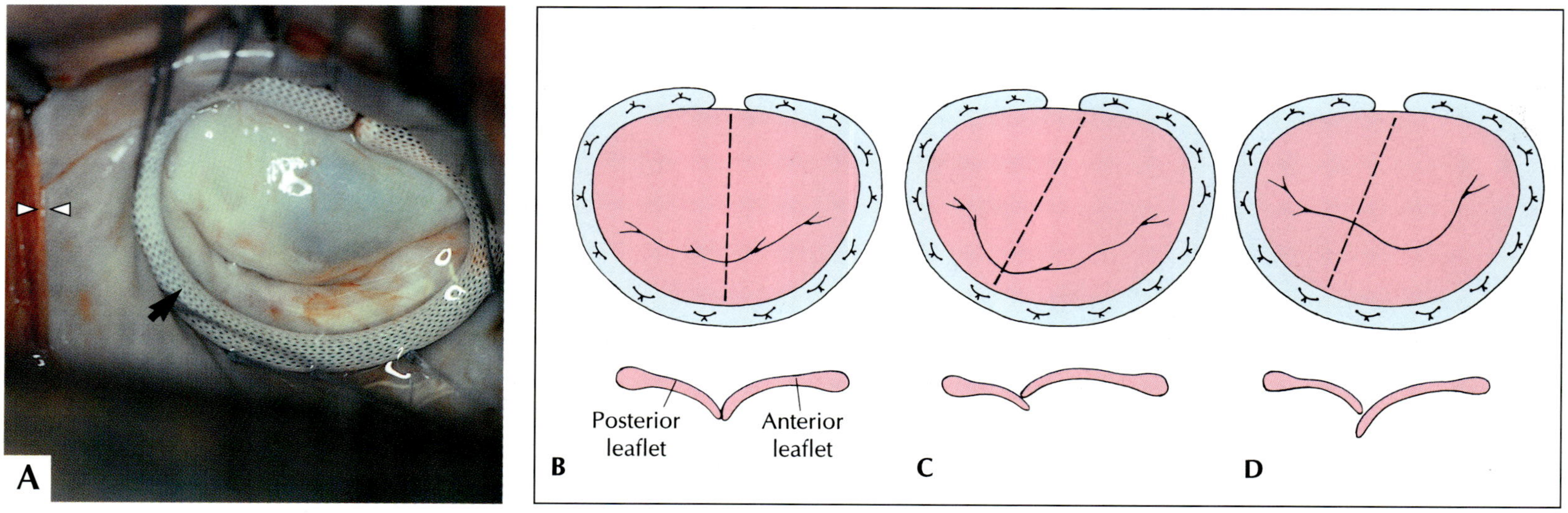

FIGURE 12-16. Test for mitral competence. **A,** After the repair is completed, the mitral valve is tested by injection of saline through an apical left ventricular cannula; this intraoperative photograph shows perfect competence. Shown here are a Carpentier-Edwards ring (*arrow*) and the line of apposition (*dotted line*). *Arrowheads* indicate the left atrial wall. In addition to assessing valve competence, this preliminary test outlines the shape of the reconstructed valve, which should be as normal as possible. **B,** The line of apposition of the two leaflets must be regular and parallel to the posterior annulus. Deviations from this pattern, even in the absence of regurgitation, are not only predictive of late problems but also diagnostic of the underlying cause, for example, insufficient (**C**) or excessive (**D**) shortening of the chordae tendineae. The necessary adjustments of the correction must be made immediately. Currently, a more definitive evaluation of valve function is the transesophageal echocardiographic evaluation performed after discontinuation of cardiopulmonary bypass [27].

REPAIR RESULTS

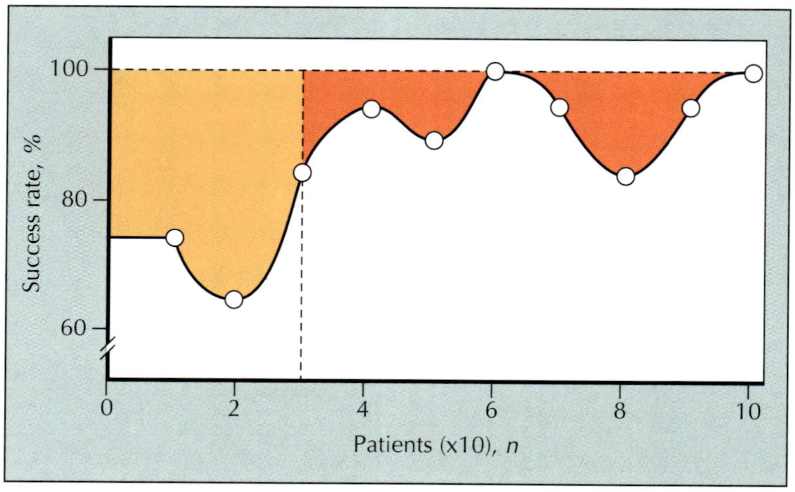

FIGURE 12-17. Valvuloplasty learning curve. Mitral valvuloplasty is subjected to a strong learning curve. This curve was constructed based on the results of the first 100 procedures performed at the author's original institution in South Africa, in patients with rheumatic regurgitation. For each consecutive group of 10 patients an arbitrary 10% for each death and 5% for each patient surviving reoperation was deducted from the maximum (100%) success rate. The *orange and red areas* in the figure thus represent the failure rate of the procedure. There is an improvement with the number of cases operated on, with a significant difference between the first 30 patients and the following 70 patients. Because valvuloplasty for patients with myxomatous disease is usually technically simpler and the immediate early and late results are much better, these are the cases that are better suited for surgeons commencing their experience. (*Adapted from* Antunes and coworkers [29].)

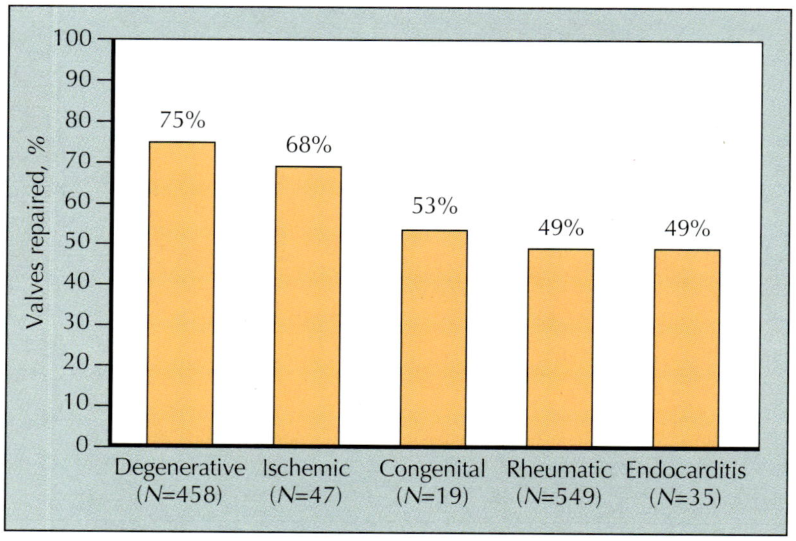

FIGURE 12-18. Feasibility of mitral valvuloplasty. In the experience of Cosgrove *et al.* [10], mitral valvuloplasty was feasible in 75% of patients with myxomatous regurgitant valves, in 68% of patients with ischemic regurgitation, and in 49% of patients with rheumatic disease. The actual figures vary from center to center, depending on the relative incidence of the different pathologies and the experience of the surgical team. In the author's most recent experience, valvuloplasty was performed in 81.4% of the more than 800 patients who had mitral valve surgery for the first time and in more than 95% of patients with myxomatous disease. By contrast, the author found valvuloplasty to be unsatisfactory or impossible in approximately 50% of the cases of regurgitation of ischemic origin. (*Adapted from* Cosgrove and coworkers [10].)

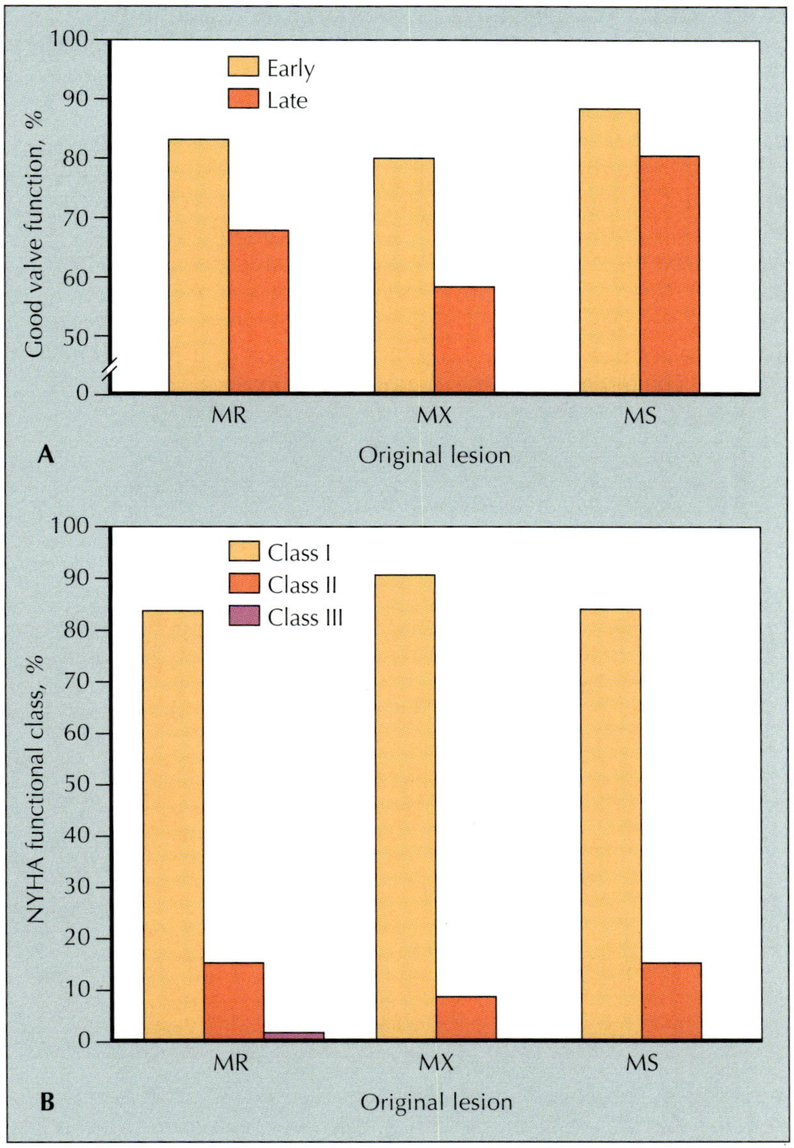

FIGURE 12-19. Valve function and patients' clinical status. **A,** Residual valve dysfunction is recognizable immediately after valvuloplasty in a number of patients, especially those with rheumatic valves. In the author's early experience, 16% of rheumatic patients had clinical signs of moderate mitral regurgitation (MR) at the time of discharge from the hospital, but after 6 years of follow-up 30% of those who had survived without reoperation had signs of moderate dysfunction. The results were better in patients with mitral stenosis (MS) and worse in those with mixed disease (MX). **B,** Nonetheless, 85% remained in New York Heart Association (NYHA) functional class I and nearly all the remainder were in class II 6 years after the operation, underscoring the importance of the complete clinical and functional evaluation of the patients. (*Adapted from* Antunes and coworkers [9].)

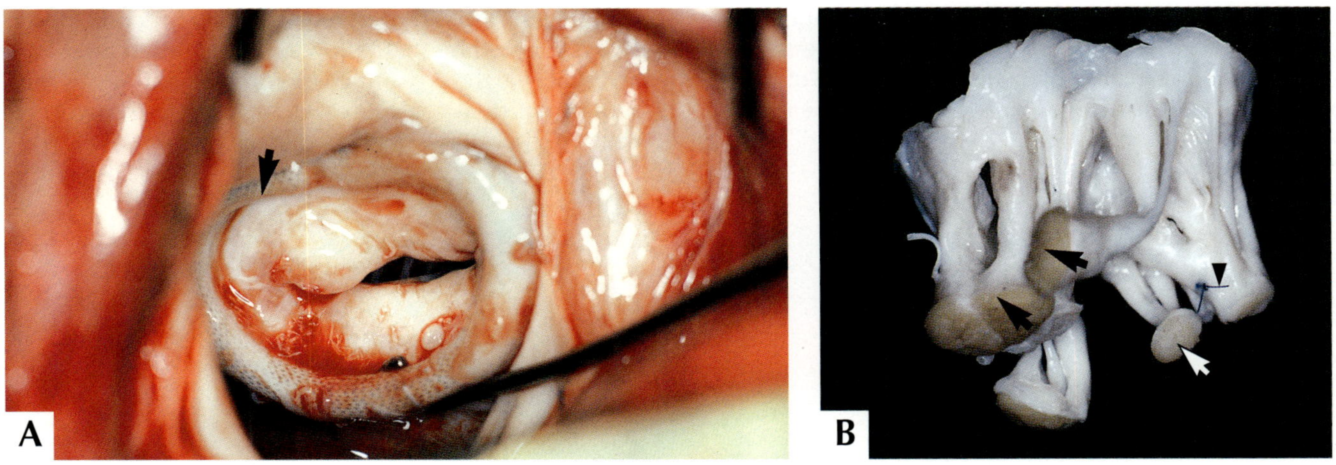

FIGURE 12-20. Late postoperative mitral regurgitation. The most important anatomic causes of regurgitation for rheumatic disease appearing late after mitral valvuloplasty are retraction of one or both leaflets and prolapse of the anterior leaflet. Retraction results mainly from progression or reactivation of the rheumatic process, which confirms the need for continued antibiotic prophylaxis to prevent recurrences of rheumatic fever. Prolapse usually results from inadequate shortening of chordae tendineae or from late rupture, some of which may have been caused by technical errors made during the procedure. In some of these cases a second conservative procedure may be performed with correction of the residual anomalies. **A,** Intraoperative photograph shows the mitral valve of a patient who had been operated on 3 years earlier for severe regurgitation during acute rheumatic carditis. Subsequent episodes of acute carditis resulted in marked retraction of the anterior leaflet and immobilization of the posterior leaflet, requiring valve replacement. The well endothelialized Carpentier-Edwards ring is denoted by an *arrow*. **B,** Ventricular aspect of the excised valve shows severe subvalvular disease. A suture from the previous chordal shortening procedure is visible (*arrowhead*). In nonrheumatic cases, such as myxomatous disease, evolution of the degenerative process, which usually affects the whole valve apparatus, accounts for most of the late failures. *Arrows* denote papillary muscle heads.

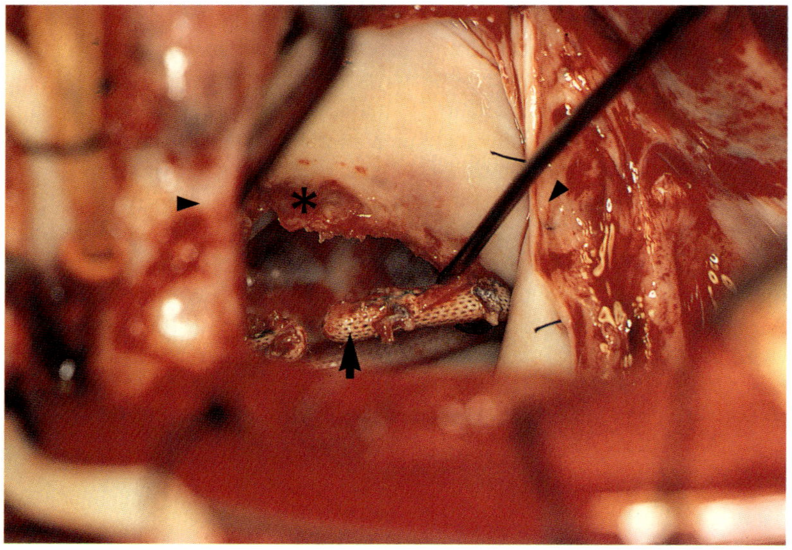

Figure 12-21. Postrepair infective endocarditis. In contrast to prosthetic mitral valve replacement, infective endocarditis occurs much less commonly after mitral valvuloplasty with implantation of an annuloplasty ring. In our experience, it occurred at a linearized rate of less than 0.4% per patient-year. In this intraoperative photograph of a patient who had had a mitral valve repair performed 2 months before, there was partial dehiscence of the infected Carpentier-Edwards ring (*arrow*). The infection (*asterisk*) was caused by a *Serratia* species and eventually resulted in the patient's death, despite mitral valve replacement. As in other cases of implanted devices, patients with prosthetic rings require adequate antibiotic prophylaxis for prevention of infective endocarditis. The left atrial wall is denoted by *arrowheads*.

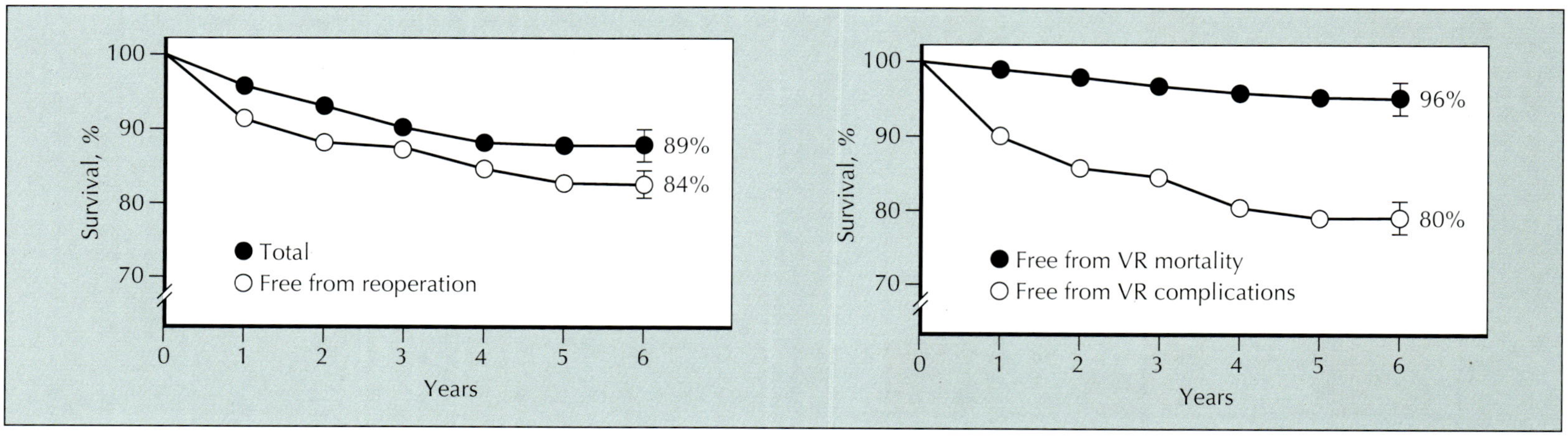

Figure 12-22. Survival rates for rheumatic patients. For our young rheumatic patients the 6-year survival rate after valvuloplasty was 89%. This value was higher than that observed in a similar group of patients who had valve replacement during the same period (82%; $P<0.05$) (not shown). More importantly, 96% of patients were free from valve-related (VR) mortality (*right panel*). Valve-related deaths are uncommon after valvuloplasty because most of the complications are not serious. The exception to this is the need for reoperation, which occurs at a linearized rate of 2% to 3% per patient year, resulting in this series in a 6-year freedom from reoperation of 84% (*left panel*). The increased need for reoperation has been the most important argument against mitral valvuloplasty. Nonetheless, the reported mortality of reoperation after repair is always lower than that following reoperation after valve replacement. Hence, the advantage of valvuloplasty over valve replacement is apparent. (*Adapted from* Antunes and coworkers [9].)

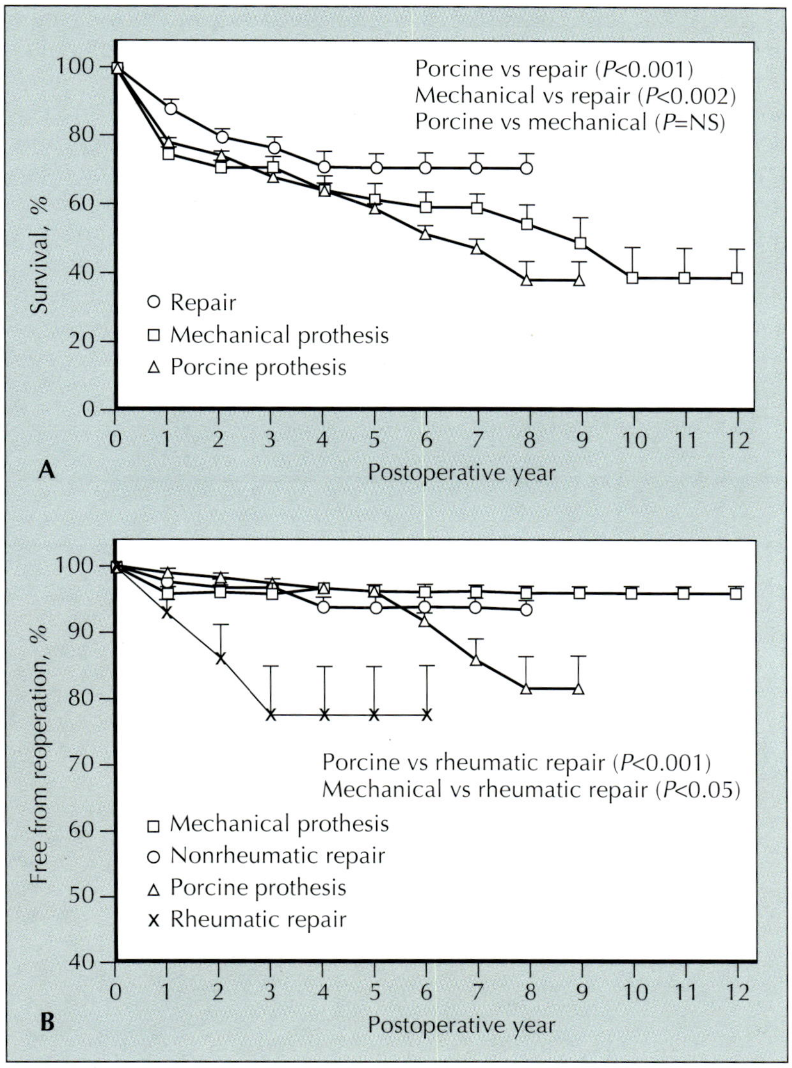

FIGURE 12-23. Comparative long-term survival in the experience at New York University. **A,** Long-term survival after mitral valve repair was much better than survival after either mechanical or biologic valve replacement. **B,** Freedom from reoperation was also better after valvuloplasty for mitral valve regurgitation of myxomatous origin but much worse after repair of rheumatic regurgitation. Similar experiences were reported from other centers. In our most recent experience reoperation was required at a rate of 0.6% per patient-year for myxomatous disease and 1.5% per patient-year for rheumatic disease. (*Adapted from* Galloway and coworkers [30].)

TRICUSPID VALVE

ANATOMY

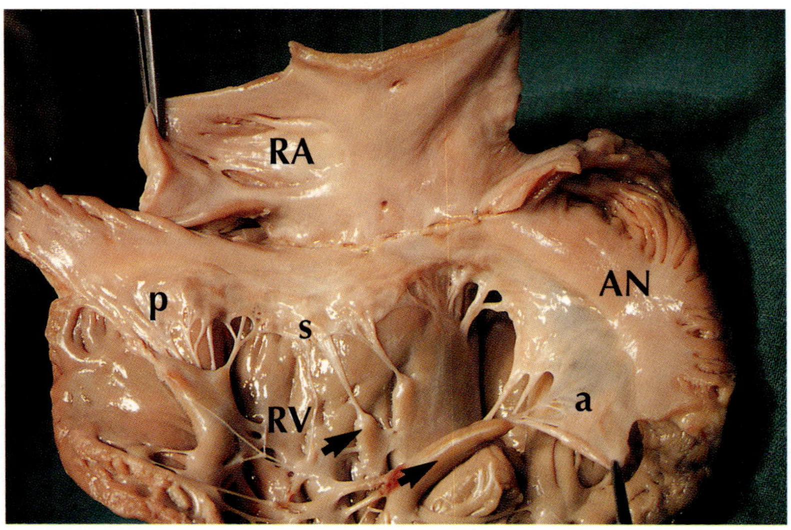

FIGURE 12-24. Tricuspid valve structure. The tricuspid valve, placed between the right atrium (RA) and the right ventricle (RV), has three leaflets, anterior (a), posterior (p), and septal (s), which are attached to the annulus (AN) at the junction of the atrial and ventricular walls. The structure of the leaflets is identical to that of the mitral valve, as is the general structure of the valve, including the annulus, the chordae tendineae, and the papillary muscles. However, the distribution of the chordae tendineae is very different [31]. Each papillary muscle (*arrows*) gives chordae essentially to the corresponding leaflet and, additionally, to the adjacent portion of the next leaflet (clockwise). The penetrating segment of the bundle of His is located in a subannular position close to the anteroseptal commissure, where it can be damaged by excessively deep sutures during annuloplasty or valve replacement. Because of the lower pressures of the right side of the heart, tricuspid valve dysfunction is much better tolerated than is mitral valve disease.

INDICATIONS FOR TRICUSPID VALVE SURGERY

DEGREE OF PULMONARY HYPERTENSION	DEGREE OF TRICUSPID REGURGITATION 1+	2+	3+
1+	N	N	N
2+	Y	Y?	N
3+	Y	Y	Y?

Figure 12-25. Indications for tricuspid valve surgery. The indications for tricuspid valve surgery in patients with significant "functional" tricuspid valve regurgitation secondary to disease of the mitral or aortic valves remain controversial. However, the majority of surgeons defend an aggressive attitude toward the tricuspid valve. The author prefers to tie the decision to intervene with the degrees of pulmonary hypertension and tricuspid regurgitation. Generally speaking, the more severe the regurgitation and the lower the pulmonary artery pressure the greater the indication for the annuloplasty. By contrast, significant pulmonary hypertension is usually a contraindication to annuloplasty, even in the unlikely coexistence of severe tricuspid regurgitation. Besides, pulmonary hypertension usually subsides after repair or replacement of the culprit left-side valve.

REPAIR TECHNIQUES

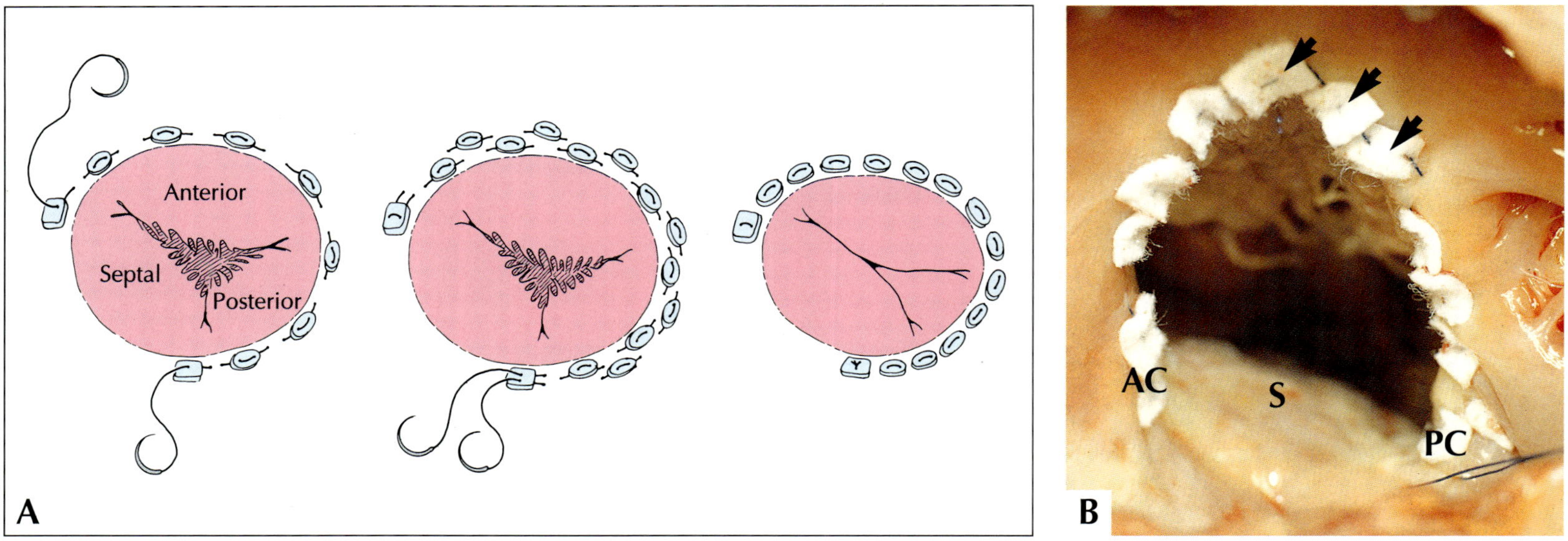

Figure 12-26. De Vega annuloplasty. Tricuspid valve surgery is required in 10% to 15% of patients undergoing mitral or aortic valve surgery, but less than 1% require tricuspid valve replacement. The De Vega tricuspid valve annuloplasty [13] is widely used for the treatment of functional tricuspid regurgitation. In this technique, a continuous suture is used to plicate the posterior and anterior portions of the annulus, from the posteroseptal to the anteroseptal commissure. The De Vega annuloplasty appears to be very effective in decreasing the tricuspid regurgitation, but the sutures may pull out of the annular tissues with a bow-string effect. For this reason, the author has modified the technique (**A** and **B**) by interposition of Teflon (Meadox Medicals, Oakland, CA) felt pledgets (*arrows in panel B*), which also have the advantage of producing an even but not excessive narrowing of the annulus [32]. AC—anteroseptal commissure; PC—posteroseptal commissure; S—septal leaflet.

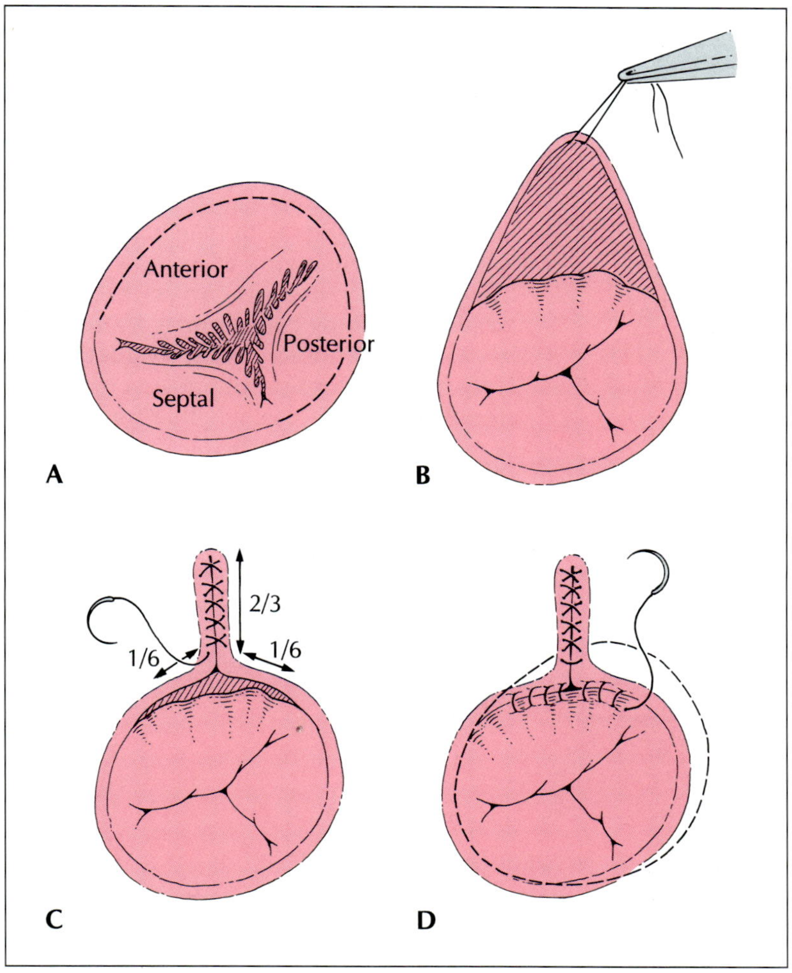

FIGURE 12-27. Alternative techniques. Other methods of annular plication, including the posterior annuloplasty developed by Kay *et al.* [33], which results in bicuspidization of the valve, are used by some surgeons. An alternative technique of selective tricuspid valve annuloplasty was described by Minale *et al.* [34]. The anterior and posterior leaflets are completely detached from the annulus, which will eventually allow them to fall to coaption with the septal leaflet (**A** and **B**). The redundant anterior and posterior annulus (approximately two thirds) is then excluded by plication with a continuous or interrupted suture (**C**). Finally, the cut edge of the leaflets is reattached to the remaining one third of the annulus (**D**). With this technique, the leaflet tissue is spared, the anterior and posterior leaflets are shifted centrally, and the circumference of the annulus is reduced. The *dotted outline* in *D* indicates the size and shape of the annulus before annuloplasty. (*Adapted from* Minale and coworkers [34].)

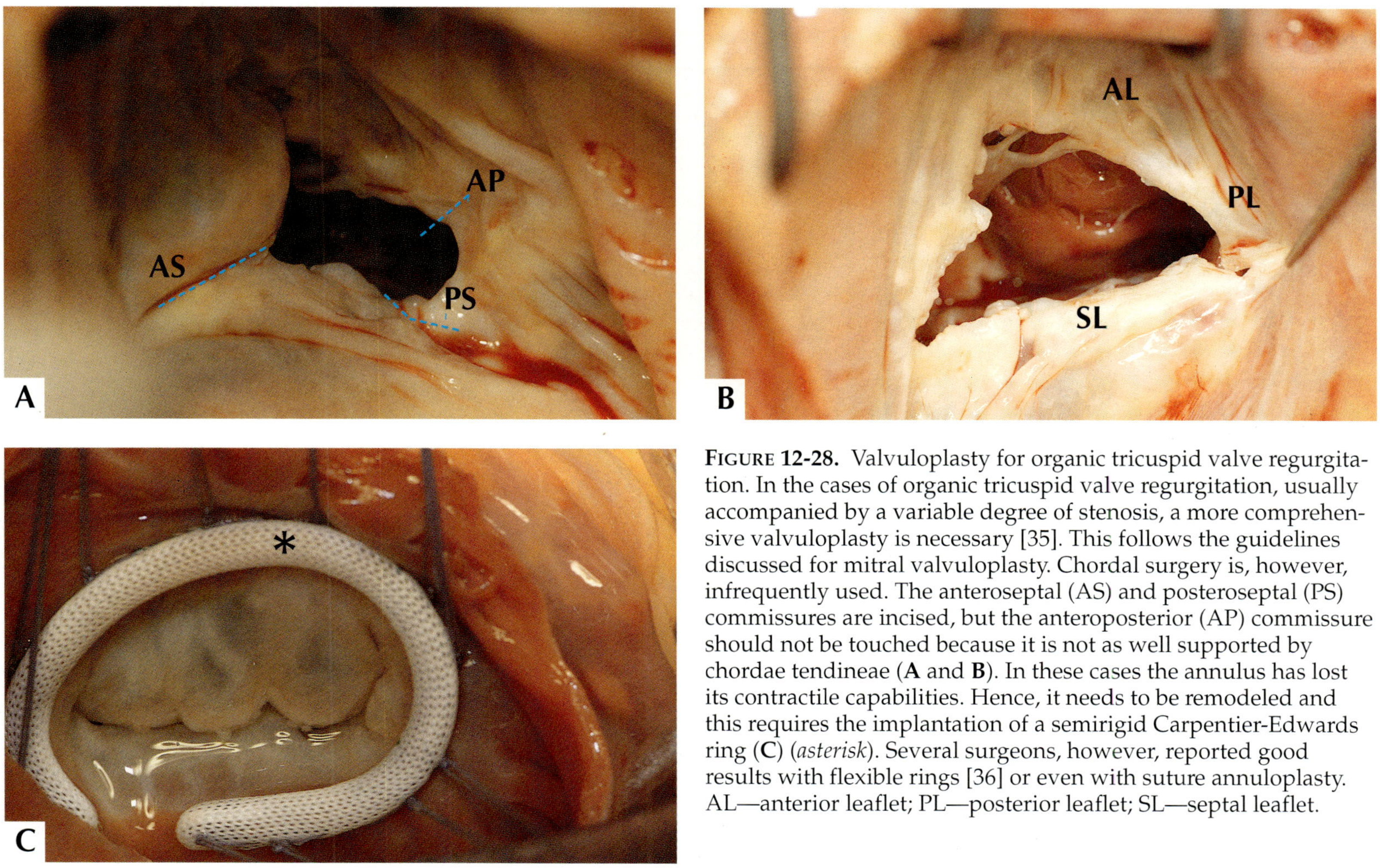

FIGURE 12-28. Valvuloplasty for organic tricuspid valve regurgitation. In the cases of organic tricuspid valve regurgitation, usually accompanied by a variable degree of stenosis, a more comprehensive valvuloplasty is necessary [35]. This follows the guidelines discussed for mitral valvuloplasty. Chordal surgery is, however, infrequently used. The anteroseptal (AS) and posteroseptal (PS) commissures are incised, but the anteroposterior (AP) commissure should not be touched because it is not as well supported by chordae tendineae (**A** and **B**). In these cases the annulus has lost its contractile capabilities. Hence, it needs to be remodeled and this requires the implantation of a semirigid Carpentier-Edwards ring (**C**) (*asterisk*). Several surgeons, however, reported good results with flexible rings [36] or even with suture annuloplasty. AL—anterior leaflet; PL—posterior leaflet; SL—septal leaflet.

REPAIR RESULTS

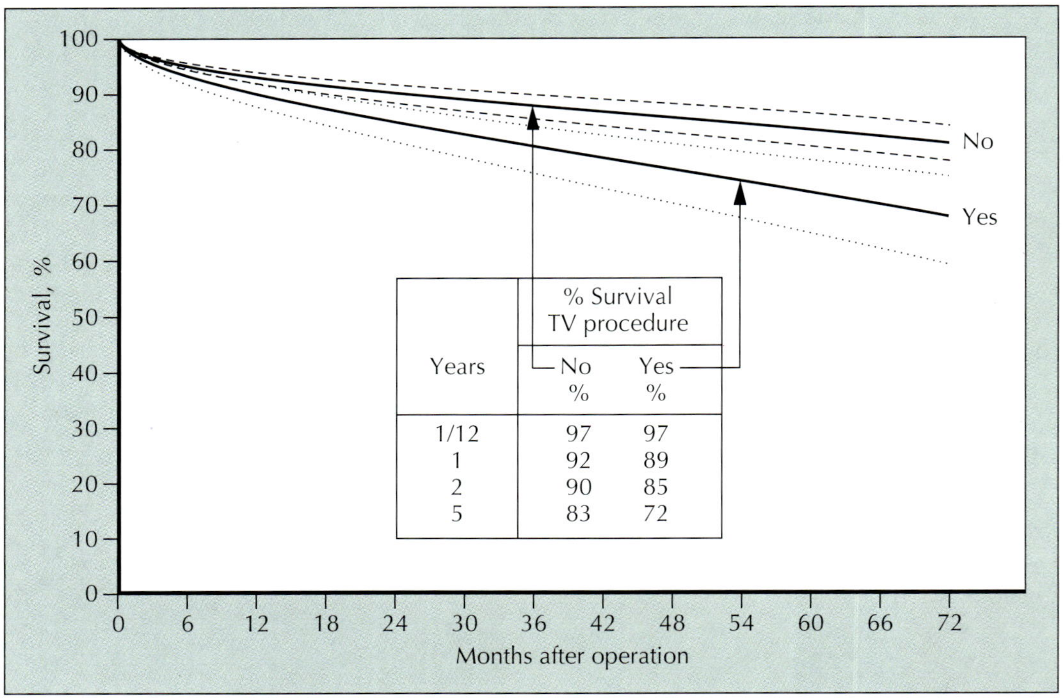

FIGURE 12-29. Survival with or without tricuspid valve (TV) surgery. Global survival after mitral or aortic valve surgery is lower in patients with than in those without accompanying tricuspid valve disease (as seen in these curves), because patients requiring concomitant TV surgery have more advanced cardiac dysfunction. Nevertheless, survival in patients with significant TV disease, whether functional or organic, is probably better in patients who have a tricuspid valve procedure performed concomitantly with surgery to the mitral valve, than in those in whom the tricuspid valve is left untouched. Hence, it is important to treat the tricuspid regurgitation. *Dashed* and *dotted lines* indicate 95% confidence levels. (*Adapted from* Kirklin and Barratt-Boyes [12].)

AORTIC VALVE

ANATOMY AND FUNCTION

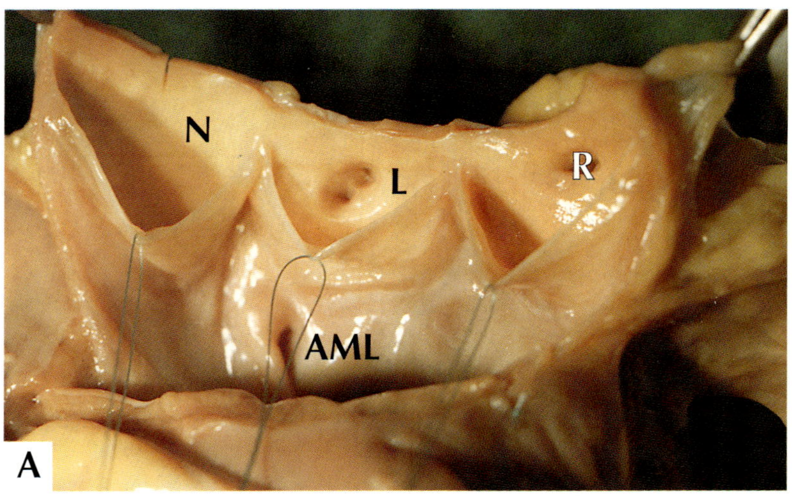

FIGURE 12-30. Aortic valve structures. The aortic valve is placed between the left ventricular outflow tract and the ascending aorta (**A**). It is formed by three cusps, each with the shape of a bird's nest with a sinusoidal attachment across the ventriculoaortic (conoarterial) junction (**B**). (*continued*)

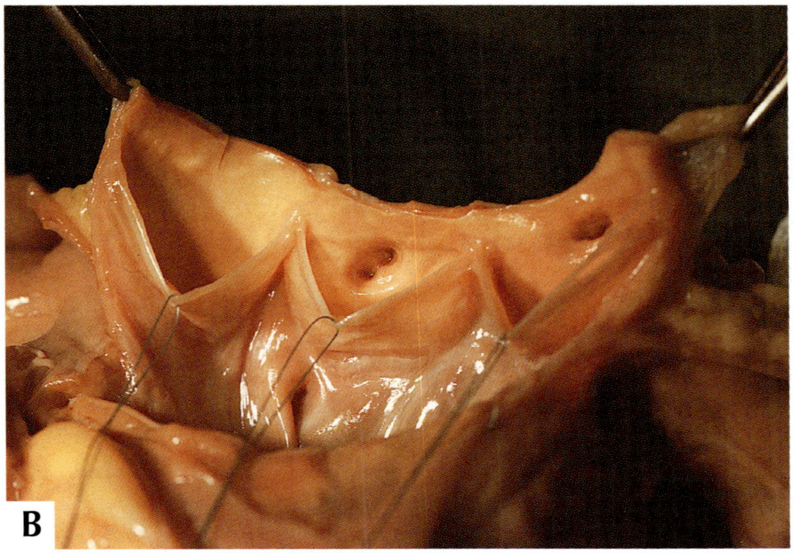

Figure 12-30. *(continued)* In this case, there is no true anatomic annulus [38]. The absence of a fibrous ring facilitates dilatation of the aortic root resulting in regurgitation. The whole length of the free edge of the cusps, reinforced in the center by the nodules of Arantius, remains in the same plane, both in diastole (closed) and in systole (open). The orifices of the coronary arteries are located in the corresponding sinuses of the aortic root, the right orifice usually somewhat higher. The sinuses are dilated portions of the aortic root where there is no contact of the cusps (open) with the arterial wall [39]. AML—anterior mitral leaflet; L—left coronary sinus; N—noncoronary sinus; R—right coronary sinus. (*Adapted from* Angelini and coworkers [38].)

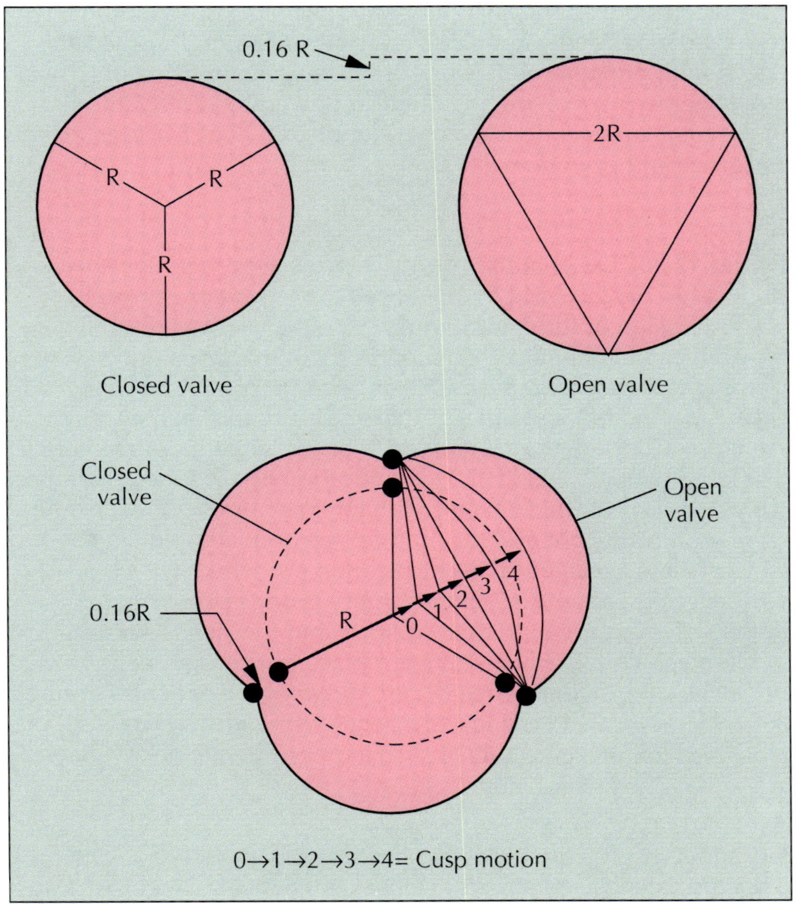

Figure 12-31. Aortic valve function. The aortic root expands during systole. The increment of 14% to 16% of the diameter (2R), commencing in the end of diastole, causes the commissural attachments to spread apart, thus initiating the opening of the valve even before systole begins. This composite movement is continued by the forward motion of the blood under the thrust of the left ventricular systole. The length of the free edge of the cusps equals the diameter of the aortic root or roughly one third of the perimeter. Hence, dilatation of the aortic root, if not accompanied by enlargement of the cusps, results in aortic regurgitation. When fully open, the cusps form a circular orifice, but they do not contact the aortic walls because of the sinusoidal dilatation that permits blood flow into the coronary orifices and facilitates the closure of the cusps in early diastole. R—radius. (*Adapted from* Brewer and coworkers [40] and Thubrikar and coworkers [41].)

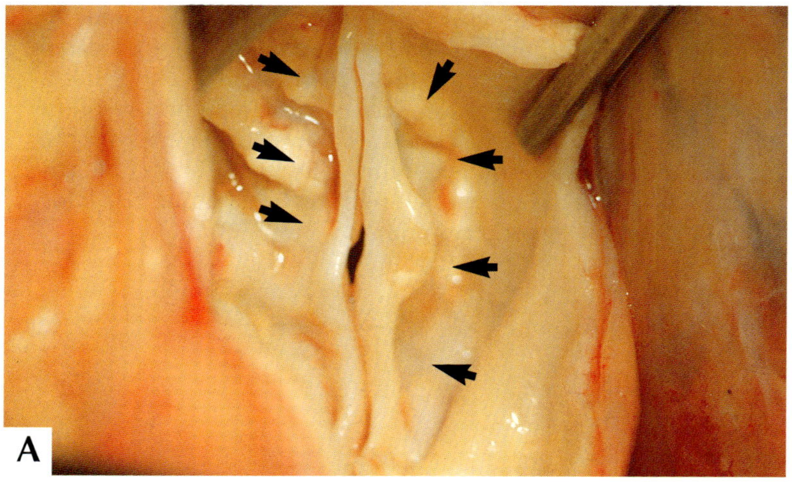

A

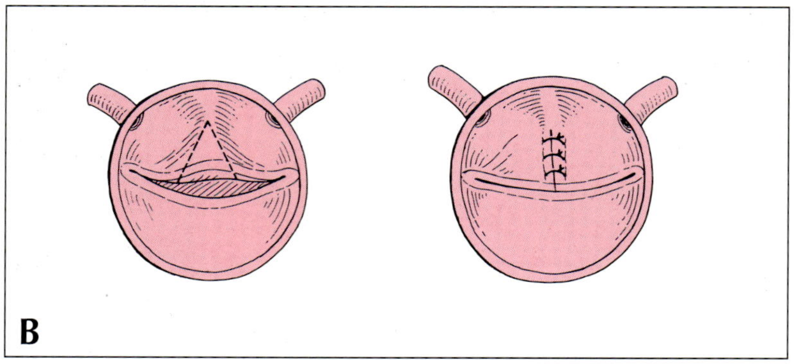

B

FIGURE 12-32. Bicuspid aortic valve stenosis. **A,** Bicuspid aortic valves are intrinsically stenotic because they cannot open completely [38]. In contrast to normal valves, in which the sum of the lengths of the free edges of the three cusps equals the circumference of the aortic root, the sum of the lengths of the free edges of the bicuspid valves is only two thirds of the perimeter. Because of this, the stress exerted on the leaflet tissue is abnormal and these valves tend to calcify early, usually in the third to fifth decade of life. Mechanical debridement of the lumps and bars of calcium (*arrows*) may restore sufficient pliability to the cusps to completely abolish transvalvular gradients. **B,** Regurgitation may result from deficient support by the raphe or from tissue redundancy with prolapse of the cusp. In these cases, excision of a triangular segment, involving the raphe, followed by reconstitution of the cusp, may render the valve competent. (Part B *adapted from* Cosgrove and coworkers [16].)

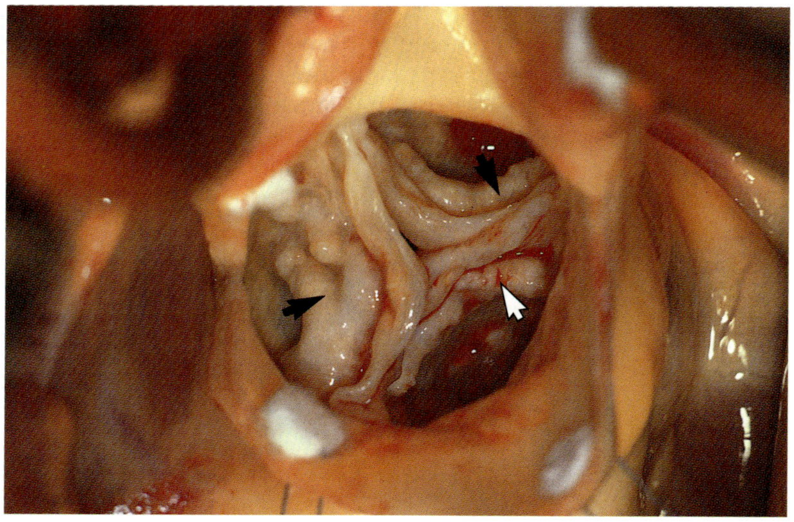

FIGURE 12-33. Degenerative aortic stenosis. Degenerative aortic stenosis is characterized by preserved leaflet anatomy, usually without fusion of the commissures. Stenosis is caused by calcification, which may involve the whole body of the cusps or be localized in the form of lumps or bars of calcium (*arrows*) that can easily be removed without significant disturbance to the leaflet structure. Contradictory results have been claimed although calcification invariably recurred. Decalcification by ultrasonic vibration (CUSA) was performed extensively for some time, but the results were uniformly poor and the method has been abandoned [14]. Nevertheless, mechanical decalcification may still have a place in very selected patients in whom surgery is done primarily for mitral valve or coronary artery disease and the stenosis is only moderate, therefore not justifying replacement of the aortic valve. It may also be an alternative in very old and sick patients because it can be performed very rapidly, hence with reduced risk [42]. However, long-term results of such a procedure are not available.

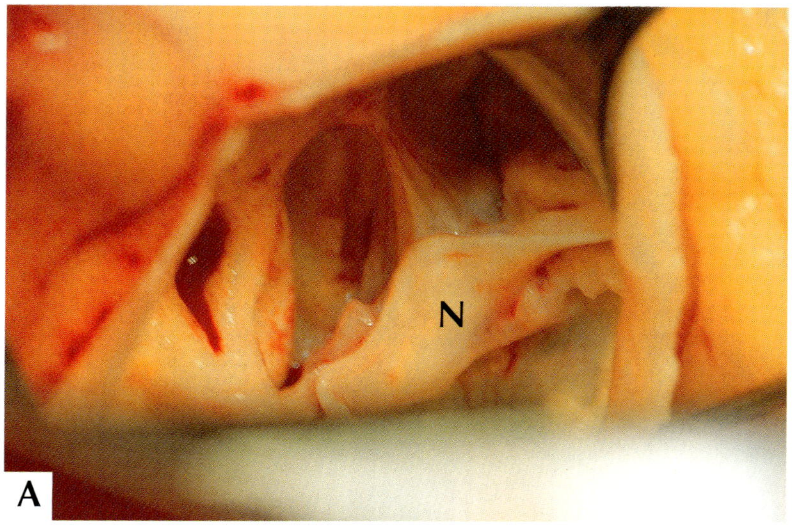

A

FIGURE 12-34. Rheumatic aortic stenosis. In contrast to degenerative aortic stenosis, rheumatic stenosis is characterized by fibrosis and distortion of the cusps, with or without calcification, and fusion of the commissures. When it is not accompanied by significant regurgitation, mild stenosis may be relieved by incision of the fused commissures with care not to interfere with the suspension of the cusps. In **A** and **B**, a rheumatic aortic valve with stenosis demonstrates isolated fusion of one commissure (*arrow* in *panel B*), which was obviously amenable to commissurotomy with an excellent result. (*continued*)

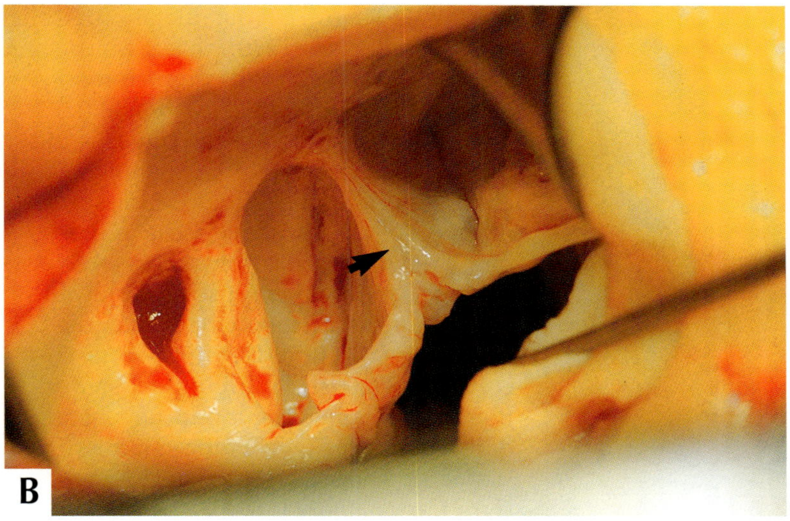

Figure 12-34. (*continued*) The author has used this procedure when the cusps are still fairly pliable, especially when the main pathology determining surgery was mitral valve disease and the aortic disease was only mild to moderate with transvalvular gradients of less than 50 mm Hg, thus probably not justifying replacement of the valve. Debridement of areas of fibrosis may enhance the mobility of the cusps improving both opening and closure. N—noncoronary cusp. (*Adapted from* Cosgrove and coworkers [16] and Duran [43]; with permission.)

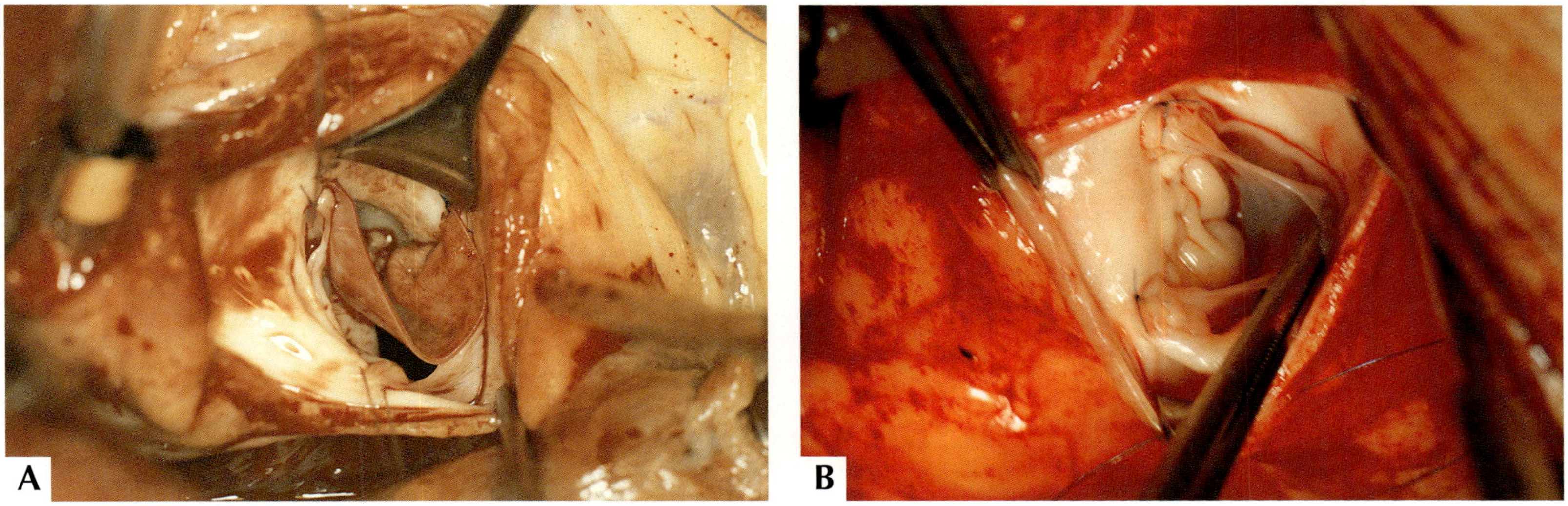

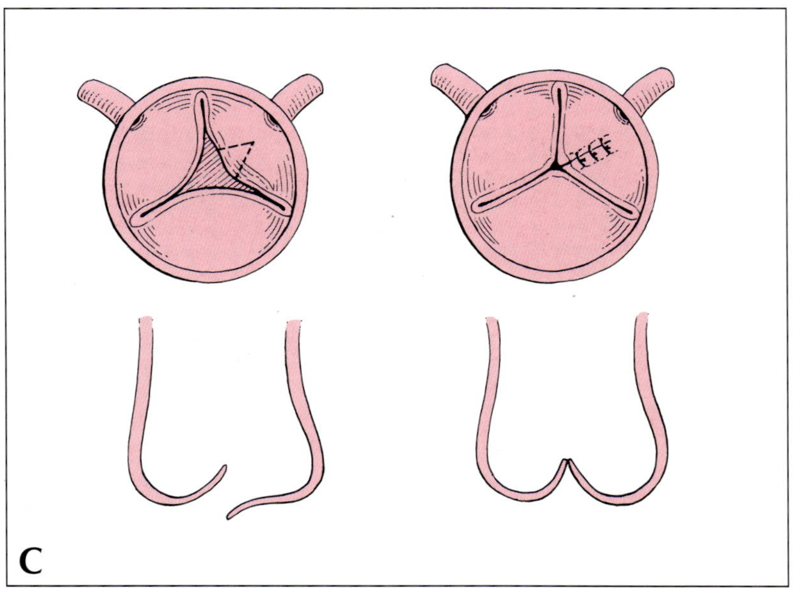

Figure 12-35. Aortic regurgitation. Aortic regurgitation may be due to cusp retraction (by fibrosis or calcification), prolapse and perforation, or by dilatation of the aortic root. Cusp retraction, especially if isolated, may be treated by extension or substitution by glutaraldehyde-treated bovine or autologous pericardium (**A**). Recently, the author has used homograft cusps for replacement of isolated diseased cusps (**B**). Substitution may also be used for treatment of a prolapsed cusp. However, commissural suspension or wedge resection of the free edge have been more frequently used. The latter is performed in the healthier, central portion of the cusp, which may better guarantee the integrity of the repair, while allowing a better reconstitution of the normal shape of the cusp (**C**). (Part C *adapted from* Cosgrove and coworkers [16].)

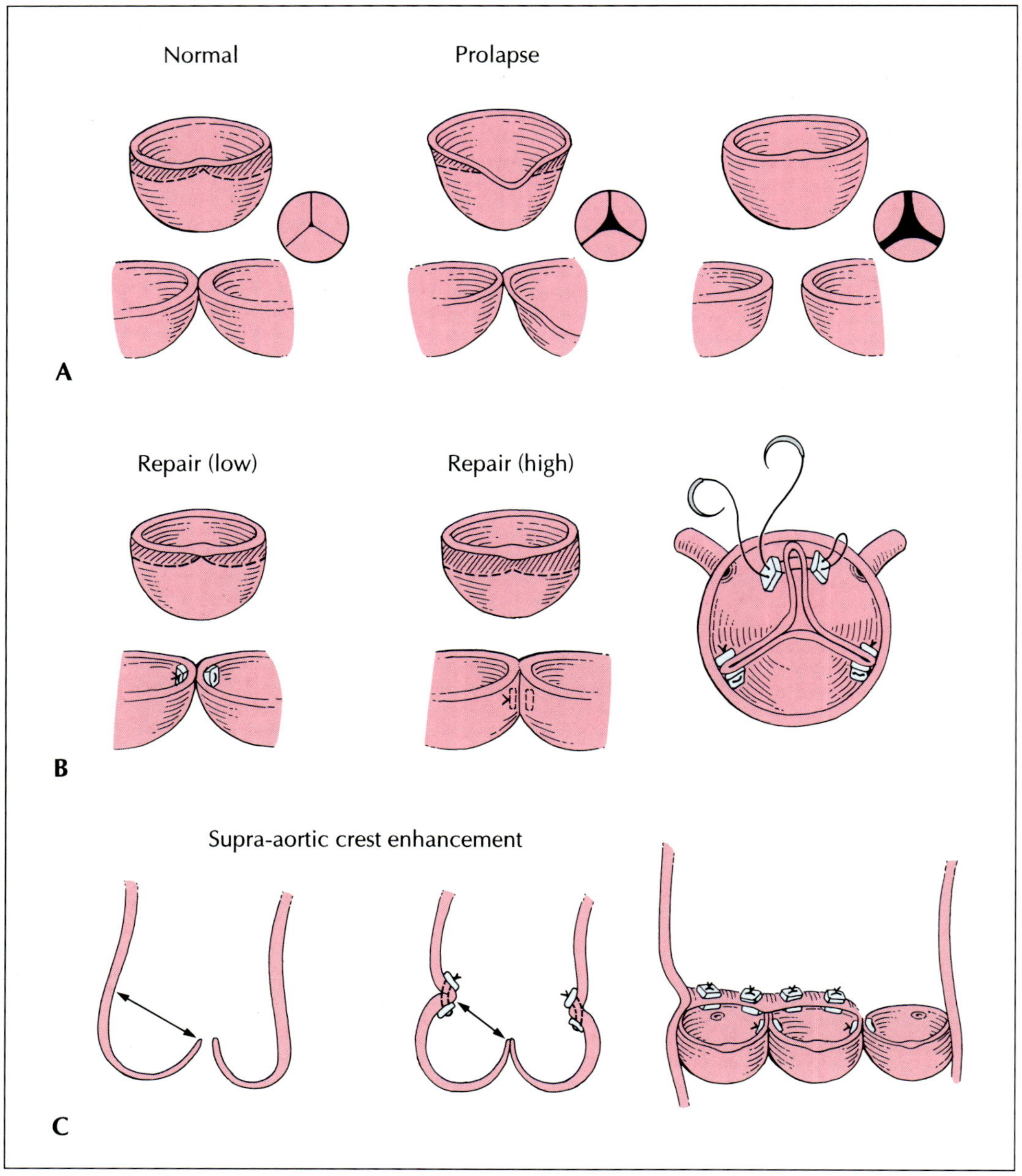

FIGURE 12-36. Aortic root dilatation. Aortic root dilatation secondary to left ventricular enlargement is one of the most common causes of regurgitation ("functional"). The cusps fail to meet in the center of the orifice and often there is separation at the commissural level (**A**). Subcommissural plication of the aortic root reduces the diameter of the orifice and increases the area of coaption of the cusps. The lower the level of the plication the greater the increase in coaption (**B**). Supra-aortic crest enhancement also contributes to a reduction in the diameter of the aortic root at or just above the level of the commissural suspension and is essential in cases with significant dilatation of the sinotubular junction [43] (**C**). These techniques have been used in isolation or in association with immediate success in patients with mild to moderate regurgitation in whom aortic valve replacement would otherwise not be justified, especially when the need for surgery is determined by predominant mitral valve disease. Intraoperative photographs show an aortic valve with moderate regurgitation because of prolapse of one cusp before (**D**) and after (**E**) repair by subcommissural plication. (Sutures are marked by *arrows* in *panel E*.) AW—aortic wall. (*Adapted from* Cosgrove and coworkers [16].)

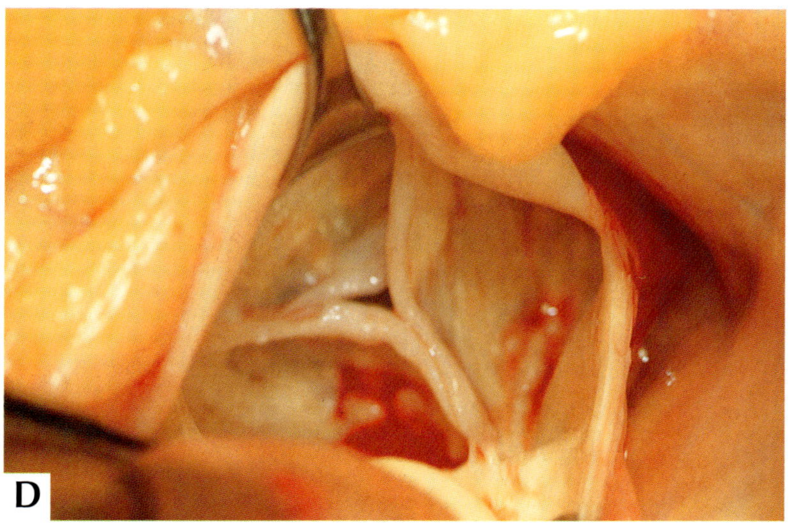

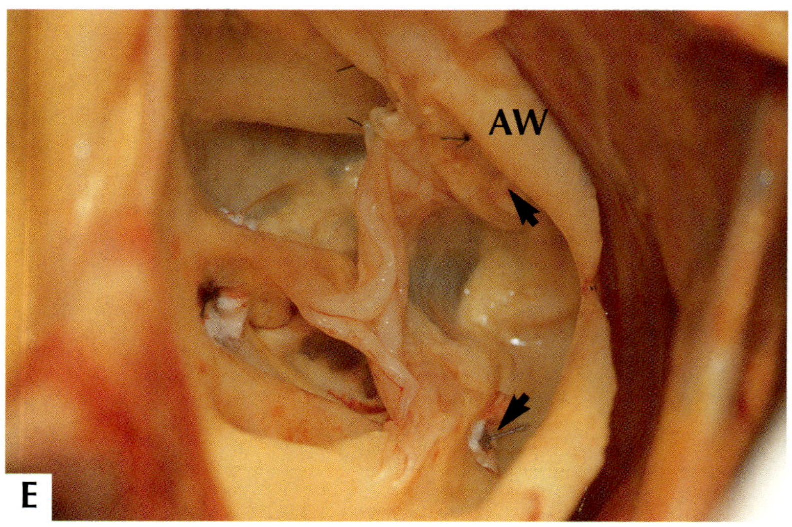

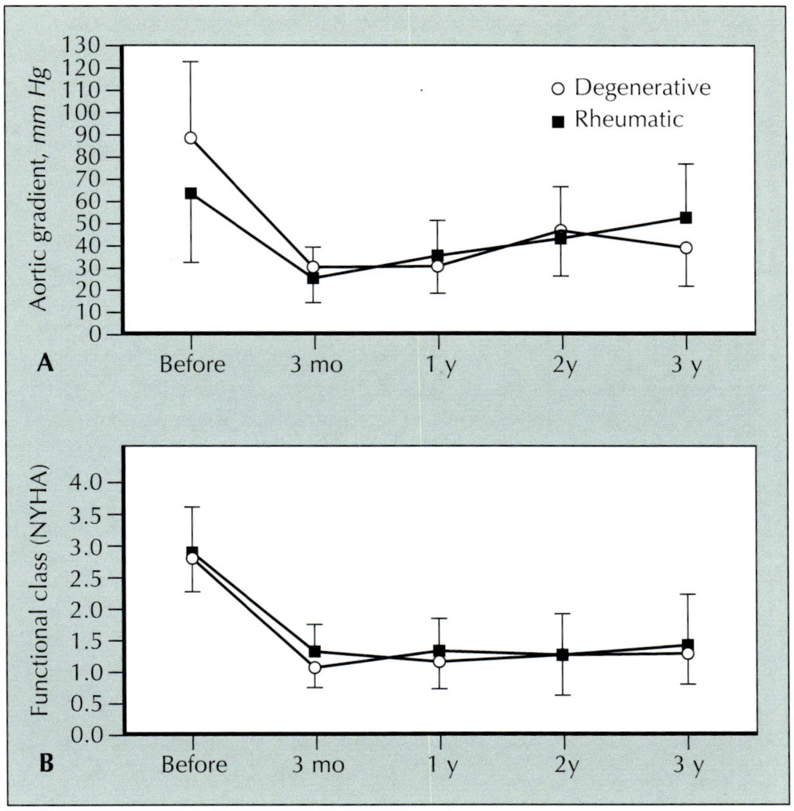

FIGURE 12-37. Postoperative gradients and functional class. **A,** Immediately after repair of aortic stenosis in 67 patients in our department (Antunes, Unpublished data) transvalvular aortic gradients decreased significantly. During the follow-up, they have increased gradually, but remained at values lower than those measured before the repair, except in the rheumatic cases in which they appear to approximate preoperative gradients.

B, Nevertheless, New York Heart Association (NYHA) functional class of the patients was much improved with only a slight deterioration during the follow-up period. The palliative nature of the procedure is obvious, but it clearly benefited a number of patients in whom it appears justified.

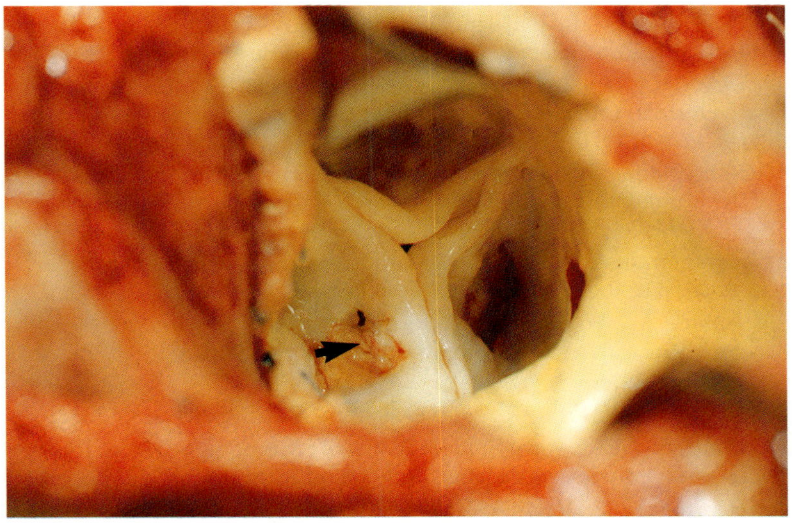

FIGURE 12-38. Intraoperative photograph of the aortic valve 3 years after extensive decalcification in a 74-year-old patient with degenerative aortic stenosis. The patient was reoperated because of acute mitral regurgitation after a myocardial infarction. The anatomic structure of the valve is well preserved and there is perfect apposition of the cusps. There are only small foci of calcification (*arrow*). The transvalvular gradient measured during reoperation was 40 mm Hg (95 mm Hg at the time of the first operation).

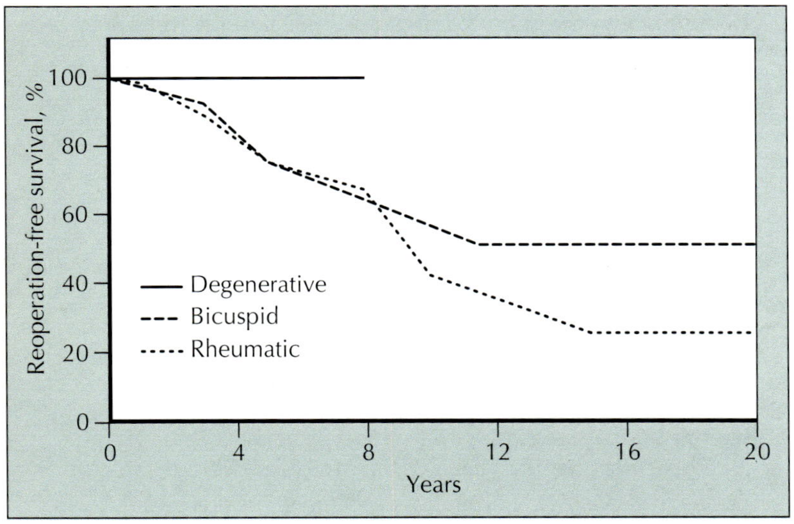

FIGURE 12-39. Long-term outcomes. Repair of aortic stenosis (AS) by decalcification, debridement, and commissurotomy has had different long-term outcomes. Rheumatic valves also had the worst results, followed by bicuspid AS. The best results are observed in patients with degenerative, calcified AS, although calcification recurred almost uniformly [44]. In the experience of King *et al.* [45], none of the surviving patients with degenerative AS required reoperation up to 8 years after repair. (*Adapted from* King and coworkers [45].)

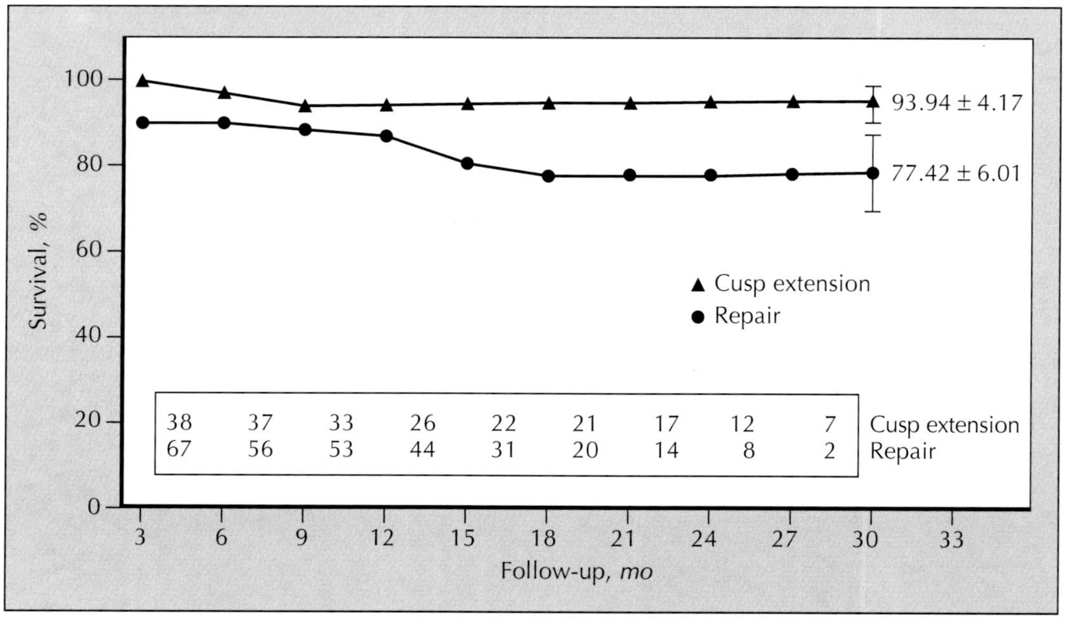

FIGURE 12-40. Aortic valvuloplasty for rheumatic disease. It is difficult to compare the results of aortic valvuloplasty because the pathologies involved in the few series published are markedly different. Duran *et al.* [15] reported on a relatively large series of rheumatic aortic regurgitation (AR) and demonstrated good medium-term results. However, the number of patients followed for more than 2 years is small. Longer periods of follow-up are required. Nonetheless, in rheumatic populations of the Third World, even relatively short (5 to 6 years) periods with a preserved natural valve may constitute a significant advantage over prosthetic valve replacement. The author's recent experience with European populations appears to confirm that valvuloplasty for treatment of AR yields good results in some subgroups of patients. (*Adapted from* Duran and coworkers [15].)

REFERENCES

1. Carpentier A: Cardiac valve surgery—the "French correction." *J Thorac Cardiovasc Surg* 1983, 86:323–337.
2. Carpentier A, Deloche A, Dauptain J, *et al.*: A new reconstructive operation for correction of mitral and tricuspid insufficiency. *J Thorac Cardiovasc Surg* 1971, 61:1–13.
3. Carpentier A, Chauvaud S, Fabiani JN, *et al.*: Reconstructive surgery of mitral valve incompetence. Ten-year appraisal. *J Thorac Cardiovasc Surg* 1980, 79:338–348.
4. Deloche A, Jebara VA, Relland JY, *et al.*: Valve repair with Carpentier techniques. The second decade. *J Thorac Cardiovasc Surg* 1990, 99:990–1001.
5. Duran CM, Gometza B, De Vol EB: Valve repair in rheumatic mitral disease. *Circulation* 1991, 84:II-125–132.
6. Lessana A, Carbone C, Romano M: Mitral valve repair: results and the decision-making process in reconstruction. Report of 275 cases. *J Thorac Cardiovasc Surg* 1990, 99:622–630.
7. Spencer FC, Colvin SB, Culliford AT, Isom OW: Experiences with the Carpentier techniques of mitral valve reconstruction in 103 patients (1980–1985). *J Thorac Cardiovasc Surg* 1985, 90:341–350.
8. Herrera JM, Vega JL, Bernal JM, *et al.*: Open mitral commissurotomy: fourteen to eighteen-year follow-up clinical study. *Ann Thorac Surg* 1993, 55:641–645.
9. Antunes MJ, Magalhaes MP, Colsen PR, Kinsley RH: Valvuloplasty for rheumatic mitral valve disease. A surgical challenge. *J Thorac Cardiovasc Surg* 1987, 94:44–56.
10. Cosgrove DM: Surgery for degenerative mitral valve disease. *Semin Thorac Cardiovasc Surg* 1989, 1:183–193.
11. Antunes MJ: Mitral valvuloplasty, a better alternative. Comparative study between valve reconstruction and replacement for rheumatic mitral valve disease. *Eur J Cardiovasc Surg* 1990, 4:257–262.
12. Kirklin JW, Barratt-Boyes B, eds: *Cardiac Surgery*, 2nd edn. New York: Churchill Livingstone; 1993.
13. De Vega NF: La annuloplastia selectiva, regulable y permanente. *Rev Esp Cardiol* 1972, 25:555–556.
14. Cosgrove DM, Ratliff NB, Schaff HV, Edwards WD: Aortic valve decalcification: history repeated with a new result. *Ann Thorac Surg* 1990, 49:689—690.
15. Duran C, Kumar N, Gometza B, Al Halees Z: Indications and limitations of aortic valve reconstruction. *Ann Thorac Surg* 1991, 52:447–454.
16. Cosgrove DM, Rosenkranz ER, Hendren WG, *et al.*: Valvuloplasty for aortic insufficiency. *J Thorac Cardiovasc Surg* 1991, 102:571–577.
17. Lam JHC, Ranganatham N, Wigle ED, Silver MD: Morphology of the human mitral valve. I. Chordae tendineae: a new classification. *Circulation* 1970, 41:449–458.
18. Ranganathan N, Lam JHC, Wigle ED, Silver MD: Morphology of the human mitral valve. II. The valve leaflets. *Circulation* 1970, 41:459–467.
19. Zimmerman J, Bailey CP: The surgical significance of the fibrous skeleton of the heart. *J Thorac Cardiovasc Surg* 1962, 44:701–712.
20. Tsakiris AG, Von Bernuth G, Rastelli GC, *et al.*: Size and motion of the mitral valve annulus in anesthetized intact dogs. *J Appl Physiol* 1971, 30:611–618.
21. Antunes MJ: *Mitral Valve Repair*. Percha, FRG: RS Schulz; 1989.
22. Hendren WG, Nemec JJ, Lytle BW, *et al.*: Mitral valve repair for ischemic mitral insufficiency. *Ann Thorac Surg* 1991, 52:1246–1251.
23. Hendren WG, Morris AS, Rosenkranz ER, *et al.*: Mitral valve repair for bacterial endocarditis. *J Thorac Cardiovasc Surg* 1992, 103:124–128.
24. Chauvaud S, Jebara V, Chachques JC, *et al.*: Valve extension with glutaraldehyde-preserved autologous pericardium. Results in mitral valve repair. *J Thorac Cardiovasc Surg* 1991, 102:171–177.
25. David TE, Bos J, Rakowski H: Mitral valve repair by replacement of chordae tendineae with polytetrafluoroethylene sutures. *J Thorac Cardiovasc Surg* 1991, 101:495–501.
26. Van Rijk-Zwikker GL, Mast F, Schipperheyn JJ, *et al.*: Comparison of rigid and flexible rings for annuloplasty of the porcine mitral valve. *Circulation* 1990, 82:IV-58–64.
27. Freeman WK, Schaff HV, Khandheria BK, *et al.*: Intraoperative evaluation of mitral valve regurgitation and repair by transesophageal echocardiography: incidence and significance of systolic anterior motion. *J Am Coll Cardiol* 1992, 20:599–609.

28. Grossi EA, Galloway AC, Parish MA, *et al.*: Experience with twenty-eight cases of systolic anterior motion after mitral valve reconstruction by the Carpentier technique. *J Thorac Cardiovasc Surg* 1992, 103:466–470.

29. Antunes MJ, Colsen PR, Kinsley RH: Mitral valvuloplasty: a learning curve. *Circulation* 1983, 68:II-70–75.

30. Galloway AC, Colvin SB, Baumann FG, *et al.*: A comparison of mitral valve reconstruction with mitral valve replacement: intermediate-term results. *Ann Thorac Surg* 1989, 47:655–662.

31. Silver MD, Lam JHC, Ranganathan N, Wigle ED: Morphology of the human tricuspid valve. *Circulation* 1971, 43:333–348.

32. Antunes MJ, Girdwood RW: Tricuspid annuloplasty. A modified technique. *Ann Thorac Surg* 1983, 35:676–678.

33. Kay JH, Maselli-Campagna G, Tsuji HK: Surgical treatment of tricuspid insufficiency. *Ann Surg* 1965, 162:53–58.

34. Minale C, Lambertz H, Nikol S, *et al.*: Selective annuloplasty of the tricuspid valve. Two-year experience. *J Thorac Cardiovasc Surg* 1990, 99:846–851.

35. Carpentier A, Deloche A, Hanania G, *et al.*: Surgical management of acquired tricuspid valve disease. *J Thorac Cardiovasc Surg* 1974, 67:53–65.

36. Duran CG, Ubago JLM: Clinical and hemodynamic performance of a totally flexible prosthetic ring for atrioventricular valve reconstruction. *Ann Thorac Surg* 1976, 22:458–463.

37. Abe T, Tukamoto M, Yanagiva M, *et al.*: De Vega's annuloplasty for acquired tricuspid disease: early and late results in 110 patients. *Ann Thorac Surg* 1989, 48:670–676.

38. Angelini A, Anderson RH, Devine WA, *et al.*: The morphology of the normal aortic valve as compared with the aortic valve having two leaflets. *J Thorac Cardiovasc Surg* 1989, 98:362–367.

39. Silver MA, Roberts WC: Detailed anatomy of the normally functioning aortic valve in hearts of normal and increased weight. *Am J Cardiol* 1985, 55:454–461.

40. Brewer RJ, Deck JD, Capati B, Nolan SP: The dynamic aortic root. Its role in aortic valve function. *J Thorac Cardiovasc Surg* 1976, 72:413–417.

41. Thubrikar M, Bosher LP, Nolan SP: The mechanism of opening of the aortic valve. *J Thorac Cardiovasc Surg* 1979, 77:863–870.

42. Baeza OR, Majid NK, Conroy DP, Donahoo JS: Combined conventional mechanical and ultrasonic debridement for aortic valvular stenosis. *Ann Thorac Surg* 1992, 54:62–67.

43. Duran CG: Reconstructive techniques for rheumatic aortic valve disease. *J Card Surg* 1988, 3:23–28.

44. Shapira N, Lemole GM, Fernandez J, *et al.*: Aortic valve repair for aortic stenosis in adults. *Ann Thorac Surg* 1990, 50:110–120.

45. King RM, Pluth JR, Giuliani ER, Piehler JM: Mechanical decalcification of the aortic valve. *Ann Thorac Surg* 1986, 42:269–272.

Prosthetic Heart Valves

13
CHAPTER

Gary L. Grunkemeier, Shahbudin H. Rahimtoola, and Albert Starr

This chapter contains an overview of current replacement heart valves and a summary of their reported clinical performance. The material is divided into seven sections.

The section on worldwide valve usage contains an outline of the valves we will review, a brief chronology of the major valves in current use, and a discussion of a few new investigational devices. It also displays the years and approximate number of valves in use. Mechanical and biologic heart valves are then described, as well as the surgical technique of aortic and mitral valve replacement with a mechanical prosthesis. The results of a recent thorough investigation and comparison of six current mechanical valves in a pulse duplication test system are also discussed and include the comparative calculations of effective orifice area and regurgitation.

The major distinguishing difference among the valves in use today involves the tradeoff between an increased risk of the thromboembolism-thrombosis-bleeding complex for mechanical valves and the structural deterioration of tissue valves. We reviewed the recently published literature and extracted the "linearized" rates of thromboembolism, thrombosis, and bleeding for major mechanical and tissue valves and compared these rates among the most popular valves in different positions. These rates are only appropriate if the time-related risk (hazard function) of these complications is constant. This is only approximately true, as a parametric fit to thromboembolism-free curves shows a declining risk over time.

We also review the published results of structural valve deterioration (SVD) for tissue valves. For homograft valves, the various methods of sterilization and preservation provide different prostheses that can be considered "models." SVD is not a constant risk event because the hazard increases dramatically over time. Thus it cannot be summarized with a simple (linearized rate) statistic but requires actuarial analysis for description and comparison. However, actuarial analysis provides the freedom from a nonfatal complication assuming the patients do not die. To determine the actual risk of SVD requires taking the rate of death into account, which decreases the actuarial estimates, especially for older patients.

Finally, recommendations with regard to selection of a prosthesis for a particular patient are given as well as speculation about the future developments in the design and manufacture of prosthetic heart valves.

Worldwide Valve Usage

MAJOR VALVES IN USE OR UNDER INVESTIGATION, 1995

MECHANICAL	BIOLOGICAL
Caged Ball	Homograft
Starr-Edwards	Autologous
Tilting/pivoting disc	Pulmonary autograft
Medtronic Hall	Stented pericardial
Omniscience/Omnicarbon	Porcine heterograft
Sorin: Monocast, Carbocast, AllCarbon, Monostrut	Medtronic: Hancock I, II, MO, MO II; Intact, Mosaic, Freestyle
Bi-leaflet	Edwards: C-E Standard, SAV, Duraflex, Primo
St. Jude	St. Jude: BioImplant, TSPV, X-Cell
Edwards TEKNA	Biocor, Bravo Cardiovascular
CarboMedics	Pericardial heterograft
Sorin Bicarbon	Carpentier-Edwards
ATS	Mitroflow
Medtronic Parallel	Sorin Pericarbon

FIGURE 13-1. Valves in use or under investigation in 1995. Heart valves can be classified into two broad categories according to the origin of their occluding mechanism: mechanical and biologic. Many valves of each category are currently in use. The first valve replacements into anatomic positions were performed by Lillehei *et al* [1]in the aortic position in 1958, and by Nina Braunwald *et al* in the mitral position in 1960 [2], both using flap valves. But the first design that led to long-term survivors was the mechanical caged-ball valve, used by Harken *et al* in the aortic [3] and Starr and Edwards in the mitral [4] position, both in 1960. Subsequently, valves with a single circular disk and, more recently, with two semicircular leaflets have been used.

The first biologic valves used were transplants from human cadavers, called homografts or allografts, pioneered by Ross [5] and Barratt-Boyes [6] in 1962. Subsequently, tissue valves of heterologous (porcine, bovine), and to a limited extent, autologous (fascia lata, pulmonary valve, pericardium) tissue have been used. Valvular devices not covered in this review are prosthetic rings used for valve repair and valved conduits (grafts).

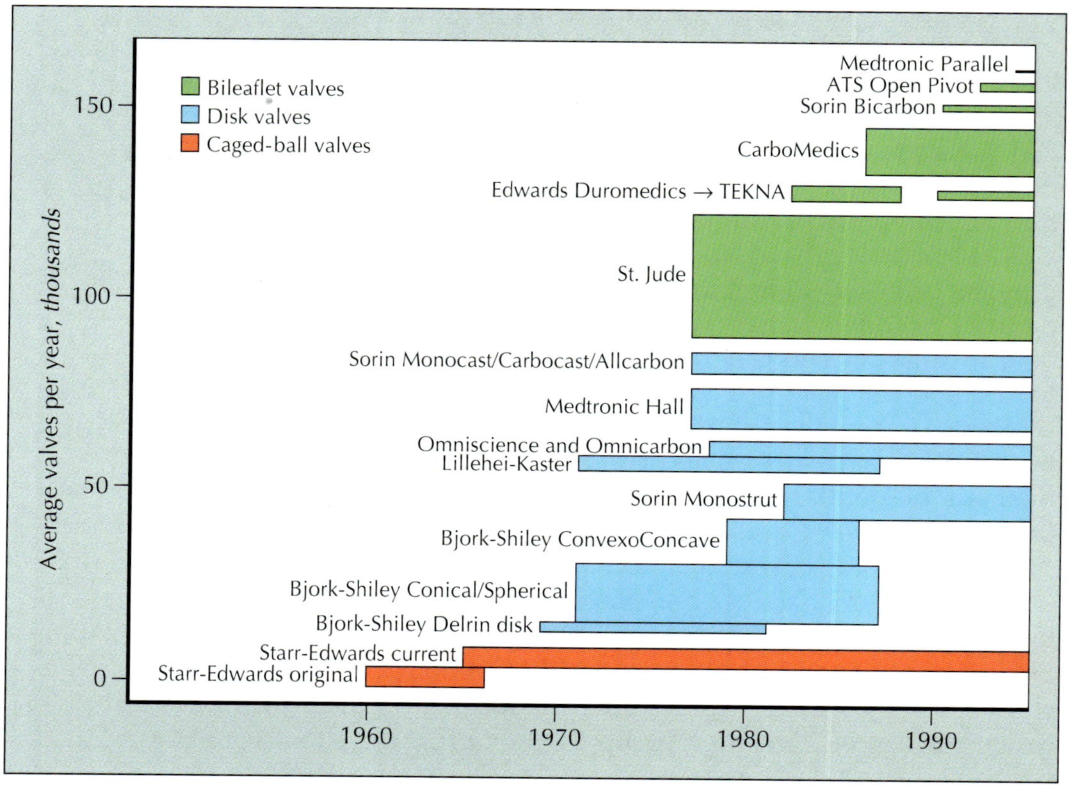

FIGURE 13-2. Mechanical valve usage. Approximate usage per year is shown for caged-ball, disk, and bileaflet mechanical valves. Only valves currently in use, or their direct predecessors, are shown. Each rectangle has its years of clinical use as its width and the average usage per year as its height. Thus the area of the rectangle equals the total number of valves implanted. However, the actual usage is not constant, rather it varies year to year for each valve. Thus the average per year (height of each rectangle) is only an approximation.

The numbers of implanted valves shown were obtained from the manufacturers and in most cases are only approximate, estimated from sales invoices or returned implant cards. Use of the Duromedics valve (Baxter Healthcare Corporation, Irvine, CA) was not constant; it was withdrawn after several valves fractured, reintroduced in a refined configuration, and subsequently renamed TEKNA (Baxter Healthcare Corporation).

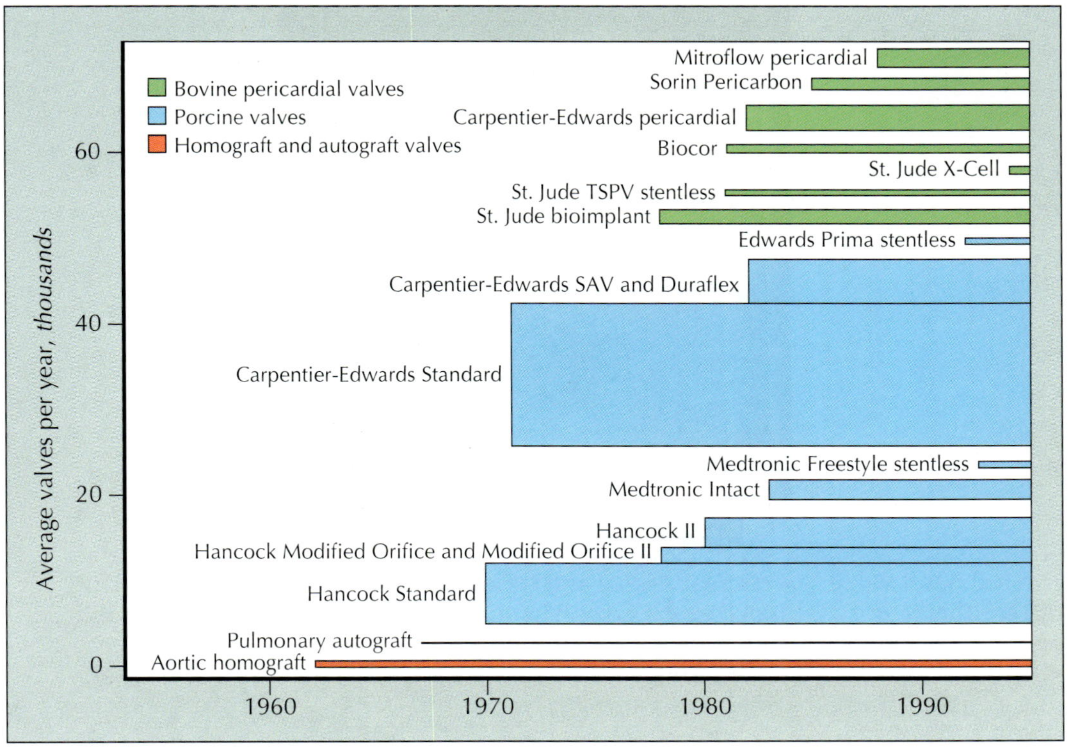

FIGURE 13-3. Biologic valve usage. Approximate usage per year of biologic valves in current use (*see* legend to Fig. 13-2). These include homografts and autografts, porcine and bovine pericardial valves.

MECHANICAL VALVE DESCRIPTIONS

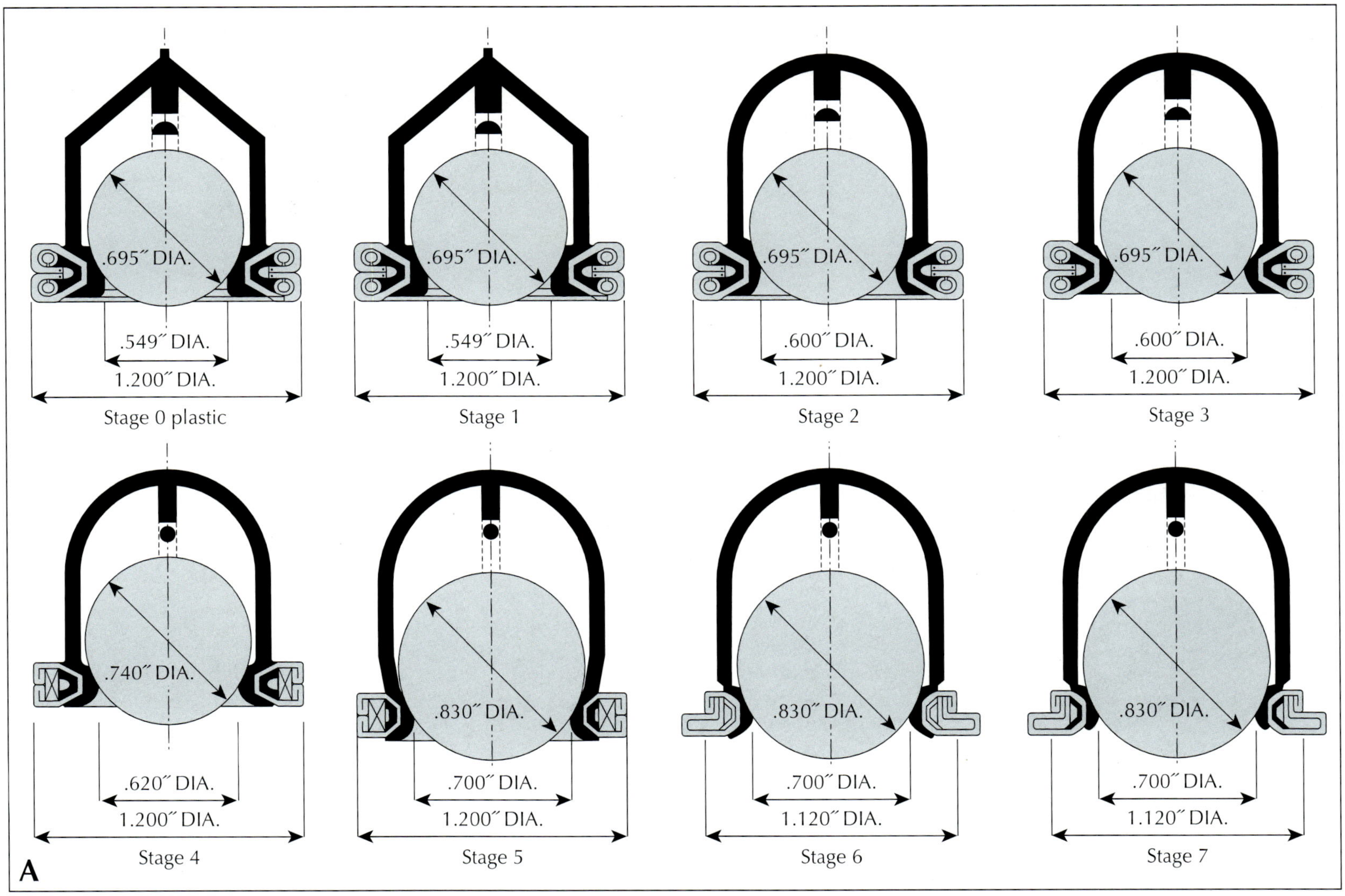

FIGURE 13-4. Starr-Edwards caged-ball valve. (*continued*)

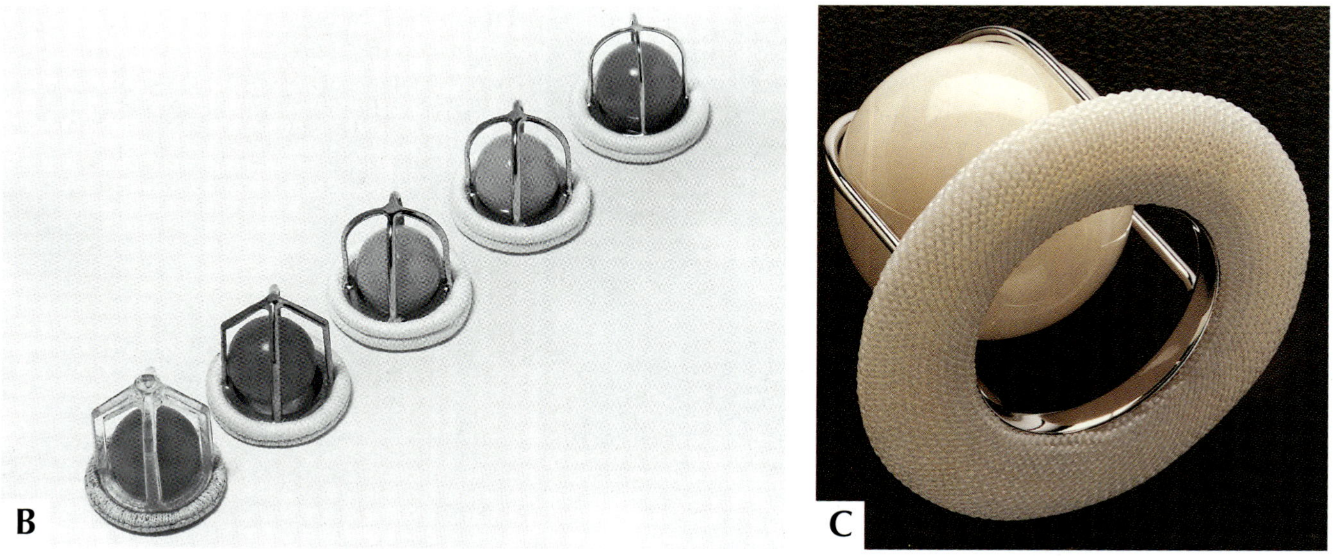

FIGURE 13-4. *(continued)* The first clinically successful heart valve was the Starr-Edwards caged-ball valve (Baxter Healthcare Corporation, Irvine, CA). The valve underwent several early design modifications (**A** and **B**), which resulted in the current Starr-Edwards ball valves (**C**). The one-piece cage consists of a circular orifice and three (aortic) or four (mitral) thin struts joined at the apex. The poppet is molded from silicone rubber and impregnated with barium sulfate for radiopacity. The sewing ring is thickly upholstered to improve coaption with irregular tissue beds.

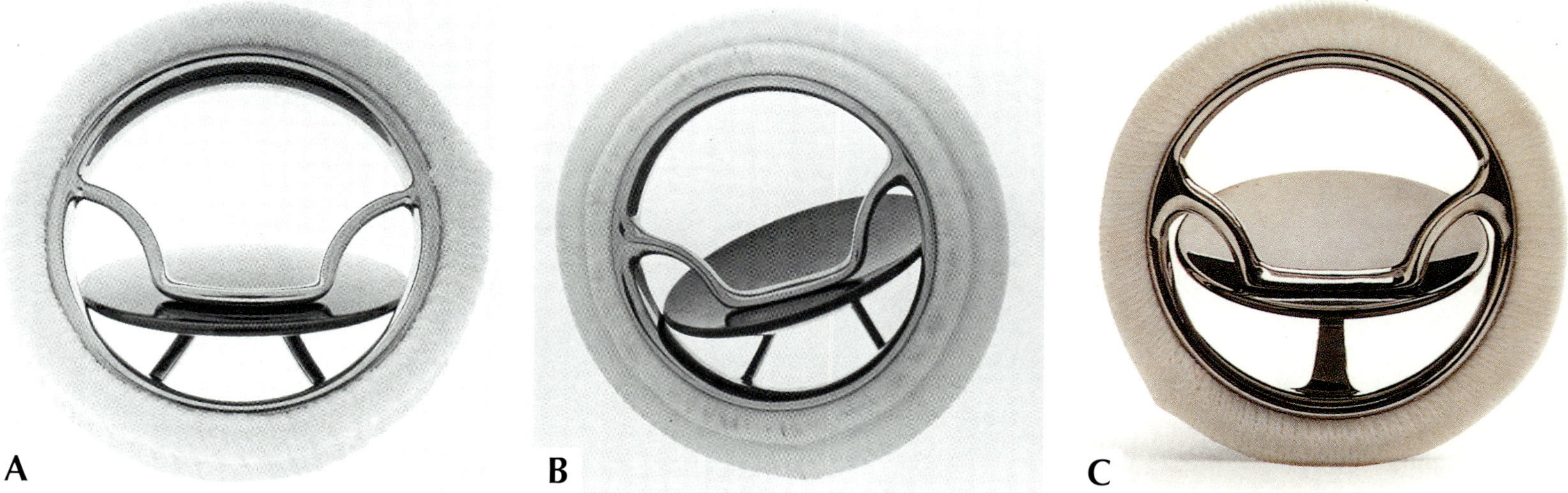

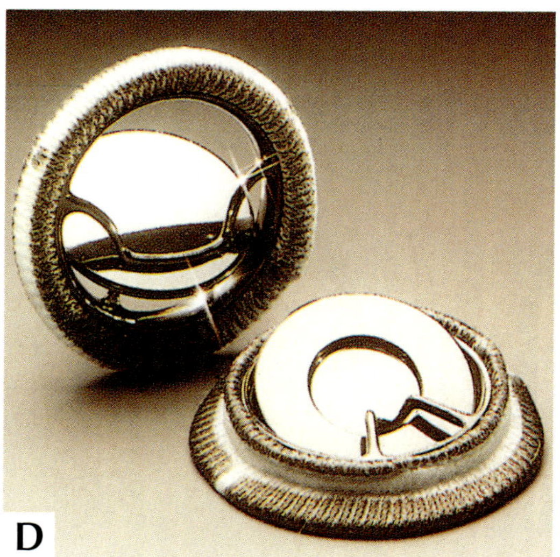

FIGURE 13-5. Bjork-Shiley and Sorin tilting disk valves. The Bjork-Shiley valve was the first successful tilting disk valve, and various modifications of it have been in use since 1969. The first model had a Delrin disk, but a pyrolitic carbon-coated (Conical) disk model became available in 1971, followed by the Spherical Disk model (**A**). The Convexo-Concave (CC) model (**B**) was designed as an improved version of the Spherical Disk valve, with a curved disk and enlarged minor orifice to improve hemodynamics and hopefully reduce thrombosis. The CC valve also had an integral (rather than welded) inflow strut to eliminate the few inflow strut fractures that had occurred with the previous models. One result of these improvements was a new failure mode caused by fracture of the remaining (outflow) welded strut. To date this has been reported in about 560 valves, or 0.7% of the 86,000 CC valves that were implanted.

The Monostrut valve (**C**) (Sorin Biomedica Cardio, Saluggia, Italy) replaced the welded strut design of the CC valve with an integral housing in which both struts are machined from a solid piece of alloy. The Monostrut valve was developed by Shiley and sold to Sorin. Shiley no longer manufactures heart valves, but their results are included because of the large number that were implanted, and the many patients alive today with these valves. Sorin also makes a tilting disk valve that is similar to the Shiley Standard disk valve, but has both struts integral to the housing (Monocast), and is available with a pyrolitic carbon-coated sewing ring (Carbocast), and also with a carbon-coated housing (AllCarbon) (**D**).

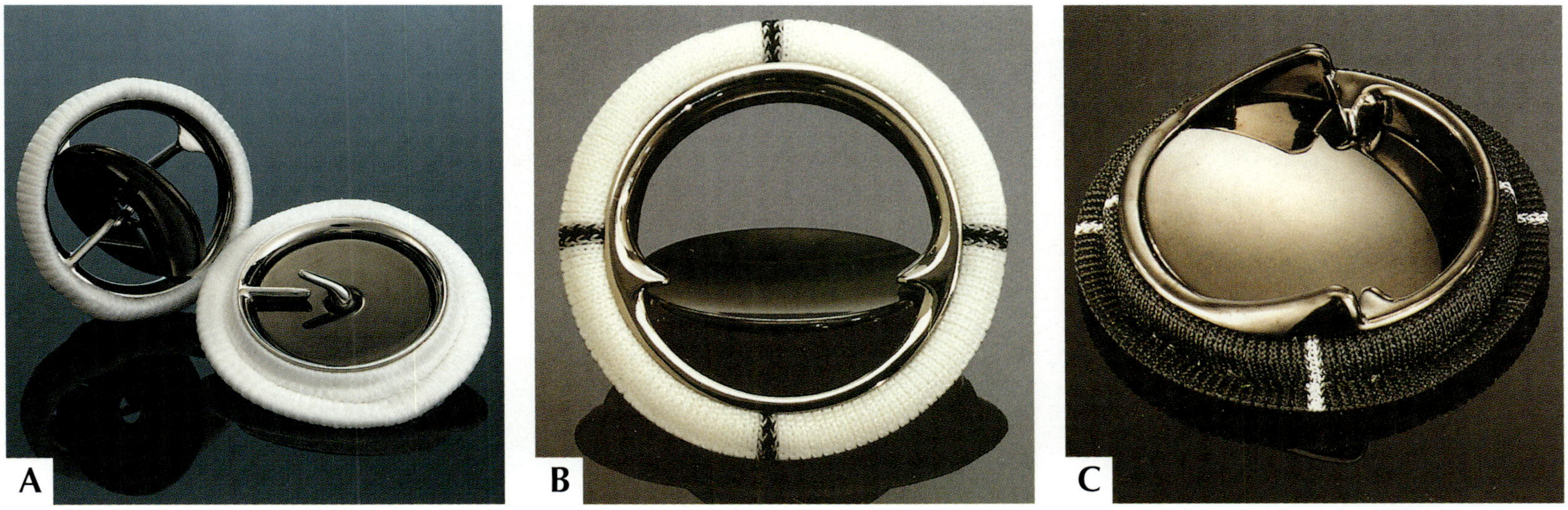

FIGURE 13-6. Medtronic Hall and Omniscience/Omnicarbon tilting disk valves. The Medtronic Hall valve (**A**) (Medtronic, Inc, Minneapolis, MN) has a Teflon sewing ring, a titanium housing machined from a solid cylinder, and a carbon-coated disk with flat parallel sides. The disk, which opens to 75° in the aortic model and 70° in the mitral, is retained by an S-shaped guide strut that protrudes through a hole in the center of the disk.

The Omniscience valve (**B**) (Medical, Inc), a successor of the discontinued Lillehei-Kaster Pivoting Disk valve, has a smoothly curved pyrolitic carbon disk, a one-piece titanium cage, and a polyester knit sewing ring. The disk opens to 80° and closes at an angle of 12° to the plane of the orifice, resulting in a 68° travel arc. The Omnicarbon valve (**C**) (Medical, Inc) is similar to the Omniscience valve, but is completely coated with pyrolitic carbon.

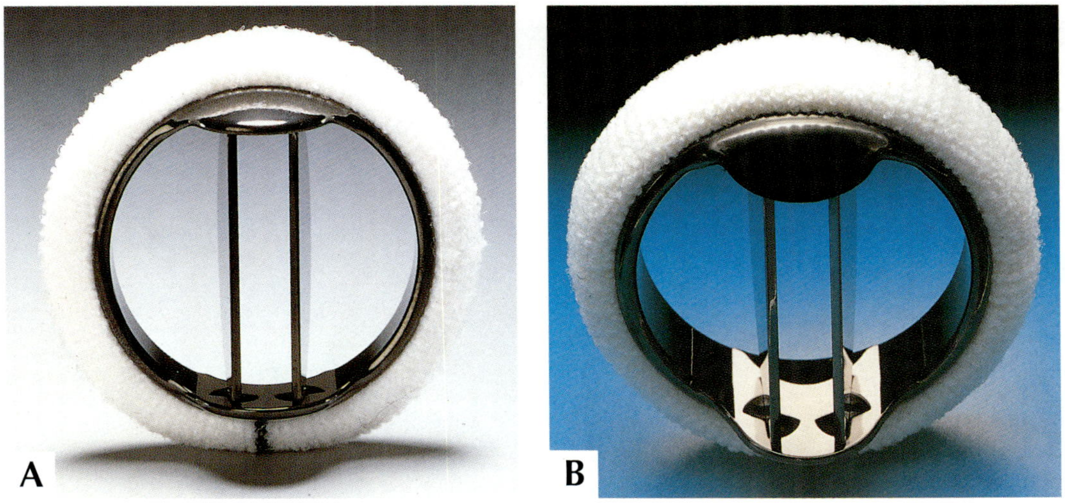

FIGURE 13-7. St. Jude bileaflet valve. The St. Jude valve (St. Jude Medical, St. Paul, MN) was the first clinically successful bileaflet valve and has been used over half a million times since its first implant in 1977. Previous bileaflet valves had been tried but were unsatisfactory; this design, with pyrolitic carbon coating and named after the patron saint of hopeless causes, led to unprecedented success and the beginning of a new family of heart valve designs.

The occluding mechanism consists of two semicircular leaflets that swing apart during opening, resulting in three separate flow areas. The housing of the valve is a cylindrically shaped piece of pyrolitic carbon with two rounded tabs, called pivot guards, which project up from the inflow side (**A**). The inside surfaces of these tabs are flat and contain two butterfly-shaped indentations that retain the leaflets (**B**). Small "ears" at the end of each diameter of the thin hemispherical leaflets fit into these indentations, which secure the leaflets in the housing and define their limits of travel.

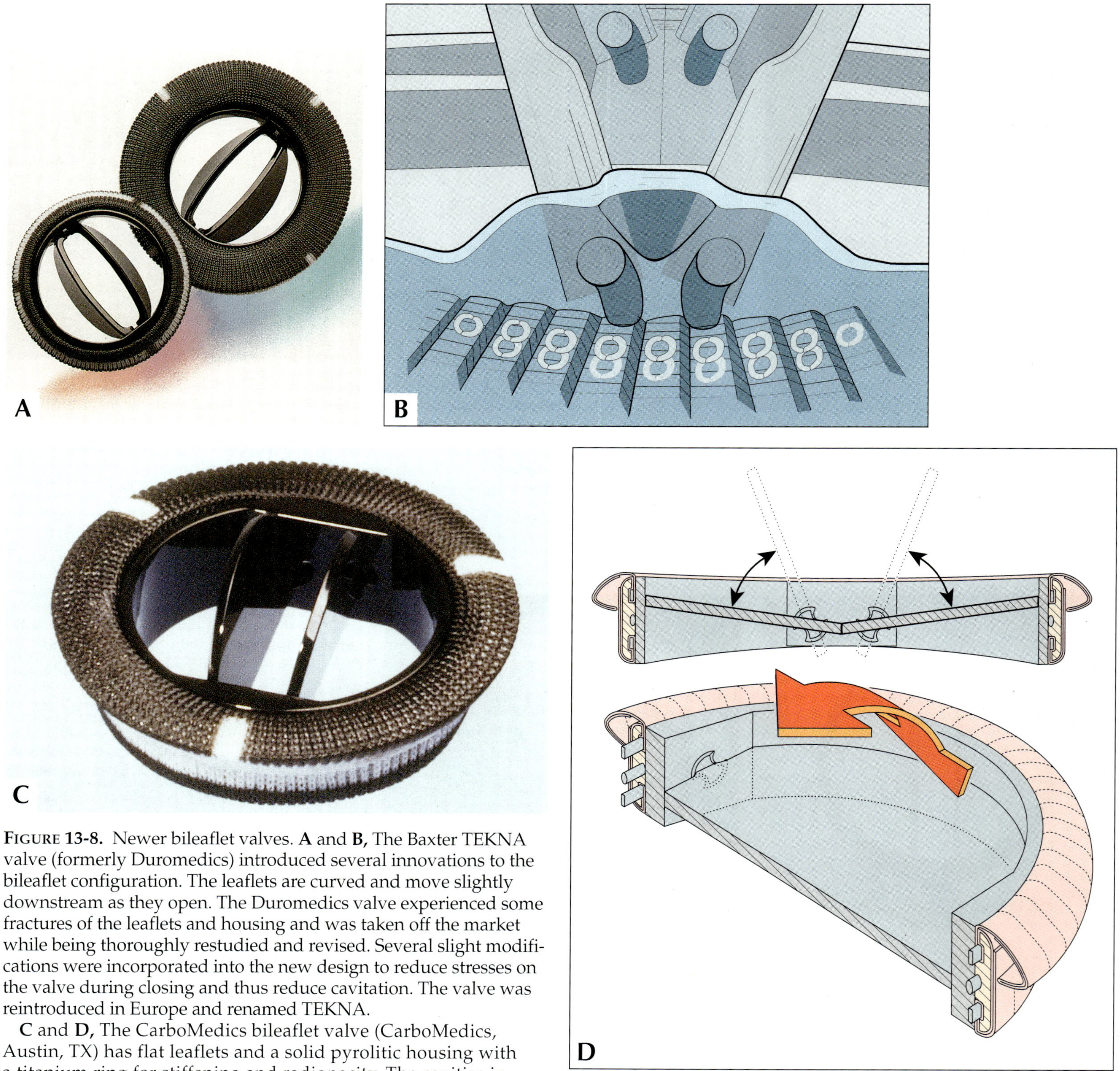

FIGURE 13-8. Newer bileaflet valves. **A** and **B,** The Baxter TEKNA valve (formerly Duromedics) introduced several innovations to the bileaflet configuration. The leaflets are curved and move slightly downstream as they open. The Duromedics valve experienced some fractures of the leaflets and housing and was taken off the market while being thoroughly restudied and revised. Several slight modifications were incorporated into the new design to reduce stresses on the valve during closing and thus reduce cavitation. The valve was reintroduced in Europe and renamed TEKNA.

C and **D,** The CarboMedics bileaflet valve (CarboMedics, Austin, TX) has flat leaflets and a solid pyrolitic housing with a titanium ring for stiffening and radiopacity. The cavities in the housing that contain the pivot recesses are located in the main body of the housing, rather than in the tabs that extend above the housing, and the leaflets themselves drop below in the open position. *(continued)*

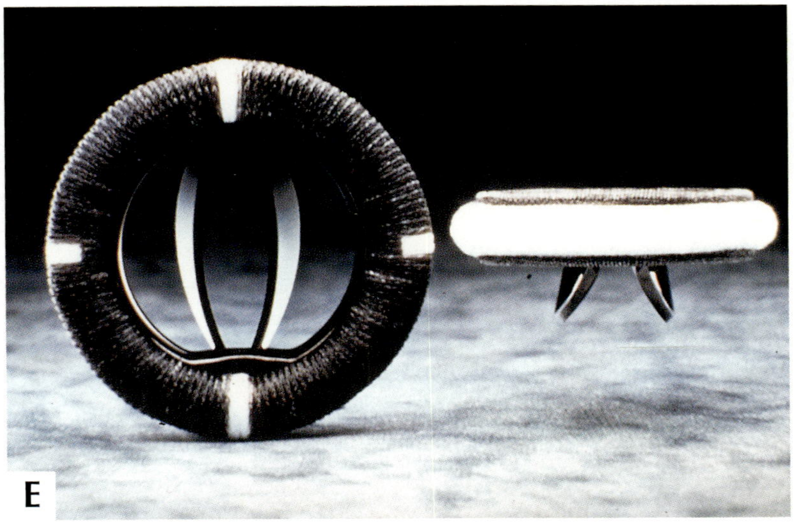

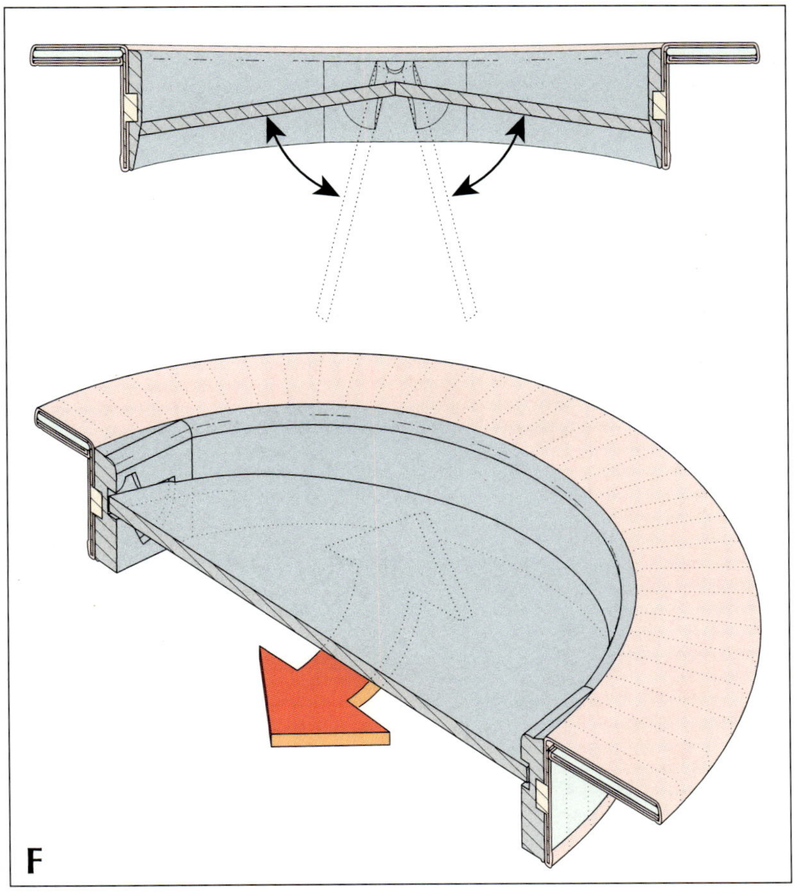

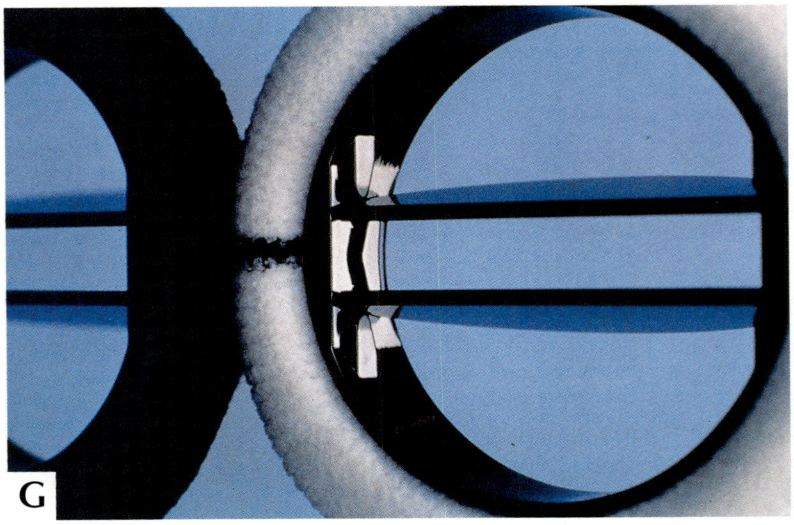

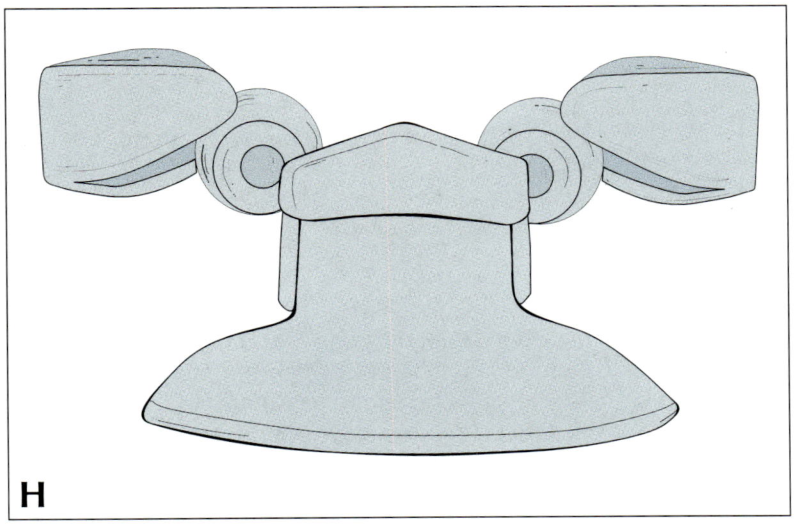

FIGURE 13-8. *(continued)* **E** and **F**, The Sorin Bicarbon bileaflet valve (Sorin Biomedica Cardio, Saluggia, Italy) has been in use for several years but not yet in the United States. It has a pyrolitic carbon-coated housing, but with a thin titanium substrate, rather than graphite, and a unique hinge mechanism that enforces a rolling, rather than sliding, motion.

G and **H**, Clinical use of the ATS Open Pivot valve (ATS Medical, Inc, Minneapolis, MN) has begun, and it is unique in that the "female" socket part of the hinge is located on the leaflet rather than in the housing. The "male" part of the hinge is a protrusion bump on the housing rather than a cavity on the leaflet. *(continued)*

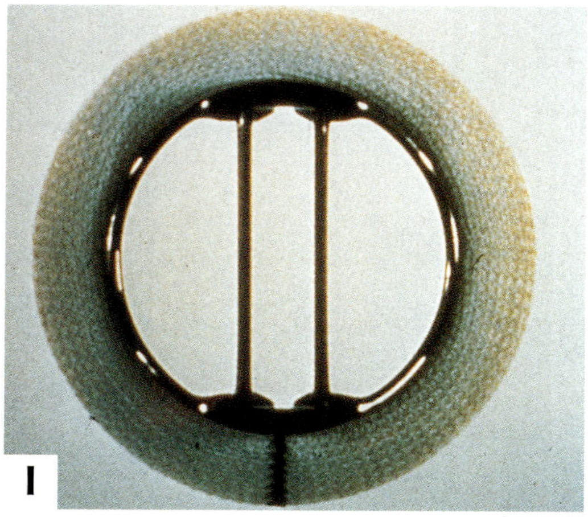

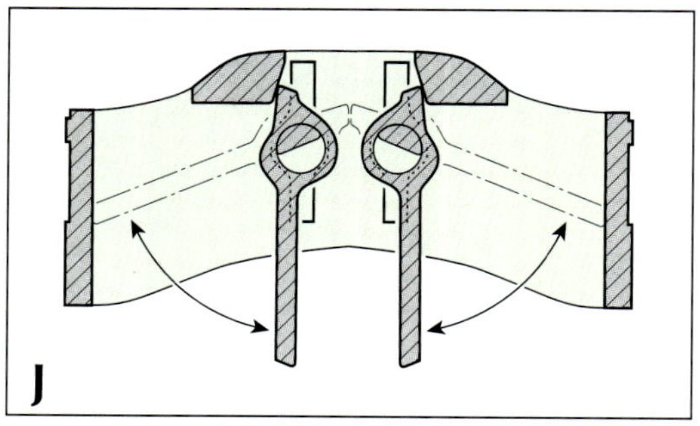

FIGURE 13-8. *(continued)* **I** and **J**, The Medtronic Parallel bileaflet valve (Medtronic, Inc, Minneapolis, MN) is unique in that the leaflets open at a 90° angle to the plane of the housing. (Note: Implants with the Medtronic Parallel valve were discontinued in January 1995, pending investigation of several cases of valvular thrombosis that occurred during the limited clinical study of this device.)

COMPARISON OF BILEAFLET VALVE FEATURES

Clinical usage	ST. JUDE	EDWARDS TEKNA	CARBOMEDICS	SORIN BICARBON	ATS OPEN PIVOT	MEDTRONIC PARALLEL
First implant	1977	1982	1986	1990	1992	1994?
Total (1000s)	500	24	78	8	1.3	0
Housing						
Solid carbon	no	yes	yes	no	yes	no
Stiffener ring	no	yes	yes	no	yes	yes
Seating lip	no	yes	no	yes	no	no
Rotatable	no	yes	yes	yes	yes	yes
Hinge socket	yes	yes	yes	yes	no	yes
Leaflets						
Curved	no	yes	no	yes	no	no
Translation	no	yes	no	yes	no	yes
Opening angle	85	77/73	80	80	85	90
Travel arc	55-60	62/58	55	55	60	50

FIGURE 13-9. Bileaflet valve comparison. The newest bileaflet valves vary with regard to several design features, and all are unique. We have included clinical performance material only for the St. Jude valve, for which a massive amount of information is available. But this table compares the design features (defined below) of the St. Jude valve with those of newer bileaflet valves. Many of these features have been associated with theoretical advantages, but they must still be proven clinically; often during the evolution of heart valve design, an "improved" version is no better and is sometimes worse, overall, than the "old" version.

The date of the first human implant was 1977. The approximate total number of valves (in thousands) implanted is usually estimated from sales figures or returned implant cards.

The housings of some bileaflet valves are solid pyrolitic carbon. Others have a core of graphite (Sorin uses a titanium alloy), which is coated with pyrolitic carbon.

The stiffener ring is either Stellite (TEKNA, Medtronic) or titanium (CarboMedics, ATS). Besides giving reinforcement to the housing, the stiffener ring also shields the housing from suture damage during implant and aids radiographic visualization. The Sorin valve has a more durable substrate material that may confer some of these advantages.

Most of the valves have a full-orifice leaflet seating design, where the leaflets fall entirely inside the housing (the projection of the closed leaflets onto the plane of the housing has a smaller diameter than the interior diameter of the housing). The TEKNA valve has a lip for the leaflets to seat against, while the Sorin leaflets seat on the outside edge of the housing, in an overlapping fashion. The full-orifice design may reduce gradients and closing impact, while the overlapping disk may produce less regurgitation and have less possibility for suture entrapment by the leaflets.

The hinge socket refers to the location of the female part of the hinge. The leaflets are a graphite substrate coated with pyrolitic carbon. The hinge mechanism of all except the ATS valve consists of a protrusion on the leaflet, which fits into a recessed cavity or socket in the housing. On the ATS valve, the housing contains the male part, and the socket is in the leaflet. In some valves, the leaflets merely pivot in the cavities, but the cavities of others (TEKNA, Medtronic) are elongated to allow a slight antegrade translation of the leaflets as they open. The Sorin valve leaflets have a "rolling" motion, which allows some translation.

The opening angle refers to the nominal degrees of maximum opening angle; the actual values for a particular valve may be 1° or 2° different. For the TEKNA valve, the aortic valve has a larger opening angle than the mitral valve. All the leaflets seat at a positive angle to the plane of the housing. Subtracting the closed angle from the fully open angle provides the degrees of arc through which the leaflet can swing from one extreme to the other. The St. Jude valve has different travel angles for different valve sizes.

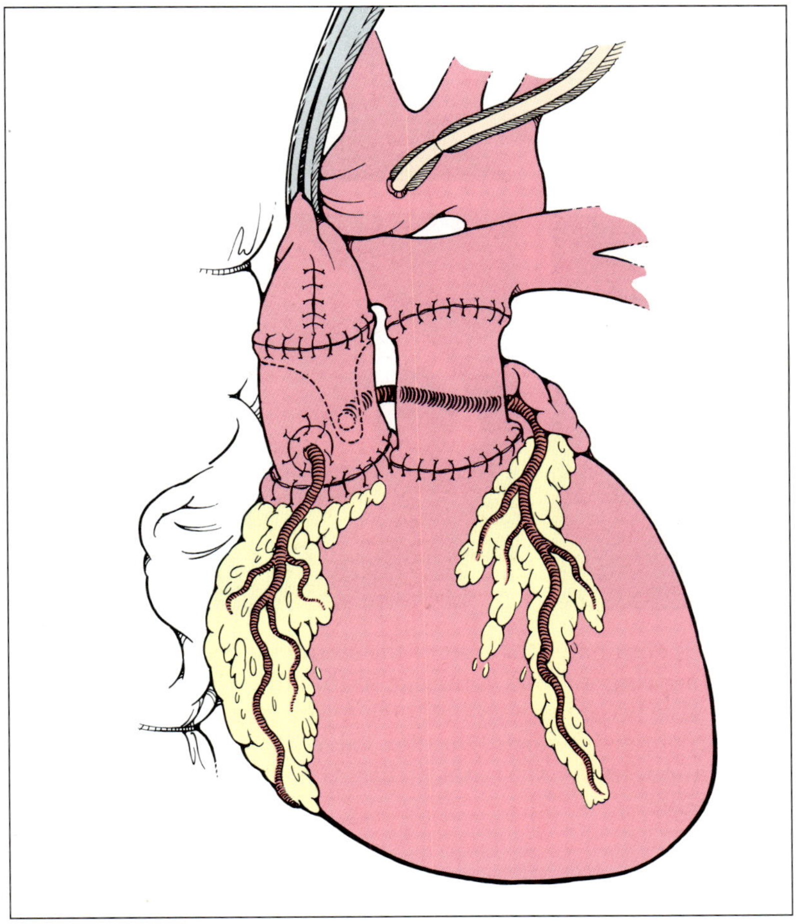

FIGURE 13-10. Homograft, autograft valves. The first successful valves of biologic origin were aortic homograft (or allograft) valves [5,6]. The homograft valve is acknowledged to be a preferred substitute for aortic valve replacement, with excellent hemodynamics, requiring no anticoagulation, and zero or low thrombogenicity. Pulmonary homografts have also been used to replace the aortic valve [7].

The pulmonary autograft aortic valve replacement (Ross) procedure was first reported in 1967 [8] and has recently undergone increased appreciation [9]. It consists of an autotransplant of the pulmonary valve to the aortic position, with the coronary arteries reimplanted into the new root, as shown. The pulmonary valve is then replaced by an aortic homograft, as shown here. A pulmonary homograft has also been used to replace the pulmonary valve [10].

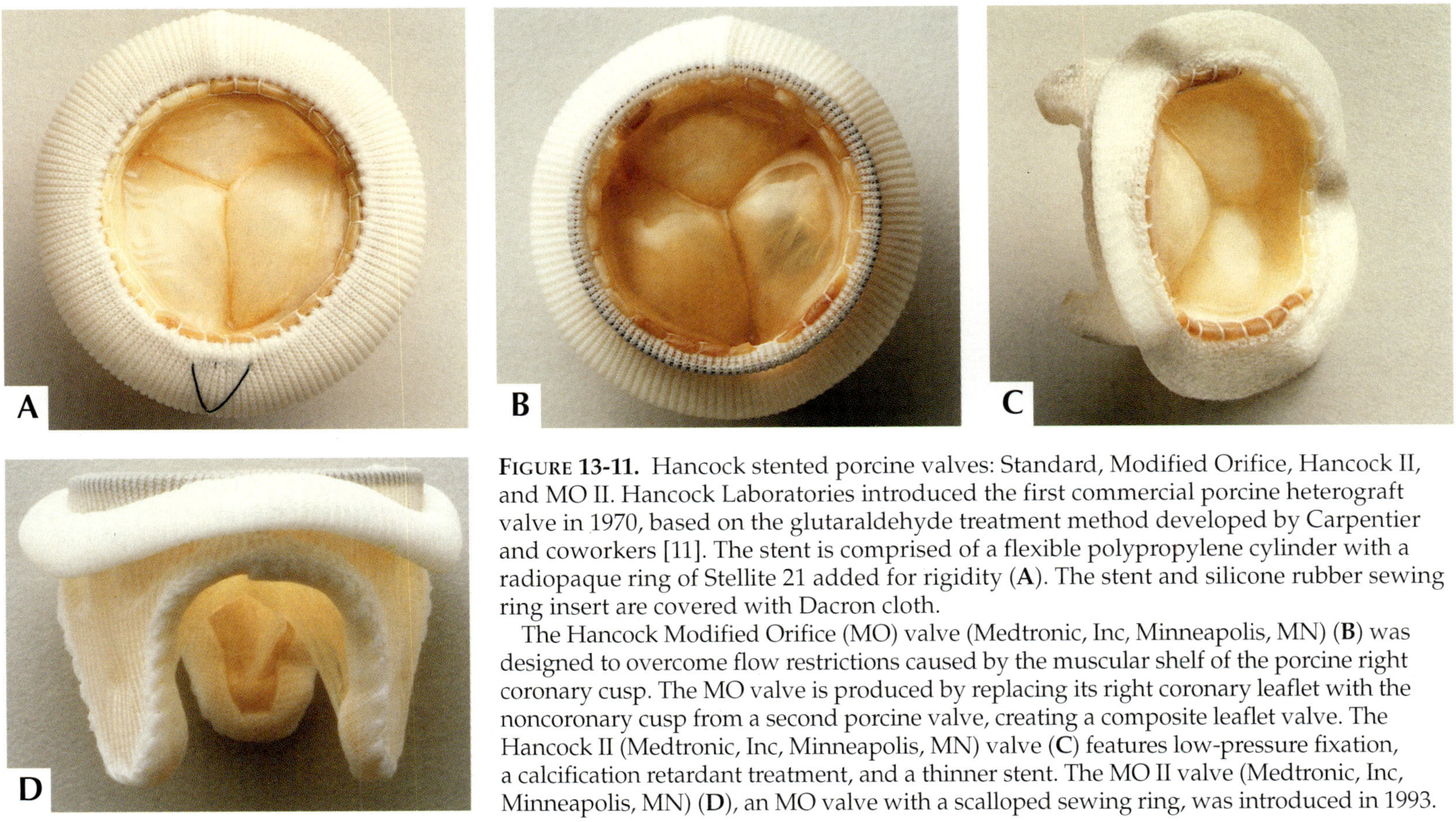

FIGURE 13-11. Hancock stented porcine valves: Standard, Modified Orifice, Hancock II, and MO II. Hancock Laboratories introduced the first commercial porcine heterograft valve in 1970, based on the glutaraldehyde treatment method developed by Carpentier and coworkers [11]. The stent is comprised of a flexible polypropylene cylinder with a radiopaque ring of Stellite 21 added for rigidity (**A**). The stent and silicone rubber sewing ring insert are covered with Dacron cloth.

The Hancock Modified Orifice (MO) valve (Medtronic, Inc, Minneapolis, MN) (**B**) was designed to overcome flow restrictions caused by the muscular shelf of the porcine right coronary cusp. The MO valve is produced by replacing its right coronary leaflet with the noncoronary cusp from a second porcine valve, creating a composite leaflet valve. The Hancock II (Medtronic, Inc, Minneapolis, MN) valve (**C**) features low-pressure fixation, a calcification retardant treatment, and a thinner stent. The MO II valve (Medtronic, Inc, Minneapolis, MN) (**D**), an MO valve with a scalloped sewing ring, was introduced in 1993.

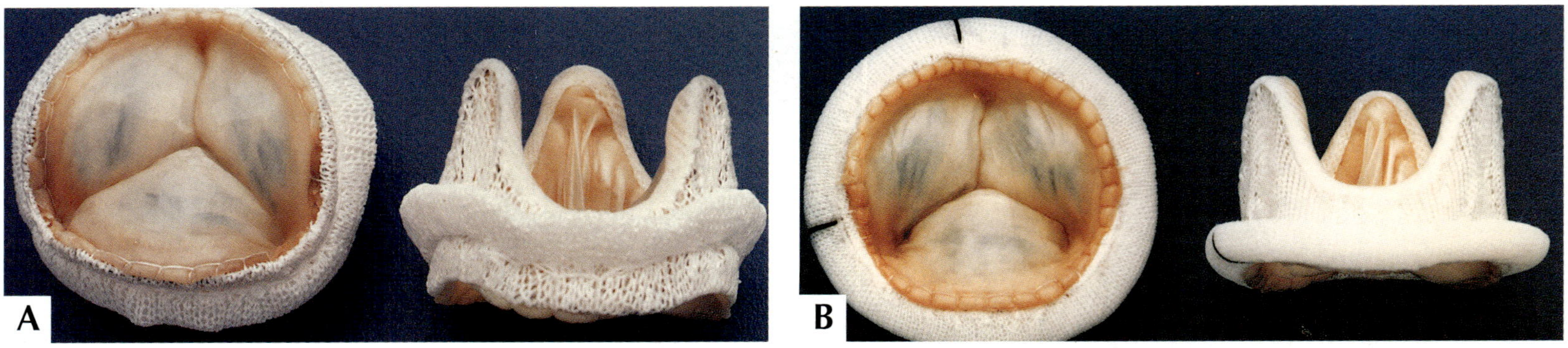

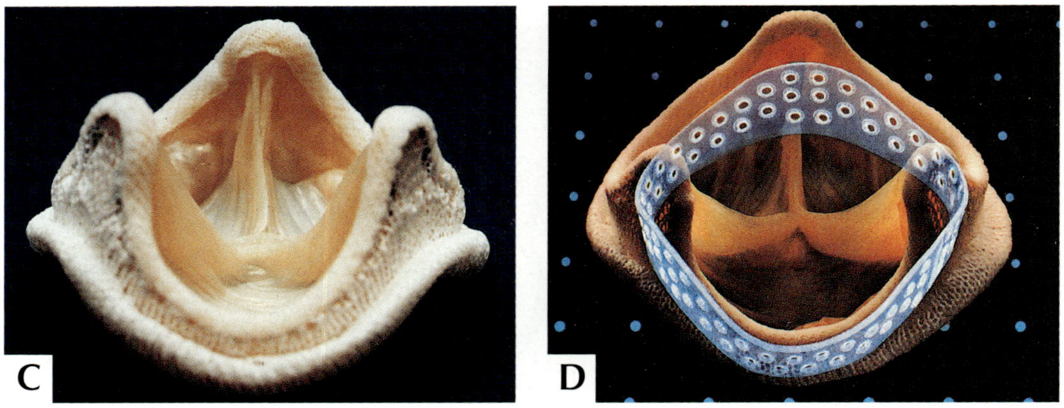

FIGURE 13-12. Carpentier-Edwards stented porcine valves: Standard, SAV, and Duraflex. The Carpentier-Edwards (Standard) (Baxter Healthcare Corporation, Irvine, CA) porcine bioprosthesis (**A** and **B**) was released for general marketing shortly after the Hancock valve. The frame of the valve is a flexible wire stent made of Elgiloy, intended to reduce stresses on the leaflets and orifice. A flexible Mylar cylinder surrounds and supports the Elgiloy frame. The annulus is asymmetrically shaped, to obliterate the septal ridge of the porcine right coronary cusp.

The sewing ring of the Carpentier-Edwards Supra Annular aortic valve (Baxter Healthcare Corporation, Irvine, CA) (**C** and **D**) has been redesigned for positioning above rather than within the annulus. Low-pressure fixation and a cone-shaped, flared stent have been used to improve leaflet durability. The sewing ring was reconfigured to originate from the bottom of the stent wall. This eliminates the part of the stent that protrudes below the sewing ring into the ventricle, so that the effective orifice of the valve becomes essentially the tissue annulus of the host. The Carpentier-Edwards Duraflex valve (Baxter Healthcare Corporation, Irvine, CA) (not pictured) is the low-pressure fixed mitral valve.

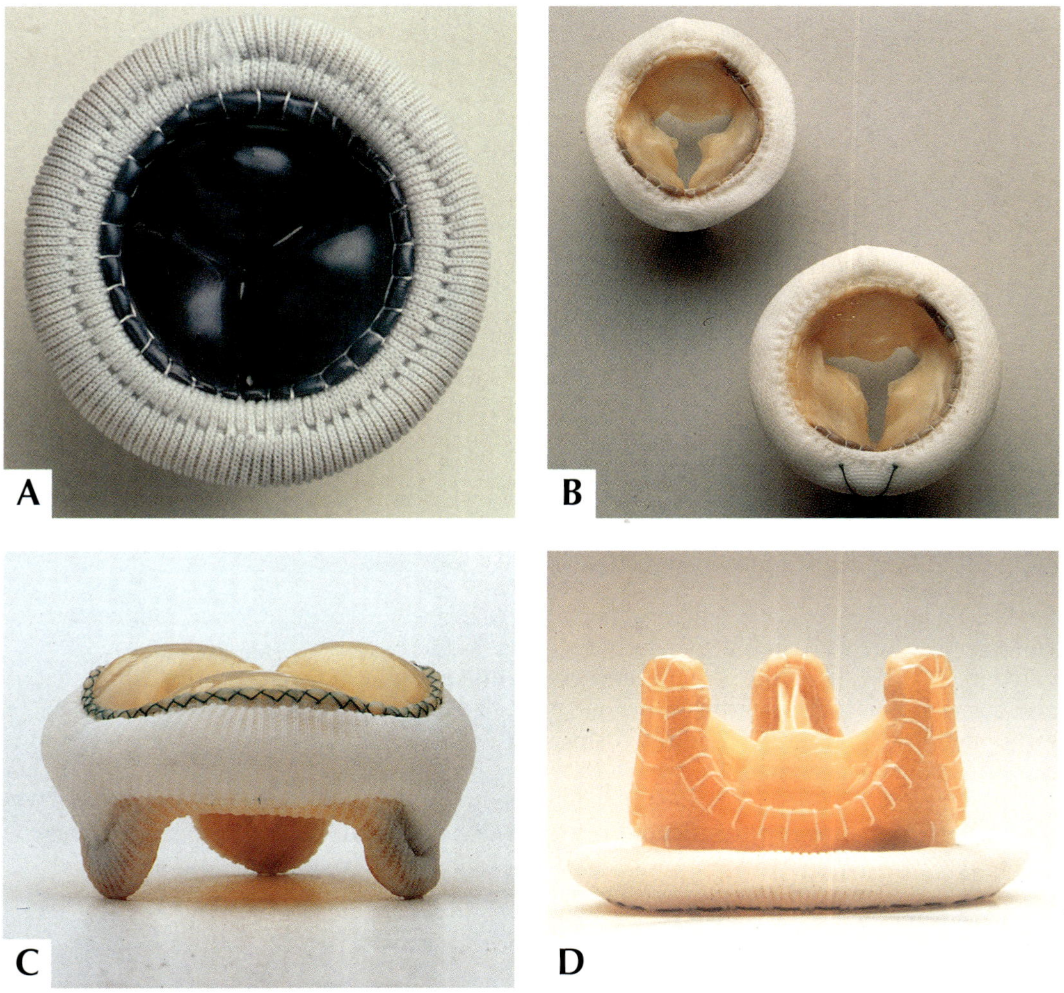

FIGURE 13-13. Other stented porcine valves: Intact, Mosaic, BioImplant, X-CELL, Biocor, and Bravo. Several other stented porcine valves are in use. The Medtronic Intact valve (Medtronic, Inc, Minneapolis, MN) (**A**) has a calcification retardant treatment that renders it blue. It is fixed at 0 mm pressure, leaving the leaflets thinner and more flexible, and sometimes causing a central hole to remain in the valve when it is in the natural, relaxed position. Medtronic has recently (1994) introduced the Mosaic valve (**B**) which features zero pressure fixation, a very thin stent, and an anticalcification treatment.

The St. Jude BioImplant valve (St. Jude Medical, Inc, St. Paul, MN) (**C**) is used internationally, and clinical investigation has begun on the X-cell porcine valve (**D**), developed jointly by St. Jude Medical and Hancock-Jaffe Laboratories. This valve incorporates an innovative process to eliminate calcification sites from the porcine tissue, sterilization by gamma irradiation, zero pressure fixation and a clothless stent. It also uses a composite leaflet arrangement in smaller sizes. (*continued*)

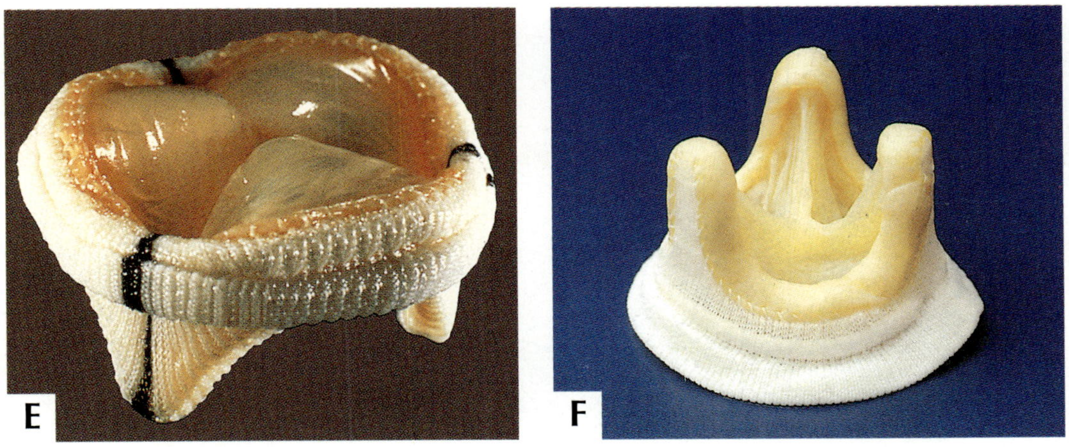

FIGURE 13-13. (*continued*) Biocor Industries of Brazil manufactures a supra-annular porcine valve with a flexible, low-profile stent (**E**). Bravo Cardiovascular (Vancouver, British Columbia) manufactures a stented porcine valve that is currently under clinical investigation (**F**).

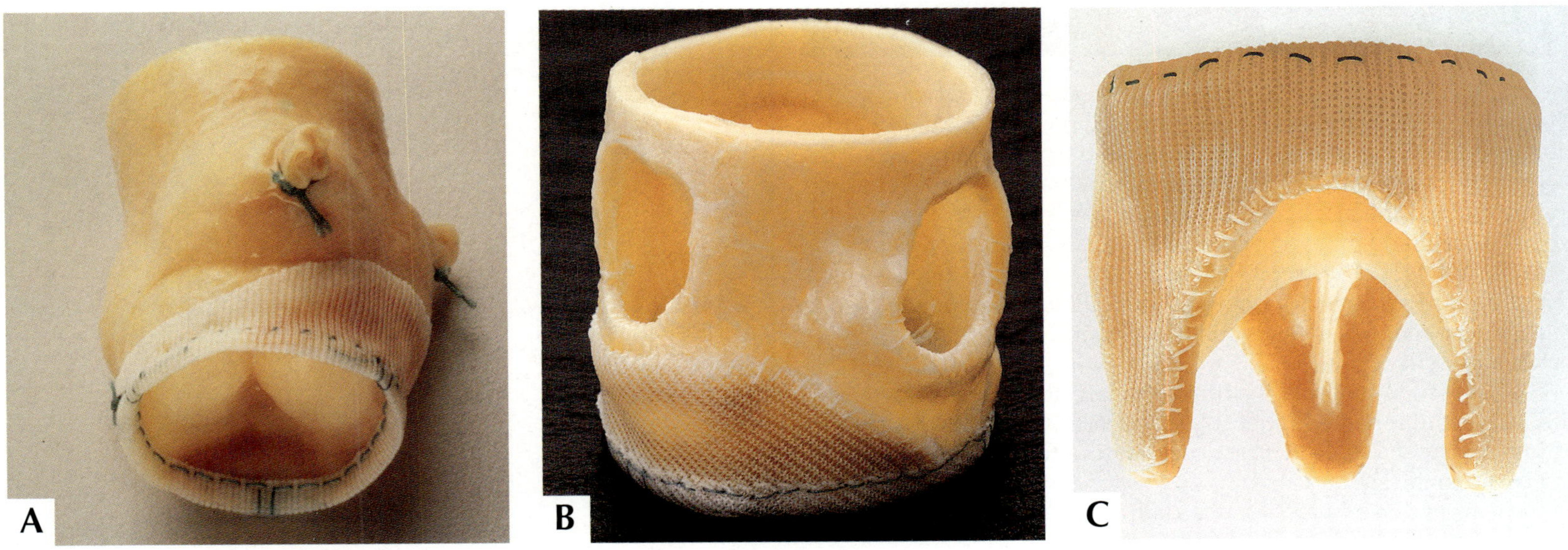

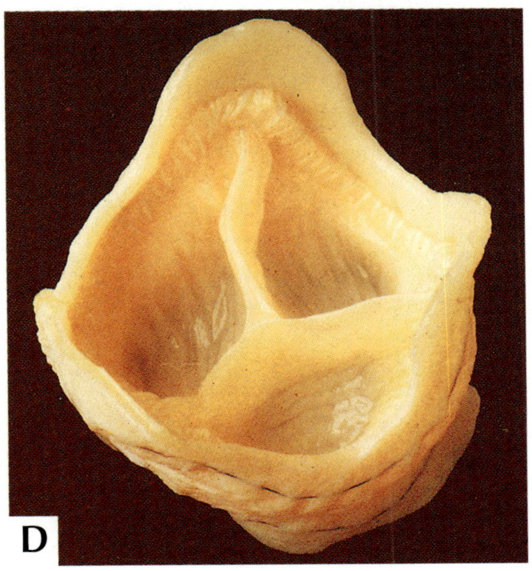

FIGURE 13-14. Stentless porcine valves: Baxter Edwards, Medtronic, St. Jude, and Biocor. To achieve some of the perceived benefits of homograft valves, but with an easily available, commercial product, stentless porcine aortic valves have been developed, and several are currently undergoing clinical testing.

The potential benefit is achieved at the expense of a more difficult implant technique compared to a stented porcine valve. There are three ways in which stentless porcine valves are used: as a conventional valve replacement, with the excised valve sewn into the subcoronary position in the host's aorta; as a mini-root replacement, with the donor aortic root inserted inside the host aorta (inclusion technique); and as a complete root replacement.

The Medtronic Freestyle (Medtronic, Inc, Minneapolis, MN) (**A**) can be implanted using any of the three techniques. The Edwards Prima (**B**) is designed for the mini-root technique, although it has been used with the other techniques. The St. Jude Medical Toronto SPV (**C**) and the Biocor stentless valve (**D**) are used only as subcoronary valve replacements. Bravo Cardiovascular has also developed a stentless aortic valve (not shown).

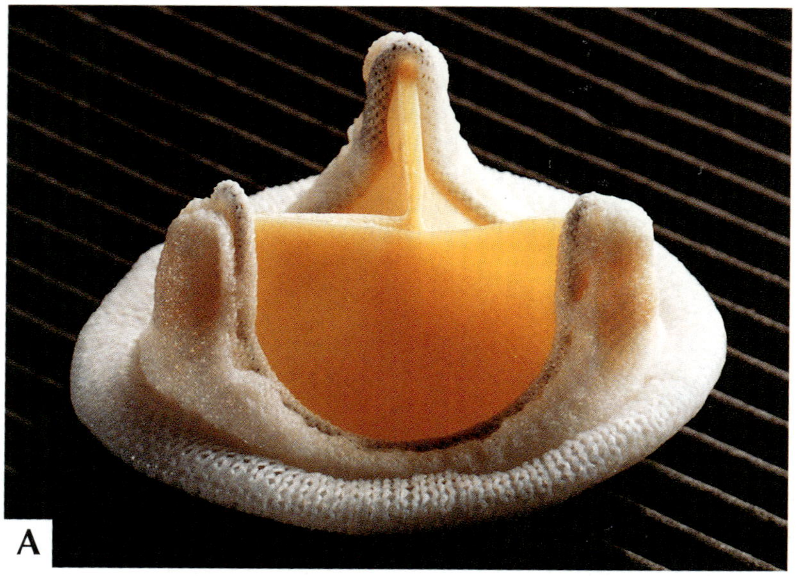

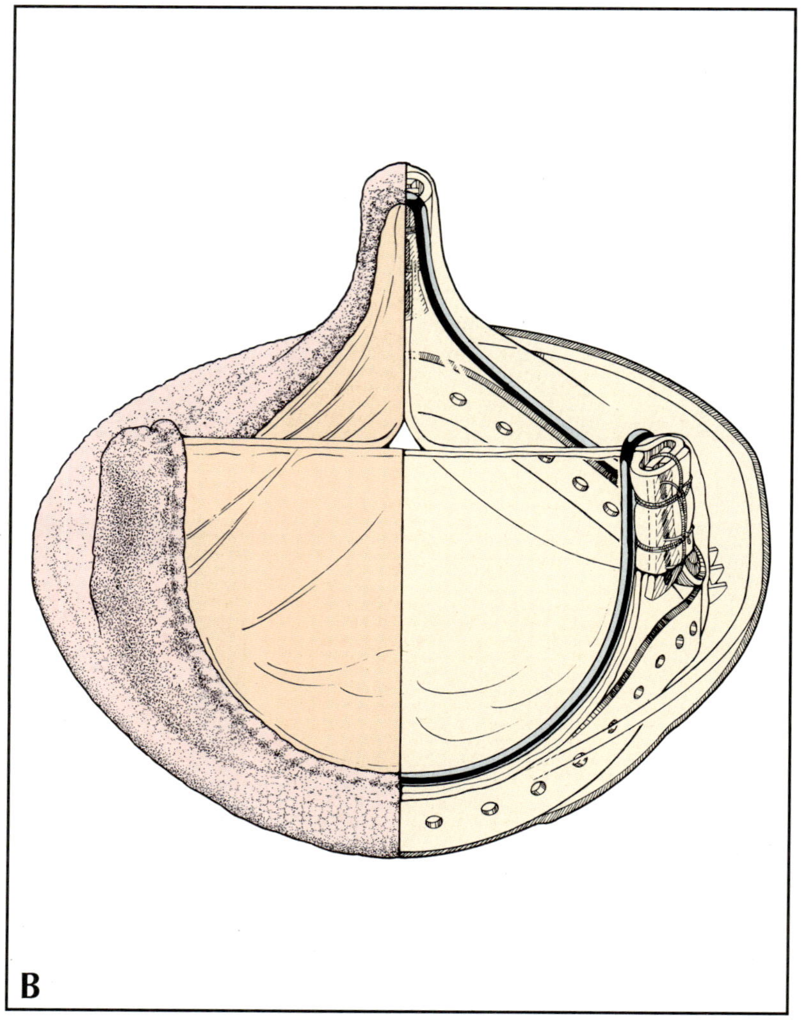

FIGURE 13-15. Bovine pericardial valves: Carpentier-Edwards, Mitroflow, and Sorin Pericarbon. Pericardial valves, unlike porcine valves, are fabricated rather than harvested directly. Although there are theoretical reasons why pericardium should be inferior to porcine leaflets [12], there are also persuasive arguments to be made in favor of pericardium as a material for valve construction [13]. The theoretical advantages include a more complete and symmetric opening, for better hemodynamics, and a higher percentage of collagen than in porcine valve tissue, for better durability.

The Ionescu-Shiley was the first commercially available pericardial valve, but it had a higher than expected rate of structural failure, partly due to leaflet tears originating from a stitch that held the tissue to the stent post.

The Carpentier-Edwards pericardial bioprosthesis (Baxter Healthcare, Inc, Irvine, CA) (**A**) received Food and Drug Administration approval in 1991, after 10 years of clinical use. It uses a method of mounting the leaflets to the stent that does not depend on retaining stitches penetrating the leaflet material (**B**).

The Mitroflow pericardial valve (Mitroflow International, Inc, Richmond, British Columbia) (**C**) also uses a method of mounting the leaflets that eliminates stitches through the leaflets. The Sorin Pericarbon valve (Sorin Biomedica Cardio, Saluggia, Italy) (**D**) has a pyrolitic-coated sewing ring and also comes in a stentless version.

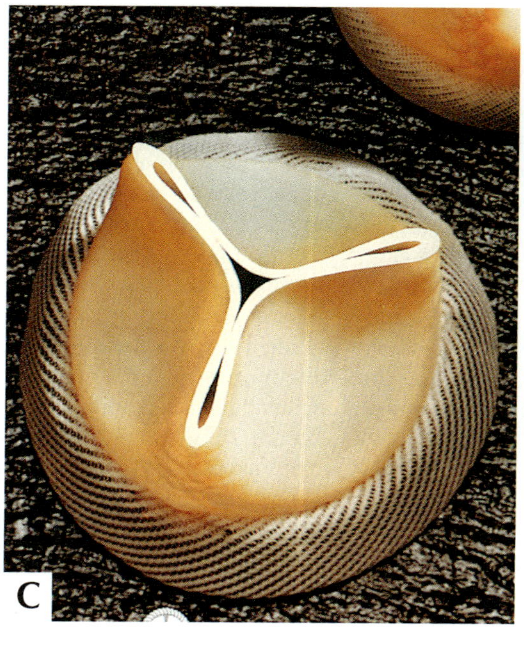

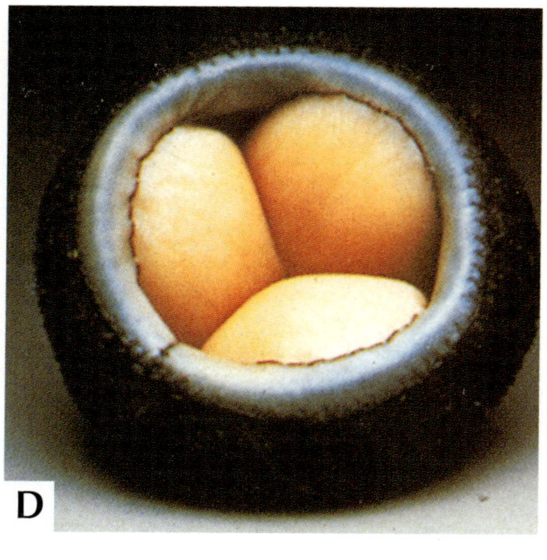

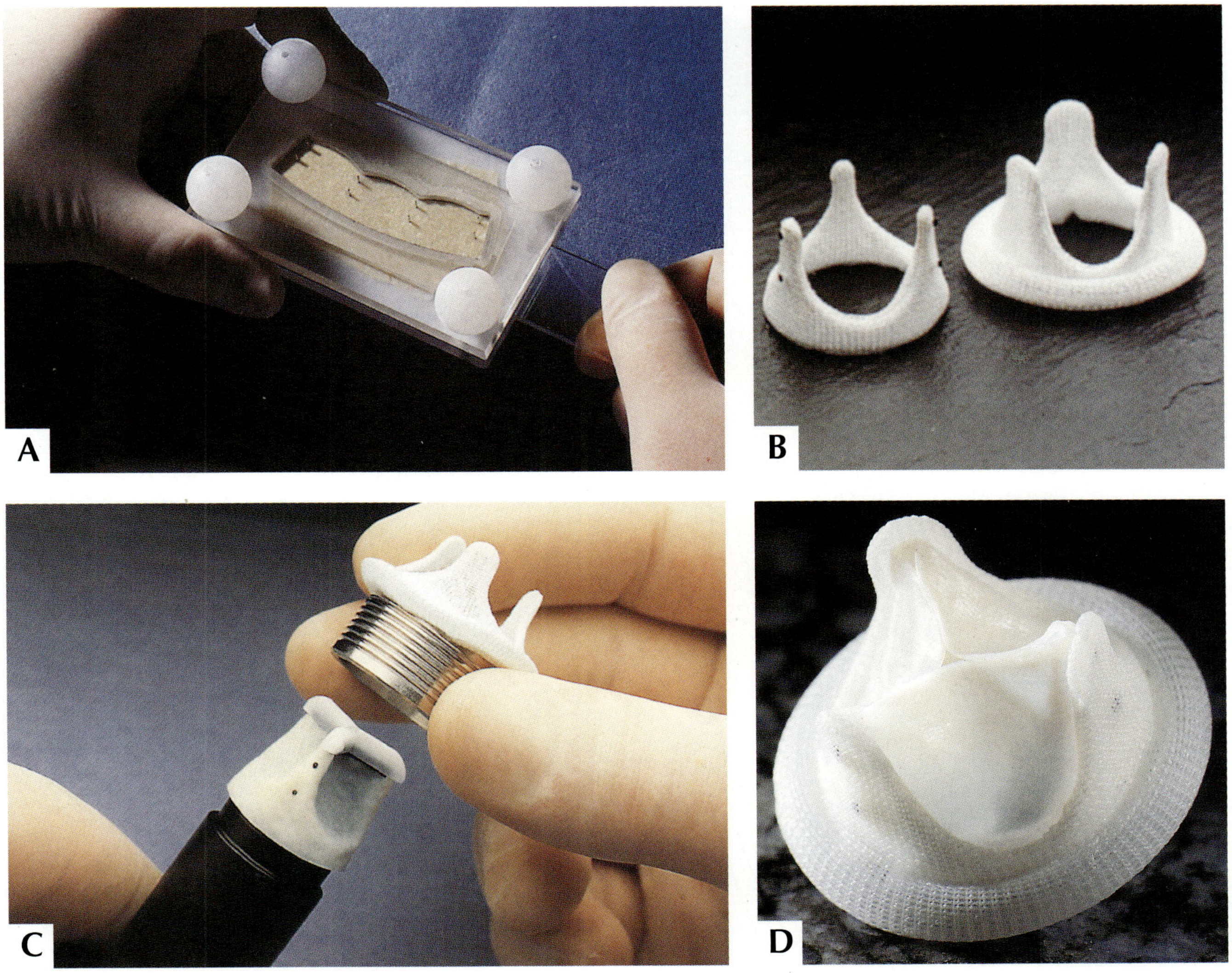

FIGURE 13-16. Autogenics autologous pericardial valve. A novel solution to aortic valve replacement has recently been developed by Love [13] and is being investigated by Autogenics. This is an attempt to combine the reproducibility and easy insertion of a commercial, stented valve, with the obvious benefits of autologous tissue: a frame-mounted autologous pericardial valve. The kit supplied contains the tools to create the valve in a few minutes: a cutting tool for obtaining a precisely shaped piece of tissue (**A**), a two-piece frame that snaps together around the tissue (**B**), and holders to align the two pieces for assembly (**C**). The completed valve is shown in **D**. The kit also contains a disposable acceptance test device (not shown) for evaluating flow and regurgitation of the valve before insertion.

Valve Replacement Procedure

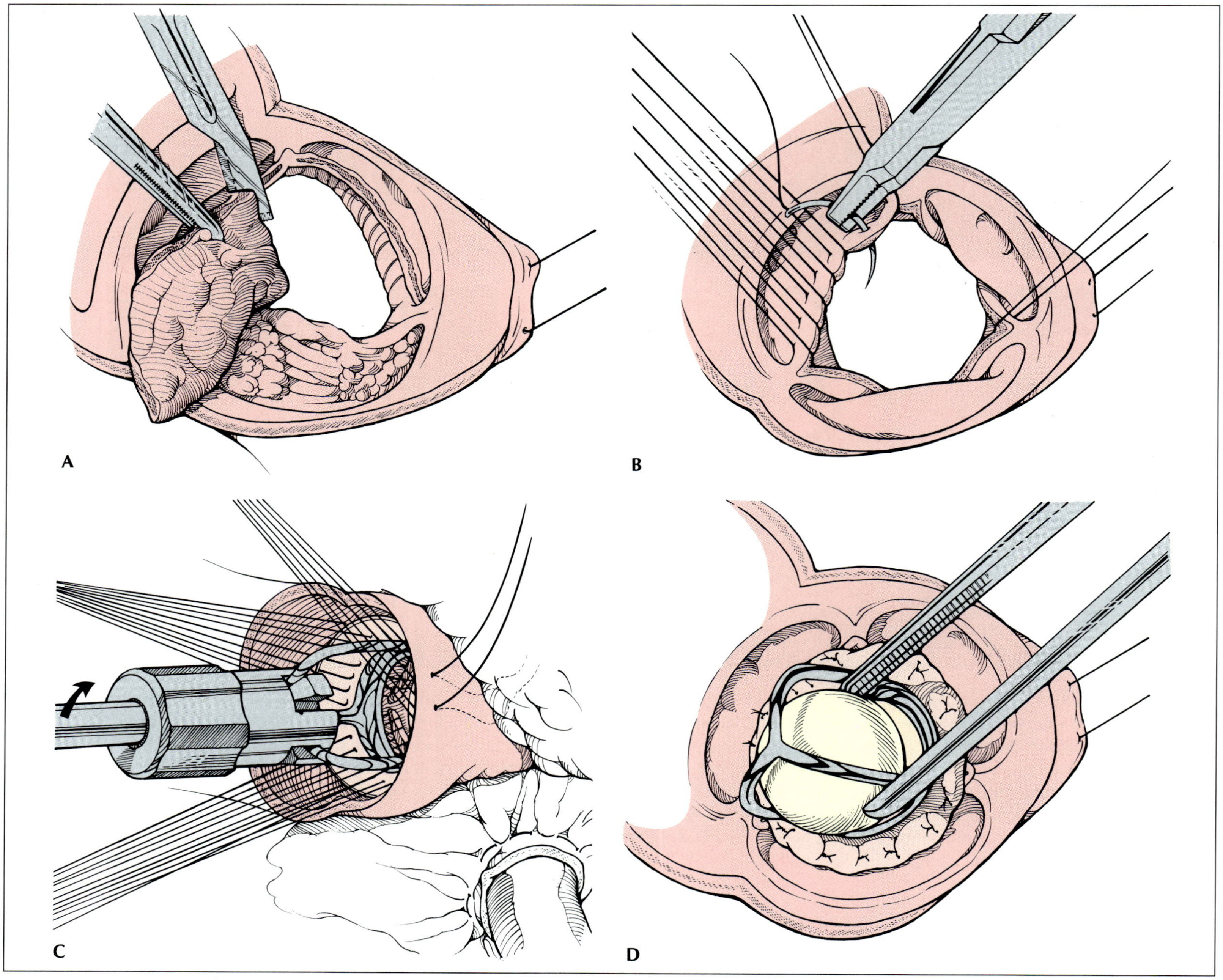

Figure 13-17. Aortic valve replacement. Valve excision. The diseased valve is exposed by a transverse aortotomy. The diseased leaflets are removed using serrated valve scissors and a no. 15 blade (**A**). Residual deposits must be carefully removed or reduced in size with a pituitary rongeur and a no. 15 blade to allow proper seating of the prosthesis.

For valve insertion, simple sutures are passed through the annulus in a clockwise direction, from six to nine sutures along each section of the annulus (**B**). The correctly sized valve, from which the Silastic ball has been removed, is attached to the holder and oriented so that the three struts of the cage align with the three commissures. The valve is seated by sliding it down the sutures. The valve is tipped forward as it slips into the aortic root (*arrow*, **C**) to avoid trauma to the cut edge of the aortotomy. Knots are tied, each in the order of placement. The ball is reinserted into its cage (**D**).

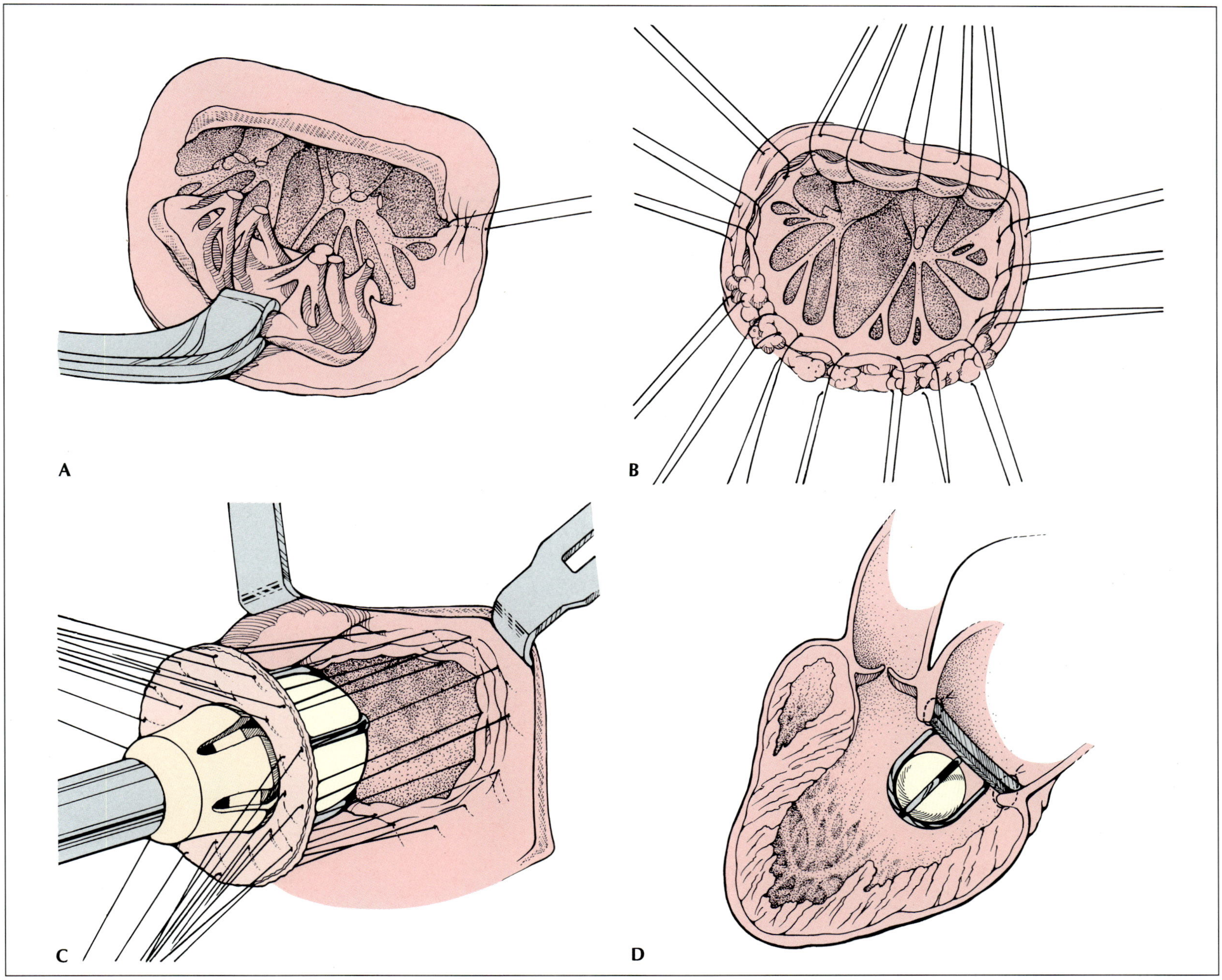

FIGURE 13-18. Mitral valve replacement. The mitral valve is always evaluated for the possibility of repair rather than replacement. When replacement is deemed necessary, a safe line of excision is identified that leaves a 5- to 10-mm margin of tissue inside the annulus to buttress the sutures. The excision is started along this line in the center of the anterior leaflet and extended in both directions. A clamp is used to grasp and invert the leaflet and allow inspection of the subvalvular structures to determine how much, if any, of the mural leaflet must be removed (**A**).

For valve insertion, the first suture is placed at the posteromedial commissure, from which two series of simple sutures are placed, first clockwise, and then counterclockwise, which meet at the anterolateral commissure (**B**). These sutures are then passed through the sewing ring of the correctly sized prosthesis, which is then lowered into position (**C**) and the knots securely tied (**D**).

In Vitro Performance of Mechanical Heart Valves

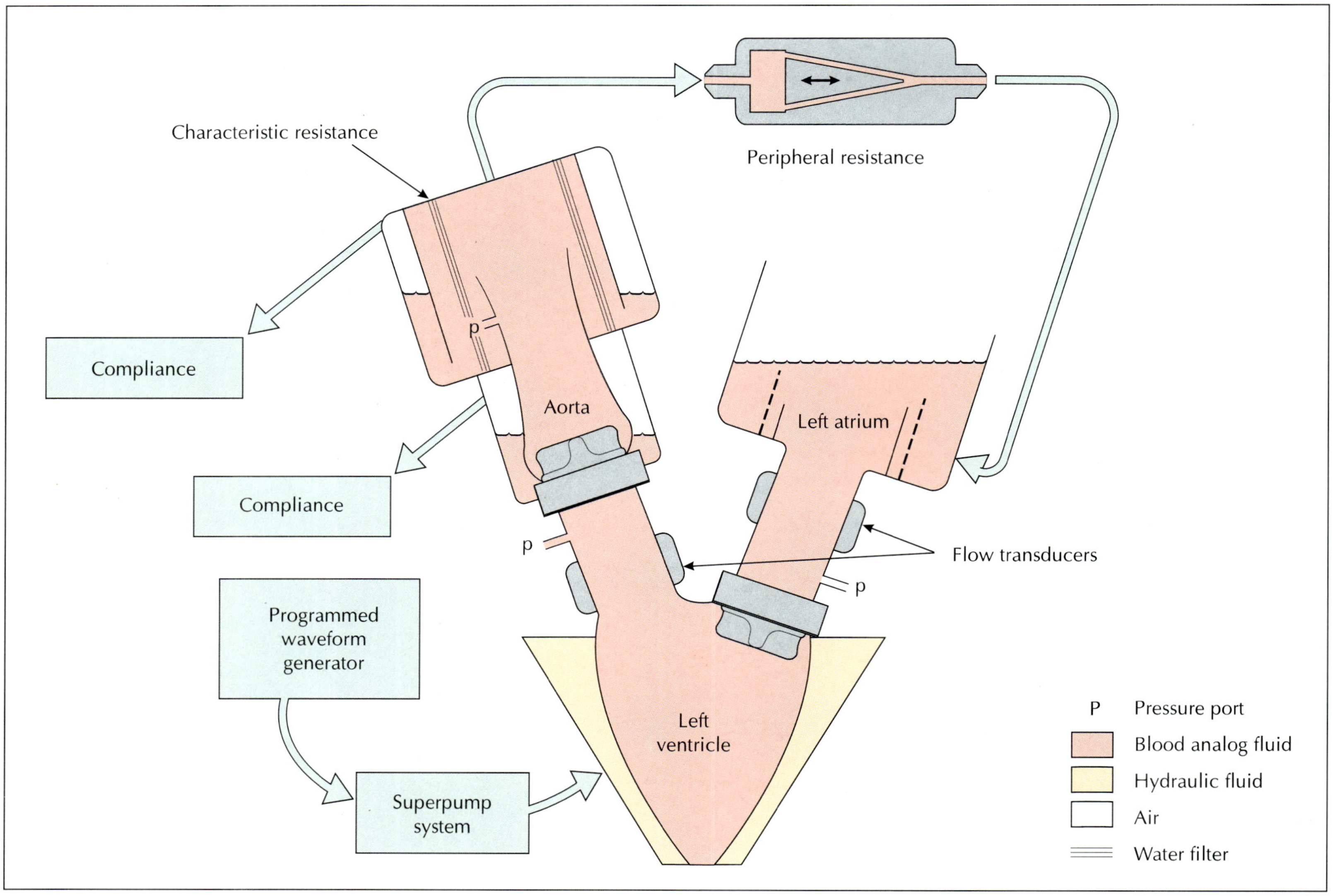

Figure 13-19. Vivitro Systems' pulse duplicator test apparatus. Vivitro Systems, Inc, in Victoria, British Columbia has for years specialized in the *in vitro* evaluation of heart valve hemodynamics. They perform valve testing for science and industry and also design and build pulse duplicators for customers around the world. Their comparative data on current mechanical valves have been put into a data base (VBase) that is commercially available as a reference tool for clinicians, valve manufacturers, valve designers, and regulatory agencies [14]. Shown is a schematic representation of their Model SD6891heart valve function test apparatus. This test system generates a range of pulsatile flows and pressures under which heart valve performance can be tested and compared. This system is computer driven and anatomically designed including simulation of a compliant aorta. Protocols for testing forward flow and closing performance and energy loss are computer programmed, and reports, including graphics, are automatically produced. *In vitro* valve performance data have the disadvantage that they may not perfectly simulate the *in vivo* performance but the advantage of a consistent testing platform for each valve.

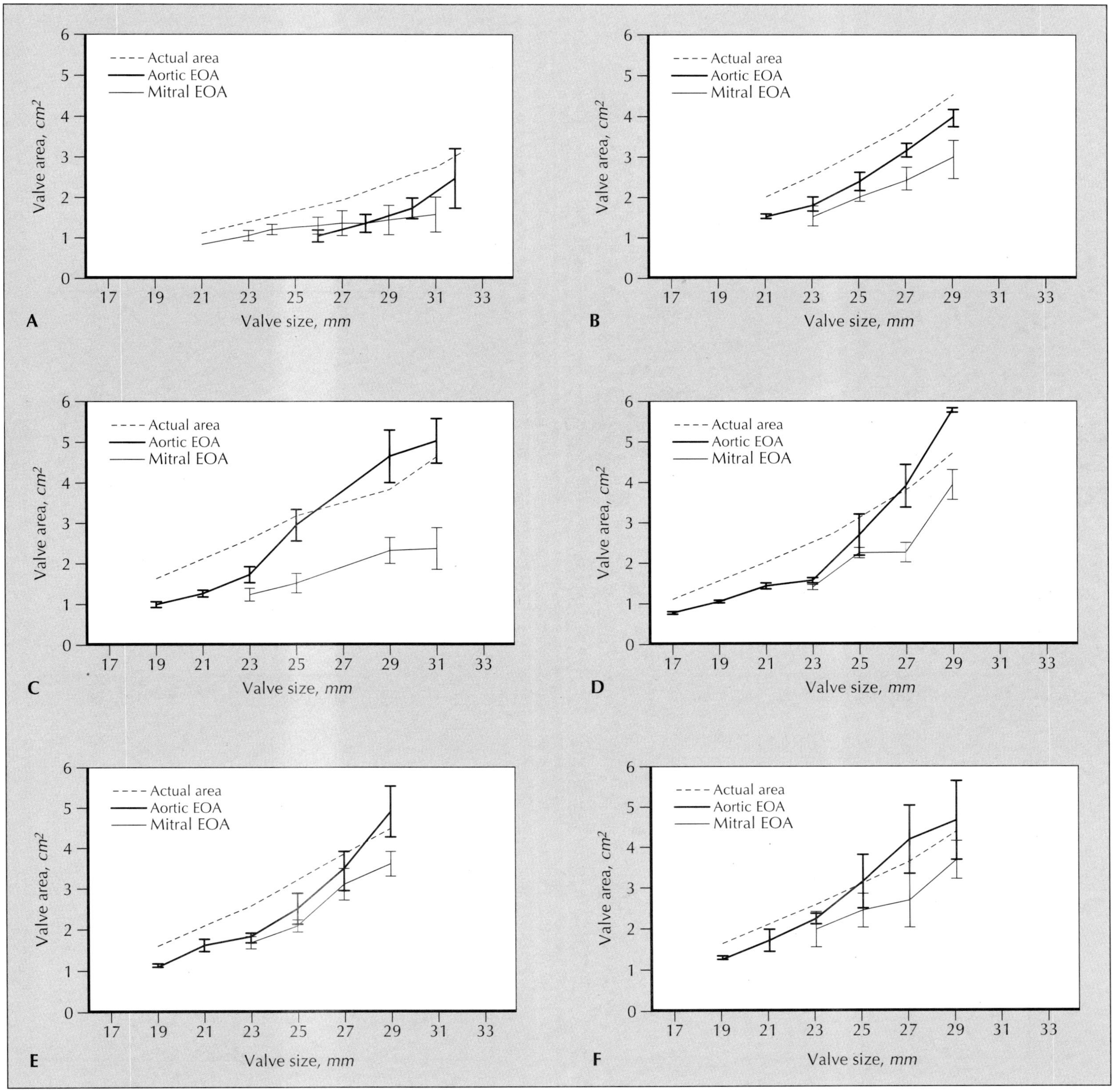

FIGURE 13-20. Forward flow comparison: effective orifice area (EOA) of mechanical prosthetic heart valves. **A** through **F** summarize the results for EOA with different sizes of mechanical valves from six manufacturers, tested in the aortic and mitral positions, over a range of test conditions.

The EOA is automatically determined using an equation analogous to the Gorlin formula. Mean EOA was calculated for 16 different flow conditions, ranging from flow rates of 2 to 9 L/min and heart rates from 45 to 160 beats/min for one valve of each size in each test position. (In some cases there were fewer than 16 valid results.) These graphs include data from more than 900 experiments. The vertical bars indicate plus and minus 1 standard deviation (SD) of the resulting EOAs for each test condition. The SDs are small for the smaller sized valves, indicating less flow and rate dependence of EOA than for larger size valves.

The manufacturers' quoted primary (geometric) orifice area is, as expected, usually greater than the EOA. For a given valve size, EOA for the mitral position is usually less than for the same valve functioning in the aortic position. This has been found to be true in other *in vitro* and *in vivo* valve studies and may be related to less pressure recovery occurring in the mitral site than in the aortic [14]. (*Adapted from* Scotten and Walker [14].)

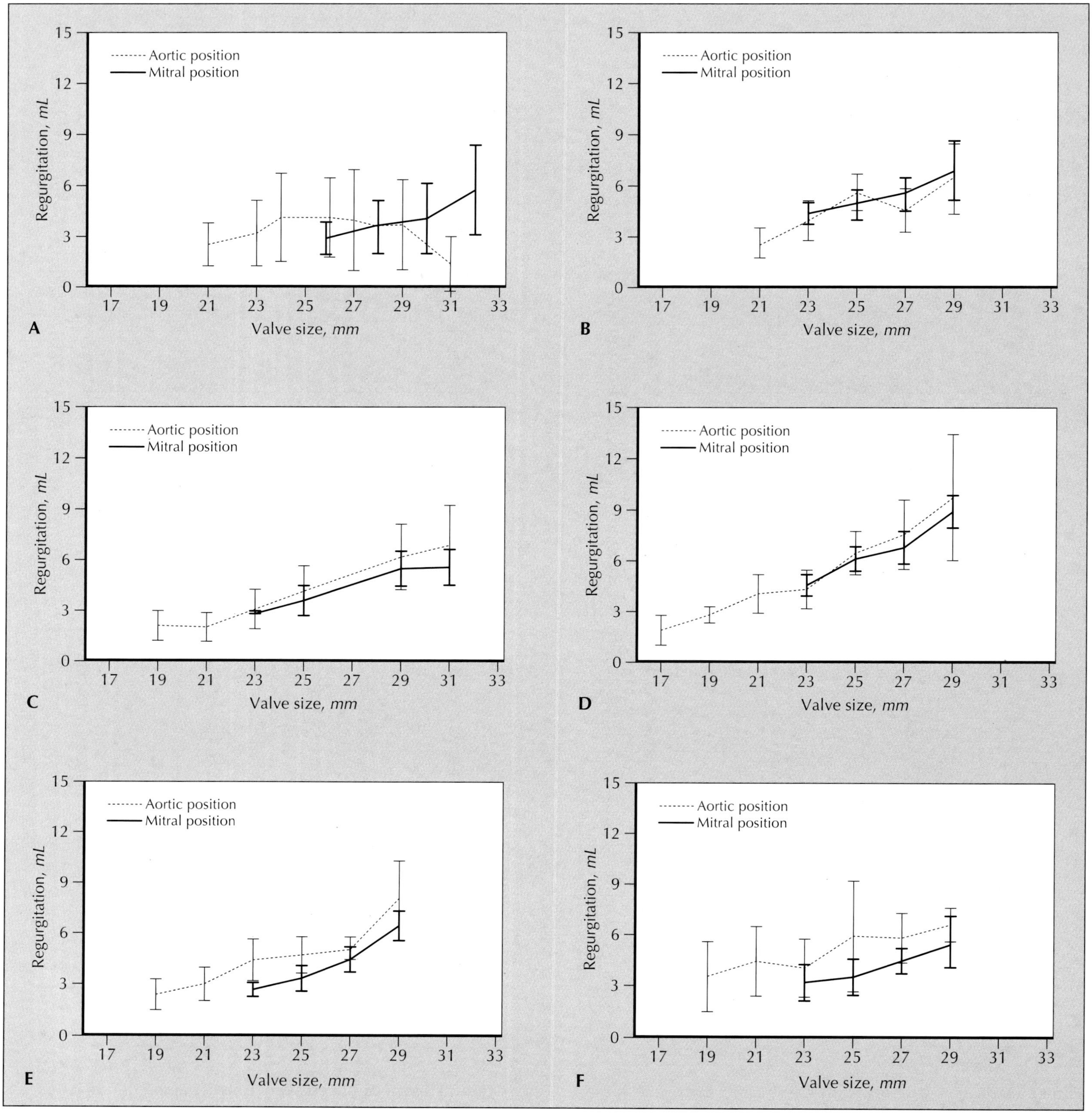

FIGURE 13-21. Total regurgitation (static and dynamic) from pulsatile flow testing. These charts summarize the results for regurgitation, static and dynamic combined, with different sizes of mechanical valves from six manufacturers, tested in the aortic and mitral positions, over a range of test conditions. (*Adapted from* Scotten and Walker [14].)

THROMBOEMBOLISM, THROMBOSIS, AND BLEEDING

CLINICAL MATERIAL FROM LITERATURE REVIEW

	POSITION*	REPORTS	PATIENTS	PATIENT-YEARS
Mechanical				
Starr-Edwards	A	6	3,609	16,876
	M	7	4,112	22,226
	D	2	503	2063
Bjork-Shiley/Sorin	A	13	3394	13,228
	M	16	3853	16,213
	D	4	1227	6364
Medtronic Hall	A	6	2193	8520
	M	6	2217	8043
	D	5	950	3748
St. Jude	A	10	3893	9374
	M	11	2524	6673
	D	3	300	956
Porcine				
Hancock	A	12	3576	11,744
	M	17	4503	17,809
	D	3	137	993
Carpentier-Edwards	A	11	3342	16,835
	M	11	3508	16,954
	D	6	761	2873

FIGURE 13-22. Total reported experience. This table summarizes comparative clinical data for a subset of the heart valves described earlier, based on a review of their long-term performance from published series [15]. Only valves currently in widespread use are included, except for the Bjork-Shiley valves, which are included because of the large amount of published data available, and the fact that a modified version (Monostrut, Sorin Biomedica Cardio, Saluggia, Italy) is in current use, but with limited available data. The results with the Bjork-Shiley Standard, Convexo-Concave, and Monostrut valves are combined in the figures, because there are relatively few reports with the latter two, and the valves are similar in design. For this same reason, reports with the Carpentier-Edwards Standard and Supra Annular porcine valves were combined. The selected series contained 44,000 valves contributing 180,000 valve-years of follow-up experience.

Summary statistics used for thromboembolism, thrombosis, and bleeding are "linearized" rates, which are based on the assumption of a constant risk. Linearized rates are widely used in the cardiac surgical literature and may be approximately valid for making broad comparisons of most of the complications reviewed here. A linearized rate is calculated as the number of events divided by total patient-years and multiplied by 100 to convert it to units of "events per 100 years" or "percent per year." Linearized rates are useful for summary and comparison; nevertheless, they must be used with caution because the risk may not be constant. A–aortic; D–double valve replacement; M–mitral. (*Adapted from* Grunkemeier and coworkers [15].)

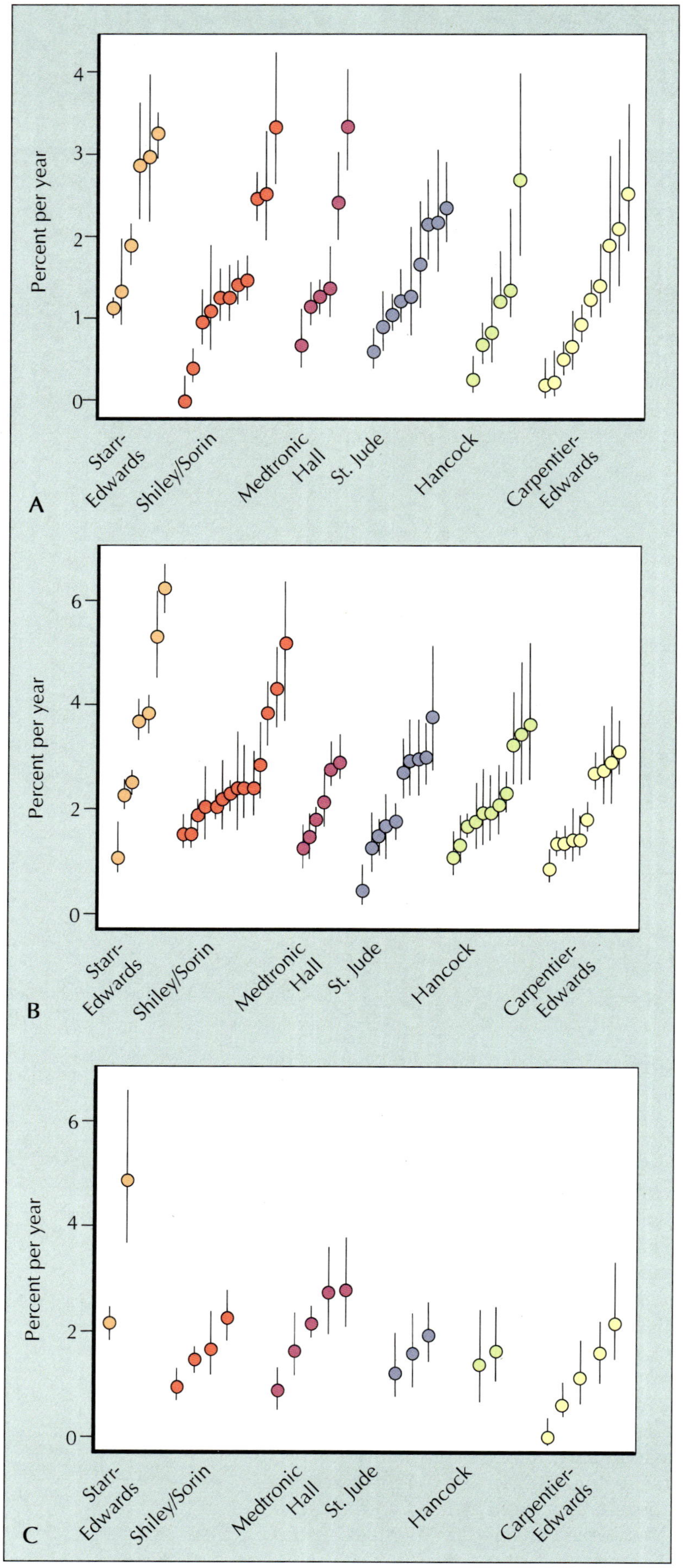

FIGURE 13-23. Comparative thromboembolism rates. Comparative thromboembolism rates are shown for isolated aortic (**A**), mitral (**B**), and double (**C**) valve replacement with mechanical and porcine valves. Each symbol represents a series, with the height of the symbol equal to the thromboembolism rate, and the vertical line indicating the 70% confidence interval. The scatter among series with each valve type is large and most valve types include series near the top and bottom of the range. This suggests that the observed rates must be largely due to factors that are not related to the valve itself, such as variability among patients, anticoagulation management, and methods of data collection and reporting. This hypothesis (that thromboembolism is not primarily device related) is further supported by the fact that embolism rates for double valve replacement are less than the sum of aortic plus mitral rates and are in fact similar to the rates with isolated valve replacement. (*Adapted from* Grunkemeier and coworkers [15].)

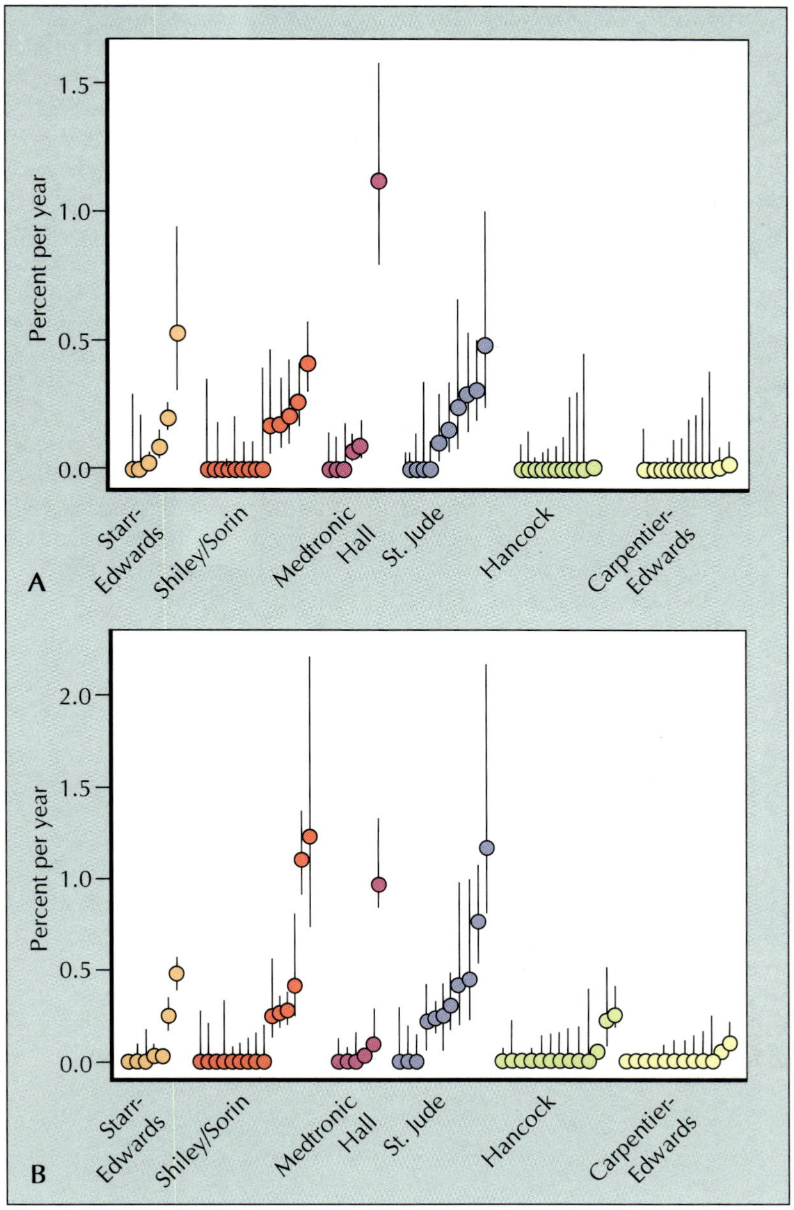

FIGURE 13-24. Comparative thrombosis rates. Comparative rates of valve thrombosis are shown for isolated aortic (**A**) and mitral (**B**) valve replacement with mechanical and porcine valves. Although thrombosis does occur with biologic valves, it is relatively rare, and the majority of series have none, especially in the aortic position. Thrombosis is a relatively rare but important complication, because it leads to reoperation or death. Its presentation varies qualitatively among valve designs: in the ball valve it is usually gradual over the course of weeks, whereas with the disk and leaflet valves it can occur suddenly. Bileaflet valves have an advantage in that one leaflet can be frozen by thrombus while the other remains movable. (*Adapted from* Grunkemeier and coworkers [15].)

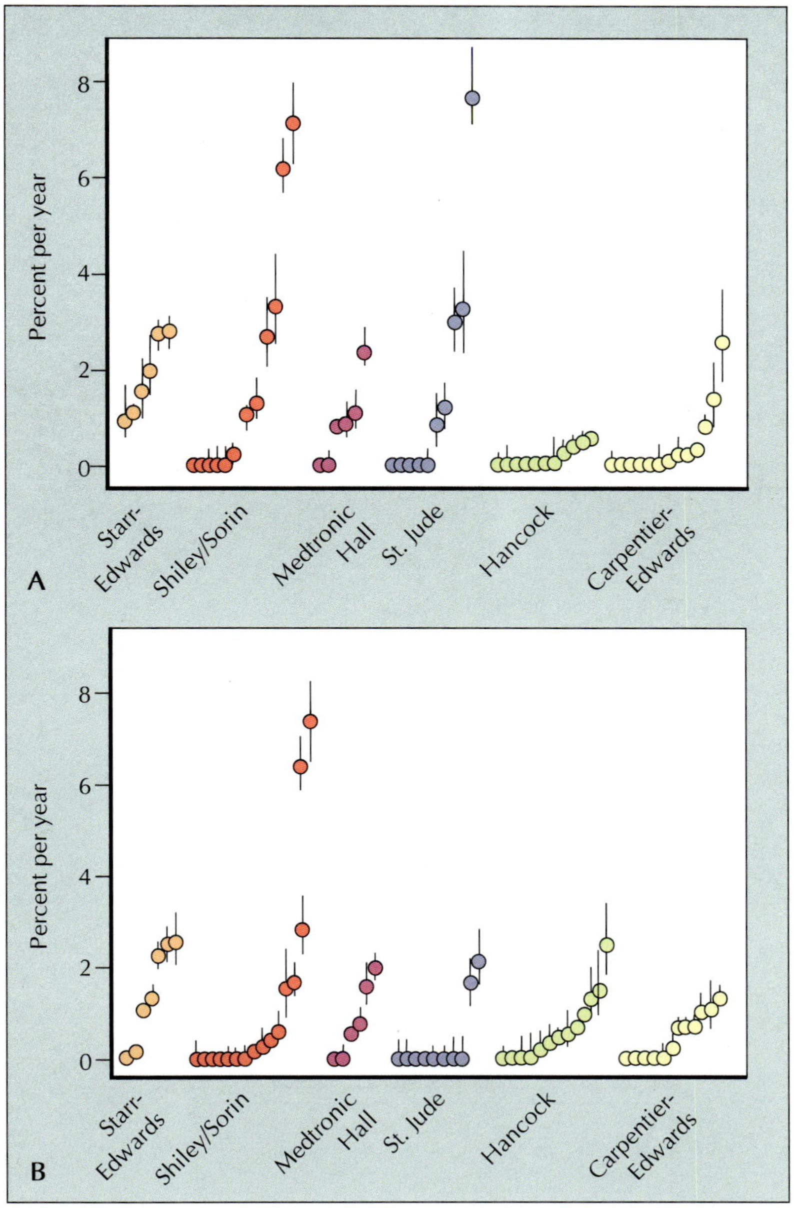

FIGURE 13-25. Comparative rates of bleeding. Comparative rates of bleeding are shown for isolated aortic (**A**) and mitral (**B**) valve replacement with mechanical and porcine valves. For comparability with mechanical series, the bleeding rate for each biologic series was computed as a weighted average for the entire series, not just for those on anticoagulation. The bleeding rates with biologic valves are thus half of those with mechanical valves (or less), approximately corresponding to the percentages of patients who require permanent anticoagulant treatment. (*Adapted from* Grunkemeier and coworkers [15].)

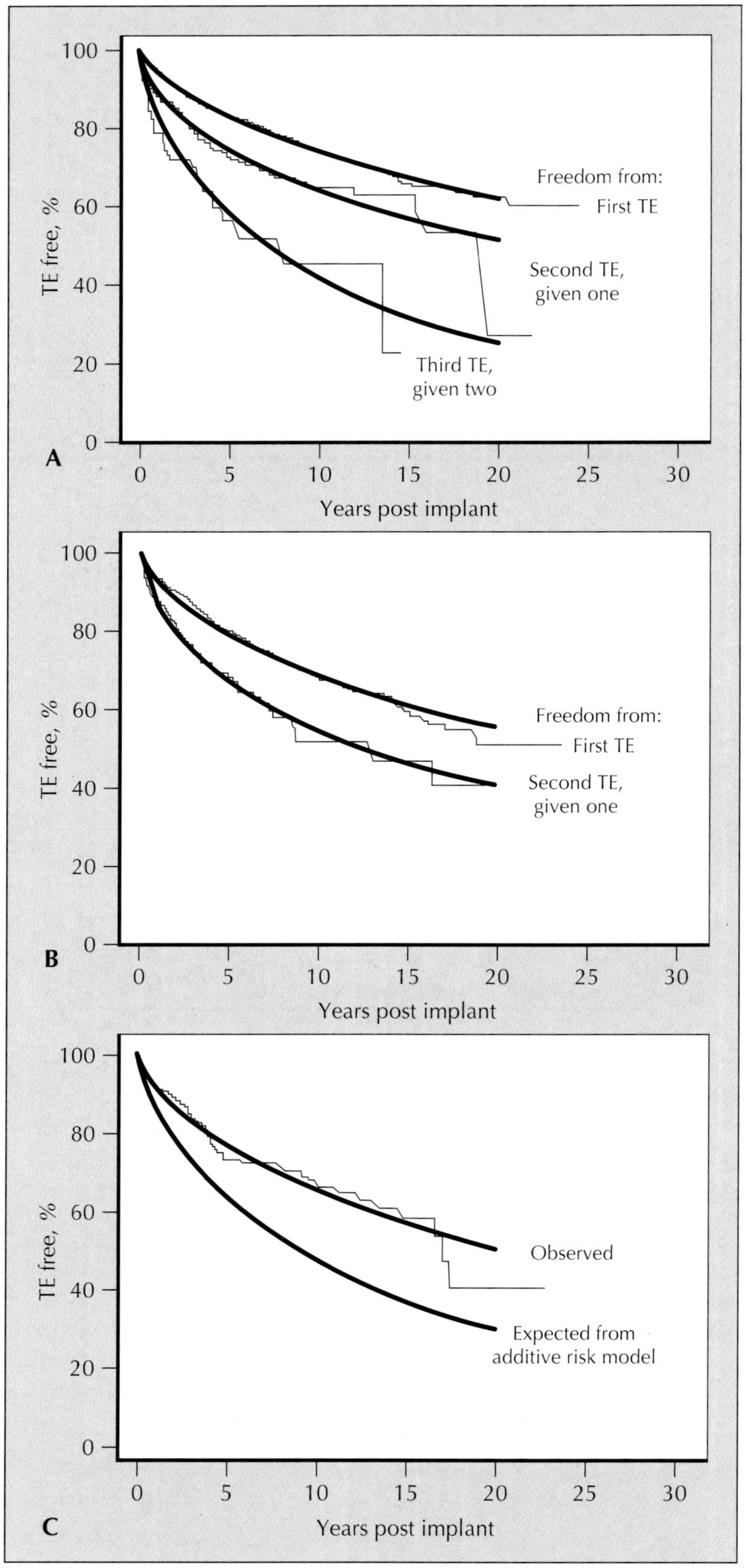

FIGURE 13-26. Recurrent thromboembolism. As mentioned previously, the linearized rate is an appropriate summary statistic only if an event has a constant risk; in that case, the event-free percentages over time form an exponential curve. We reviewed our thromboembolism (TE) experience with isolated caged-ball valve replacement to examine constancy of the risk over time, to compare the risks of recurrent versus initial TE, and to compare TE risk of isolated versus double valve replacement [16]. A total of 1593 aortic (**A**) and 1032 mitral (**B**) Starr-Edwards caged-ball valves were implanted from 1965 through 1988 and followed continuously since implant. This includes the cloth-covered valves (1968–1980) and the current silastic ball valves. TE was defined according to the published guidelines for reporting [17].

The jagged lines are the actuarial (Kaplan-Meier) TE-free estimates, and the smooth fit is not an exponential, which describes a constant risk over time, but rather a Weibull distribution [18], which describes a decreasing risk over time. That the *population* risk of TE decreases with time can be explained by a mixture of constant, but different, individual *patient* risks [19]. This is consistent with the theory that the majority of TE risk may be due to the patient or factors other than the prosthesis itself.

The top curve in each graph is the (usual) freedom from first TE. The next lower curve measures the freedom from a second TE, starting from the time of the first. Thus, the risk of a second TE, given the occurrence of a first, is greater than the risk of the first. For the aortic series, there were enough cases to see a continuance of this trend, by determining freedom from a third TE given that a second has occurred (*panel A*).

Double valve replacement was performed in 267 patients (C). The empiric TE curve for these valves was compared to that based on the Weibull models for the aortic and mitral valves, assuming an additive risk. The observed risk of TE was less than that predicted by adding the risk for each position, again consistent with the concept of patient-specific, rather than valve-specific risk. (*Adapted from* Starr and Grunkemeier [16].)

COMBINATIONS OF STERILIZATION/PRESERVATION METHODS FOR HOMOGRAFT VALVES*

	METHOD OF STERILIZATION		
METHOD OF PRESERVATION	ANTIBIOTIC	CHEMICAL	IRRADIATION
Cryopreservation	AC	CC	IC
Freeze-drying	AF	CF	IF
Nutrient at 4°C	AN	CN	IN

*Homovital valves have neither.

Figure 13-27. Combinations of sterilization and preservation methods for homograft valves. Homografts are affected by many variable factors, creating as much variability within the genus of homografts as among different models of mechanical or bioprosthetic valves. These variables include the method of procurement, the donor and time lapse from donor to host, and the insertion method, whether freehand, root replacement, or inclusion inside the aortic root. Especially important may be the methods of sterilization [20].

Because of these many factors, often not mentioned in clinical reports, comparison among series is difficult. The factors that are usually mentioned, the methods of sterilization and preservation, have been used to classify reported series. This figure contains a proposed classification scheme for the combinations of sterilization and preservation, inspired by a recent review article [20]. The two-letter abbreviations contain a code for the methods of sterilization (first letter) and preservation (second letter). The only homografts not represented in this figure are the "homovital" valves used immediately from transplant patients, which are neither sterilized nor preserved. A—antibiotic; C—chemical; Cr—cryopreservation; F—freeze-drying; I—irridation: N—nutrient at 4° C. (*Adapted from* Bodnar and Ross [20].)

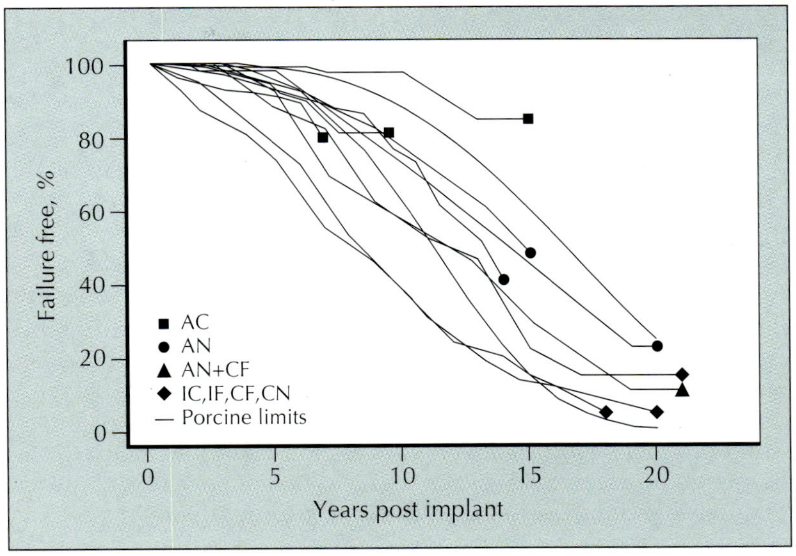

Figure 13-28. Comparison of structural failure by homograft "models." Structural failure of reported series of homograft valves [21], placed primarily in the aortic position, are compared in this figure. For structural failure of biologic valves it is necessary to use such time-related statistical methods as these actuarial failure-free curves because the risk of biologic valve failure increases with time. We used these curves for qualitative comparison only and did not compute comparative statistics (*P* values) because raw data for the curves were not available.

The "models" of the homograft valves are indicated, according to the methods of sterilization and preservation, using the two-letter codes introduced in Fig. 13-27. The definitions of structural valve deterioration (SVD) usually included only death or reoperation secondary to structural failure, but sometimes included significant regurgitation or reoperation for endocarditis. Mean age at operation for these series reviewed ranged from 47 to 52 years and the percent follow-up from 95% to 99%.

It appears that the series that used a chemical (C) or irradiation (I) process for sterilization have the highest rates of failure, about 40% SVD-free at 10 years. Those sterilized by antibiotic (A), whether stored in nutrient (N) solution or cryopreserved (Cr), are more durable, about 75% SVD-free at 10 years (an exception is the single cryopreserved series with the highest curve). The smooth lines labeled "porcine limits" are for visual comparison with aortic porcine valves (*see* Fig. 13-29).

The pulmonary autograft used as an aortic valve replacement is considered a permanent valve [22], especially appropriate for very young patients. Freedom from replacement for all reasons, including endocarditis, has been reported as high as 85% at 20 years [22], but has also been found to be 48.5% at 19 years [23]. To fully assess this procedure, complications of the valve that replaces the pulmonary valve must be combined with those of the pulmonary autograft. F—freeze-drying. (*Adapted from* Grunkemeier and Bodnar [21].)

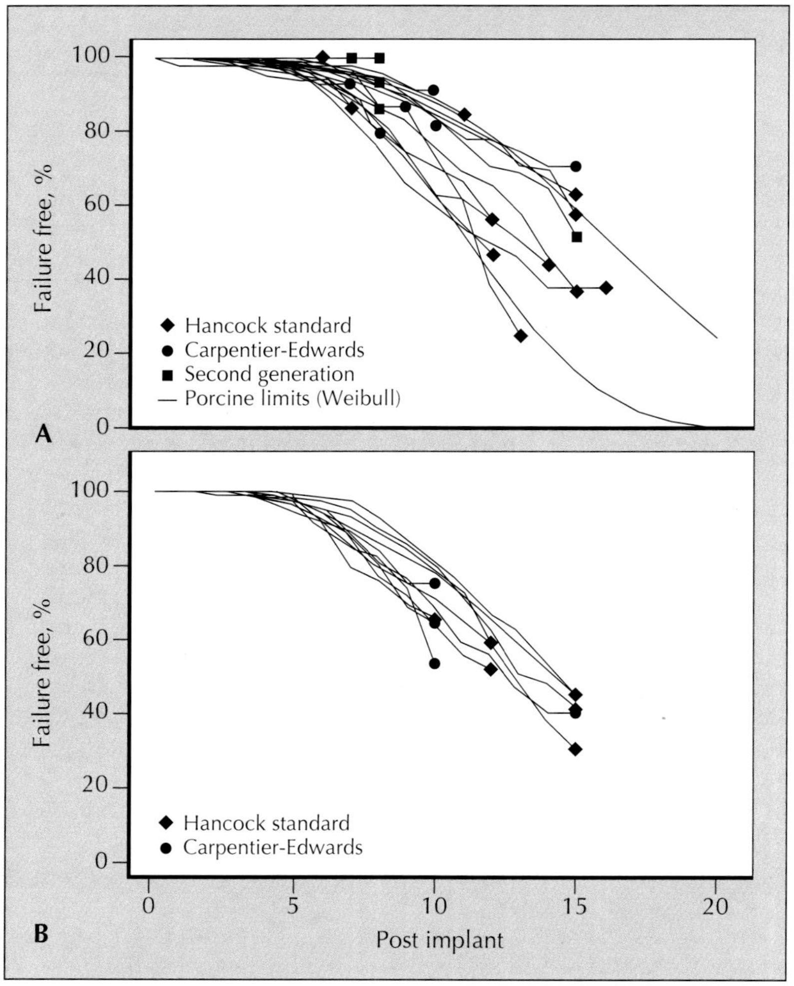

FIGURE 13-29. Structural failure of porcine valves. In analyzing the structural failure of aortic (**A**) and mitral (**B**) porcine valves, the mitral series contains only those with 10 or more years of follow-up [15]. The aortic series contains those with less than 10 years as well and includes a set of smooth curves (from the Weibull distribution), which encompasses the range of observed failure curves [24].

The rate of failure increases with time, being low (but not zero) for the first 5 years and then increasing. Because these series are not matched, it is not possible to draw conclusions regarding the relative performance of the two types of bioprostheses. These series with the longest follow-up include the earliest patients, who received biologic valves before young age was determined to be a significant risk factor. Thus most of these series have patients with a mean age of around 50 years. Because the rate of structural failures declines in older patients, the long-term results in current series, with older patients and with newer generations of porcine valves, should be better than those shown in these figures. (*Adapted from* Grunkemeier and Bodnar [24].)

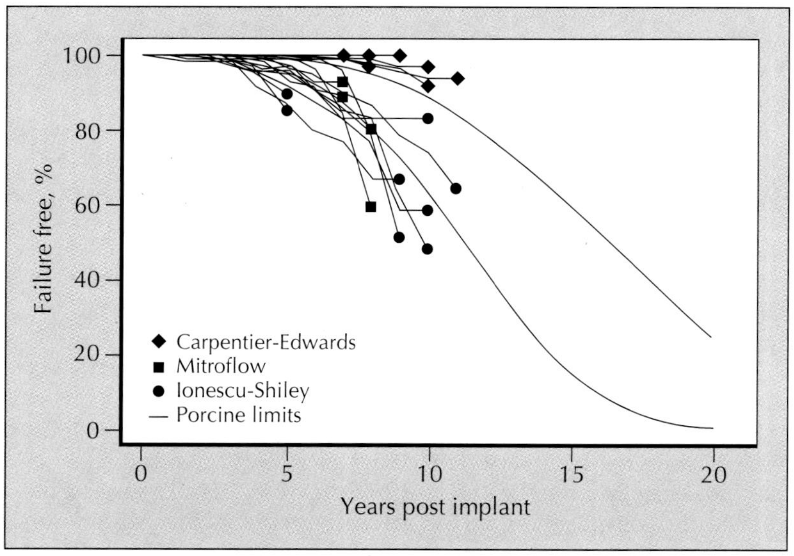

FIGURE 13-30. Structural failure of aortic pericardial valves. Ionescu-Shiley pericardial valves, discontinued in 1987, are included here for comparison purposes. The results up to 10 years with Carpentier-Edwards valves are encouraging, with all the series reported so far surpassing the Ionescu-Shiley durability and also the upper limit of the porcine valve durability curves, represented by the smooth (Weibull) curve (*see* Fig. 13-29) [24].

Patient selection is a confounding factor in the comparison of durability between tissue valve series. For example, older age is known to be associated with a reduced risk of structural failure. The Ionescu-Shiley series had mean ages generally below 60 years; the porcine series reported in Fig. 13-29 had mean ages generally below 60 years, and sometimes below 50; and the Carpentier-Edwards series have mean ages generally over 60 years, and sometimes over 70. Thus, a comparison between these results and those with porcine valves may be misleading. (*Adapted from* Grunkemeier and Bodnar [24].)

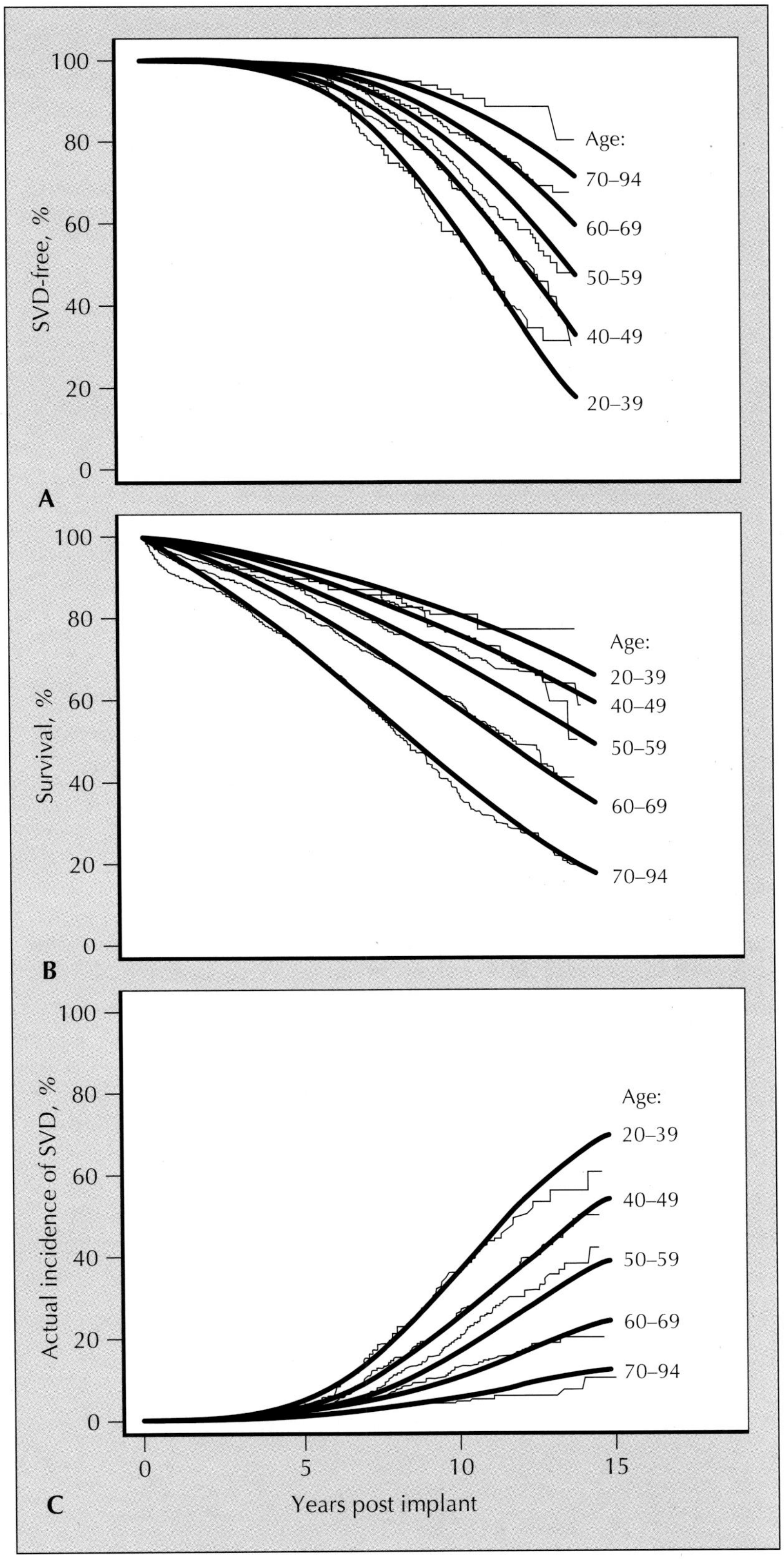

FIGURE 13-31. Actual versus actuarial freedom from structural valve deterioration (SVD). Time-related curves are required for the comparisons of biologic valves to incorporate the nonconstant risk of structural failure. It is important to understand that the usual actuarial curve gives the percentage free of an event at a given time, provided that the patients do not die (*ie*, that the risk of death has been eliminated). But many patients will die before their valve would have failed, so that the percent of patients who *actually* experience tissue failure will be lower than the usual *actuarial* estimates [25].

A, The usual *actuarial* failure-free curves for 4910 operative survivors of isolated aortic or mitral replacement with Hancock or Carpentier-Edwards porcine valves from two centers (Stanford and Vancouver), followed up to 15 years, for a total of almost 30,000 valve-years [26]. The curves are stratified by age group, and a Weibull regression model based on patient age and valve position (*smooth lines*) was used to fit the actuarial Kaplan-Meier curves (*jagged lines*). Older patients have a much lower risk than younger patients.

B, Patient survival by age group for isolated valve replacement. Actuarial curves (*jagged lines*) and Gompertz model (*smooth curves*) are based on a model that incorporates patient age and gender and valve position. Older patients have much higher risk than younger patients.

C, The *actual* risk of valve failure by age group. Again, the *jagged lines* are the observed, nonparametric estimates, and the *smooth curves* are a predicted fit based on integrating the two models developed from actuarial SVD and patient survival. Older patients have the lowest risk, but this effect is more amplified than in the upper graph because older patients, in whom the intrinsic life of the valve may be greater, will also have a lower incidence of actual failure because of their shorter expected lifetime. Appreciation of this effect could cause one to lower the recommended age for consideration of tissue valves.

An additional 164 patients with double valves from these same institutions were not used in the modeling above, but their risk of valve failure was as predicted based on the model for isolated valves only. Thus, the risk for a valve to fail does not seem to be influenced by the existence of a comparison valve in the same patient. (*Adapted from* Grunkemeier and coworkers [26].)

Patient Selection and Future Developments

VALVE SELECTION FOR AN INDIVIDUAL PATIENT

RELATIVE INDICATIONS FOR A MECHANICAL VALVE

Long expected lifetime (age <40 years)
Previous dysfunctional tissue valve
Anticoagulation required anyway
Double valve replacement
Conposite graft needed
Renal failure, dialysis

RELATIVE INDICATIONS FOR A BIOPROSTHESIS

Short expected lifetime (age ≥65 years)
Unreliable anticoagulant risk
Previous thrombosed valve
Anticoagulant intolerance
Pregnancy anticipated

FIGURE 13-32. Selection of prosthesis for a particular patient. The general principles in valve selection derive from the fundamental difference between the mechanical and biologic valves. Mechanical valves are extremely durable yet require lifetime anticoagulation to mitigate thromboembolic complications. Biologic valves have not eliminated thromboembolism, but they achieve rates comparable to those of mechanical valves without anticoagulation; however, they have limited lifetimes. Beyond this fundamental difference between types of valves, patient-specific factors influence the results as much as valve-specific factors.

Valve repair (not covered in this review) should be considered preferable to replacement for the mitral position [27,28]. Repair can also be considered for the aortic position [29]. Homografts or the Ross procedure may also be considered, especially for very young patients. However, the vast majority of patients requiring replacement will be served by one of the commercially available prostheses.

When prosthetic replacement is necessary, some general recommendations can be made with regard to valve selection, based on the above fundamental difference between valve types. A biologic valve would be preferred for a patient who cannot, or does not want to take, anticoagulants, who desires pregnancy, or who has a short life expectancy. A mechanical valve would be preferred for a patient who will be receiving anticoagulants for another reason (*eg*, previous stroke or infarction, atrial fibrillation, mechanical valve in another position), who is in renal failure or on dialysis, or who has a long life expectancy.

FUTURE DEVELOPMENTS IN PROSTHETIC HEART VAVLES

REDUCTION OF THROMBOEMBOLISM BY:

Less thrombogenic protheses
Better anticoagulant management
Identification of embolism-prone patients

IMPROVED TISSUE VALVE DURABILITY BY:

New sterilization/preservation methods
Calcification mitigation treatments
Reducing immunologic response
Low stress design configurations

FIGURE 13-33. The ongoing search among mechanical heart valve designers is for ways of reducing the complex of thromboembolism-thrombosis-bleeding complications. Potential improvements may come from achieving better hemodynamic flow patterns [30], reduced thrombogenicity via thromboresistant surfactant coatings [31], and individualized anticoagulant management strategies [32]. Identifying markers of thrombogenicity preoperatively [33] would allow preferential use of tissue valves in higher risk patients and mechanical valves in lower risk patients.

The goal of newer designs for biologic valves is to improve structural durability. The move has been toward very low or zero pressure fixation, which allows the valve leaflets to be fixed in the neutral (slightly open) position, and to retain more of the natural flexibility. Anticalcification (surfactant) treatments may help improve durability. The current experiments with nonstented valves should result in improved hemodynamics and possibly improved durability as well. Development of valves incorporating autologous tissue [13] could eliminate complications associated with an autoimmune reaction.

The authors wish to thank the valve manufacturers and their representatives (ATS Medical, Inc, Autogenics, Baxter Healthcare Corporation, Biocor Institute, Bravo Cardiovascular Inc, CarboMedics, Cryolife, Inc., Medical Incorporated, Medtronic Inc., Mitroflow International, Inc., Sorin Biomedica Cardio, St. Jude Medical, Inc.), who kindly contributed photographs and information; Larry Scotten and David Walker of Vivitro Systems for their valuable hydrodynamic data; Joanie Livermore for suggestions regarding graphic presentation of the material; and Glenda Farrell, Maria Wesley, Elaine Inman, and Maryam Ahmad for logistic support.

References

1. Lillehei CW, Barnard CN, Long DM Jr, *et al.*: Aortic valve reconstruction and replacement by total valve prostheses. In *Prosthetic Valves for Cardiac Surgery*. Edited by Merendino KA. Springfield, IL: Charles C. Thomas; 1961:527–575.
2. Braunwald NS, Cooper T, Morrow AG: Complete replacement of the mitral valve: successful clinical application of a flexible polyurethane prosthesis. *J Thorac Cardiovasc Surg* 1960, 40:1–11.
3. Harken DE, Soroff HS, Taylor WJ, *et al.*: Aortic valve replacement. In *Prosthetic Valves for Cardiac Surgery*. Edited by Merendino KA. Springfield, IL: Charles C. Thomas; 1961:508–526.
4. Starr A, Edwards MS: Mitral replacement: clinical experience with a ball-valve prosthesis. *Ann Surg* 1961, 154:726–740.
5. Ross DN: Homograft replacement of the aortic valve. *Lancet* 1962, 2:487.
6. Barratt-Boyes BG: Homograft aortic valve replacement in aortic incompetence and stenosis. *Thorax* 1964, 19:131–135.
7. Gerosa G, Ross DN, Brucke PE, *et al.*: Aortic valve replacement with pulmonary homografts. *J Thorac Cardiovasc Surg* 1994, 107:424–437.
8. Ross DN: Replacement of aortic and mitral valves with a pulmonary autograft. *Lancet* 1967, 2:956–958.
9. Oury H, Angell WW, Eddy AC, Cleveland JC: Pulmonary autograft—past, present, and future. *J Heart Valve Dis* 1993, 2:365–375.
10. Kay PH, Livi U, Robles A, Ross DN: Pulmonary homograft. In *Biologic and Bioprosthetic Valves*. Edited by Bodnar E, Yacoub M. Stoneham, MA: Yorke Medical Books; 1986:58–63.
11. Carpentier A, Lemaigre G, Robert L, *et al.*: Biological factors affecting long-term results of valvular heterografts. *J Thorac Cardiovasc Surg* 1995, 58:467–483.
12. Barratt-Boyes BG, Christie GW: What is the best bioprosthetic operation for the small aortic root? Allograft, autograft, porcine, pericardial? Stented or unstented? *J Card Surg* 1994, 9:158–164.
13. Love JW: *Autologous Tissue Heart Valves*. Austin: R.G. Landes Company; 1993.
14. Scotten LN, Walker DK: A database obtained from in vitro testing of mechanical prosthetic heart valves. *J Heart Valve Dis* 1994, 3:561–570.
15. Grunkemeier GL, Starr A, Rahimtoola SH: Prosthetic heart valves: long-term follow-up. *Cur Prob Cardiol* 1992, 17:329–406.
16. Starr A, Grunkemeier GL: Recurrent thromboembolism: significance and management. In *Proceedings of Symposium on Thrombosis, Embolism and Bleeding*. London: ICR Publishers, 1991: 402–415.
17. Edmunds LH, Clark RE, Cohn LH, *et al.*: Guidelines for reporting morbidity and mortality after cardiac valvular operations. *Ann Thorac Surg* 1988, 46:257–259.
18. Aitkin M, Clayton D: The fitting of exponential, Weibull, and extreme value distributions to complex censored survival data using GLIM. *Appl Statist* 1990, 29:156–163.
19. Jewell NP: Mixture of exponential distributions. *Ann Stat* 1982, 10:479–484.
20. Bodnar E, Ross DN: Valvular homografts. In *Replacement Cardiac Valves*. Edited by Bodnar E, Frater RMW. New York: Pergamon Press; 1991:287–306.
21. Grunkemeier GL, Bodnar E: Comparison of structural valve failure among different "models" of homograft valves. *J Heart Valve Dis* 1994, 3:556–560.
22. Ross D, Jackson M, Davies J: Pulmonary autograft aortic valve replacement: long-term results. *J Card Surg* 1991, 6:529–533.
23. Matsuki O, Okita Y, Almeida RS, *et al.*: Two decades' experience with aortic valve replacement with pulmonary autograft. *J Thorac Cardiovasc Surg* 1988, 95:705–711.
24. Grunkemeier GL, Bodnar E: Comparative assessment of bioprosthesis durability in the aortic position. *J Heart Valve Dis* 1995, 4:49–55.
25. Starr A, Grunkemeier GL: The expected lifetime of porcine valves. *Ann Thorac Surg* 1989, 48:317–318.
26. Grunkmeier GL, Jamieson WRE, Miller DC, Starr A: Actual vs. actuarial risk of structural valve deterioration. *J Thorac Cardiovasc Surg* 1994, 108:709–718.
27. Duran C: Mitral reconstruction in predominant mitral stenosis. In *Recent Progress in Mitral Valve Disease*. Edited by Duran C, Angell WW, Johnson AD, Oury JH. London: Butterworths; 1984:255–264.
28. Carpentier A: Mitral reconstruction in predominant mitral incompetence. In *Recent Progress in Mitral Valve Disease*. Edited by Duran C, Angell WW, Johnson AD, Oury JH. London: Butterworths; 1984:265–276.
29. Cosgrove DM, Rosenkranz ER, Hendren WG, *et al.*: Valvuloplasty for aortic insufficiency. *J Thorac Cardiovasc Surg* 1991, 102:571–576.
30. Nygaard H, Paulsen PK, Hasenkam JM, *et al.*: Turbulent stresses downstream of three mechanical aortic valve prostheses in human beings. *J Thorac Cardiovasc Surg* 1994, 107:438–446.
31. Horbett TA, Grunkemeier JM, Lew KR: Fibrinogen orientation on a surface coated with a GPIIb/IIIa peptides detected with monoclonal antibodies. Transactions of the 20th Annual Meeting of the Society for Biomaterials, April 5, 1994, Boston, MA.
32. Butchart EG: Thrombosis and anticoagulation in heart valve disease: towards a rational approach (editorial). *J Heart Dis* 1993, 2:1–6.
33. Gough SCL, Prentice CRM: The investigation of a heart valve patient with suspected hypercoagulability. *J Heart Valve Dis* 1993, 2:7–17.

Antibiotic Prophylaxis for Rheumatic Fever and Endocarditis

14

CHAPTER

Kathryn A. Taubert, Adnan S. Dajani, and Shahbudin H. Rahimtoola

Bacterial infections can cause serious cardiac disease. Two examples are rheumatic fever and bacterial endocarditis, both of which can often be prevented by antibiotic prophylaxis. Antibiotics can prevent rheumatic fever by eradicating group A streptococci from the throat. Likewise, antibiotic prophylaxis given before certain surgical or dental procedures can decrease the likelihood of endocarditis in individuals at risk.

Rheumatic Fever

Rheumatic fever is relatively uncommon in the United States today although local outbreaks have been reported in several areas since the mid-1980s [1–10]. Worldwide, however, rheumatic fever remains a major cause of heart disease in developing countries [11].

Prevention of acute rheumatic fever depends on the proper diagnosis and control of the antecedent group A streptococcal pharyngitis. Certain common symptoms and signs are associated with streptococcal pharyngitis, including sudden-onset sore throat, pain on swallowing, and fever and headache. Common signs include tonsillopharyngeal erythema and exudate and soft palate petechiae. Although these may be helpful clues, a definitive diagnosis can be established only after a throat culture or rapid antigen detection test. The available rapid antigen detection tests can provide results in minutes rather than the 24 to 48 hours required for a throat culture. These tests are generally specific (specificity rates 88% to 100%) but are not very sensitive (sensitivity rates 55% to 95%) [12]. If the rapid antigen test is positive, antibiotic treatment should be started. If the test is negative, a throat culture should be processed. The 24- to 48-hour delay before beginning antibiotics does not increase the risk of developing rheumatic fever. Antibiotic treatment of streptococcal tonsillopharyngitis typically requires penicillin. The primary aim of therapy is eradication of group A streptococci from the throat and thus prevention of an initial attack of rheumatic fever. Individuals are considered to be noncontagious 24 hours after beginning therapy [13].

An individual who has had one attack of rheumatic fever is inordinately susceptible to a second attack and therefore needs continuous prophylaxis, usually with penicillin, to prevent a recurrence. The proper diagnosis of an initial attack of acute rheumatic fever must have been made for secondary prevention to be initiated. The Jones criteria for the diagnosis of rheumatic fever were initially written in 1944 [14] and have been updated by the American Heart Association [15]. The likelihood of a recurrent attack of rheumatic fever is influenced by several factors, such as the interval since the most recent attack, the number of previous attacks, and whether the individual is in an environment where he or she is often exposed to streptococcal infections. The duration of secondary prophylaxis is determined by the presence or absence of carditis.

Bacterial Endocarditis

Bacterial endocarditis is a relatively uncommon but serious disease. It occurs when certain blood-borne bacteria lodge on damaged endocardial (endothelial) surfaces of the heart, usually an abnormal valve or a congenital cardiac defect. Certain cardiac conditions predispose the patient for the development of endocarditis. Risk categories vary and have been subdivided into high, medium, and low (or negligible) risk. Patients at high or medium risk are those who routinely need endocarditis prophylaxis. Patients with mitral valve prolapse are among the most problematic for whom to choose prophylaxis. For those with no murmur, the incidence of endocarditis is no greater than that in the general population, although one study has shown that for patients with a mitral regurgitant murmur, the incidence of endocarditis is about 10-fold greater [16]. A frequent clinical problem is that the mitral regurgitant murmur may be present only intermittently. In most cases of endocarditis, an antecedent medical procedure that can lead to bacteremia cannot be identified.

Nonetheless, certain surgical and dental procedures are more likely to induce bacteremia. If the bacteria have a propensity for adherence to damaged endothelium (usually alpha-hemolytic streptococci), then endocarditis may ensue. In the absence of prospective clinical trials, recommendations for prevention of endocarditis are based on experimental animal data, *in vitro* studies, and clinical experiences. The standard antibiotic prophylaxis for dental/oral/upper respiratory procedures is amoxicillin. All patients at high to medium risk are eligible for this regimen, unless they are allergic to penicillins or cannot take oral medications. Oral prophylaxis for high-risk patients has been a part of the recommendations from the American Heart Association [17] and the British Endocarditis Working Party [18] for several years, and an increased incidence of prophylaxis failures has not been reported. In some high-risk patients, however, the practitioner may choose to use a parenteral regimen (*ie*, a patient with a prosthetic heart valve and a history of endocarditis). Prophylaxis recommendations for patients undergoing genitourinary/gastrointestinal tract procedures are directed against enterococci and require intravenous or intramuscular antibiotic administration. Some special situations, such as a patient already taking an oral penicillin or a patient on anticoagulant therapy, may alter the usual prophylaxis regimen.

Streptococcal Tonsillopharyngitis

SYMPTOMS AND SIGNS IN STREPTOCOCCAL TONSILLOPHARYNGITIS

COMMON FINDINGS	FINDINGS NOT SUGGESTIVE OF GROUP A STREPTOCOCCAL INFECTION
Symptoms	
Sudden onset sore throat	Coryza
Pain on swallowing	Hoarseness
Fever	Cough
Headache	Diarrhea
Abdominal pain	
Nausea and vomiting	
Signs	
Tonsillopharyngeal erythema	Conjunctivitis
Tonsillopharyngeal exudate	Anterior stomatitis
Soft palate petechiae	Discrete ulcerative lesions
Beefy red, swollen uvula	
Anterior cervical adenitis	
Scarlatiniform rash	

Figure 14-1. Common and less common signs and symptoms of tonsillopharyngitis described by the patient and encountered by the practitioner. The findings are seen primarily in individuals older than 3 years. These are useful adjuncts in establishing a diagnosis of streptococcal throat infection, although a throat culture or rapid antigen test is needed for a definitive diagnosis. (*Adapted from* Dajani and coworkers [19].)

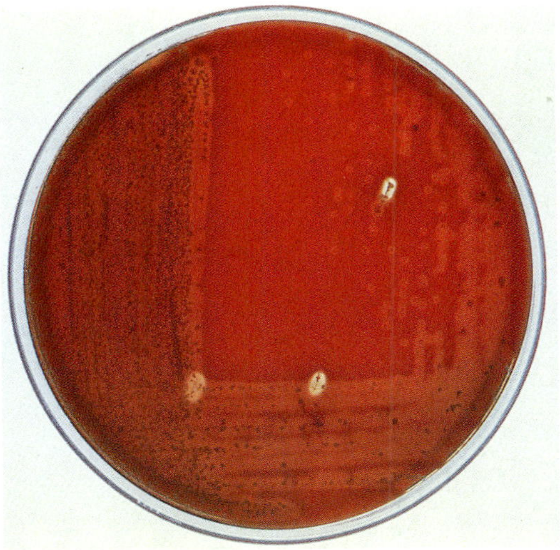

FIGURE 14-2. Blood agar plate showing group A streptococcal colonies. To obtain a throat culture, 1) depress tongue; 2) rub sterile swab vigorously over each tonsillar area and the posterior pharynx, 3) streak swab onto sheep blood agar plate, covering about one sixth of plate, 4) streak sterile wire loop through primary inoculum onto one third of plate, streak loop through this secondary area onto rest of plate, make two to three stabs into the agar, and 5) incubate plate at 37°C for 18 to 24 hours.

Group A streptococcal colonies are usually small, colorless, or slightly whitish and surrounded by a halo of complete beta hemolysis. Hemolysis sometimes occurs only in the stabs or is accentuated in the stabs. Definitive identification of group A streptococci is achieved by serologic means.

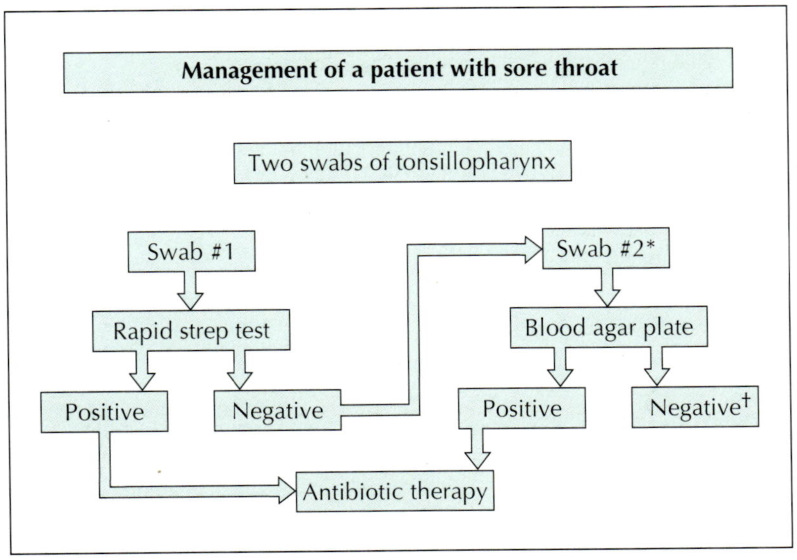

FIGURE 14-3. Algorithm for the management of the patient with a sore throat. Two tonsillopharyngeal swabs should be taken. One swab is used for a rapid antigen detection test. If this test is positive, the other swab is discarded (*asterisk*) and antibiotic treatment for streptococcal infection is begun. If the rapid antigen detection test is negative, the second swab should be processed onto a blood agar plate. If the plate is positive, antibiotic therapy for streptococcal infection is begun. If the blood agar plate is negative (*dagger*), consider other causes such as viruses, chlamydia, and so forth.

PREVENTION, DIAGNOSIS, AND PATHOGENESIS

PRIMARY PREVENTION OF RHEUMATIC FEVER (TREATMENT OF STREPTOCOCCAL TONSILLOPHARYNGITIS)

AGENT	DOSE	MODE	DURATION
Benzathine penicillin G	600,000 U for patients ≤ 27 kg 1,200,000 U for patients > 27 kg	Intramuscular	Once
	or		
Penicillin V (phenoxymethyl penicillin)	Children: 250 mg 2–3 times daily Adolescents and adults: 500 mg 2–3 times daily	Oral	10 d
For patients allergic to penicillin:			
Erythromycin estolate	20–40 mg/kg 2–4 times daily (maximum 1 g/d)	Oral	10 d
	or		
Ethylsuccinate	40 mg/kg 2–4 times daily (maximum 1 g/d)	Oral	10 d

FIGURE 14-4. Primary prevention of rheumatic fever (treatment of streptococcal tonsillopharyngitis). Prevention of rheumatic fever requires eradication of group A streptococci from the throat. Penicillin is the drug of choice unless the patient is allergic to it. Treatment should be begun as soon as the diagnosis of streptococcal pharyngitis is made. If oral treatment is used, treatment must continue for the full 10 days.

The following agents are also acceptable: amoxicillin, amoxicillin/clavulanate, cephalosporins, other macrolides, and clindamycin [20]. The following agents are not acceptable: sulfonamides, trimethoprim, tetracyclines, and chloramphenicol. (*Adapted from* Dajani and coworkers [19].)

SECONDARY PREVENTION OF RHEUMATIC FEVER (PREVENTION OF RECURRENT ATTACKS)

AGENT	DOSE	MODE
Benzathine penicillin G	1,200,000 U	Intramuscular every 4 wks*
	or	
Penicillin V	250 mg twice daily	Oral
	or	
Sulfadiazine	0.5 g once daily for patients ≤ 27 kg 1.0 g once daily for patients > 27 kg	Oral
For patients allergic to penicillin and sulfadiazine:		
Erythromycin	250 mg twice daily	Oral

*In high-risk situations, where the patient is exposed to streptococcal infection often (health care providers, parents of young children, schoolteachers), administration every 3 weeks is advised.

FIGURE 14-5. Secondary prevention of rheumatic fever (prevention of recurrent attacks). Individuals with a history of rheumatic fever are at high risk for a recurrent attack should they develop streptococcal pharyngitis. Asymptomatic infections can trigger a recurrence. Therefore, continuous long-term prophylaxis is needed. This prophylaxis should be begun as soon as the primary prevention course of antibiotics (one injection of benzathine penicillin G or 10 days of penicillin V or erythromycin—*see* Fig. 14-4 for dosages) is completed. (*Adapted from* Dajani and coworkers [19].)

GUIDELINES FOR THE DIAGNOSIS OF INITIAL ATTACK OF RHEUMATIC FEVER (JONES CRITERIA, UPDATED 1992)

MAJOR MANIFESTATIONS	MINOR MANIFESTATIONS	SUPPORTING EVIDENCE OF ANTECEDENT GROUP A STREPTOCOCCAL INFECTION
Carditis	Clinical	Positive throat culture or rapid streptococcal antigen test
Polyarthritis	Arthralgia	Elevated or rising streptococcal antibody titer
Chorea	Fever	
Erythema marginatum	Laboratory	
Subcutaneous nodules	Elevated acute phase reactants	
	Erythrocyte sedimentation rate	
	C-reactive protein	
	Prolonged PR interval	

FIGURE 14-6. Guidelines for the diagnosis of initial attack of rheumatic fever (Jones criteria, updated 1992). No single symptom, sign, or laboratory test is pathognomonic of acute rheumatic fever. These criteria are designed to establish an *initial* attack of acute rheumatic fever. If supported by evidence of preceding group A streptococcal infection, the presence of two major manifestations or of one major and two minor manifestations indicates a high probability of acute rheumatic fever. (*Adapted from* Dajani and coworkers [15].)

FACTORS INVOLVED IN THE PATHOGENESIS OF RHEUMATIC FEVER

GROUP A STREPTOCOCCUS

Tonsillopharyngeal infection (not skin or other route)
Intensity of antibody response
Rheumatogenic streptococci
- Limited serotypes (M 1, 3, 5, 6, 14, 18, 19, 24, 27, and 29)
- M protein has long terminal antigenic domain
- M protein contains epitopes that are shared with human heart tissue (sarcolemmal membrane and cardiac myosin)
- Heavily encapsulated, forming mucoid colonies on blood agar
- Strains resist phagocytosis
- Strains do not produce opacity factor

SUSCEPTIBLE HOST

Familial predisposition
Presence of specific B-cell alloantigen
Association with class II HLA antigens

ENVIRONMENT

Crowded living conditions
Low income
Poor medical care

FIGURE 14-7. Factors involved in the pathogenesis of rheumatic fever. Certain characteristics of the infectious agent and of the host and host environment increase the likelihood of the development of rheumatic fever. For example, certain serotypes of group A streptococci are considered to be rheumatogenic serotypes. Some individuals appear to be more susceptible to the development of rheumatic fever than others. Rheumatic fever is classically associated with certain environments of the host.

Rheumatic Fever: Recurrence and Prophylaxis Duration

FACTORS INFLUENCING RISK OF RHEUMATIC FEVER RECURRENCE

Interval since most recent attacks—the longer the interval the less the likelihood of recurrence
Number of previous attacks—risk increases with increasing number of previous attacks
Individual profile
- Parents of young children
- Teachers
- Health professionals
- Military recruits
- Crowded living situations
- Economically disadvantaged
- Younger age groups
- Previous rheumatic carditis

FIGURE 14-8. Factors influencing risk of rheumatic fever recurrence. For the individual profile category, most profiles relate to situations in which the individual will be placed in an environment of increased exposure to streptococcal infections. Patients with previous rheumatic carditis are at relatively high risk for recurrences of carditis with reinfection and are likely to sustain serious cardiac complications.

DURATION OF SECONDARY RHEUMATIC FEVER PROPHYLAXIS

CATEGORY	DURATION
Rheumatic fever without carditis	5 y or until age 21, whichever is longer
Rheumatic fever with carditis but no residual heart disease (no clinical or echocardiographic evidence of valvular disease)	10 y or well into adulthood, whichever is longer
Rheumatic fever with carditis and residual heart disease (clinical or echocardiographic evidence of persistent valvular disease)	At least 10 y since last episode and at least until age 40, sometimes lifelong prophylaxis

FIGURE 14-9. Duration of secondary rheumatic fever prophylaxis varies depending on the situation. In the second and third categories, prophylaxis may be stopped and then reinstated at a later time if a situation deems it necessary. For example, a person could become a grandparent or day care center worker, and thus be placed in a situation of increased exposure to streptococcal infection. (*Adapted from* Dajani and coworkers [19].)

ENDOCARDITIS PROPHYLAXIS: CARDIAC CONDITIONS

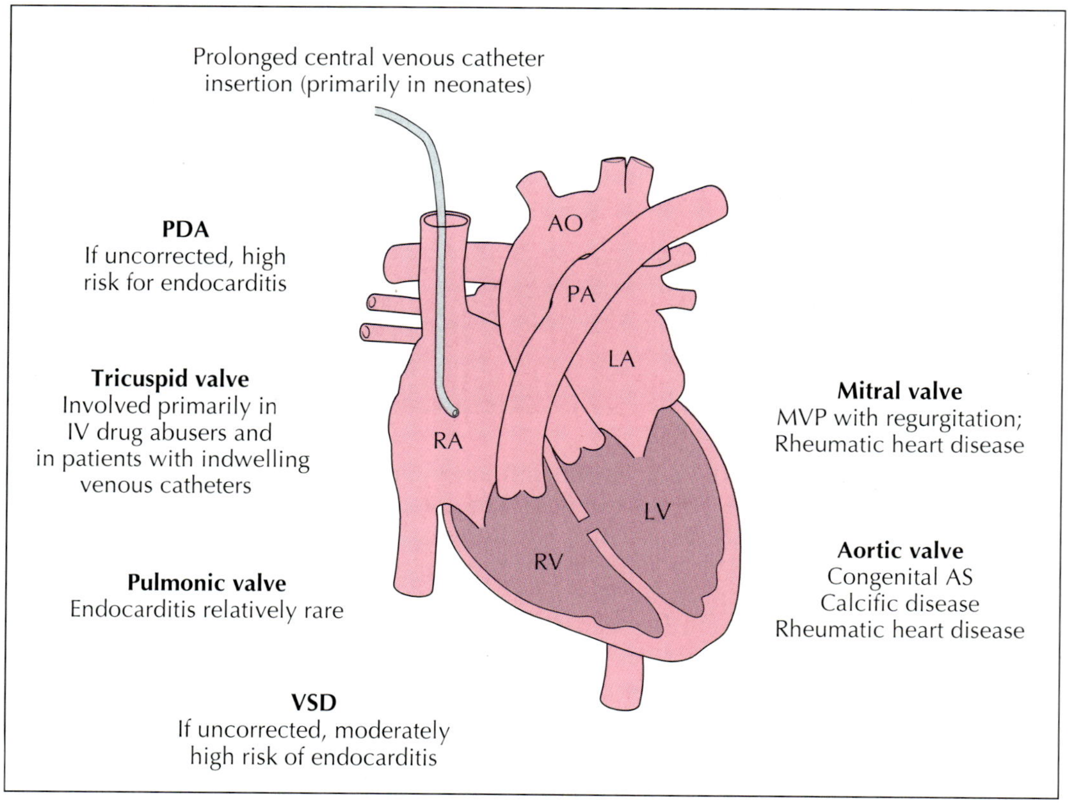

FIGURE 14-10. Some common conditions for, and sites of, endocarditis infection. This figure is *not* meant to be all-inclusive.

The mitral valve is a site for endocarditis in patients with mitral valve prolapse (MVP) who have regurgitation; patients who have never had a murmur are at no greater risk for the development of endocarditis than the general public [10]. Although rheumatic fever can lead to valvular damage of any of the valves, the mitral or aortic valves are the usual sites of endocarditis, with the mitral valve being involved most frequently. Right-sided endocarditis is rare except in intravenous (IV) drug abusers or in patients with indwelling venous catheters. Most uncorrected congenital cardiac defects (except isolated secundum atrial septal defect) are potential sites for endocarditis. Any prosthetic cardiac valve is a high-risk site for the development of endocarditis. AO—aorta; AS—aortic stenosis; LA—left atrium; LV—left ventricle; PA—pulmonary artery; PDA—patent ductus arteriosus; RA—right atrium; RV—right ventricle; VSD—ventricular septal defect.

CARDIAC CONDITIONS REQUIRING ENDOCARDITIS PROPHYLAXIS

HIGH RISK

Prosthetic cardiac valves, including bioprosthetic and homograft valves

Previous bacterial endocarditis, even in the absence of heart disease

Surgically constructed systemic-pulmonary shunts or conduits

MEDIUM RISK

Most congenital cardiac malformations

Acquired valvular dysfunction, including rheumatic valve disease

Hypertrophic cardiomyopathy

Clinical mitral valve prolapse with valvular regurgitation

FIGURE 14-11. Certain cardiac conditions require prophylaxis for endocarditis. The murmur of mitral valve prolapse may not be heard at every examination. If the murmur has been detected, patients with intermittent mitral valve murmurs should be included in the category of those needing prophylaxis. Individuals who have a mitral valve prolapse associated with thickening or redundancy of the valve leaflets may be at increased risk for bacterial endocarditis, particularly men 45 years of age or older.

For patients with a cardiac transplant, data are insufficient to make specific recommendations. Surveys of transplant centers, however, indicate that these patients are recommended to receive antibiotics before procedures likely to cause a bacteremia.

CARDIAC CONDITIONS NOT REQUIRING ENDOCARDITIS PROPHYLAXIS

LOW OR NEGLIGIBLE RISK

Isolated secundum atrial septal defect

Surgical repair without residua beyond 6 mo of secundum atrial septal defect, ventricular septal defect, or patent ductus arteriosus

Previous coronary artery bypass graft surgery

Mitral valve prolapse without valvular regurgitation

Physiologic, functional, or innocent heart murmurs

Previous Kawasaki disease without valvular dysfunction

Previous rheumatic fever without valvular dysfunction

Cardiac pacemakers and implanted defibrillators

FIGURE 14-12. Cardiac conditions that do not require endocarditis prophylaxis. These conditions have not been shown to place patients at increased risk, *ie*, above that of the general population, for the development of endocarditis. The conditions described for mitral valve prolapse (*see* Fig. 14-11) apply here also.

ENDOCARDITIS PROPHYLAXIS: DENTAL AND SURGICAL PROCEDURES

DENTAL OR SURGICAL PROCEDURES FOR WHICH ENDOCARDITIS PROPHYLAXIS IS RECOMMENDED

DENTAL/RESPIRATORY TRACT

Dental procedures known to induce gingival or mucosal bleeding, including professional cleaning

Tonsillectomy or adenoidectomy

Surgical operations that involve respiratory mucosa

Bronchoscopy with a rigid bronchoscope

GASTROINTESTINAL TRACT

Sclerotherapy for esophageal varices*

Esophageal stricture dilation*

Endoscopic retrograde cholangiography*

Gallbladder surgery

Surgical operations that involve intestinal mucosa

GENITOURINARY TRACT

Urinary tract surgery if urinary tract infection is present

Prostatic surgery

Incision and drainage of infected tissue†

Vaginal hysterectomy

Vaginal delivery in the presence of infection†

Cystoscopy

Urethral dilation

Urethral catheterization

*Prophylaxis is recommended for high-risk patients; optional for medium-risk patients.

†Antibiotic therapy should be directed against the most likely bacterial pathogen.

FIGURE 14-13. Endocarditis prophylaxis is recommended for certain dental or surgical procedures, although this list is not all-inclusive. (*Adapted from* Dajani and coworkers [17].)

DENTAL OR SURGICAL PROCEDURES FOR WHICH ENDOCARDITIS PROPHYLAXIS IS NOT RECOMMENDED
Dental procedures not likely to induce gingival bleeding, such as simple adjustment of orthodontic appliances or fillings above the gum line
Injection of local intraoral anesthetic (except intraligamentary injections)
Shedding of primary teeth
Tympanostomy tube insertion
Endotracheal intubation
Bronchoscopy with a flexible bronchoscope, with or without biopsy
Cardiac catheterization
Endoscopy with or without gastrointestinal biopsy
Cesarean section
In the absence of infection for urethral catheterization, dilatation and curettage, uncomplicated vaginal delivery, therapeutic abortion, sterilization procedures, or insertion or removal of intrauterine devices

FIGURE 14-14. Dental or surgical procedures for which endocarditis prophylaxis is not recommended. Patients who have prosthetic heart valves, a previous history of endocarditis, or surgically constructed systemic-pulmonary shunts or conduits are at highest risk for endocarditis. Physicians may choose to administer prophylactic antibiotics for procedures involving the lower respiratory, genitourinary, or gastrointestinal tracts that do not require antibiotics. Surgery on the skin does not normally require prophylaxis because the procedure is performed in a sterile environment. If an infection is present, prophylaxis should be directed toward the pathogen. This list is not meant to be all-inclusive. (*Adapted from* Dajani and coworkers [17].)

ENDOCARDITIS PROPHYLAXIS: ANTIBIOTIC RECOMMENDATIONS

RECOMMENDED STANDARD PROPHYLACTIC REGIMEN FOR DENTAL, ORAL, OR RESPIRATORY TRACT PROCEDURES IN PATIENTS AT HIGH AND MEDIUM RISK OF ENDOCARDITIS

DRUG	DOSING REGIMEN
Amoxicillin	Adult: 3.0 g orally 1 h before procedure; then 1.5 g 6 h after initial dose
	Pediatric: initial dose, 50 mg/kg; follow-up dose 25 mg/kg. *The total pediatric dose should not exceed the total adult dose.*

FIGURE 14-15. Recommended standard prophylactic regimen for dental, oral, or respiratory tract procedures in patients at high and medium risk of endocarditis. This antibiotic regimen is directed toward alpha-hemolytic streptococci. All patients at high and medium risk are eligible for this regimen unless allergic to penicillins (or cannot take oral medications). Oral prophylaxis for high-risk patients has been recommended in the United States and Britain for several years, and an increased incidence of prophylaxis failures has not been reported. In some high-risk patients, however, the practitioner may choose to use a parenteral regimen (*ie*, a patient with a prosthetic heart valve and a history of endocarditis).

If a patient has been treated and it is then discovered that the patient forgot to take the antibiotic, the dose should be administered as soon as possible, if within 6 to 8 hours of the procedure.

One recent study compared 2- and 3-g doses of amoxicillin and found that adequate serum levels of amoxicillin were obtained and maintained with the 2-g regimen [21]. IM—intramuscular; IV—intravenous. (*Adapted from* Dajani and coworkers [17].)

ALTERNATE PROPHYLACTIC REGIMENS FOR DENTAL, ORAL, OR RESPIRATORY TRACT PROCEDURES IN PATIENTS AT HIGH AND MEDIUM RISK OF ENDOCARDITIS

DRUG	PATIENT GROUP	DOSING REGIMEN
Ampicillin	Patients unable to take oral medications	IV or IM administration of ampicillin, 2.0 g within 30 min before procedure; then IV or IM administration of ampicillin, 1.0 g, or oral administration of amoxicillin, 1.5 g 6 h after initial dose
Clindamycin	Amoxicillin/penicillin–allergic patients	300 mg orally 1 h before procedure and 150 mg 6 h after initial dose
Clindamycin	Ampicillin/amoxicillin/penicillin–allergic patients unable to take oral medications	IV administration of 300 mg within 30 min before procedure and an IV or oral administration of 150 mg 6 h after initial dose
Ampicillin, gentamicin, and amoxicillin	High-risk patients not candidates for standard regimen	IV or IM administration of ampicillin, 2.0 g, plus gentamicin, 1.5 mg/kg (not to exceed 80 mg), within 30 min before procedure; followed by amoxicillin, 1.5 g orally, 6 h after initial dose; alternatively, half the parenteral regimen may be repeated 8 h after initial dose
Vancomycin	Ampicillin/amoxicillin/penicillin–allergic patients considered high risk	IV administration of 1.0 g over 1 h, starting 1 h before procedure; no repeated dose necessary

FIGURE 14-16. Alternate prophylactic regimens for dental, oral, or respiratory tract procedures in patients who are at high and medium risk of endocarditis. This table lists antibiotic regimens for those patients who cannot take the standard oral amoxicillin regimen. In some situations, patients requiring intravenous vancomycin will be unable to receive their medication at the same site where their dental procedure will be performed. In this case, the dental procedure can be started within 1 hour of the end of the vancomycin administration.

In the patient allergic to penicillin known to be able to take cephalosporins, 1.0 g of a first-generation cephalosporin 1 hour before the procedure and 500 mg 6 hours after the first dose may be used.

Initial pediatric doses are as follows: ampicillin, 50 mg/kg; clindamycin, 10 mg/kg; gentamicin, 2.0 mg/kg; and vancomycin, 20 mg/kg. Follow-up doses should be one half the initial dose. *Total pediatric dose should not exceed total adult dose.* No initial dose is recommended in this table for amoxicillin (25 mg/kg is the follow-up dose). IM—intramuscular; IV—intravenous. (*Adapted from* Dajani and coworkers [17].)

REGIMENS FOR GENITOURINARY/GASTROINTESTINAL PROCEDURES

DRUG	DOSAGE REGIMEN
Standard regimen	
Ampicillin, gentamicin, and amoxicillin	IV or IM administration of ampicillin, 2.0 g, plus gentamicin, 1.5 mg/kg (not to exceed 80 mg), within 30 min before procedure; followed by amoxicillin, 1.5 g, orally 6 h after initial dose; alternatively, half the parenteral regimen may be repeated once 8 h after initial dose
Ampicillin/amoxicillin/penicillin-allergic patient regimen	
Vancomycin and gentamicin	IV administration of vancomycin, 1.0 g, over 1 h beginning 1 h before procedure plus IV or IM administration of gentamicin, 1.5 mg/kg (not to exceed 80 mg), within 1 h of procedure; half the original dose may be repeated once 8 h after initial dose

FIGURE 14-17. Regimens for genitourinary/gastrointestinal procedures. This table lists antibiotic regimens for patients at medium to high risk for endocarditis. Regimens are directed toward enterococci. Procedures for which prophylaxis is recommended are listed in Fig. 14-13. In high-risk patients (prosthetic heart valves, previous history of endocarditis, and surgically constructed systemic-pulmonary shunts), physicians may choose to administer prophylactic antibiotics for gastrointestinal/genitourinary procedures in which prophylaxis is not normally recommended.

Initial pediatric doses are as follows: ampicillin, 50 mg/kg; amoxicillin, 50 mg/kg; gentamicin, 2.0 mg/kg; and vancomycin, 20 mg/kg. Follow-up doses should be half the initial dose. *Total pediatric dose should not exceed total adult dose.* (*Adapted from* Dajani and coworkers [17].)

SPECIAL SITUATIONS IN PATIENTS NEEDING ENDOCARDITIS PROPHYLAXIS

Patients with previous penicillin administration

If patient has taken a course of an oral penicillin within the past month and requires prophlaxis for dental/oral/upper respiratory tract procedures, clindamycin (300 mg orally 1 h before procedure and 150 mg 6 h after initial dose) or vancomycin (1.0 g intravenously administered over 1 h, starting 1 h before procedure; no repeat dose is necessary) should be used. **This includes patients on oral penicillin for secondary prevention of rheumatic fever.**

Patients on anticoagulation drugs

In these patients, one should avoid intramuscular antibiotic administration.

Patients with renal dysfunction

In patients with compromised renal function, it may be necessary to modify or omit the second dose of gentamycin or vancomycin.

Patients undergoing cardiac surgery

Prophylaxis is primarily against staphylococci (coagulase positive and negative). A first-generation cephalosporin is most often used. Alternatively, vancomycin can be used in situations where a high prevalence of methicillin-resistent staphylococci is noted. Prophylaxis should be started immediately before surgery, given every 4–6 h, and discontinued 24 h postoperatively.

FIGURE 14-18. Special situations in patients needing endocarditis prophylaxis. Some patients needing antibiotic prophylaxis before undergoing dental, oral, respiratory tract, genitourinary tract, or gastrointestinal tract procedures have special situations (first three in list) for which regular prophylactic regimens need to be changed or adjusted. Patients with cardiac conditions in the high- or medium-risk categories of Fig. 14-11 are at risk for developing endocarditis when undergoing cardiac surgery. (*Adapted from* Dajani and coworkers [15].)

REFERENCES

1. Veasy LG, Wiedmeier SE, Orsmond GS, *et al.*: Resurgence of acute rheumatic fever in the intermountain area of the United States. *N Engl J Med* 1986, 316:421–427.
2. Congeni B, Rizzo C, Congeni J, Sreenivasan VV: Outbreak of acute rheumatic fever in northeast Ohio. *J Pediatr* 1987, 111:176–179.
3. Wald ER, Dashefsky B, Feidt C, *et al.*: Acute rheumatic fever in western Pennsylvania and the tristate area. *Pediatrics* 1987, 80:371–374.
4. Hosier DM, Craenen JM, Teske DW, Wheller JJ: Resurgence of acute rheumatic fever. *Am J Dis Child* 1987, 141:730–733.
5. Westlake RM, Graham TP, Edwards KM: An outbreak of acute rheumatic fever in Tennessee. *Pediatr Infect Dis J* 1990, 9:97–100.
6. Wallace MR, Garst PD, Papadimos TJ, Oldfield EC: The return of acute rheumatic fever in young adults. *JAMA* 1989, 262:2557–2561.
7. Centers for Disease Control: Acute rheumatic fever at a Navy training center—San Diego, California. *MMWR* 1988, 37:101–104.
8. Centers for Disease Control: Acute rheumatic fever among army trainees—Fort Leonard Wood, Missouri, 1987–1988. *MMWR* 1988, 37:519–522.
9. Dajani AS: Current status of nonsuppurative complications of group A streptococci. *Pediatr Infect Dis J* 1991, 10:S25–S27.
10. Veasy LG, Tani LY, Hill HR: Persistence of acute rheumatic fever in the intermountain area of the United States. *J Pediatr* 1994, 124:9–16.
11. World Health Organization Study Group: Rheumatic fever and rheumatic heart disease. Geneva, Switzerland: World Health Organization; 1988. [Technical Report Series #764.]
12. Lieu TA, Fleisher GR, Schwartz JS: Clinical evaluation of a latex agglutination test for streptococcal pharyngitis: performance and impact on treatment rates. *Pediatr Infect Dis* 1988, 7:847–854.
13. Snellman LW, Stang HJ, Stang JM, *et al.*: Duration of positive throat cultures for group A streptococci after initiation of antibiotic therapy. *Pediatrics* 1993, 91:1166–1170.
14. Jones TD: Diagnosis of rheumatic fever. *JAMA* 1944, 126:481–484.
15. Dajani AS, Ayoub E, Bierman F, *et al.*: Guidelines for the diagnosis of rheumatic fever (Jones criteria, updated 1992). *JAMA* 1992, 268:2069–2073.
16. MacMahon SW, Roberts JK, Kramer-Fox R, *et al.*: Mitral valve prolapse and infective endocarditis. *Am Heart J* 1987, 113:1291–1298.
17. Dajani AS, Bisno AL, Chung KJ, *et al.*: Prevention of bacterial endocarditis. *JAMA* 1990, 264:2919–2922.
18. Simmons NA, Ball AP, Cawson RA, *et al.*: Antibiotic practice and infective endocarditis. *Lancet* 1992, 339:1292–1293.
19. Dajani A, Taubert K, Ferrieri P, *et al.*: Treatment of acute streptococcal pharyngitis and prevention of rheumatic fever. *Pediatrics* 1995, 96;758–764.
20. Pichichero ME: Group A streptococcal tonsillopharyngitis: cost-effective diagnosis and treatment. *Ann Emerg Med* 1995, 25:390–403.
21. Dajani AS, Bawdon RE, Berry MC: Oral amoxicillin as prophylaxis for endocarditis: what is the optimal dose? *Clin Infect Dis* 1994, 18:157–160.

INDEX